The Columbia Manual of Dermatologic Cosmetic Surgery

The Columbia Manual of Dermatologic Cosmetic Surgery

Emil Bisaccia, M.D., F.A.C.P.
Clinical Professor of Dermatology
Columbia University
College of Physicians and Surgeons
New York, New York

Dwight A. Scarborough, M.D.
Assistant Clinical Professor of Medicine
Dermatology Division
Ohio State University Hospital
Columbus, Ohio

McGraw-Hill
Medical Publishing Division

New York   Chicago   San Francisco   Lisbon   London
Madrid   Mexico City   Milan   New Delhi
San Juan   Seoul   Singapore   Sydney   Toronto

McGraw-Hill

A Division of The McGraw·Hill Companies

THE COLUMBIA MANUAL OF DERMATOLOGIC COSMETIC SURGERY

1 2 3 4 5 6 7 8 9 0 KGPKGP 0 9 8 7 6 5 4 3 2

ISBN 0-8385-1626-2

This book was set in Palatino by V&M Graphics, Inc.
The editors were Darlene Barela Cooke, Susan R. Noujaim, and Lester A. Sheinis.
The production supervisor was Catherine H. Saggese.
The text designer was Robert Freese.
The cover designer was Eve Siegel.
The indexer was Alexandra Nickerson.
Quebecor World/Kingsport was printer and binder.

This book is printed on acid-free paper.

Library of Congress Cataloging-in-Publication Data is on file for this title at the Library of Congress.

This book is dedicated to the dermatologic cosmetic surgeons who continue to advance their training and experience and who use sound medical judgment to enhance their patients' quality of life.

Emil Bisaccia, M.D.
Dwight Scarborough, M.D.

Contents

Contributors

Authors

Emil Bisaccia, M.D., F.A.C.P.
Clinical Professor of Dermatology
Columbia University
College of Physicians and Surgeons
New York, New York

Dwight A. Scarborough, M.D.
Assistant Clinical Professor of Medicine
Dermatology Division
Ohio State University Hospital
Columbus, Ohio

Major Contributions by Present and Former Fellows

Ingrid P. Warmuth, M.D.
Columbia University
College of Physicians and Surgeons
New York, New York

Michael A. Radonich, M.D.
Affiliated Dermatology
Dublin, Ohio

Contributions by Present and Former Fellows

Gwen O. Abeles, M.D.
Dermatology Center of Rockland
Orangeburg, New York

Robert Bader, M.D.
Deerfield Beach, Florida

Deborah J. Daly, D.O.
Affiliated Dermatology
Dublin, Ohio

Audrey F. Echt, M.D.
Raleigh, North Carolina

Eyal Levit, M.D.
Affiliated Dermatology
Morristown, New Jersey

Mario Sequeira, M.D.
Brevard Skin and Cancer Center
Rockledge, Florida

Mona Zaher, M.D.
Mount Pleasant, South Carolina

Foreword

The clinical practice of dermatology has undergone a revolution in recent years and has expanded from a largely medical focus to one that embraces an ever-expanding range of surgical modalities. This evolution of the specialty is in many respects a natural one because for dermatologists the skin has always been their major organ of interest. Furthermore, the field of dermatology encompasses cutaneous biology in which basic research has helped to expand our base of knowledge regarding the structure and function of the skin. These advances have allowed dermatologists to be well positioned to exploit the latest advances and apply them to better patient care.

The Columbia Manual of Dermatologic Cosmetic Surgery written by Dr. Bisaccia and Dr. Scarborough is a superb and comprehensive compendium of information addressing the major aspects of cosmetic surgery as performed by two outstanding and experienced practitioners. They have also made the material extremely readable and provided a tremendous amount of very practical information both about surgical procedures and the requirements for the facilities in which to perform them.

The material is organized into 20 chapters of which the first few address important issues related to ambulatory surgical units and their accreditation, credentialing and hospital staff privileges, as well as marketing. The remaining chapters address the principles of cosmetic surgery, including facial and body analysis, anesthesia, soft tissue augmentation, use of botulinum toxin, clinical peels, microdermabrasion, dermabrasion, laser surgery, scar revision, liposuction, face-lift, blepharoplasty, hair restoration, and otoplasty. The authors have shared their vast experience in all aspects of cosmetic surgery and offer a balanced perspective concerning their approaches. Extensive practical information is provided in virtually all areas. Detailed information for patients is presented and should prove to be very useful in the practice setting.

The practice of cosmetic surgery in dermatology is expanding rapidly, and this book will serve as a basic reference for both the novice and the experienced cosmetic dermatologic surgeon. The detailed practical information included assures that this is a text that will not simply sit on the shelf but rather will prove to be a remarkably useful resource. Dr. Bisaccia and Dr. Scarborough have produced an important new contribution to the field of cosmetic dermatologic surgery.

David R. Bickers, M.D.
Carl Truman Nelson Professor and Chair
Department of Dermatology
Columbia University College of Physicians and Surgeons
New York, New York

Preface

There can be no argument with good work. Amid the cacophony of claims arising from interspecialty rivalry, the only credible voice is that of competence. Dermatologists possess a rich and substantive history in developing the field of contemporary cosmetic surgery. Expertise acquired through training and experience is the unassailable high ground that positions dermatologic cosmetic surgeons to best serve the cosmetic surgical patient. The purpose of this book is to further the clarity by which cosmetic dermatologic surgeons may address their patients who seek assistance with their restoration or enhancement of appearance.

This book offers a deliberative method of approaching the cosmetic surgical patient based on tiered strategies for intervening in the aging process. Relevance and practicality were the foremost intent in composing this book, translating our past 15 year experience of surgical practice and mentoring of fellows into a useful format. Through a systematic approach to facial and body analysis as presented in Chapters 6 and 7, aesthetic maintenance and rejuvenation goals can be accomplished in accord with the patient and surgeon's level of comfort. Understanding the often complex framework from which to position a practice can be challenging. Included are the very basics of office surgery setup and simple ethical marketing strategies to help those starting out, to delineating some of the intricacies in a more sophisticated ambulatory surgery center, intended for the established dermatologic cosmetic surgeon. Chapters 1, 2, and 3 address the thought processes and actions associated with various credentialing and office surgical setup issues we belive will be beneficial to the practitioners in the field of dermatologic cosmetic surgery at each level.

The core of the book is aimed toward comprehensively defining the patient's concern(s), then laying out treatment algorithms from which to mediate improvement. Various cosmetic surgical procedures are outlined to highlight the technical components involved with each specific intervention. Added to these procedural chapters are the practical elements of patient information sheets, consent forms, specific pre- and postoperative instructions for patients, and setup materials that support outpatient surgical patient care. The ability to offer the patient a range of treatment options based on the degree of improvement desired, cost, duration of correction, and recovery time available is highly useful in building and maintaining a successful dermatologic cosmetic surgical practice.

Clearly this is not a "how-to" book. The acquisition of good surgical technique, mature judgment, superior hand skills, and the ability to safely and effectively manage complications comes with appropriate training and experience. This book is, however, intended to serve as a significant aid to furthering one's cosmetic dermatologic surgical knowledge. We trust that the interventional algorithms and procedure outlined herein, supporting the surgeon's thoughtful assessment and leading to a satisfactory patient outcome, will serve as a helpful guide in the busy dermatologic cosmetic surgical practice.

Emil Bisaccia, M.D.
Dwight A. Scarborough, M.D.

Acknowledgments

This book is in honor of the memory of Dr. Edmund Lowney, who brought us into the field of dermatology. We should like to express our sincere appreciation to our entire office staffs for their support during the writing of this book. A special thanks goes to Rob Lombardi, Steve Morales, Ellen Kole, Laurie Johannsen, and Marsha Morgan.

CHAPTER 1

Office-Based Surgery

Within the past decade, the demand for office-based surgery has increased at a staggering rate. This is largely due to increased demands by managed care organizations and patients to reduce costs. Insurance companies are increasingly less likely to precertify ambulatory surgery in a hospital operating room (OR) as their guidelines hold that such procedures can be performed in an office-based setting. Because cosmetic surgery has become increasingly popular, the competitiveness of pricing has become stiffer, further shifting procedures from the hospital to the office or ambulatory surgery center.

Advantages and Disadvantages of Office-Based Surgery

There are both advantages and disadvantages to performing office-based surgery; these need to be considered in terms of the scoped procedure to be performed, the patient's underlying health, the office's proximity to emergency medical services (EMS) and hospitals, state regulations, the physician's training and experience, and the equipment available in the office setting (Table 1-1).

By defining the standards for and requirements of the procedures to be performed, the practitioner can help to ensure optimal results.[1–3] The guidelines presented at the end of this chapter should serve as an example.

Regulations and Restrictions

In the past, office-based surgery has typically been performed at the physician's initiative; it was largely unmonitored and more or less unregulated. Recently, however, regulatory agencies in some states have begun to place restrictions on office procedures: who can perform them, what procedures can be performed, which type of anesthesia can be used, and how long a patient may stay in the facility to recover. Over the past decade, some state medical boards—including those of California, Florida, and New

Table 1-1
Office-Based Surgery

Pros	Cons
Less cost	Potentially fewer safeguards than with hospital-based surgery
More comfortable surroundings for patients	Depending upon the facility/office, possibly less emergency/resuscitation equipment
Good overall track record	Fewer resources available
More flexible scheduling	Higher cost to physician initially due to the need for equipment, instruments, and supplies
More physician control of scheduling	State mandates as to quality control and procedures performed
More specialized training for staff on specific procedures	Perhaps less breadth of background and experience of staff
More physician control over the process, greater staff accountability	Less ancillary staff available for backup

Jersey—have implemented regulations regarding office-based surgery. It is therefore essential to check with one's local regulatory agencies before planning to perform any procedures in the office.

Currently, many states are implementing significant regulations and some, including Florida, have temporarily banned some office-based surgeries as a result of problems with elective, mainly cosmetic procedures. The rapid growth of office-based surgery is dramatic, currently encompassing more than 15 to 20 percent of all elective surgeries. Clearly these regulatory efforts may be opposed for economic reasons, but the state boards of medicine have put them in place in order to provide for patient safety and protection. It is incumbent on office-based surgeons to make patient safety and well-being their top priorities in planning facilities for office-based surgery.

For example, in New Jersey, for any surgery performed in an office setting, the surgeon must have hospital privileges for the procedure as well as the method of anesthesia used in the hospital (see Chap. 3). Meanwhile, the Florida Board of Medicine has instituted its own requirements for simple surgical procedures, including excisions performed entirely under local anesthesia. For procedures involving any degree of altered consciousness, the Florida Board of Medicine requires that the office be inspected and accredited by an authorized agency. Many of Florida's standards revolve around a three-tiered classification system based on the level of anesthesia given.

Level I Procedures

Under this system, level I procedures are defined by the standard as "minor procedures," such as excision of skin lesions, moles, warts, cysts, and lipomas as well as repair of lacerations or surgery limited to the skin and subcutaneous tissue performed under topical or local anesthesia; such surgery does not involve drug-induced alteration of consciousness other than minimal preoperative tranquilization of the patient. Under level I, liposuction involving the removal of less than 4000 mL of supernatant fat is allowed.

Level II Procedures

Level II procedures are defined as those "in which the patient is placed in a state which allows the patient to tolerate unpleasant procedures while maintaining adequate cardiorespiratory function and the ability to respond purposefully to verbal command and/or tactile stimulation."

Level III Procedures

Level III surgeries are the most highly regulated procedures in the state of Florida. This level is defined as "surgery, which involves, or reasonably should require, the use of general anesthesia or major conduction anesthesia and preoperative sedation. This includes the use of intravenous sedation beyond that defined for Level II office surgery."

Among the aspects of the Florida regulations that stand to impact dermatologists most is the requirement for inspection/accreditation of facilities where level II or III procedures are performed.

Accreditation and Inspection

While undue regulation is burdensome, office-based surgeons should welcome the current climate as an opportunity to assure that they are providing the best possible care for their patients. They should also become involved at the state level to develop the model that best suits their regional area, without unnecessary intrusion. Under the Florida standard, physicians can choose either accreditation or inspection in order to remain in compliance. The rule states that unless the physician has provided written notification of accreditation—by either a nationally recognized accrediting agency or an accrediting organization approved by Florida's Board of Medicine—the office will be subject to inspection by Florida's Department of Health in order to verify compliance with the standards.

The accrediting process is discussed in more detail in Chap. 2, "Creating an Accredited Ambulatory Surgery Facility." The first step in establishing the design should be based on the types of procedures to be performed in this facility. Depending on the state, it is advisable to have written policies concerning the procedures that may be performed in the office, the specific anesthesia services, the responsibilities of the health care personnel, infection control policies, procedures to be followed if a patient experiences complications, and with procedures to be followed if a patient requires transport to the hospital. The duties of the personnel throughout the transfer should also be specified. In addition, procedures for following a patient who is recovering in the office need to be detailed. Also required are criteria for discharging patients, along with a means for reviewing records and ensuring follow-up on complications and outcomes. There should be a transfer agreement with the local hospital to cover cases of untoward reactions or complications requiring hospitalization. These procedures and responsibilities, along with discharge criteria and monitoring, appear in Chap. 2.

The surgical suite may be planned in any of a variety of shapes and designs. Unless one is creating an ambulatory surgical center, dermatologic surgical rooms generally serve as minor surgical procedure rooms as well as office examining rooms. Their size can vary depending on the procedures to be performed; however, adequate access to the patient, 360-degree access around the operating tables, as well as surgical assistance and surgical equipment all require at least a 10- by 12-ft room; many textbooks suggest a minimum of 20 by 20 ft. Again, it is important to have enough space to allow for full resuscitation code procedures; optimal illumination of the surgical field should also be provided. A powered, foot-controlled operating table with multiple joints best ensures patient comfort and safety. The interior design aspects generally include a vinyl wall covering over sheetrock and vinyl flooring, all of which are easily sanitized. The electrical panel for room lighting should provide for emergency lighting and emergency power. Fluorescent lights may have battery packs so as to remain illuminated in case of a power outage. A battery pack for power ensures against outages with no need for expensive generators (Fig. 1-1).

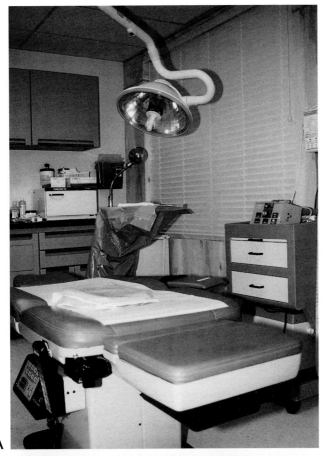

A

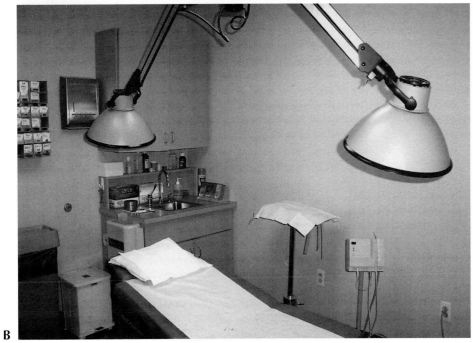

B

Figure 1-1 (*A*) An office surgical room. (*B*) A variation of this design.

Staff Training

Even though the office setting may strike the patient as less threatening, it remains essential to train the staff to interact well with the patients. All surgical staff should be trained in basic life support and advanced cardiac life support if possible. Nursing staff should be adequately trained in instrument identification, handling, and care; use of surgical dressings; charting; delivering pre- and postoperative instructions to patients; conducting telephone triage and differentiating between routine, urgent, and emergent phone calls; and handling emergency office protocols—i.e., fire drills, loss of power, patient medical emergencies. It is well to remember that each member of the office staff is an extension of and reflection of the surgeon.

Office Setup

EQUIPMENT

Sterilization

In getting started, one must consider what method of sterilization to use. Each method has advantages and disadvantages.

Most offices that perform surgery use steam sterilizers, as they are fast, easy to operate, easy to install, and cause minimal wear and tear on most instruments. As not all equipment can be sterilized by steam sterilization, cold sterilization can be used for instruments or equipment not able to tolerate steam or dry-heat sterilization. Newer steam sterilizing equipment is fully automated, thus reducing demands on staff time (Table 1-2).

Monitoring Equipment

Some states—depending mainly on the level of anesthesia to be used—now have specific requirements for a "crash cart" and emergency equipment. Therefore it is vitally important to check with local regulatory agencies before planning to perform any surgical procedures in the office.

If any degree of sedation (i.e., altered consciousness) is to be utilized, additional monitoring equipment should be considered—i.e., noninvasive blood pressure monitoring, electro-cardiography (ECG), oxygen saturation, and defibrillation (Table 1-3) (Fig. 1-2). Under current standards of care, the minimum recommended equipment for office-based surgery is based on level of anesthesia.

ROOM DESIGN

Before the office is designed, the procedures to be performed in each of the rooms must be decided upon. For example, a room in which level II anesthesia for laser resurfacing is to be administered must be designed differently than one which would be used only for simple excisions, flaps, and grafts. All of the possible equipment, number of personnel, and electrical needs for each type of procedure must be taken into consideration.

Hallways should be at least 4 ft wide so as to accommodate wheelchairs and EMS equipment. Rooms, as well, should be large enough to accommodate this traffic, to handle all necessary personnel and equipment, and, to let the surgeon maneuver around the patient with ease.[4,5]

Table 1-3
Minimum Recommended Equipment for Office-Based Surgery Based on Level of Anesthesia

	Level I	Level II	Level III
Manual BP cuff	Yes	Yes	Yes
Oxygen	Yes	Yes	Yes
NIBP* monitoring	No	Yes	Yes
Oxygen saturation	No	Yes	Yes
ECG	No	Yes	Yes
Defibrillator	See note	Yes	Yes
Full crash cart	See note	Yes	Yes
Injectable Benadryl, Solu-Medrol, epinephrine	Yes	Yes	Yes

Note: Depending upon proximity to EMS.
*NIBP = noninvasive blood pressure.

Table 1-2
Sterilization Methods

	Steam	Gas	Dry Heat	Cold
Time needed for adequate sterilization	Fast	Fast	Slow	Slowest
Instrument wear and tear	Minimal	Least	Moderate	Moderate
Equipment cost/installation	Moderate/expensive	Expensive	Inexpensive/moderate	Little or none
Cost to run	Moderate	Moderate	Little	Least
Maintenance/repair costs	Some	Some	Little	None

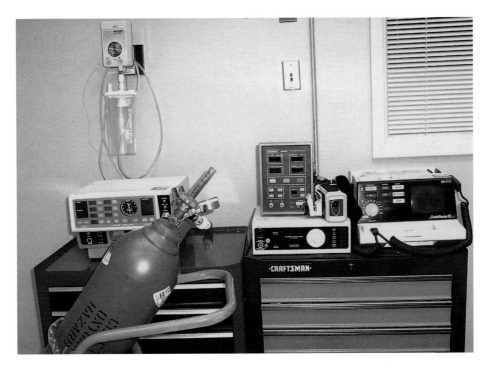

Figure 1-2 Emergency equipment: crash cart, monitoring equipment, oxygen.

General Guidelines for Surgical Care

Many specialty groups, such as the American Academy of Dermatology, have developed specific guidelines for office-based surgery. It is good practice to put such guidelines to use in any office-based surgical practice. In fact, in some states, it is mandatory to have such guidelines in place. The following may serve as a general model for such guidelines.

I. Introduction

This office has developed guidelines for the care of its surgical patients. These guidelines will promote the delivery of quality care and the boundaries of surgical care within this office.

II. Rationale

A. Scope

All staff of this office are expected to adhere to the guidelines described herein.

B. Practitioner qualifications

1. Practitioners may perform only those surgical procedures in which they have been appropriately trained during residency or postgraduate training with hands-on experience.

a. Practitioners who perform cosmetic procedures must have documentation of training in such procedures. It is expected that practitioners will be able to document both didactic and hands-on training for any procedures that will be performed within the office, and this will be reviewed prior to the performance of such procedures.

b. Practitioners who perform cosmetic surgery must be able to demonstrate participation in continuing medical education activities related to cosmetic surgery.

C. Other criteria

1. Physicians who perform any procedure using level II anesthesia must have a transfer agreement with a local hospital.

2. All procedures using level II anesthesia must be performed with a board-certified anesthesiologist and/or certified registered nurse anesthetist (CRNA).

3. No level III anesthesia procedures should be performed in the office.

III. Diagnostic criteria

A. Clinical

Patient selection and evaluation are critical in determining the feasibility of procedure to be performed. Patients undergoing any surgical procedure within this office must have an appropriate history and physical examination performed and documented within his or her record.

1. History should include:

a. General medical history as appropriate

b. Condition or area being treated

c. Duration of condition

d. Location

e. Precipitating event(s)

f. Previous treatment(s)

g. Patient's expectations, desires, and tolerance of side effects

h. Conditions that may be absolute or relative contraindications to performing the surgical procedure for which the patient is being evaluated

2. Physical examination should include:
   a. General physical examination as appropriate
   b. Evaluation of the areas to be treated to assess likelihood of improvement with the surgical procedure for which the patient is being evaluated
   c. Inspection of skin for the presence of findings that might be predisposing factors for complications, such as infection, active disease processes, and other preexisting conditions

3. Additional requirements for patients undergoing level II anesthesia include the following:
   a. A complete physical examination, including examination of the heart and lungs, must be performed and documented by the surgeon or other qualified practitioner with written clearance for surgery by the surgeon, anesthesiologist, or other qualified practitioner.
   b. For all patients over 40 years of age, an electrocardiogram must be obtained within 3 weeks of surgery and placed in the patient's record.
   c. For all patients over 40 years of age, a complete blood count must be obtained.
   d. For all patients over 65 years of age, a Chem 7 (chemistry profile metabolic panel) and chest x-ray must be performed.
   e. For all female patients who have not had a total hysterectomy, a pregnancy test is required within 2 weeks of surgery.
   f. The surgeon must review all of the above information 48 h prior to surgery.
   g. All patients undergoing elective cosmetic surgery must be judged to be medically stable based on their history and physical examination as well as other laboratory data as necessary.

IV. Recommendations
   A. Medical
      1. All patients who are cleared for surgery will have been judged to be medically stable based on their pre-operative history and physical examination.
      2. Patients who are not judged to be medically stable will be required to obtain a letter of medical clearance from their primary care physician prior to undergoing any surgical procedure within the office.
   B. Surgical
      1. Preoperative
         a. Informed consent will be obtained from the patient prior to any surgical procedure. Such consent will include a verbal discussion of the risks, benefits, and possible complications of such a procedure as well as other therapeutic options. Such consent should be documented in the patient's record.
         b. Prophylactic antibiotics
            Use of antibiotics is at the discretion of the physician and depends upon the surgical site, the length of time the wound will be open before repair, the patient's immune status and history of infection, heart valve disease, valve or joint replacement, and other underlying medical conditions. The use of antibiotics should be strongly considered for patients who are diabetic or immunosuppressed, patients with a prolonged operative time, surgical sites with a compromised vascular supply, or contamination of the wound during surgery. Patients with a history of valve replacement, rheumatic fever, or joint replacement should receive a prescription for prophylactic antibiotics preoperatively. If there is uncertainty regarding whether antibiotics are required, the patient's primary care physician should be consulted.
         c. Anticoagulants
            1. Patients taking warfarin (Coumadin) may be asked to discontinue this medication 48 to 72 h preoperatively and resume 24 h postoperatively, but only when written clearance is obtained from the primary care physician.
            2. Patients taking aspirin may be asked to discontinue this medication 10 days before surgery and may resume it 2 days after surgery, but only with written clearance from their primary care physician (if that physician has recommended that they take this medication). Patients who are taking aspirin of their own volition may be asked to discontinue this medication without medical clearance.
            3. Patients taking nonsteroidal anti-inflammatory drugs (NSAIDs) may be asked to discontinue these medications 2 to 5 days before surgery
            4. Patients who drink may be asked to refrain from drinking alcohol for 48 h before and after surgery.
            5. Postoperative activity restrictions should be discussed with each patient prior to surgery.
            6. It is strongly suggested that all patients undergoing elective surgical procedures follow the above recommendations.
         d. Nothing by mouth (NPO) status
            1. For local anesthetic procedures, the patient may be allowed to eat and drink normally with the exception of alcohol.
            2. Patients undergoing level II anesthesia will be given appropriate instructions by their supervising anesthesiologist or CRNA.
      2. Surgical setting
         a. The surgical facilities of the office will conform to the standards set forth in the guidelines.

3. Monitoring
   a. Monitoring of patients will be performed in accordance with standards generally recognized as appropriate for the type of anesthetic employed, the medical condition and age of the patient, and the type and duration of the surgical procedure.
4. Aseptic technique
   a. All instruments and materials in contact with the surgical field will be adequately sterilized.
   b. Sterile gloves will be worn by staff during all excisions of lesions greater than 6 mm in size requiring sutures as well as reconstructive and cosmetic procedures.
   c. Masks and eye protection will be worn by staff during all excisional, reconstructive, and cosmetic procedures.
   d. Sterile gowns and/or surgical scrubs will be worn as appropriate during all excisional, reconstructive, and cosmetic procedures.
   e. The operative site will be prepped with an antibacterial agent before any surgical procedure is performed.
   f. The operative site will be draped in an aseptic fashion before any surgical procedure is performed.
   g. An aseptic postoperative dressing will be applied after surgery.
5. Procedure
   a. All surgical procedures will be performed in accordance with appropriate standards of care.
   b. All laser users will adhere to the safety standards of the American National Standards Institute for the safe use of lasers in health care facilities.
   c. An operative note will be generated after each surgical procedure, documenting in detail the procedure performed and staff present during it.
   d. An operative log will be maintained by each practitioner, documenting the patient's name, procedure, and the date of procedure.
   e. A medication and narcotics log will be maintained by the practitioner and anesthesiologist and/or CRNA.
6. Postoperative care
   a. Postoperative dressings should be placed appropriately.
   b. When necessary, analgesics may be recommended.
   c. Postoperative restrictions may be given when appropriate.
   d. All postoperative instructions must be be both verbal and written. Instructions should be discussed thoroughly with the patient before he or she leaves the office. These discussions should be documented in the patient's record.
   e. The practitioner should be available to manage any complication that may arise. At the discretion of the practitioner, patients will be called at home the evening of surgery to make sure that all is well, to discuss postoperative care, and to deal with any questions. The practitioner should be immediately available for at least 48 h after surgery. Then, in the event that the surgeon is unavailable, a covering physician must be on call. Both staff and the patient should be told who will be covering.
7. Equipment
   a. All equipment and instruments should be properly maintained by the physicians and staff.
   b. Any device or equipment that is broken, defective, or malfunctioning should be set aside for proper servicing, repair, or replacement; its condition should be reported to the head nurse.

V. Emergency protocols
1. In the event of fire
   a. All patients and staff are to be removed from danger immediately. The front-desk staff will bring all patients out through the two exits and have them wait across the street.
   b. The fire alarm will be activated and the office manager told to call 911.
   c. The fire may be contained by closing all doors.
   d. The fire may be extinguished by using one of the fire extinguishers located [state locations].
2. In the event of a medical emergency
   a. All BLS/ACLS procedures will be followed. The oxygen tank and crash cart is located in the surgical room. Copies of the BLS/ACLS procedures are located in the top drawer of the crash cart.
   b. The office manager will be notified of the problem and will call 911.
   c. The office manager will instruct the check-out staff to bring all other patients and their companions away from the area in which the emergency exists. The check-out staff will bring the patient's family members into the doctor's office to calm them and explain what is going on.
   d. The office manager will then oversee the movement of all patients away from the area and clear a path for EMS personnel. They will use the back door. The office manager will instruct the check-in staff member to wait outside for the EMS personnel and direct them to the office.

VI. Room maintenance
1. The room will be mopped after each surgical case.
2. The counters and examination table will be cleaned between cases using a bleach/water mixture that is stored under the sink.
3. The red garbage bags containing biohazard material will be closed and thrown in the large red garbage container located in the lab
4. The white garbage bags containing regular garbage will be closed, put in the lab, and thrown out in the proper receptacle outside when time permits.

References

1. Drake LA, Deilley RI, Cornelison RL, et al. Guidelines of care for office surgical facilities. Part I. *J Am Acad Dermatol* 1992; 25(5):763–765.

2. Elliott RA. The design and management of an aesthetic surgeon's office and surgery suite. In: Tegnault P, Daniel R, eds. *Aesthetic Plastic Surgery: Principles and Techniques.* Boston: Little, Brown; 1984:45–73.

3. Gilbert Da, Adamson JA. Procedure manuals in office surgery. *Clin Plast Surg* 1983; 10:269.

4. Klebanoff G. Operating room design. *Am Coll Surg Bull* 1979; 64:6–10.

5. Stegman SJ, Tromovitch RA, Glogau RG. *Basics of Dermatologic Surgery.* Chicago: Yearbook; 1982:1–22.

CHAPTER 2

Creating an Accredited Ambulatory Surgical Facility

Background

For many decades, dermatologists have performed surgical procedures and have been at the forefront in developing and pioneering cosmetic and surgical techniques. They have performed and perfected these procedures primarily in office-based facilities. Given the escalating costs of in-hospital surgery, many physicians who used to be based in hospitals have now converted to office-based facilities. In recent years, state medical boards and governmental regulatory committees have sought to hold outpatient surgical facilities to the same standards and regulations as hospitals. This has created increased pressure on outpatient facilities that are currently adhering to office-based surgical policies to become accredited ambulatory surgical facilities. In addition, many insurance carriers and managed care organizations are requiring accreditation of the affiliated facilities with which they contract.[1]

As dermatologic surgery has undergone increasing levels of sophistication, many dermatologic and cosmetic surgeons have adopted various anesthetic techniques. Conscious sedation is a form of monitored anesthesia that is widely used for outpatient surgical procedures, including (but not limited to) dermatologic and cosmetic surgery.[2] General anesthesia and unconscious sedation are considered appropriate in either a hospital or an ambulatory surgical facility, and conscious sedation has been considered appropriate in office settings if certain guidelines are followed.[3] Many office-based dermatologic surgeons are experiencing increasing pressure to perform procedures that entail the use of conscious sedation in accredited ambulatory surgical facilities. As a result, many dermatologic and cosmetic surgeons are seeking to comply with current recommendations for ambulatory health care accreditation.

WHAT IS ACCREDITATION?

Accreditation represents the highest form of public recognition that a health care organization can receive. The process of accreditation is designed to verify that an organization meets specified criteria that are assumed to indicate quality care. In general, accreditation allows an organization to compare the quality of its services and performance to nationally recognized standards.[4]

The concept of accreditation originated in hospitals, with organizations such as the Joint Commission for Accreditation of Health Care Organizations (JCAHO). The major focus of the JCAHO remains the accreditation of hospitals. The three main organizations that certify ambulatory surgical units are the Health Care Financing Administration (HCFA) (usually via the applicable state department of health), the JCAHO, and the Accreditation Association for Ambulatory Health Care (AAAHC). The HCFA remains the major organization for Medicare service and reimbursement certification. The AAAHC and the JCAHO have been considered the major organizations certifying ambulatory health care centers. As of 1996, the AAAHC was granted deemed status for Medicare certification by the HCFA; therefore, ambulatory health care centers now have the option to pursue an AAAHC-Medicare survey if they wish to be Medicare-certified.

ACCREDITATION ASSOCIATION FOR AMBULATORY HEALTH CARE

Established in 1979, the AAAHC is a private, not-for-profit organization whose purpose is to improve the quality of care that ambulatory surgical facilities provide for patients. The AAAHC has specific standards, including (but not limited to) standards that regulate the physical environment, quality of care, medical staff, medical records, and facility management and administration. These standards that have been developed over a 20-year period and have been adapted to reflect current changes in medicine and health care. Updates have been instituted as deemed necessary. The AAAHC strives to set standards among ambulatory surgical facilities, helps to measure the performance of these facilities, and provides consultation and education to continually advance such facilities.

Surveyors for the AAAHC are health care professionals that represent at least 13 of the nation's leading health care associations. These associations include the American Society for Dermatologic Surgery (ASDS), American Academy of Cosmetic Surgery, American Academy of Facial Plastic and Reconstructive Surgery, Outpatient Ophthalmic Surgery Association, and American Association of Oral and Maxillofacial Surgeons. The ASDS became a sponsoring society in 1993.

PRESURVEY CRITERIA

The types of organizations that may seek accreditation via the AAAHC are varied, ranging from dental and birthing facilities to ambulatory surgical centers. Certain eligibility criteria must be met before the AAAHC surveyors may consider an organization. First, the organization must have provided health care for at least 6 months before the on-site survey or evaluation can be done. An exception occurs for an organization that applies for the AAAHC Early Options Survey. Next, the organization must be in compliance with federal, state, and local laws and must be state-licensed (if required by the state). The organization must share facility, equipment, business management, and patient care records with the AAAHC. Finally, before the on-site survey, the organization must supply a signed Application for Accreditation Survey and a completed Pre-Survey Questionnaire and pay the appropriate fees.[5] Only after these eligibility criteria have been met can the AAAHC determine whether or not the AAAHC standards can be applied to a given institution and whether that institution may undergo an on-site survey.

The remaining portion of this chapter focuses primarily on AAAHC certification. Most of the information has been adapted from AAAHC materials and handouts. This is not meant to substitute for any of the AAAHC materials; rather, it is meant to provide guidelines for a better understanding of the process of accreditation for physicians who may be interested in beginning the accreditation process.

Getting Started

First, the applicant must contact the AAAHC either by writing to the AAAHC (9933 Lawler Avenue, Skokie, IL 60077-3708) or by calling 847-676-9610 and requesting the accreditation material. For a fee, the *Self-Assessment Manual*, Pre-Survey Questionnaire, and *Accreditation Handbook for Ambulatory Health Care* will be provided. The *Self-Assessment Manual* enables an organization to prepare for the survey by evaluating its current level of compliance with the AAAHC standards. To further assist in this preparation, the manual is in a format similar to that which the AAAHC surveyors will use. The checklist allows an organization to determine its current status regarding each of the accreditation standards.

Upon receiving the Pre-Survey Questionnaire, the AAAHC will assess the organization's current level of health care services and management structure. Several supporting documents must be submitted with this questionnaire. These include a description of the organization's ownership, a description of the history of the organization, and a mission statement of the organization's future goals. Specific credentialing materials concerning current hiring practices and administration policies are also requested.

After review by the AAAHC, the information provided by the organization allows the AAAHC surveyors to determine the exact details of each individual survey and how to most closely match the surveyor to the type of organization being evaluated.

The Accreditation Survey Process

The on-site Accreditation Survey may vary depending on the type of organization being evaluated. The number of days and the number of surveyors are decided based on information from the Pre-Survey Questionnaire and supporting documents. The AAAHC has certain "core standards" that all health care organizations must meet in order to become accredited. Other "adjunct standards" are relevant only to certain types of facilities.

Each core standard is clearly delineated in the *Accreditation Handbook for Ambulatory Health Care*. The core standards are as follows:

1. **Rights of patients:** An accreditable organization recognizes the basic human rights of patients.

2. **Governance:** An accreditable organization has a governing body that sets policies and is responsible for the organization.

3. **Administration:** An accreditable organization is administered in a manner that assures provision of high-quality health services and that fulfills the organization's mission, goals, and objectives.

4. **Quality of care provided:** An accreditable organization provides high-quality health care service in accordance with the principles of professional practice and ethical conduct and with concern for the costs of care and for improving the community's health status.

5. **Quality management and improvement:** In striving to improve the quality of care and to promote more effective and efficient use of facilities and services, an accreditable organization maintains an active, integrated, organized, peer-based program of quality management and improvement that links peer review, quality improvement activities, and risk management in an organized, systematic way.

6. **Clinical records:** An accreditable organization maintains a clinical record system from which information can be retrieved promptly.

7. **Professional improvement:** An accreditable organization strives to improve the professional competence, skills, and quality of performance of the health care practitioners and other professional personnel it employs.

8. **Facilities and environment:** An accreditable organization provides a functionally safe and sanitary environment for its patients, personnel, and visitors.[5]

A manual called the *Physical Environment Checklist for Ambulatory Surgical Centers* is included in the AAAHC materials. This checklist is based on National Fire Protection

Association (NFPA) code and standards. Organizations are encouraged to conform to as many of the items as possible, especially those required by state law, Medicare, and local building codes.

Certification of the Operating Room

Over the years, the movement toward outpatient surgery and cost control has led to the certification of ambulatory surgical facilities, which must meet the standard of outpatient hospital operating rooms (ORs). Medicare, the AAAHC, and other organizations are certifiers of these facilities. For these facilities to qualify for fee reimbursements from Medicare and other insurers, the centers must comply with HCFA-mandated standards. The AAAHC and JCAHO also conduct surveys and accrediting programs to promote and identify high quality and recognize compliance with these standards. AAAHC issues a certificate of accreditation.

The accreditation process of Medicare represents the highest standard and allows for Medicare reimbursement. In addition, the achievement of these criteria assures patient safety and recognizes the surgical dermatologist as meeting the highest standards for surgical procedures. Moreover, with the accreditation of their facilities it recognizes dermatologic cosmetic surgeons as providing the highest quality in their work and deserving the greatest public and peer recognition.

MEDICARE CERTIFICATION

Certification may be obtained from an individual state department of health, the AAAHC, and the JCAHO. The policy and procedure characteristics vary by state with respect to the requirements of licensing the facility, while in certain states an OR waiver from this licensing requirement is available. The facility issues are mainly based on safety and sanitation. In terms of design, requirements include a separate waiting room, recovery room, and surgical suite, which should be equipped to support the types of surgery conducted in the facility (see Table 2-1, Figs. 2-1, 2-2, 2-3, and 2-4). The halls must be wide enough to transport patients and must have two alarmed exit doors. The floors must be vinyl, welded for sanitation.

As a safety sanitary requirement, emergency equipment to handle cardiac and respiratory emergencies must be

Table 2-1
Standard Medicare-Approved Surgical Suite

Monitoring equipment	Power table
Respirator oxygen	Emergency lighting
Defibrillator	Emergency power
Pulse oximeter	Emergency call alarm
Crash cart	Wall suction

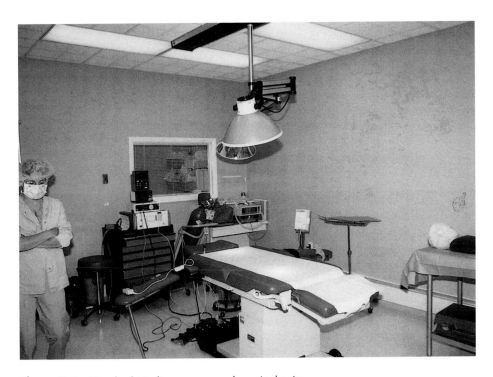

Figure 2-1 Standard Medicare-approved surgical suite.

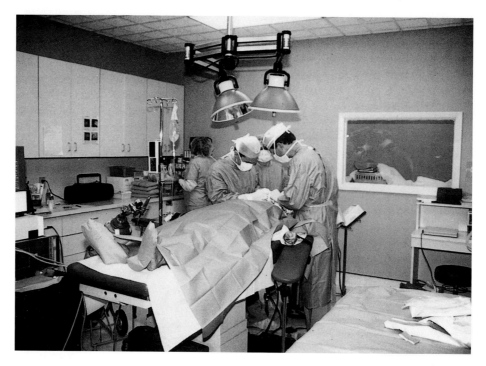

Figure 2-2 Ambulatory surgery suite.

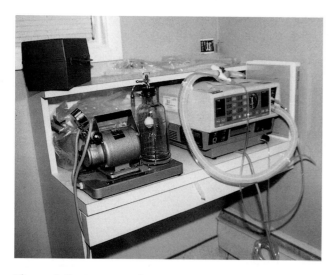

Figure 2-3 Suction and respirator are available in the surgical suite.

provided, including cardiac defibrillation and monitoring equipment, oxygen, laryngoscope, endotrachial tubes, crash cart, mechanical ventilators, assistance equipment, tracheotomy set, and an emergency call system and transportation agreement to the nearest hospital. Policy and procedure requirements based on safety require the surgical services to be performed by qualified physicians who have privileges granted by the governing body. These privileges are detailed

at the specific surgical site, but specific legislative issues vary from state to state with respect to the need for hospital credentialing for these procedures.

Guidelines include everything from aseptic techniques to OR attire. The facilities must meet certain physical plant requirements published by Medicare; however, each state may apply these differently. The HCFA has published interpretive guidelines that detail the HCFA's overview with respect to the mandated policies and procedures.

The issues fall into several categories. The survey, depending on the organization certifying, involves an architect, nurse, physician, pharmacist, and sanitarian. Each individual oversees the specific area of his or her expertise, tours the facility, and reviews policy and procedural manuals.

CERTIFICATION REVIEW

The architect reviews the physical plant with respect to conformance with required HCFA environmental issues. The fire rating must be in accordance with state regulations as well as the 1985 National Fire Prevention Association (NFPA) regulations. Many of these physical plant requirements appear in an HCFA publication. The ambulatory surgery center is to be used exclusively for the purpose of providing surgery to patients not requiring hospitalization. It requires physical separation by semipermanent walls and doors from any other clinic facility. It also requires a separate space for records, a waiting area, and an operative recovery room. The environment must be safe, constructed properly, adequately equipped, and appropriately maintained. The architect reviews in great detail the facility's occupancy separation,

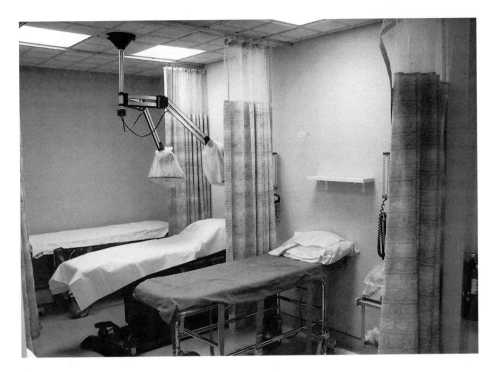

Figure 2-4 Recovery room.

smoke compartmentalization, smoke and fire detectors, and fire alarms and their locations. The facility must have at least two exits that are separate and distinct, an emergency generator, portable fire extinguishers, and a nurse call system.

The nurse or physician, sanitarian, and pharmacist review the facility's governing body, which is responsible for total management of the facility. In so doing, they review corporate documents, contracts, and letters of agreement. The facility must provide for immediate transfer to a local hospital where surgeons have admitting privileges. The reviewers examine the credentials of the physicians in order to be certain that all of them have been qualified by the governing body to perform surgery. In addition, they review the policies on equipment, supplies, space, aseptic technique, and surgical sterilization equipment and even the sterilization tapes. Additionally, they review the maintenance and care of surgical specimens and the handling of infected and contaminated cases. They review anesthetic risk and evaluation, the method of discharge, the type of anesthesia used, laboratory tests ordered, pre- and postoperative physician evaluations, and the qualifications of the person who administers anesthesia. If an anesthetist must be supervised by a qualified physician (as in New Jersey), the physician must have similar privileges in a hospital setting. These surveyors also evaluate the quality of the facility in terms of quality assurance (QA). They review the physicians' involvement in QA and the medical necessity of procedures with chart review. They also consider the procedure from incision to specimen management, especially a review of attendant complications. They review training of personnel for emergencies, including Advanced Cardiac Life Support

(ACLS) and the availability of these personnel from incision to discharge.

The medical records are reviewed for completeness and accuracy. The pharmacy services review the drug provided and the guidelines with respect to accepted standards of procedure, including the records of receipt and disposition labels. The policy and procedures for disposal of outdated drugs, handling of drugs, and proper administration are reviewed as well.

Accreditation by the AAAHC, HCFA, or JCAHO is also a mechanism a surgeon can use. These organizations provide accreditation documentation after audit and review that is recognized by the ambulatory care industry, managed care industry, and insurance carriers.

Protocol Forms

Policy and procedure documentation is very important in applying for accreditation as well as in maintaining an ambulatory surgery center after it is established. These documents are maintained and kept on hand for quick reference. They include a listing of procedures done at the ambulatory surgery center (Table 2-2); patient rights (Table 2-3); general staff responsibilities (Table 2-4A) and staff responsibilities during an emergency (Table 2-4B); anesthesia policies (Table 2-5A to E); and conscious sedation evaluation forms. In the area of QA, the policies include a form for QA indicators (Fig. 2-6A), QA audit form (Fig. 2-6B), and procedures for QA meetings (Table 2-6). The policies also spell out infection control policies, including procedures for the infection control committee

(Table 2-7*A*), infection control education (Table 2-7*B*), and general infection control procedures (Table 2-7*C*).

The prevention of blood-borne diseases is also spelled out in these documents, including general procedures concerning gowns, masks, and gloves (Table 2-8*A*) as well as an impact list for preventing blood-borne diseases (Table 2-8*B*). Also included are policies on aseptic technique (Table 2-9), storage of sterile supplies (Table 2-10), instrument decontamination (Table 2-11), contamination control in the OR suite (Table 2-12), and cleaning procedures for the surgical suite (Table 2-13).

Also included are postoperative procedures, comprising a document concerning the recovery room (Table 2-14*A* to *C*); a surgical outcome reporting form (Fig. 2-7); a postoperative checklist (Fig. 2-8*A*) and a postoperative patient evaluation form (Fig. 2-8*B*); autoclave monitoring procedures (Table 2-15); and a form for recording autoclave cleaning (Fig. 2-9). Last, patient discharge instructions (Fig. 2-10) and policies for hospital transfers of patients (Table 2-16) are laid out in the documents.

All of these procedural documents are essential to establishing—and, thereafter, maintaining—the smooth functioning of an ambulatory surgery center. They must be maintained and kept handy for easy access to the information.

Table 2-2
Procedures Done in the Ambulatory Surgery Center

Excision: lesions of the mouth and nose

Excision: lesions of the skin, subcutaneous and excess breast tissue (gynecomastia), lipomas

Vein ligation (one leg)

Excision of ganglion

Z-plasty

Blepharoplasty

Hair transplantation

Otoplasty

Excision of malignant or benign lesions of the face, lip, scalp, and body

Revision of scars

Laceration repair

Dermabrasion

Facial plasty and rhytidectomy

Skin grafts

Scalp reduction

Liposuction

Advancement flaps

Mohs' surgery

Sebaceous cysts of scrotum

Laser resurfacing

Table 2-3
Patient's Rights

The ambulatory surgery center (ASC) and medical staff have adopted the following list of patient's rights:

1. These rights will be exercised without regard to gender; cultural, economic, educational, religious background; or the source of payment for the patient's care.

2. The patient will be provided with considerate and respectful care.

3. The patient will be told the names of the physicians who have primary responsibility for coordination of his or her care and the names and professional relationship of other physicians who will see the patient.

4. The patient will receive information from the physician about his or her illness, course of treatment, and prospect for recovery in terms that he or she can understand.

5. The patient will receive as much information about any proposed treatment or procedure that he or she may need to have in order to give informed consent or to refuse. Except in emergencies, this information shall include a description of the procedure or treatment, medically significant risks involved, and the name of the person who will carry out the procedure or treatment.

6. The patient will actively participate in decisions regarding his or her medical care to the extent permitted by law. This includes the right to refuse treatment.

7. The patient will be given full consideration of privacy concerning his or her medical care program. Case discussion, consultation, examination, and treatment are confidential and will be conducted discreetly. The patient has the right to be advised as to the reason for the presence of any individual.

8. Confidential treatment of all communications and records pertaining to his or her care and stay in the ASC. The patient's written permission shall be obtained before his or her medical records can be made available to anyone not directly concerned with the patient's care.

9. The patient will receive a reasonable response to any reasonable requests for service that he or she may make.

10. The patient is permitted to leave the ASC even against the advice of his or her physician.

11. The patient will be given reasonable continuity of care and will be able to know in advance the time and location of appointments as well as the physician providing the care.

12. The patient will be advised if the ASC or personnel propose to engage in or perform human experimentation affecting the patient's treatment. The patient has the right to refuse to participate in such research projects.

13. The patient will be informed by his or her physician or a delegate of the physician of his or her continuing health care requirements after discharge from the ASC.

14. The patient will be able to examine and receive an explanation of his or her bill regardless of source of payment.

15. The patient will be informed about which ASC rules and policies apply to his or her conduct as a patient.

16. The patient will have the right to apply to the person who may have legal responsibility to make decisions regarding medical care on behalf of the patient.

Table 2-4*A*
Staff Responsibilities

Title: Supervising Registered Nurse
Responsibilities:
1. Interviews, evaluates, and supervises nursing personnel.
2. Develops nursing personnel's schedules and ensure sufficient nursing coverage on a daily basis.
3. Provides administrator with pertinent performance information that will assist in arriving at salary adjustments of nursing personnel.
4. Implements personnel policies and procedures.
5. Supervises inventory; orders and maintains medical supplies, instruments, and equipment to ensure their appropriate utilization.
6. Orders drugs and pharmaceutical agents and supervises their inventory and maintenance to ensure appropriate utilization.
7. Develops and implements QA program.
8. Develops and implements in-service training program.
9. Coordinates maintenance of nursing log book.
10. Conducts nursing staff meetings on a regular basis.
11. Participates in practice development and marketing.
12. Performs special projects as required.
13. Performs general nursing duties as required.
14. Performs other related duties as requested by the administrator and physician.
Reports to: Administrator (administrative matters); physicians (clinical matters)

Title: Registered Nurse
Responsibilities:
1. Maintains a safe perioperative environment.
2. Escorts patients into changing room; interviews and prepares patients for physician (e.g., undressing); identifies each patient verbally.
3. Verifies patient consent form.
4. Assesses chart findings and physical status of each patient; confirms knowledge of abnormal findings with surgeon or anesthetist or anesthesiologist.
5. Consistently applies principles of appropriate body alignment and proper functioning of required instrumentation and equipment.
6. Anticipates, provides, and assumes responsibility for instrumentation and proper functioning of required instrumentation and equipment.
7. Follows established policies and procedures regarding counts, aseptic technique, and physical monitoring of patients during surgery.
8. Delivers quality patient care.
9. Competent in the delivery of drugs and solutions.
10. Participates in QA activities by assisting in the development of plans of action for resolving problems.
11. Conducts QA studies for solving problems.
12. Provides psychosocial support to perioperative patients.
13. Provides for privacy through physical protection and maintaining confidentiality.
14. Assesses patients' reactions.
Reports to: Director

Title: Staff Registered Nurse
Responsibilities:
1. Maintains a safe perioperative environment.
2. Escorts patients into changing room; interviews and prepares patients for physician (e.g., undressing); identifies each patient verbally.
3. Verifies patient consent form.
4. Assesses chart findings and physical status of each patient. Confirms knowledge of abnormal findings with surgeon or anesthetist or anesthesiologist.
5. Consistently applies principles of appropriate body alignment and proper functioning of required instrumentation and equipment.
6. Anticipates, provides, and assumes responsibility for instrumentation and proper functioning of required instrumentation and equipment.
7. Follows established policies and procedures regarding counts, aseptic technique, and physical monitoring of patients during surgery.
8. Delivers quality patient care.
9. Competent in the delivery of drugs and solutions.
10. Participates in QA activities by assisting in the development of plans of action for resolving problems.
11. Conducts QA studies for resolving problems.
12. Provides support to perioperative patients.
13. Provides for privacy through physical protection and maintaining confidentiality.
14. Assesses patients' reactions.
15. Identifies and is supportive of family understanding and reactions to surgical procedures.
16. Acts as patients' advocate.
17. Participates in daily operation of the OR.
18. Communicates effectively to schedule coordinator as to the progress of care in the OR.
19. Organizes responsibilities and activities in an effective manner.
20. Assures efficient turnaround of room between procedures.
21. Sets up cases in an effective manner.
22. Does procedure preps appropriately.
23. Maintains stock supplies to the surgical suite.
24. Reports stock deficiencies to appropriate personnel.
25. Performs competently in emergency situation.
26. Participates in continuing education and in-service programs to maintain and develop skills.
27. Offers constructive suggestions to leadership staff.
28. Seeks assistance from appropriate sources when necessary.
29. Maintains composure during stressful situations.
30. Performs assigned activities in a self-directed and cooperative manner.
31. Uses time constructively and organizes assignments to maximize productivity.
32. Coordinates handling of biopsy specimens, including maintenance of biopsy log book.
33. Accurately completes intraoperative records and all additional reports.

Table 2-4*A*
Staff Responsibilities (*continued*)

34. Maintains confidentiality.
35. Sterilizes instruments.
36. Submits current state license to administrator.
37. Completes annual cardiopulmonary resuscitation (CPR) review.
38. Adheres to standards and facility policies and procedures.
39. Gives postoperative instructions to patients.
40. Demonstrates an active interest in the growth and management of OR area through participation in committees, orientation of new staff, and in-service meetings.
41. Develops knowledge and skills to scrub and circulate.

Reports to: Nursing Supervisor

Title: Reception Registered Nurse
Responsibilities:

1. Acts as liaison to alert medical director, anesthetist or anesthesiologist, or other designated person of any problems related to conflicts of policy and procedure during patients' admission or discharge.
2. Conducts assessment interview of patients.
3. Oversees and coordinates interviews conducted by LPN and relief RN.
4. Formulates an audit for medical records by adding preoperative diagnosis to operative schedule.
5. Functions within the framework of the ambulatory surgery facility department policies and procedures and maintains a professional manner.
6. Supports goals and objectives of ambulatory surgery facility.
7. Accountable for own conduct.
8. Maintains patient information confidentiality.
9. Promotes positive working relationships.
10. Attends in-service and continuing education programs and shares knowledge.
11. Demonstrates responsibility toward punctuality and attendance.
12. Contributes to data collection and problem identification for QA activities.

Reports to: Nursing Supervisor

Title: Receptionist, Ambulatory Surgery
Responsibilities:

1. Creates and maintains patient data and information for assemblage of complete patient charts.
2. Coordinates chart assembly of ancillary area to ensure 48-h preoperative completion time of chart.
3. Assists in patient preparation for surgery.
4. Greets patients and assists them when necessary.
5. Arranges patient interviews with assigned RNs.
6. Communicates with patients' family members as to the progress of patients' surgery and recovery.
7. Processes charge routing forms assigning appropriate diagnosis and procedure codes.
8. Transports patients if requested.
9. Communicates pertinent patient information to appropriate personnel.

10. Promotes a positive working environment.
11. Demonstrates punctuality.
12. Performs other duties as indicated by coordinator.

Reports to: Nursing Supervisor

Title: Scrub Assistant
Responsibilities:

A. Reports on duty and check assignment.
B. Checks doctor's preference card and helps circulatory to prepare the room.
C. Scrubs according to scrub routine and puts on sterile gown and gloves.
D. Sets up case:
   1. Breaks down and arranges pack.
   2. Drapes Mayo stand.
   3. Separates and arranges basin set.
   4. Places drapes, gowns, and gloves on right-hand corner of the table.
   5. Washes powder off gloves.
   6. Takes instrument, sponge, and needle counts (PRN).
   7. Arranges instruments on back table and Mayo stand in the standard manner. Checks that all needed instruments are available.
   8. Prepares suture material.
E. Establishes a sterile field for surgery:
   1. Gowns and gloves surgeon and assistants.
   2. Drapes surgical field in proper manner and with the assistance of the surgeon.
   3. Hooks up cautery cords and suction (PRN).
   4. Positions Mayo stand, table, and so on.
F. During the procedure:
   1. Watches and listens closely.
   2. Anticipates surgeon's needs.
   3. Keeps a neat Mayo stand and field.
   4. Maintains good technique.
   5. Asks for supplies quietly.
   6. Works quickly without sacrificing accuracy and technique while passing instruments, sutures, and so on.
   7. Takes care of the specimen carefully.
   8. Is ready with the sutures for closing.
   9. Is ready with dressing.
   10. Removes drapes from the patient.
G. At the end of the procedure:
   1. Assists in the moving of the patient to the recovery room.
   2. Removes light handles.
   3. Prepares instruments and basins for cleanup. Cleans all instruments after surgery and places them in baskets ready for sterilization. Disposes of blades and sharps in a needle protector.
   4. Wraps instruments accordingly and sterilizes. Helps circulating nurse to prepare for the next procedure.
H. Remembers:
   1. To use good sterile technique at all times.

Table 2-4*A*
Staff Responsibilities (*continued*)

a. Always to face the sterile field and pass another sterile person back to back.

b. If there is any chance of contamination, considers the area unsterile.

c. Does not argue.

d. Always passes supplies in front of the surgeon.

e. Always protects gloves while draping.

f. Does not reach across an unsterile field.

g. Considers only arms and front of gowns above waist to be sterile.

2. Knows that a good job can be performed only if there is good teamwork between the scrub assistant and circulator.

Reports to: Surgeon; Head Nurse

Title: Desk Charge
Responsibilities:

1. Checks for call-ins.

2. Makes adjustments to assignments.

3. Surveys schedule for changes (if added cases, picks cards and notifies technician of needed equipment).

4. Initiates written morning report with above information and supplies it to the director or assistant director upon his or her arrival.

5. Counts narcotics with nurse.

6. Has continuous interaction with those in the main OR.

7. Makes the following notations on the working schedule:

   a. Personnel in each room

   b. Physicians' beeper numbers

   c. OR cases with doctors scheduled in the ASC so that any time difficulties can be checked on during the day

8. Makes calls to physicians regarding difficulties in charts or orders for first procedures and any subsequent ones.

9. Notifies instrument tech of any additional instruments or equipment needed for first procedures.

10. Adjusts case arrangements to fill in cancellations.

11. Creates lunch schedule. Uses natural breaks in schedule or adjusts times of procedures if the ASC is short on personnel for relief. Verifies delays with anesthesia and physicians. Adjusts relief schedule in accordance with schedule delays or changes.

12. Initiates tasks or assigns them to the waiting circulating nurse.

Reports to: Faculty Manager

Title: Circulating Nurse
Responsibilities:

Objective: The first responsibility of the circulating nurse is to the patient, who is completely dependent on the nurse. The nurse in the OR is the patient's advocate.

I. Preparation of the patient

A. Schedule

1. Checks the schedule to see where he or she is posted and what personnel are assigned to him or her.

2. Knows the procedure and is able to give a brief synopsis of what will occur.

3. Assigns personnel to tasks for which they are best suited (e.g., technician to scrub, to run errands).

4. Consults with the charge nurse regarding schedule problems.

B. Instruments and supplies

1. Obtains as much information as possible from the schedule.

2. The first case should have been placed in the assignment room.

3. Checks the doctor's preference cards.

4. Picks up additional supplies if needed.

5. Places instruments in autoclave at required type of sterilization if needed.

C. Checks OR suite

1. Makes sure the surgical light and center spot are working.

2. Makes sure that the cautery machine is complete.

3. Sets up catheter and urimeter if necessary.

4. Pours povidone/iodine (Betadine) for prep or sets up Betadine scrub or patient prep.

II. Preoperative care of the patient

A. Upon arrival

1. Calls for patients approximately 20 min before scheduled operation time.

2. In the holding area, greets the patients by name and introduces himself or herself.

3. Verifies five important items:

   a. Checks patient's identification for correct name.

   b. Checks the chart for consent, laboratory work, electrocardiogram (ECG), radiographs, preoperative checklist, allergies, doctor's order for premedication, and nurse's note.

   c. Notifies the surgeon or anesthesiologist or anesthetist of any problem, such as elevated temperature or incorrectly signed or incomplete operating permit.

   d. Explains procedures to the patient—that the anesthesiologist or anesthetist will be in to place the blood pressure (BP) cuff and ECG leads and start an IV (if not already done).

   e. Meets the comfort needs of the patient. Helps him or her onto the OR table. Supplies a pillow and blanket as needed.

4. Makes a note of the time entering the room and records it on the perioperative record.

5. Assesses the patient's level of consciousness and emotional state.

6. Reassures patient and supports his or her needs at this time.

7. Connects the suction and cautery as they are passed off.

8. Positions buckets for the scrub nurse.

B. During the procedure

1. Pays close attention to procedure so that the needs of the surgical team can be anticipated.

2. Provides additional supplies as necessary.

Table 2-4*A*
Staff Responsibilities (*continued*)

3. Cleans up prep set or any other tables no longer in use.
4. Keeps all trash and sponges off the floor, using gloves for handling.
C. Documentation
1. Completes the operative sheet, making sure the patient's name and number are legible. Accurately records pre- and postoperative diagnosis and operative procedure without the use of abbreviations. Accurately records the members of the surgical team in the correct order.
2. Completes the specimen labels and heading of the pathology sheet.
3. Fills out the appropriate requisitions; labels each specimen, places it at the nurses' station, and records them in the book.
D. As surgery ends

1. Checks with the anesthesiologist or anesthetist about premedicating the next patient (about 1 h before).
2. If cases are going as scheduled, sends for next patient about 20 min before the scheduled time. Prepares the environment, instruments, and supplies as needed.
3. If the case is not running on schedule, notifies the charge nurse, because he or she may wish to move the next case; informs the surgeon of the change.
4. Counts instruments according to policy.
5. Supplies dressing materials and assists with application as necessary.
6. Keeps suction available and functioning until the patient is out of room.
7. Provides warm gown and blanket to cover the patient.
8. Assists with transfer of the patient.

Reports to: Surgeon; Head Nurse

Table 2-4*B*
General Responsibilities of Staff During Emergency Situations

Procedures:

Registered nurse

1. In case of cardiac arrest in the OR, the RN pulls the emergency signal cord, which alerts the receptionist, who, in turn, calls 911. If the cardiac arrest is not in the OR, the RN determines the location of the arrest, notifies the receptionist and the physician, and readies the crash cart, oxygen, suction, defibrillator, and emergency drugs. *The RN records the time of the cardiac arrest.*
2. Appoints the recorder.
3. States out loud the drug and times given so that the recorder can hear and document them. Also monitors the rhythm and type of ventilation.
4. Assists the anesthesiologist or anesthetist.
5. Accompanies the patient to the hospital.

Anesthetist (ACLS-certified anesthesiologist, MD, or anesthetist):

The anesthetist runs the emergency situation in the OR.
He or she releases the patient to the hospital when the crisis is stable.

Doctor:

1. Maintains CPR.
2. Gives instructions on drugs to be given.
3. Accompanies the patient to the hospital if necessary.

Scrub RN:

1. Aids in preparing drugs.
2. Relieves member of CPR team.
3. Takes and delivers messages.

Administrator:

1. Alerts all personnel that there is an emergency.
2. Directs all personnel to clear the hallways of visitors and patients.
3. Unlocks the doors.
4. Directs a front staff member to show paramedics to the OR or to the site of the crisis.
5. Directs family members to private waiting room and stays with them until further orders from the doctor.
6. Sends copy of emergency record with the patient to hospital.

Table 2-5*A*
Department of Anesthesia

An assistant medical director shall be assigned and shall assume the duties of the medical director in his absence.

Physicians, anesthesiologists, and certified registered nurse anesthetists (CRNAs) must meet the qualifications of their respective qualifying board and be duly licensed and insured.

Duties: Physicians are responsible for the preoperative evaluation, operative management, and postoperative follow-up of patients assigned to their care. They shall meet their obligations to the OR schedule. They will perform such teaching duties and other functions as the medical director may assign them.

Nurse anesthetists:

1. Qualifications: Nurse members of the ambulatory surgery center anesthesia department must be CRNAs and must meet the other qualifications of being properly licensed and insured.

2. Duties and functions: Nurse members of the ambulatory surgery center anesthesia department may administer local with monitored anesthesia control (L/MAC) and may attend patients under regional anesthesia. Their performance will be under the overall supervision of the medical director or his or her designee, who will also assign patients to their care as needed. In addition, each patient assigned to a nurse will be under the direct supervision of the attending physician, who will be available in the operating suite of the ambulatory surgery center and will supervise.

Intraoperative:

Each patient having general anesthesia, L/MAC, or regional anesthesia will be attended during the entire procedure by a physician, anesthesiologist, or CRNA.

An anesthesia record will be completed for each patient and will be part of the permanent records. The records will indicate anesthetic agents, doses, techniques, and all adjunctive medication and fluids. They will also show the types of monitoring used and a graphic record of the patient's vital signs.

All patients under the care of a physician/anesthetist or CRNA will have the following monitoring:

1. ECG
2. BP
3. Pulse oximetry

Postoperative:

At the end of surgery, the anesthesiologist or anesthetist will decide when the patient to whom he or she has rendered care may be placed under the care of the postanesthesia care unit (PACU) staff.

Meetings:

The patient care committee of the ambulatory surgery center will hold meetings quarterly or as deemed necessary.

Table 2-5*B*
Quality of Anesthesia Care

A. Preoperative
1. The health screening survey form will be reviewed before surgery. When indicated, the physician will call the patient whose screening yields matters of concern.
2. A physician, anesthesiologist, or CRNA will make a preoperative evaluation of each patient in the holding area of the ambulatory surgery center and record this on the patient's chart before preoperative sedation is given and before the patient is transferred to the OR.

B. Preinduction
1. Before induction, the physician, anesthesiologist, or CRNA must, after reviewing the patient's chart, ascertain any last-minute changes in patient evaluation.
2. The physician, anesthesiologist, or CRNA must check all equipment and be sure that everything is in proper working order and all necessary supplies are present before induction of anesthesia.
3. The surgeon is responsible for the administration of the location anesthetic.
4. The RN monitor can only administer sedatives, relaxants, tranquilizers, or analgesics by direct order from the surgeon.
5. The RN monitor should be able to assess and react appropriately to emergency situations and be qualified to administer appropriate medications to stabilize the patient as per a physician's direct order.
6. Preadmission testing is ordered at the surgeon's discretion based on the patient's physical condition.
7. All patients undergoing local anesthesia have venous access established preoperatively in accordance with the scope of the planned procedure according to the physician or surgeon's instructions.
8. All patients having local anesthetic are accompanied to the PACU by the surgeons and the RN monitor.
9. Duration of stay of the local patient depends on the type of medication administered and is the responsibility of the surgeon according to the discharge criteria.

Table 2-5*C*
Local Anesthesia in the Ambulatory Surgery Center

"Local cases" are procedures that use infiltration of anesthetic agents, with or without the additional administration of relaxants sedatives, tranquilizers, or analgesics (e.g., Versed, Valium, Demerol).

Ambulatory patients receiving local anesthesia with or without administration of sedatives, tranquilizers, or relaxants may be monitored by a qualified RN.

All "local cases" are performed in the specific OR designated for these procedures.

Safety rules:

A. Anesthesia equipment, if relevant to the procedure
   1. Oxygen tanks may be stored. No flammable gases or vapors are stored but other nonflammable gases may be.
   2. All reusable anesthetic equipment (e.g., laryngoscopes, airways, masks) in direct contact with patients are properly cleaned after each use.
   3. No flammable anesthetics are used. All former rules related to their use are null and void, including the need

for conductive flooring and the avoidance of certain fabrics. Sign posted on the OR door: "AREA RESTRICTED TO NONFLAMMABLE ANESTHETICS."

B. Electrical safety
   1. All new electrical equipment is checked and certified safe before it is sent to the OR for use.
   2. When a piece of electrical equipment malfunctions, it is tagged as broken and removed from the area. The biomedical engineer is notified and arrangements made for its repair.

C. Power failure
   1. Monitors are equipped with an automatic battery power pack.
   2. Lighting in the OR is secured with the use of an automatic power pack.

D. Telephone failure
   1. An emergency telephone backup unit is located in the telephone room of the doctor's office in case a telephone power failure occurs.

Table 2-5*D*
Rules and Regulations for the Anesthesia Patient

I. General Considerations
   A. The ambulatory surgery facility is to provide an arrangement for the safe administration of anesthesia for appropriate surgical procedures that can be conveniently and safely performed in an ambulatory setting. This saves the cost of hospitalization and affords a greater convenience to patients.
   B. The primary concern must be the type of patient selected. For general anesthesia, the patient should be an American Society of Anesthesiologists (ASA) class I or II anesthesia risk, preferably with no serious uncontrolled cardiac, respiratory, renal, or metabolic abnormalities.
   C. Medications and allergies should be recorded on the history sheet. Class II patients are acceptable for local anesthesia.
   D. The patient is treated in the same way as any pre-operative in-hospital patient—that is, nothing by mouth past midnight except for medicine taken with a sip of water, before medications are taken per anesthesiologist or anesthetist or surgeon, reviews operative request, and history and physical examination.
   E. Indicated laboratory studies are done and recorded before surgery and should be done within 14 days of surgery.
   F. Chest radiographs and ECGs are ordered if clinically indicated according to the following guidelines listed under class I.
   G. The necessary paperwork and consent must be in the ambulatory surgery office by 24 h before surgery.
   H. Laboratory work for preadmission testing for ambulatory surgery patients must be done within 2 weeks before surgery at any licensed laboratory or physician's office laboratory provided that the results are available by 24 h before surgery.
   I. Chest radiographs or their reports are acceptable if they are done in licensed facilities. ECGs are acceptable

from any doctor's office or laboratory provided that a reading of the ECG is available 24 h before surgery.
   J. Failure to obtain the history and perform the physical examination on time will result in notification to the surgeon and cancellation of the case.
   K. The supervising nurse is afforded the power to reschedule or cancel appointments if a surgeon is more than 15 min late for his or her scheduled appointments.
   L. The surgeon sees each patient immediately before surgery.

II. Anesthesia criteria
   A. The anesthetics are short-acting with minimal or no preoperative sedation. The patient remains in the recovery room until he or she has recovered satisfactory motor and cerebral function. Then, in the case of local anesthetics, the patient is discharged by the physician.
   B. In order to use intravenous (IV) conscious sedation as a modality in the ambulatory surgery OR, the physician must be credentialed.
   C. Further requirements include mandatory monitoring with continuous ECG pulse oximetry and taking the BP by a certified RN, as well as having an ACLS-certified physician present in the facility until all patients are discharged. The surgeon may not administer the drug or do the procedure but he or she may order the nurse to administer sedation.
   D. All patients attended in the OR are discharged from the ambulatory surgery center by the patient's attending surgeon, who signs the chart.
   E. The following methods of discharge may be used:
      1. The physician may see the patient and sign the chart.
      2. The physician may take a verbal report from the nurse and sign the chart. If the verbal report is by telephone, a verbal order may be given and the chart signed later.
      3. The physician may give a written or verbal order for the patient to be discharged later when certain criteria are met.

Table 2-5*D*
Rules and Regulations for the Anesthesia Patient (*continued*)

F. At the times of discharge, the PACU nurse will sign a note that the criteria are met.

III. Discharge Criteria

A. Standard discharge criteria include separate criteria for ambulatory patients. The physician, anesthesiologist, or anesthetist may specify additions or exceptions to the standard discharge criteria in any case. These criteria are not intended to prevent a physician from discharging a patient who fails to meet them when the physician has evaluated the patient and the individual circumstances. This evaluation may be by discussion with the PACU nurse. The criteria are as follows:

1. The patient is awake or easily aroused, oriented, and coherent and is appropriately responsive to verbal stimuli. Mild sedation caused by narcotic or antiemetic drugs is acceptable.

2. Pain or nausea is reasonably controlled.

3. Heart rate and BP are stable for 30 min and within normal limits for the patient. No vasopressor or antihypertensive drugs are used for 30 min. The skin is warm and dry.

4. The patient does not have respiratory depression or respiratory distress but does have good respiratory rate and excursion, good color (no cyanosis or severe pallor), and good swallowing. The gag and cough reflexes are present. There is no dyspnea, tachypnea, wheezing, excessive cough, stridor, retractions, or flaring.

5. No narcotic drugs have been given during the 30 min before discharge. No narcotic antagonists or agents for muscle relaxant reversal have been given in the 60 min before discharge.

6. All dressings are dry and intact and all tubes, lines, and drains are secure.

7. The patient is able to understand the discharge instructions.

8. The patient is able to retain oral fluids.

9. The patient is able to void.

10. The patient is able to ambulate with minimal assistance (if surgery permits).

11. A responsible adult is available to accompany the patient home and provide care.

12. Minimum PACU stay: 30 min after local with monitored anesthesia control (L/MAC) or regional anesthesia; 1 h after general anesthesia; or 2 h after endotracheal anesthesia.

13. Anesthesia discharge instructions are provided. These are given verbally to the patient by the physician, anesthesiologist, or anesthetist at the preanesthesia interview before sedation is administered. A written copy is given to the patient and responsible adult companion at the time of discharge and reviewed with them by the PACU nurse.

IV. Requirements for laboratory data and anesthesia status

A. Local cases are unique in that all levels of anesthesia risk may be considered for this approach. The ambulatory surgery center allows for a cleaner environment with more equipment, anesthesia standby if necessary, and assistants. These points essentially determine whether a surgeon chooses the outpatient department of a hospital or the ASC for his or her local cases. Laboratory data required for local cases should be determined by the physician's evaluation of the patient.

B. For patients undergoing anesthesia or local anesthesia with IV sedation and L/MAC, the following guidelines for minimal preoperative laboratory tests should be followed:

1. Otherwise healthy patient younger than age 40 years: Hb and Hct

2. Otherwise healthy patients age 40 to 60 years: Hb, Hct, and ECG

3. Otherwise healthy patient older than age 60 years: Hb and Hct, ECG, CXR, blood urea nitrogen (BUN), and blood sugar

C. Duration of validity of laboratory results (if the patient's medical condition is unchanged and results are within normal range): Hb and Hct for 1 month; CXR for 1 year; ECG for 6 months; electrodes for 1 month.

D. For subsequent or follow-up procedures, the requirements for repeat CXR and ECG may be waived if the patient has continued good health status and no hospitalizations.

E. The need for a preoperative CXR in younger patients is left to the discretion of the attending physician. It is based on the patient's past medical history and coexisting disease (e.g., chronic obstructive pulmonary disease, asthma, smoking history). Regardless of age, patients with other medical problems (e.g., renal, hepatic, pulmonary, or cardiac diseases) need appropriate laboratory tests pertaining to the specific disorders (e.g., electrolytes, liver function tests, pulmonary function tests).

F. Appropriate medical consultations, access to old charts, or previous medical or anesthesia records facilitate a complete preoperative evaluation. All local cases with IV sedation or L/MAC have the same requirements as those for general anesthesia

V. Monitoring and recovery

A. All patients have IV access (IV or heparin lock) and ECG monitoring with the exception of those with minor skin excisions of benign or malignant lesions as ordered by the attending physician. They are admitted to the recovery room and released by the attending physician. They are admitted to the recovery room by the usual recovery room policies.

B. Whenever a nurse is monitoring a patient under local anesthesia and believes there is sufficient concern, he or she is empowered to involve a member of the medical staff.

C. The physician, anesthesiologist, or anesthetist will monitor patients with anesthesia standby (L/MAC) if deemed necessary by ASA classification or by the attending physician.

D. In case of adverse reaction to surgery or anesthesia, the patient may be admitted directly to the associated hospital.

VI. Postdischarge

A. Postoperatively, the patient must be accompanied by a responsible adult.

B. The patient should not make any important decisions, drink alcohol, or attempt to drive for 24 h after discharge.

C. Unless contraindicated, the patient is called the day after discharge to ascertain his or her postoperative status.

Table 2-5D
Rules and Regulations for the Anesthesia Patient (*continued*)

D. Patients who have undergone strictly local anesthesia with no sedation need not be held to these restrictions.
VII. Classes of risk
  A. Class II risk for general anesthesia includes patients with well-controlled diseases with only mild manifestations, such as
    1. Controlled hypertension
    2. Controlled diabetes mellitus
    3. Controlled asthma (i.e., symptom-free)
    4. Controlled seizure disorder (i.e., no seizures for the past year)
    5. Obesity with no other system diseases
    6. Mild anemia (i.e., HCT, 30 to 10 g;. Hb dialysis and gynecology patients may be understandably lower)
  B. Many ophthalmology patients are classified in class III and may have surgery in this setting with appropriate care and precautions. They should be allowed to take their usual cardiac medications on the morning of the surgery and should have had appropriate medical clearance and liberal use of recovery arrangements.
  C. If any questions arise relating to the risk classification, consultation with a member of the medical staff is appropriate. Class III patients done under lock may occasionally require anesthesia standby, which should be used with discretion and appropriate indications.
  D. Anesthesiologists or anesthetist physical status scale
    1. Class I: A normal, healthy individual
    2. Class II: A patient with mild systemic disease
    3. Class III: A patient with severe systemic disease that is not incapacitating
    4. Class IV: A patient with incapacitating systemic disease that is a constant threat to life.
    5. Class V: A moribund patient who is not expected to survive 24 h with or without an operation

E. Wound Classifications
  1. Class I
    a. Wound description: Clean
    b. Examples: Nontraumatic, uninfected operative wounds in which the respiratory, alimentary, or genitourinary tract is not entered; usually closed without drains
  2. Class II
    a. Wound description: Clean or contaminated
    b. Examples: Operative wounds in which the respiratory, alimentary, or genitourinary tract is entered with only minimal contamination
  3. Class III
    a. Wound description: Contaminated
    b. Examples: Fresh, traumatic wounds; wounds with a major break in the sterile technique; wounds encountering nonpurulent inflammation; wounds made in or near contaminated skin
  4. Class IV
    a. Wound description: Infected
    b. Examples: Wounds in which purulent infection is encountered
VIII. Reservations
  A. A physician wishing to reserve time for an operation must call and request the ambulatory surgery center OR time. The hours for the ambulatory surgery center are from 7:45 A.M. to 2:00 P.M. daily. Cases are limited to operating time of 8:00 A.M. to 4:00 P.M.
IX. Supervision
  A. The overall supervision of the ambulatory surgery center is under the direction of the medical director. The administrative supervision is the responsibility of the administrative director.
  B. The ACS OR is supervised by the nursing supervisor.

Table 2-5E
Patient's Anesthesia Discharge Instructions

When you get home, rest. Do not plan any activities for the rest of the day.

Consider yourself under the influence of drugs for the next 24 hours.

Your reflexes and judgment may be impaired.

Do not drive.

Do not use knives or tools or operate any machinery; doing so could cause injury to you or others.

Do not make any important decisions.

Avoid alcohol. Do not take tranquilizers, sleeping pills, antihistamines, or muscle relaxants unless specifically ordered by your doctor.

Drink fluids freely, but eat cautiously until you are sure that food will not upset your stomach.

Start with small amounts of light foods and increase gradually.

If you have any problems, contact your surgeon.

PATIENT INTERVIEW   CHART REVIEW

DATE: _____

Medical History: _____

_____

Allergies:_____

_____

_____

Medications:_____

_____

Previous anesthesia or conscious sedation complications: _____

_____

_____

Condition of teeth:

_____

Pertinent physical findings:

_____

Pertinent laboratory findings:

_____

ECG:

_____

Conscious sedation procedure, risks and options discussed:

_____

_____

Signature: _____

Presedation assessment:

_____

_____

_____

CRNA administering conscious sedation:

_____

Figure 2-5A Ambulatory surgery center conscious sedation evaluation.

Date: _____

Postprocedure note:_____

1. Vital signs stable:_____

_____

2. Responding to spoken voice: _____

_____

3. Conditons:_____

_____

_____

Attending physician: _____

_____

Date: _____

DISCHARGE NOTE: _____

Condition of patient:

_____

_____

_____

Complications:

_____

Attending physician:

_____

Figure 2-5*B* Ambulatory surgery center conscious sedation evaluation.

DATE OF PROCEDURE:_____
                                                    Patient's Name

Quality assurance indicators:

[ ] CNS complications occurring within 24 h

[ ] Peripheral neurologic deficit occurring within 48 h

[ ] Unexpected cardiac arrest occurring within 24 h

[ ] Acute myocardial infarction occurring within 48 h

[ ] Unplanned respiratory arrest occurring within 24 h

[ ] Unplanned admission of ambulatory patient

[ ] Death within 48 h of anesthesia

[ ] Pulmonary edema occurring within 24 h

[ ] Aspiration pneumonitis occurring within 48 h

[ ] Postural headache within 96 h (after spinal)

[ ] Postural headache within 96 h (after epidural)

[ ] Dental injury during anesthesia

[ ] Ocular injury during anesthesia

[ ] Other unusual incident (if more room is needed, use other side)

_____

_____

_____

_____

Date: _____

Attending Physician or Anesthetist: _____

Figure 2-6A   Ambulatory surgery center department of anesthesia.

DATE OF MEETING: _____

QUALITY ASSURANCE COMMITTEE

Medical Director

OR Supervisor

Administrator

A total of _____ local and _____ IV sedation cases were performed in the ambulatory surgery facility.

For the period of _____ through _____, charts of _____ patients were selected at random. Compliance with the highest standards of care was found during the audit review.

There were _____ untoward incidents observed. Charts were found to contain pertinent information but were incomplete in the following areas:

Report of findings will go to the OR committee members and the ambulatory surgery center's board of directors.

The following action was deemed necessary.

Respectfully submitted,

Committee Member

Figure 2-6*B* Quality assurance audit.

Table 2-6
Quality Assurance Meetings

These meetings are held in order to assure quality patient care to all patients treated in the ambulatory surgery center through periodic evaluations and conducted audits.

1. The OR committee receives appropriate reports from the medical director concerning QA results affecting the function of the unit.
2. The medical director and members of the QA committee review and evaluate the care of all patients who require hospitalization after ambulatory surgery. Identification of common factors is attempted and reported to the OR committee and the board of directors of the ambulatory surgery center.
3. The nursing supervisor ensures the conduct of environmental and nursing process audits for review by the medical director.
4. The medical director ensures the conduct of a retrospective (recurrent) chart audit with specific criteria performed quarterly consisting of review of five random charts. Results are communicated to staff members, along with recommendations for correcting areas of deficit.
5. The medical director takes all reasonable measures to assure the quality, safety, and appropriateness of services are monitored and evaluated and that appropriate action follows up on findings.

Table 2-7*A*
Infection Control Committee

Policy: An infection control committee shall be maintained to review and direct the infection control mechanism of the ambulatory surgery facility to maintain a safe, infection-free environment for staff members and patients.

Procedures

1. The Committee members will consist of:
   a. Medical director
   b. Consultant as required
   c. Registered nurse or disaster nursing chairperson
   d. Administrator
2. Consultation will be rendered by an infectious disease consultant.
3. The committee will meet to review any and all surgery-related infections. All infections thought to be related to surgery performed in the facility will be recorded in writing by the medical director or his or her designee as to the site of the infection, the organism involved, and the result of appropriate medical treatment.
   a. In addition, the attending physician will see patients 1 and 3 weeks after surgery to determine if an infection has occurred that has not been reported by the patient.
   b. Such infections will be tabulated as above and discussed at each of the committee's meetings. In addition, all infection control procedures will be evaluated and rewritten on a yearly basis. The minutes of each meeting will be prepared in writing and maintained in the facility by the designee of the medical director and reviewed by him or her at each committee meeting.
   c. The medical director of the ambulatory surgery center shall be responsible for maintenance and OR discipline. He or she shall be empowered to temporarily suspend the privileges of any member who does not adhere to the regulations of the OR or in any manner jeopardizes the safety and welfare of a patient.
   d. The medical director is also the supervisor of pharmaceutical services for the ambulatory surgery center.
4. The minutes of each meeting and any problems discussed therein will be brought to the attention of all staff members by the medical director so appropriate follow-up measures can be instituted immediately.
5. The committee will review all updated educational material on new procedures on infection control and ensure that infection control education is provided for all employees during a period of orientation and on a routine basis.

Table 2-7*B*
Infection Control Education

PURPOSE: To inform employees of potential dangers and protective measures needed to maintain the safety of staff members and patients.

1. All employees will go through a period of orientation in working in a potentially contaminated environment and the procedures for isolation precautions. Review of Occupational Safety and Health Administration (OSHA) standards by all employees will be required on yearly basis.
2. Updates on new policies and procedures will be presented to all employees at in-service education meeting.
3. All in-service programs that are applicable to the department must be attended.
A. Standard surgical preparation shall be used for all patients.
   1. Surgical scrubs shall initiate from the incision site to the periphery large enough to include the entire incision and adjacent area wide enough for the surgeon to work during surgery without contacting unprepared skin. Circular strokes are used to prep.
   2. The prep sponge is never returned to clean areas; new sponges are used.
   3. Prepping sponges are discarded in the trash, never to the prep tray.
   4. A sterile towel is placed over the prepped area and patted (not moved) over the area.
   5. An antimicrobial skin preparation is applied from the operative site to the periphery.
   6. An antimicrobial prep may be substituted as a combined method of pre-using small circular strokes from the incision to the periphery.
B. The patient is draped in surgical manner.
   1. Draping material shall be an impervious type and disposable.
   2. No part of the patient is left uncovered by sterile drapes except the operative field and the parts necessary for anesthesia to be administered and maintained.
   3. For conscious patients, draping around the face will be curtailed except when the face is the operative site.
C. Responsibilities to operative technique
   1. It is the responsibility of the scrub and circulating nurse to ensure the integrity of an open sterile field by not leaving the setup unattended after it is opened.
   2. Equipment, instruments, and supplies are organized in advance to prevent inefficient use of operating time.
D. Instrument sterilization
   1. All instrument sets, power equipment, and equipment sets are decontaminated.
   2. Only essential nonreplaceable instruments may be flashed.
E. Surgical scrubs
   1. The surgical scrub is the removal of as many bacteria as possible from the hands and arms by mechanical washing and antimicrobial disinfection before participating in the surgical procedure.

Table 2-7 *B*
Infection Control Education *(continued)*

2. All team members who will touch the sterile field, sterile instruments, or an incisional wound will perform surgical scrub with antimicrobial skin preparation from the fingertips to 3 in. above the elbow taking 5 min of scrubbing before the first procedure of the day.

3. Subsequent scrubs may be of a 3-min duration.

4. When using chlorhexidine, a 3-min hand wash followed by a 3-min scrub is required at all times.

5. Procedure for complete scrub

   a. Put several drops of antimicrobial agent into the palm of the hand and add enough water to make a lather. Wash to about 3 in. above the elbow.

   b. Rinse from the hands to the elbows.

   c. Using sterile disposable brush, apply the antimicrobial agent to the brush and scrub the nails and hands for 0.5 min for each hand.

   d. With a brush in hand, clean the nails with nail cleaner under running water. Discard the nail cleaner.

   e. Again, scrub the nails and hands with brush for 0.5 min for each hand.

   f. Rinse the hands.

   g. Using the sponge side, add enough soap and water to make a lather. Turn and scrub the hands and arms for 3 min beginning with the hands and scrubbing between fingers. Then scrub the sides of the hands and end with the arms.

   h. Rinse the hands and arms, starting with the hands. Keep the water running down toward the elbows.

   i. During and after scrubbing, keep the hands higher than the elbows so that the water running from the marginal areas of the upper arm will drip.

Table 2-7 *C*
Infection Control Procedures

1. The door to the OR suite and to the individual OR will be kept closed at all times.

2. Persons wearing scrub suits outside the OR suite must change them before reentering the OR suite. An exception is recommended in the case of orderlies who have no contact with other patients while outside of the OR, provided they wear buttoned white coats over their scrub suits and remove their OR booties on reentering the OR.

3. All exposed hair is to be covered with proper or disposable caps. The scalp and face should be covered.

4. It is recommended that all shoes be covered with OR booties.

5. Masks must not be worn for more than one procedure. Masks should be removed when not in place. They should not be allowed to dangle from the neck.

6. In any case in which the potential danger of the spread of infection from transferring an infectious patient to the OR suite comes into question, the infection control committee chairman or the attending surgeon will be consulted. His or her decision will be final.

7. Eating, drinking, and smoking are not permitted in the OR.

Table 2-8A
Prevention of Bloodborne Diseases

I. General policy statements
  A. All health care workers should routinely use appropriate barrier precautions to prevent skin and mucous membrane exposure when in contact with blood or other body fluids or any patient is anticipated.
  B. Hands should be washed before and after contact with every patient.
  C. Hands and other skin surfaces should be washed immediately and thoroughly if contaminated with blood or other body fluids.

II. Gowns
  A. Policy statement: Caps, gowns, and aprons should be worn during procedures that are likely to generate splashes of blood or other body fluids.
  B. Procedural steps
    1. Gowns shall be removed and disposed of according to procedural steps in the Centers for Disease Control and Prevention (CDC) manual.
    2. If clothing becomes soiled with blood or body fluids, the clothing must be changed.
    3. Hands should be washed immediately after removing gowns and immediately after contact with each patient.

III. Masks
  A. Policy statement: During procedures that are likely to aerosolize droplets of blood or other body fluids, masks and protective eyewear should be worn to prevent exposure of mucous membranes of the mouth, nose, and eyes.
  B. Procedural steps
    1. Masks shall be removed and disposed of according to procedural steps in the CDC manual.
    2. Eyewear and goggles should be washed with alcohol after patient contact.
    3. Eyewear and goggles visibly contaminated with blood or body fluids shall be disposed of in containers designated for contaminated refuse.

  4. Hands shall be washed immediately after removing protective eyewear and after contact with each patient.

IV. Gloves
  A. Policy statement: Gloves shall be worn for touching blood and body fluids, mucous membranes, or nonintact skin of all patients; for handling all surfaces soiled with blood or body fluids; and for performing venipuncture and other vascular access procedures.
  B. Procedural steps
    1. Gloves shall be removed and disposed of according to procedural steps in the CDC manual.
    2. Gloves shall be changed after contact with every patient.
    3. Gloves visibly contaminated with blood or body fluids shall be disposed of in containers designated for contaminated refuse.
    4. Hands shall be washed immediately after gloves are removed.
  C. Gloves should be worn when:
    1. Performing arterial or venous puncture
    2. Discontinuing arterial or venous lines or catheters
      a. Holding digital pressure on arterial or venous bleeding sites
    3. Performing perinatal care and checking perinatal pads
    4. Handling newborns covered with amniotic fluids and vernix
    5. Performing oral hygiene or nasal, oral, or gastric suctioning
    6. Performing and discarding chemical sticks
    7. Changing dressing or performing wound care
    8. Performing procedures related to hemodialysis and apheresis
    9. Handling specimens of blood or body fluids
    10. Measuring or emptying urine or other drainage containers and any other situation when exposed to blood or body fluids

Table 2-8*B*

Impact List to Implement Prevention of Bloodborne Disease Transmission to Ambulatory Surgery Employees

I. Medical waste containers

Large, covered, labeled medical waste containers are available in the dirty utility room.

II. Needle disposal

To carry out existing policies regarding destruction of needles and syringes, employees will not recap needles; rather, they will place them into the labeled rigid waste sharps containers immediately after use. Locked syringe and needle disposal containers are placed in the OR utility rooms. Additional containers are in the recovery area and dirty utility room.

III. Gloves

Inventory of properly fitting latex, vinyl, and powder-free gloves shall be increased for performing procedures.

IV. Protective eyewear

Goggles (disposable or reusable) and face shields are provided for ambulatory surgery personnel when aerosolizing blood or body fluids is anticipated.

V. Masks and alcohol swabs

The inventory of masks and alcohol swabs must be increased.

VI. Disposable garb

Gowns and hats are provided for performing procedures likely to generate splashes of blood or body fluids.

Table 2-9

Aseptic Technique

Policy: To maintain a sterile and safe environment for the patient.
Procedure

1. Scrubbed personnel must wear sterile gowns and gloves.
2. Shoe covers must be worn.
3. Sterile drapes should be used to establish a sterile field.
4. All items introduced into a sterile field should be dispensed by methods that maintain sterility of the item and integrity of the sterile field.
5. A sterile field should be constantly monitored and maintained.

Table 2-10

Storage of Sterile Supplies

Policy: To keep all sterile supplies separate from nonsterile supplies.

Procedure: Upon completion of the sterilization process, sterile supplies shall be stored in a closed, separate area from the nonsterile supplies.

Table 2-11

Instrument Decontamination Policy and Procedures in the Operating Room

Policy: All surgical and special tray instrumentation must be properly cleaned to ensure the effectiveness of the sterilization process.

Procedure: This procedure is to be followed for resterilization of imminently needed instruments or for instruments being returned to packs after a procedure.

1. At the end of the procedure, instruments shall be contained in basin on the back table.
2. Initial cleansing is to begin with enzymatic detergent and 2 oz presoak added to 1 gal of water, which is provided by the circulating nurse.
3. After removing the gown and changing gloves from a previous procedure, instruments are brought to the soiled utility room. The scrub tech will don apron and goggles in preparation for washing soiled instruments. Disposable examination gloves are worn.
4. Using enzymatic detergent and presoak with a brush available at the sink in the soiled utility room, instruments are washed thoroughly. If cannulae and suction tips are to be cleaned, pipe cleaners are available at the sink for evacuating blood and other material from inside the instrument. At this time, instruments are to be checked for broken tips, scratches, missing screws, and other defects.
5. For maximum cleansing, serrated instruments are to be scrubbed with the brush end of the scrub brush.
6. All instruments leaving the sterile field during the course of the procedure will be cleaned according to the applicable procedure before flashing.
7. After instruments have been thoroughly washed, they are to be rinsed for 30 seconds and left in the open position. *No instrument is to be clamped shut during the sterilization process.* They are then put into full-strength Madacide solution in the ultrasound machine and processed for 10 min for disinfection. They are rinsed again and dried on thickened toweling and then packed in appropriate color-coded packs (see Setups at the end of each surgical procedure chapter). Sterilization monitoring strips are placed in wrapped packs. All are marked and dated with expiration dates:
   a. See-through seal packs: 6-month expiration
   b. Double-green wrap packs: 1-month expiration
8. After cooling, packs are returned to appropriate cabinets in the OR. Broken instruments are to be removed and reported to the OR supervisor.

Table 2-12
Infection Control Contamination Containment of the Operating Room Suite

Purpose: To maintain a contamination-free environment

Procedure:

1. After surgery, instruments, equipment, and the surgical room are all to be treated as contaminated.

2. The scrub nurse may clean any obvious contamination.

3. The circulating nurse uses disposable gloves or a sponge stick when handling any sponges or patient-contaminated items.

4. The scrub nurse opens all instruments in the fully open position. Instruments are placed in the basket at the end of the case with other instruments from the same tray. If possible, separate trays should be maintained.

5. To enable faster assembly, dispose of all gauze and applicators (closed and sealed). All linens are placed in the linen hamper in the dirty utility room. Injectable needles and syringes should be discarded in the dirty utility room in a rigid medical waster container. Solutions from the case will be s1uctioned into autoclavable containers. Basins and trays are put in clean plastic bags and plastic baskets are covered with clean plastic bag with ends twisted and tucked under. All table linens are placed in the dirty utility room's rigid medical waste container along with the scrub nurse's gown, gloves, and mask.

6. Instruments and basins are taken to the dirty utility room. Specimens are placed in containers with screw-cap lids, and specimen slips are logged and placed in the laboratory for courier pickup to the respective laboratory.

7. Floors are to be cleaned with Madacide solution and wet-mopped at the end of each case.

8. Solutions are discarded down a clinical sink.

9. Linens are to be closed and removed from the dirty utility room at the end of each case and must be properly laundered.

Table 2-13
Cleaning Procedures for the Surgical Suite

There are three separate cleaning procedures for the surgical suite: between-case cleaning, terminal cleaning, and periodic projects.

Note: Anesthesia equipment is traditionally cleaned by the anesthesia staff because of the sensitivity of the equipment.

I. Between-case cleaning

  A. Frequency: After each procedure.

  B. Protective apparel: A scrub unit is worn to protect clothing, as are shoe covers, cap (which covers all scalp hair), and gloves.

  C. A phenolic germicidal solution is used for all cleaning; the solution is discarded at the end of each cleaning procedure.

  D. Steps

    1. "Wet Floor" signs are posted.

    2. Soiled linen is removed and liners are replaced.

    3. Trash and debris are removed, containers are washed, and liners replaced.

    4. The light over the surgical table is cleaned.

    5. Stools, Mayo tables, utility tables, IV poles, and surgical table are cleaned.

    6. Walls are spot-washed for blood splashes and other stains.

    7. Floor is mopped with germicidal solution after each procedure. If gross soiling has occurred, floor is flooded with germicidal solution and wet-vacuum is used to remove it.

    8. OR furnishings are restored to prearranged setup.

    9. Area is inspected for any cleaning errors.

II. Terminal cleaning

  A. Frequency: Daily after last procedure.

  B. Protective apparel: A scrub unit is worn to protect clothing, as are shoe covers, cap (which covers all scalp hair), and gloves.

  C. A phenolic germicidal solution is used for all cleaning; the solution is discarded at the end of each cleaning procedure.

  D. Steps

    1. "Wet Floor" signs are posted.

    2. Soiled linens are removed and liners replaced.

    3. Trash and debris are removed; containers are washed and liners replaced.

    4. Walls and doors are spot-washed.

    5. Dust vents are damped.

    6. Surgical lights are cleaned.

    7. All ledges are damp-wiped.

    8. Drop hoses are damp-wiped.

    9. Ceiling is spot-cleaned.

    10. All furniture, tables, IV poles, and surgical tables (including casters) are thoroughly cleaned.

    11. Floor is wet-mopped using germicidal solution. If gross soiling has occurred, floor is flooded with germicidal solution and wet-vacuum is used to remove it.

    12. Work area is inspected.

    13. All work tools are cleaned.

III. Periodic projects

  A. Frequency: Once per week

  B. Protective apparel: A scrub unit is worn to protect clothing, as are shoe covers, cap (which covers all scalp hair), and gloves.

  C. A phenolic germicidal solution is used for all cleaning; the solution is discarded at the end of each cleaning procedure.

  D. Steps

    1. "Wet Floor" signs are posted.

    2. Linen hampers are washed.

Table 2-13
Cleaning Procedures for the Surgical Suite *(continued)*

---

3. Trash containers are washed inside and outside.

4. Walls are washed completely, top to bottom and edges.

5. Vents are washed and cleaned thoroughly, including vacuuming.

6. Surgical lights are thoroughly washed.

7. Complete washing at ceiling and tracks are thoroughly washed.

8. Floor is flooded and rotary-scrubbed, then wet mopped.

9. The area is inspected.

10. Clean all equipment.

IV. Recommendations for equipment, supplies, and chemicals

A. All cleaning of surfaces contaminated with blood or body fluids must be done with a phenolic germicidal solution, per OSHA guidelines. To keep procedures simple, all surfaces can be cleaned with this same solution. Because of the nonneutral nature of phenolic agents, contact with a concentrate may cause irritation. It is therefore recommended to use a phenolic agent that can be dispensed through a proportioning system.

B. All equipment and supplies used in the surgical area should be used *only* in that area in order to prevent cross-contamination.

C. Disposable or launderable supplies (e.g., mops, rags) as well as cleaning solutions must be changed after each procedure.

D. Equipment should be stainless steel where possible. The following equipment and supplies should be available:

1. Mop bucket on casters

2. Mop wringer

3. Nonporous ladder tall enough to allow for cleaning of ceiling

4. Looped-end wet mops (sufficient quantity to change after each case)

5. Nonporous wet mop handle

6. Portable vacuum with disposable gags and wand attachments

7. 10-quart bucket with handle

8. Wipe cloths (sufficient quantity to change after each case)

9. Disposable gloves (nonsterile examination type)

10. Isolation gowns or coveralls, shoe covers, and hair cover

11. Trash liners

12. Scrub pads (hand size)

13. "Wet Floor" signs

V. Worker safety

A. Workers' "right to know" mandates that material safety data sheets (MSDS) for all substances be available to workers. MSDS are available from chemical suppliers.

B. Employees must wear gloves whenever they are working with cleaning solutions, handling waste, or performing any cleaning activity. Other protective clothing should be worn as deemed necessary. These steps are known as universal precautions.

C. Eye protection must be worn whenever cleaning solutions are being prepared or when splashing may occur.

D. "Wet Floor" signs must be posted whenever cleaning activities are in progress in order to prevent slips and falls.

E. All products must be labeled, including repackaged products from bulk (e.g., spray bottles). Labels must include the product name, ingredients, uses, and antidote. Labels are available from chemical suppliers.

F. Cleaning chemicals should never be used in a manner inconsistent with the manufacturer's instructions. Fatal chemical interactions have been known to occur when two or more cleaning products were mixed together.

G. OSHA regulations regarding blood-borne pathogens call for any spill of blood or body fluid to be cleaned up and disinfected by use of a phenolic germicidal solution.

H. Any unsafe condition should be immediately reported to a management representative.

VI. Handling of Regulated Medical Waste

1. Responsibility for regulated medical waste (RMW) and hazardous waste is *forever*.

2. Anticipated amount of RMW to be generated is first determined. RMW is categorized under the following headings:

a. Class I waste: Culture and stocks

Class 1 cultures and stocks of infectious agents and attenuated biological agents, including specimen cultures, culture dishes and devices, wastes from the production of biological agents, and discarded live and attenuated vaccines.

b. Class 2 waste: Pathologic wastes

Class 2 human pathologic wastes, including tissues, organs, body parts, and fluids that are removed during surgery or autopsy or other medical procedures and specimens of body fluids and their containers.

c. Class 3 waste: Human blood and blood products

Class 3 liquid waste and human blood and products of blood, including items saturated or dripping with human blood; items that were saturated or dripping with human blood that are now caked with human blood, including serum, plasma, and other blood components and the containers that were used or intended for use in either patient care, testing, and laboratory analysis or the development of pharmaceutical agents. IV bags are also included in this category.

d. Class 4 waste: Sharps

Class 4 sharps that have been used in animal or human patient care or treatment in medical research or industrial laboratories, including hypodermic needles, syringes (with or without the attached needle), Pasteur pipettes, scalpel blades, blood vials, needles with attached tubing, and culture dishes (regardless of presence of infectious agents). Also included are other types of broken glassware that were in contact with infectious agents, such as used slides and cover slips.

Table 2-13
Cleaning Procedures for the Surgical Suite (*continued*)

    e. Class 5 waste: Animal waste

       Class 5 contaminated animal carcasses, body parts, and bedding of animals that were known to be exposed to infectious agents during research, production of biological agents, or testing of pharmaceutical agents.

    f. Class 6 waste: Isolation waste

       Class 6 biological waste and discarded materials contaminated with blood, excretion, exudates, or secretions from humans who are isolated in order to protect others from certain highly communicable diseases or isolated animals known to be infected with highly communicable diseases (e.g., Ebola, Marburg, Lassa, or smallpox viruses).

    g. Class 7 waste: Unused sharps

       The following unused, discarded sharps: hypodermic needles, suture needles, syringes, and scalpel blades.

3. Generator ID number should be obtained if it has not already been noted.
4. Contract arranged with a licensed hauler
5. Set up of internal system:

    a. RMW segregated from general waste at generating source.

    b. Covered trash containers with "Bio Hazard" symbol or wording "Regulated Medical Waste" to be used.

    c. Red liners with same wording or symbol to be used.

    d. Complete monthly records made using generator log.

    e. Accurate tracking of forms from hauler maintained.

Table 2-14*A*
The Recovery Room

Objective:

A. To ensure the safety and well being of all patients

B. To follow *Standards of Nursing Practice: Recovery Room* as developed by the American Nursing Association and the Association of Operating Room Nurses to guarantee high quality of service

C. Assurance that ambulatory surgical patients receive the same quality of pre- and postoperative care as in-hospital patients

D. Continual advancement of professional and technical expertise of staff for improved nursing care

Table 2-14*B*
Recovery Room Protocol

Objective: To provide a workable guideline for the staff to care for patients by acceptable standards of aseptic practice

Policy

A. Personnel must wear scrub clothing. If they leave the recovery room area, buttoned laboratory coats must be worn within the confines of the surgery center.

B. Hand-washing shall be carefully done before and after every contact with a patient.

C. Aseptic technique is used in handling dressings.

D. Infected patients are isolated from the other patients to ensure protection.

E. Clean linen is stored in a covered area. Soiled linen is stored in a covered cart.

F. Stretchers are stripped and washed between patients with an appropriate disinfectant solution.

G. Suction equipment and connecting tubing are discarded after each patient use.

H. Oxygen equipment and supplies are discarded after each patient use.

I. BP cuffs are wiped weekly when soiled with an appropriate cleaning solution and allowed to dry before use.

J. All contaminated dressing, tissues, IV tubing and catheters, and so on are discarded in the regulated waste container to ensure proper disposal.

Table 2-14C
Recovery Room Patient Care Policy and Procedures

I. Recovery room
  A. Policy: To provide optimal nursing care for all patients admitted to the recovery room.
  B. Procedure
    1. The initial assessment of each patient is done after receiving the surgeon's report and is charted on the recovery room records. This includes the vital signs and all dressings and surgical areas to be checked.
    2. Vital signs are taken and recorded at specific intervals every 5 min if patient is unstable. When patient is stable, vital signs are taken every 15 min for 1 h and every 30 min thereafter.
    3. Doctor's orders are checked and initialed.
    4. Any significant changes in the patient's status (e.g., bleeding, vital signs, pain, drainage) are reported to the surgeon immediately and charted.
    5. Use of oxygen nasal cannula will continue until no longer deemed necessary by the anesthetist.
    6. When the patient regains full consciousness, with no complaints of nausea, sips of water or ice chips are offered for the patient's comfort and to initiate nutrition. The diet then progresses according to the patient's tolerance.
    7. Medication is given as per surgeon's orders and recorded immediately on appropriate forms.
    8. Dressings are routinely checked every 15 min.
II. Specific nursing functions to prevent complications
  A. Policy: Knowledge of the following procedures is necessary for all recovery room personnel so as to ensure successful postoperative recovery of the patient.
  B. Procedure
    1. Basics
      a. Cause: The tongue falling back into the throat or a collection of mucus, vomitus, or blood in the posterior pharynx.
      b. Symptoms: Breathing becomes uneven and the patient struggles for air. A "crowing" sound is made on inspiration.
      c. To maintain airways: Extend head and pull lower jaw forward; oropharyngeal suctioning is used to remove excess secretions from mouth and pharynx. A mechanical airway may be needed.
    2. Turning and coughing
      a. This is not encouraged until BP is stable.
      b. Deep breathing is begun as soon as the patient has reacted.
      c. When BP is stable, the patient is encouraged to cough.
      d. The patient is placed in the semi-Fowler's position after he or she has reacted.
      e. The patient is turned from side to side after the vital signs are stable.
    3. Pain
      a. Relieved: Nursing intervention and medication are used if necessary.
    4. Apprehension
      a. Relieve apprehension by explaining to patient that the procedure is over and his or her condition is satisfactory.
      b. If the condition is not satisfactory, assure the patient that he or she will improve. Tell the patient that someone will be in constant attendance.
III. Criteria for discharge from the recovery room
  A. Policy: These criteria are followed for each patient unless otherwise ordered by the surgeon.
  B. Procedure
    1. No excessive bleeding or drainage is present.
    2. The chart has been reviewed and the recovery room records have been completed and signed by recovery room nurse.
    3. The IV line may be terminated in the recovery room, making sure that the angiocatheter is intact.
    4. The patient is escorted to the rest room, where he or she may void and get dressed with the assistance of the recovery room nurse.
    5. After reviewing the chart and orders, a final postoperative assessment (including vital signs and dressing check) is done by the nurse and recorded appropriately.
    6. Postoperative teaching is continued and reemphasized during this phase of recovery. Discharge instructions are read and explained to the patient and companion, including prescriptions and possible side effects or complications. The patient and companion are asked to verify that they understand the instructions. They receive a copy of the instruction sheet.
    7. Specific instruction sheets from individual surgeons are also provided.
IV. Discharge from the Surgery Center
  A. Policy: Safe discharge from the surgery center is made upon completion of the discharge criteria and surgeon approval for the patient who has had local or local IV sedation.
  B. Procedure
    1. All patients are escorted from the surgery center by the recovery room nurse in charge of the patient.
    2. The patient must have a responsible person available to drive him or her home.

Date of surgery: _____

Total number of patients called: _____

Patient interviewed with postops: _____

Left message machine with postoperative instructions: _____

Spoke with significant other: _____

Unable to reach: _____

PROBLEMS:

Discomfort:_____

Swelling: _____

Bleeding:_____

Other: _____

_____

_____

_____

_____

RN's signature:

_____

Figure 2-7   Ambulatory surgery center surgical outcome reporting form.

Patient's name: _____

ID#: _____ Phone #:_____

MOHs ( ) AS ( ) SX DATE:_____

CALL-BACK DATE:_____

First-day postop call: _____ Site _____

Date: _____

[ ] Dressing change   [ ] Type of dressing

[ ] Discomfort

[ ] Meds required:

_____

_____

_____

[ ] Swelling:

_____

_____

[ ] Bleeding:

_____

_____

[ ] Reinforce postoperative instructions:

[ ] SO appointment date: _____

Office location: _____

RN INITIALS: _____

(If not scheduled at AS location, copy and fax this page + AS, doctor, and

RN notes)

SO appointment in _____ days

Date of appointment: _____

[ ] Clean (if not, explain):

_____

_____

_____

[ ] Intact

[ ] # _____ staples removed

[ ] Healing well

[ ] Untoward reaction:

_____

_____

[ ] RTC–CSE

[ ] Biopsy report PRN

Recall Date: _____

RN's initials: _____

Figure 2-8A   Ambulatory surgery center postoperative checklist.
Abbreviations: MOHs = a specific type of surgery; AS = ambulatory surgery; SO = sutures out; RTC–CSE = return to clinic for complete skin examination.

Postoperative patient

___ 1. Check patient's vitals when entering recovery room and at 15 min

    A. BP _____

    B. Pulse _____

    C. Alertness_____

2. Keep patient warm

3. Offer a hot drink (coffee, tea)

4. Check IV. If nearly finished, ask anesthetist or physician to remove IV.

5. Check surgery site for excessive drainage.

6. Ask patient if he or she needs to use the bathroom.

BEFORE a surgery patient is discharged:

1. Discharge BP _____ Pulse _____ Time _____

2. Time voided: _____

3. Oriented to person, place, and time

4. Discharged to responsible adult

5 Checked by physician.

RN's signature: _____

Figure 2-8*B* Ambulatory surgery center postoperative patient evaluation form.

Table 2-15
Policies and Procedures

Subject: Autoclave monitoring

Purpose: To provide a mechanism for monitoring and maintaining autoclave performance to ensure the sterility of processed items and maintain retrievable data relating to patient care.

1. Sterilization monitoring is conducted weekly using the dated chemical indictor system. Records of tests are kept in the appropriate log.

2. Sterilization records are kept in the appropriately labeled binder along with load monitor strips and chemical indictors. Biological strip test monitoring is performed on-site using the 3M Biological Monitoring System.

3. Maintenance is performed on an as-needed basis and the machine is tagged to indicate the need for repair. A record of this maintenance is kept in the equipment log.

4. Minimum requirements:

    a. Temperature should attain 250°F (121°C).

    b. Chamber pressure should reach 15 to 33 psi.

5. Exposure times (automatic settings appear in digital screen):

    a. Three min for one to three unwrapped instruments; 275°F (135°C)

    b. Ten min for more than three unwrapped instruments; 275°F (135°C)

    c. Thirty min for any wrapped instrument tray; 250°F (121°C)

    d. Thirty min for any fabrics and dressings; 250°F (121°C)

6. The cleaning of the autoclave is documented.

7. OSHA standards are maintained with regard to biological monitoring. In the event of a positive culture result, the following procedures are undertaken:

    a. Records are reviewed to determine if the processing was completed correctly.

    b. A list is compiled of the physicians who used the potentially nonsterile items.

    c. The nursing supervisor and attending physician are advised. The infection control committee is advised along with the names and addresses of the patients involved.

    d. An incident report is filed for each patient and is indicated in the patient's chart.

    e. Proper medical treatment is rendered by the attending physician.

8. In the event that daily sterilization monitoring indicates an incomplete sterilization cycle, the resterilization with new, dated, itemized sterilization monitoring strips is performed.

Month: _____ 200 _____

Day/Date   Solution used   Name of person cleaning autoclave

Figure 2-9   Ambulatory surgery center record of autoclave cleaning.

1. Immediately after your surgery and for the first day after, *relax*. Keep all activities to a minimum of 24 hours. *Refrain from any vigorous activity.* Do not jog, do not bend over, do not engage in sexual intercourse, and so on.

2. You can expect soreness after surgery, which can be relieved by pain medication. Take medications as prescribed. Do not skip or double up on medications. *Do not take aspirin or aspirin-containing products for 2 weeks.* Tylenol may be used. During the surgery, you may be given an IV antibiotic, which is used to reduce the chances of infection that might retard healing.

   ____ Yes, you were given pain medication while in recovery. Should you experience pain and need additional medication, you may take it at _____.

   ____ No pain medication was given to you.

3. You can expect some swelling after surgery, which may last approximately 6 to 8 weeks. This will gradually decrease by itself.

   ____ Use of dry, cold compresses or ice packs and avoiding dietary salt will help.

   ____ To sleep, elevate your head using either extra pillows on the bed or a recliner.

4. For emergencies, you may reach _____ tonight at _____.

   You may also call _____ during office hours.

5. Other information: _____

6. Discharged ambulatory in good condition with _____

                                                   Driver's name

   To (circle one):

      Home   Friend's home   Parent's home

   _____   _____   _____
   Physician's signature   RN/Recovery Room   Patient's signature
                            Tech's signature

Figure 2-10 Ambulatory surgery center patient discharge instructions.

Table 2-16
Policy and Procedures for Hospital Transfer of Patient

Policy: It is the policy of the ambulatory surgery center to transfer patients requiring overnight hospital admission to the closest facility.

Procedure

1. When determined by the patient's surgeon that the patient's condition requires overnight hospitalization, the circulating nurse will contact 911 to alert the rescue squad of the need for patient transportation to the hospital.

2. The attending surgeon will contact the hospital emergency department physician apprising him or her of the imminent arrival of the patient. The hospital's admitting department will also be advised that the transportation is under way and be told the reason for the hospital admission.

3. The patient's ambulatory surgery chart will accompany the patient to the hospital.

4. An RN will accompany the patient to the hospital if deemed necessary by the attending physician.

5. The attending physician will accompany the patient to the hospital if deemed necessary by the physician.

6. The patient's family will be advised of the patient's status and of the need for overnight admission to the hospital.

References

1. Hanke CW, Coleman WP. Accreditation of the office surgical facility. In: Coleman WP, Hanke CW, Alt TH, et al, eds. *Cosmetic Surgery of the Skin, Principles and Techniques*, 2d ed. St. Louis, Mosby-Year Book; 1997:81.

2. Abeles G, Warmuth IP, Sequeia M, et al. The use of conscious sedation for outpatient dermatologic surgical procedures. *Dermatol Surg* 2000; 26:121–126.

3. Higgins T, Hearn CJ, Manurer WG. Conscious sedation: What an internist needs to know. *Cleve Clin J Med* 1996; 63:355–361.

4. Joint AAD/ASDA Committee. Current issues in office-based surgery. *Dermatol Surg* 1999; 25:10:806–815.

5. Accrediation Association for Ambulatory Health Care. *Accreditation Handbook for Ambulatory Health Care*. Skokie, IL: The Association; 1999.

CHAPTER 3

Credentialing and Hospital Staff Privileges

I t is common knowledge that the general population has been bombarded with news stories reporting surgical mishaps that have occurred in an outpatient setting. As a result, there have been growing efforts on the part of state medical boards to regulate outpatient surgery. The assumption being advanced is that surgeries performed in a hospital setting are safer than those done in physicians' offices. One such example cited is that of ambulatory liposuction. Because certain groups have economic gain at stake, little is done to correct this misconception. It has been suggested that if anyone is to perform an in-office procedure, he or she should have such privileges in a hospital.[1] Hospitals, however, become hamstrung when asked to credential physicians for procedures normally done out of the hospital setting. They cannot be expected to serve as a quasi-quality control agencies for procedures normally done beyond their precincts. Yet groups with competitive economic interests continue to push the point beyond a reasonable limit in hope of achieving a competitive advantage. Rivalry being what is is, this trend continues. Certain specialties have been affected by this trend, particularly those that are non-hospital based, such as dermatology. In an effort to comply with changing regulations as well as the many new demands from patients for cosmetic procedures, many members of these specialties have felt impelled to seek such privileges. As this situation concerns dermatologists, their applications are often delayed, restricted, or denied based on the hospital surgical committee's preconceived misconceptions of what a dermatologic surgeon can or cannot do. It is a fact that the field of dermatology has progressively become a more surgically oriented specialty. Regrettably, many of our surgical colleagues in other specialties are not aware of the procedures performed by the surgical dermatologist.[2] In order to avoid delays in the granting of clinical privileges, it is the duty of the applicant to educate his or her fellow hospital staff members on the range of procedures encompassed by our specialty while also being much involved during the different steps of the application process.

This chapter outlines the typical procedure for appointment of privileges; it also recommends supporting materials that will enhance an application. An example of a prototype credentialing committee with its rules and regulations is presented. Many states have pending legislation to limit the scope of surgical practice without hospital operating room (OR) privileges. New Jersey passed such legislation in 1998, requiring that a practitioner who performs in-office surgery (other than minor surgery) or special procedures such as cosmetic surgery calling for the administration of anesthesia (including parental, intramuscular, intravenous, and/or inhalational anesthesia) shall not only be credentialed to perform that surgery or special procedure by a hospital but shall also have privileges for the anesthesia to be utilized. If a practitioner is not credentialed but wishes to perform surgery or special procedures in an office, the practitioner shall apply to the New Jersey State Medical Board to seek board-approved credentialing. Before a credentialed practitioner may perform surgery (other than minor surgery) or special procedures, he or she must meet an extensive list of requirements, which include monitoring, anesthesia privileges, transfer agreements, and policies and procedures (see Chap. 2). Other states are currently reviewing similar legislation; e.g. California, Florida, New York, Ohio, and Texas.

The Credentialing Process

It is imperative that every applicant understand the medical staff bylaws of the hospital in which privileges are being sought. Typically, a completed application is delivered to the credential committee or designee, who will verify the applicants' references, training, board certification, and the truthfulness of the supporting documentation. When this step is completed, the information is sent to the department chairperson, who further reviews the application and schedules an interview with the applicant, possibly in the presence of the department advisory committee during its monthly scheduled meeting. The department typically will have 1 month to make its recommendations known to the medical staff credentials committee. Eventually, the department chairperson will issue a report to the credentials committee supporting or declining the applicant's requested privileges and giving the rationale for this decision. The credentials committee may choose to follow the recommendations of the department chairperson or may reverse his or her decision. In many cases, a less biased judgment is rendered by this committee, as multiple specialties, surgical and nonsurgical, are represented. The applicant should seek to meet with this committee, if possible, to state his or her position.

The credential committee will transmit its decision to the general medical staff, whose members will vote on the recommendations at their monthly meeting. The applicant may again request to address the medical staff prior to their vote. The decision will then be transferred to the hospital president, who will supply it to the hospital's board of directors. They, in turn, will adopt or reject the application or return it to the general medical staff for further consideration. If the board's decision opposes that of the general medical staff, a committee of equal members of the board of directors and general staff will reach a final decision, which will be given to the applicant, the hospital president, and various committees. Some variation on this sequence of events is typical in most hospitals.

As is evident, the application process is lengthy. Dermatologists are generally assigned to the department of medicine, yet surgical privileges are handled by the surgery department. Historically, dermatology has been a nonsurgical specialty, and this view is still upheld by many physicians. Requests for liposuction privileges as well as advanced flap-and-graft repairs are viewed with suspicion. Some surgeons are sternly opposed to the granting of such privileges, and this is understandable given our specialty's lack of involvement in medical staffs and the generally poor understanding of dermatologists' skills. The first step in the achieving the granting of privileges is to be actively involved throughout the entire process and to document the dermatologist's skills in every procedure for which privileges are being sought. It is important to have a surgical log of all cases performed as well as to document all postgraduate courses attended. The core curriculum of the applicant's training program must also be described. Position statements of our societies and academy on the different procedures should be included. The American Academy of Dermatology and American Society for Dermatologic Surgery have guidelines of care for liposuction and laser surgery that should accompany every application.[3–5] The safety of tumescent liposuction as performed by dermatologists should be emphasized.[6] Any publications in scientific journals related to the privileges applied for should always be furnished.

Dermatology training is mostly based in an outpatient setting. Therefore, since many dermatologic surgeons are unfamiliar with the inner workings of hospital credentialing processes, an overview is in order.

The Hospital Credentialing Process

The credentials committee generally consists of attending physicians of varied specialties with a broad experience in and understanding of credentialing matters as well as famil-iarity with the hospital medical staff bylaws and the leadership service within the hospital. The credentials committee usually meets several times yearly. Their purpose is to determine if the applying practitioners have the level of competence and corresponding credentials required and are qualified to perform their surgical procedures according to the generally accepted standards of care. This committee should also ensure that each practitioner has already been appointed to the medical staff and that those who, in addition, have already been granted surgical privileges have attained and/or continue to attain the expected level of competence.

The credentials committee therefore examines all requests for surgical privileges with care, whether they are for new applicants or for present members of the medical staff. It requires all applicants for surgical privileges to resolve any doubts concerning their competence, ethics, training, ability to fulfill the obligations of membership, and any other matter bearing upon suitability for surgery privileges. The credentials committee actively seeks the ability to perceive distinctions and the information it requires in the execution of its task and requires that service chiefs send to the applicants all needed information. It then makes recommendations concerning the granting or denial of dermatologic privileges to the executive committee of the hospital.

SURGICAL CASE REVIEW/ INVASIVE PROCEDURES COMMITTEE

There is also usually a surgical case review of procedures. The surgical case review committee usually consists of the surgeons of the surgical service, and this committee will make recommendations to the chief of service and to the credentials committee.

The committee usually meets at least quarterly to ensure that the work of the surgeons is of the highest quality. The surgical case review committee is primarily concerned with the appropriateness and quality of advanced surgical procedures and appropriateness regarding removal of tissue. It usually has the authority to review any invasive procedure whatsoever in order to ascertain the quality of care. Generally a member of this committee, often a plastic surgeon, may be chosen as a surgical supervisor if privileges are granted. He or she reports deficiencies to the service chief, generally for 1 year, and where necessary propose corrective actions with regard to newly privileged physicians.

ELIGIBILITY REQUIREMENT FOR APPOINTMENT AND SURGICAL PRIVILEGES

Candidates for membership on the surgical staff are qualified practitioners who meet the clinical standards established by the surgical credentials committee, having a plenary license from the state and a level of malpractice insurance commensurate with the procedures performed and the requirement set by the medical board and/or the board of trustees of the hospital. Candidates must be "qualified" by the surgical credentials committee and approved by the service chief and the executive committee. The possession of the specified qualifications is necessary but not sufficient for membership.

"QUALIFIED"

In general, in order to be qualified, the candidates must usually have certain forms: board certification, letters of recommendation, and a documented specific training and malpractice history.

The service chief first reviews each application and determines whether it is complete and appropriate. Next, the application for the requested privileges is referred to the credentials committee. The credentials committee usually considers the application, accompanying documentation, and letters of recommendation and any opinions elicited from members of the department or the service chief(s) concerned. The credentials committee considers evidence concerning the ability of the applicant to fulfill his or her commitments to the service. The credentials committee then submits a written report and recommendation to the executive committee.

Many times, a practitioner who presents clear and convincing evidence (including the recommendation of the department chairperson) demonstrating, in the opinion of the surgical credentials committee, that he or she possesses the degree of knowledge, expertise, and judgment considered necessary requires the affirmative vote of those voting on a motion at both the surgical credentials committee and two-thirds of the executive committee.

The executive committee has the authority to enact appropriate policies and procedures to provide for consideration of exceptional classes of individuals, which is important to the dermatologic surgeon. If the executive committee approves the request, a surgical supervisor is appointed and privileges are granted. In the event that the credentials committee recommends denial of privileges, the practitioner usually receives written notice the request is denied. It is here that the applicant can request a meeting with the committee, surgical staff representatives, and/or executive committee.

FAILURE TO SUPPLY INFORMATION

The credentials surgical committee will usually make an adverse inference and enter its recommendation accordingly if, during its inquiry, a concerned practitioner fails to provide, obtain, or authorize information required by the application (e.g., case logs, specific training, proctored cases, letters of recommendation from the training program or proctor).

Submission of an application for appointment or privileges that, in the opinion of the credentials surgical committee and chairperson, contains a material omission or misstatement can result in denial of the requested privileges. In the event that an appointment or privileges have been granted on the basis of such false or misleading information, the chairperson can order emergency revocation of privileges. Therefore very detailed documentation with accurate dating and history of remuneration is required.

For the practitioner who already has certain privileges but desires to add additional privileges, his or her experience can be indicated on a form submitted through the department chairperson to the surgical credentials committee. The department chairperson usually can append his recommendation (and those of other concerned department or section chairperson) concerning whether the privileges should be granted, whether supervision should be required, and if so by whom. The credentialing committee usually considers the material presented and formulates its recommendation to the executive committee. Here is where a dermatologist with mostly medical privileges can have problems, because aside from skin biopsy, such practitioners are considered by most hospitals to be members of the department of medicine. This issue generally requires an interdepartmental discussion with resolution of the appropriateness of the request for privileges in another department; it can frequently lead to disputes.

DISPUTES AMONG MEMBERS/PRIVILEGES

A private complaint of one staff practitioner against another shall be presented to the department chairperson, who shall satisfy himself or herself that intradepartmental or other informal means of resolution have been exhausted. Such matters are usually referred to the credentials committee, which is made up of various specialists and will convene to consider the matter within a specified time. Usually, in an attempt to allow for fair examination, the affected individual is entitled to appear before any of the committee members reviewing the information in order to clarify any discrepancies. It is therefore critical that the dermatologist applying for surgical privileges supply a detailed history of his or her training, case log, pre- and postoperative photos, and letters from preceptors/fellowship directors. It is especially helpful to try to attend all meetings that pertain to obtaining privileges. It is also helpful to have an informal meeting with the chairs of medicine and surgery to try to determine what obstacles there may be to obtaining these privileges and the possible methods of resolving of these issues.

Table 3-1 provides an example of the criteria reviewed in application for hospital privileges.

Table 3-1
Format for Request for Privileges or Expanding New Clinical Privileges

Person Seeking Privileges _____

Privileges Sought or Expanded _____
_____
_____

Present Privileges Relevant to Those Sought if Applicable _____
_____

Basis for Granting PROPOSED Privileges (Specific training dates, sites, extent of course work, and program syllabus—fill in as appropriate):

Specific Training and Extent of Training (show dates):
_____
_____
_____
_____
_____
_____
_____
_____
_____
_____
_____
_____
_____
_____
_____

Preceptorship (site, name of institution (show dates):
_____
_____
_____
_____
_____
_____
_____
_____
_____

Proctored or Supervised:
Experience_____
(Show how, where, when, by whom proctored, outcomes):
_____
_____
_____
_____
_____
_____
_____
_____
_____
_____
_____
_____

Table 3-1
Format for Request for Privileges or Expanding New Clinical Privileges (*continued*)

List Criteria Used to Gauge Result (include before and after photographs and other relevant information):

_____

SIGNATURE OF APPLICANT: _____ DATE: _____

_____ _____
Signature, Department Chairperson   Date

_____ _____
Signature, Surgical Credential Committee   Date

_____ _____
Signature, Executive Committee   Date

References

1. Coleman WP, Hanke CW, Lillis P, et al. Does the location of the surgery or the specialty of the physician affect malpractice claims in liposuction? *Dermatol Surg* 1999; 25(5):343–347.
2. Roth R. Hospital staff privileges for dermatologists. *Dermatol Clin* 1993; 11(3):273–279.
3. Drake LA, Ceiley RI, Cornelison RL, et al. Guidelines of care for liposuction. *J Am Acad Dermatol* 1991; 24(3):489–494.
4. The American Society for Dermatologic Surgery. Guiding principles for liposuction. *Dermatol Surg* 1997; 23:1127–1129.
5. Lawrence N, Clark RE, Flynn TC. American Society for Dermatologic Surgery guidelines of care for liposuction. *Dermatol Surg* 2000; 26(3):265–269.
6. Hanke CW, Bernstein GB, Bullock S. Safety of tumescent liposuction in 15,336 patients. *Dermatol Surg* 1995; 21:459–462.
7. Herbich G. Dermatology and hospital liposuction privileges. *J Dermatol Surg Oncol* 1993; 19:1132.
8. Firstone MH, Shur R. Malicious deprivation of hospital staff privileges. *Legal Med* 1996; 199–215.

CHAPTER 4

Marketing Your Practice

The importance of marketing a medical practice is often misunderstood and neglected. Marketing is much more than selling oneself. Perhaps another and more constructive view would be to consider marketing as a "practice-building tool." With that attitude, one should actively try to serve the patient and tailor the practice to the needs and wishes of patients and referral sources. This chapter is intended to serve as a guide for such practice promotion.

Practice Location

The office should be easy to find and in a convenient location for your patients. The area should be within a viable growing market to further enhance practice growth. Parking should be adequate and convenient; if possible, public transportation should be readily accessible. Close proximity to a major highway may be beneficial. Being on the ground floor is an added convenience to both patients and staff.[1]

Strip malls tend to have a lot of traffic, which may help to draw patients, but such a location may seem less professional than a medical building. Medical complexes can have the benefit of including potential referral sources, although there may also be competitors. Additionally, some medical complexes have ambulatory surgical centers—possibly an added convenience.

PARKING LOT

Believe it or not, the parking lot will determine the patient's second impression of the practice, the first being the scheduling of the appointment. The parking lot should be clean and in good condition. There should be adequate parking close to the building.

BRANCH OFFICE

Occasionally, it may be beneficial to open one or more smaller branch offices to increase the area from which to draw patients. Initially, it would be most cost-effective to sublease space on a per diem basis. For most solo practitioners, the need for an additional practice location will diminish with time unless additional practitioners are brought into the practice. In many instances, branch locations increase travel time and staff fatigue. For larger groups, it may be necessary to open an additional office.

Office Environment

The office should have been redecorated within the last 3 to 5 years and be clean at all times. The reception room should be large enough to accommodate all patients and those accompanying them. The temperature should be comfortable, and reading materials, such as magazines, should be current, neat, and available to patients in both waiting and examination rooms (Fig. 4-1).

SEATING

There should be adequate seating to easily accommodate all patients and those accompanying them. The waiting room should have chairs with arms to accommodate elderly patients or those with disabilities. Cosmetic-oriented practices may want to consider using sofas and/or loveseats—in addition to armchairs—to create a more refined look. If space permits, one or two wingback chairs may be added for dramatic effect. If possible, it is recommended that all fabrics be Teflon-coated to resist staining.

CARPETING

Carpeting must be practical, as it must handle the wear and tear of heavy traffic. There are newer types of commercial carpeting that look neat and clean, resist staining and wear, and are more attractive than previously available commercial carpets. Darker carpets are often more dramatic, although they tend to show more dust and lint, while lighter carpets tend to stain more easily. Most offices use a carpet that is neither too light nor too dark and usually has a pattern, which helps to camouflage any dust or lint.

WALLS

Wallpaper tends to be more resistant than paint to scuffs and scratches, although it can tear. Any wallpaper chosen should be tough (resistant to wear) as well as washable and

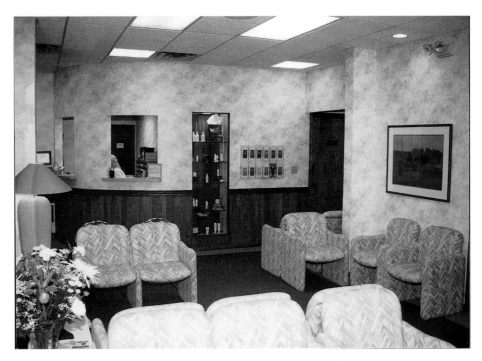

Figure 4-1 A stylish, comfortable, well-kept reception area reflects the physician's professionalism. Fresh flowers add a nice touch.

scrubbable. Freshly painted walls can provide a clean, crisp look, although it will scuff easily, thus requiring frequent touch-ups. Consider adding painted or stained chair rails.

LIGHTING

Most offices utilize a drop ceiling with fluorescent lighting. Instead of fluorescent tube lighting, consider high-hat lighting in the waiting rooms, which can be installed in a drop ceiling or sheetrock. Such lighting will look much more subtle and elegant than standard fluorescent lighting. Floor and table lamps can be provide as well, but these can be damaged, especially by children, and broken lamps can cause injuries. A few well-placed wall sconces may be an attractive option and can brighten dark areas.

HALLWAYS/DOORS/WALLS

In most cases, carpeting in the hallways is the most practical option. Carpets must be able to handle the daily wear and tear of busy traffic. If hallways are long, chair rails can be added. Examination room doors should be made of solid wood. Consider adding decorative moldings to doors to create a more sophisticated look, or doors incorporating designs may be chosen. Consider insulating the walls between the examination rooms to reduce noise and ensure patient privacy.

MUSIC/ENTERTAINMENT SYSTEMS

Most patients appreciate soft background music while they wait. Typically, light music is best suited for the waiting room and examination rooms, while classical might be even more relaxing for procedure rooms. Speakers should be built into the ceilings or walls so as not to look obtrusive.

Inexpensive sound systems can be purchased at almost any electronics store.

PERIODICALS

Periodicals should be up to date. Many offices keep the last 3 months of any given magazine issue available. Periodicals can be placed on coffee tables or end tables. If space is limited, Lucite or wood wall-mounted and free-standing racks are available. Periodicals should be straightened up by office staff at least once or twice daily so as to look clean and neat. Magazine covers may be employed if theft of magazines becomes problematic.

FLOWERS

Some practices may choose to have fresh flowers in the waiting room, which most patients find both pleasing and calming. A few small arrangements strategically placed in the nursing, check-in, and checkout areas will add a cheering touch for both staff and patients.

FISH TANKS/FOUNTAINS

Some practices may wish to have a fish tank or fountain in the waiting room or entrance foyer. Many patients find these soothing and relaxing. It may be best to have fish tanks or fountains professionally maintained.

CREDENTIALS

Credentials and diplomas should be displayed in areas where patients can see them (Fig. 4-2). Most practices display credentials in the reception room and/or examination rooms. Make sure that any continuing medical education (CME) recognition awards are up to date.

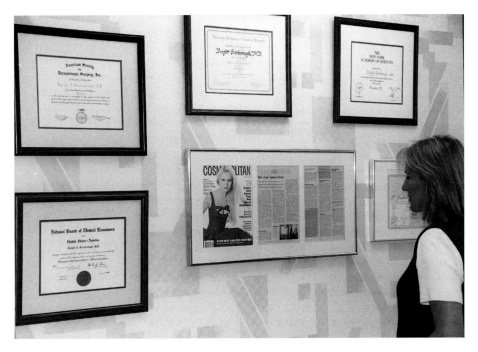

Figure 4-2   Credentials and media attention can be displayed to reenforce the patient's confidence in the practice.

EXAMINATION ROOMS

Examination rooms should be adequate (about 10 by 20 ft) and brightly lit; they should have a comfortable feel yet be clinically oriented. Oversized rooms are less efficient, while undersized ones cramp movement (Fig. 4-3).

Product

It is essential for all staff to be friendly and courteous at all times. Physicians and staff should smile, maintain eye contact when speaking with patients, and have a reassuring touch.

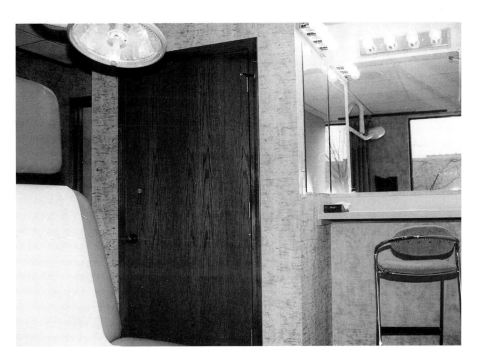

Figure 4-3   Examination rooms should be well lit, with enough space to accommodate patient and staff movement.

OFFICE STAFF

All staff should have written guidelines explaining all aspects of patient contact, from scheduling an appointment to checkout. Staff should never argue or discuss patients in the hearing of others, whether patients, friends, or relatives. Private conversations are to be kept private. Instruct office staff not to make negative remarks to patients. The following serve as examples:

> *Instead of saying*, "I'm sorry the doctor cannot speak with you."
> *Say*, "The doctor is currently in surgery. Can I have the doctor call you back in the late afternoon or evening?"
> *Instead of saying*, "I don't know."
> *Say*, "I'm not certain, but let me see if [name], our [title] can help you with that."

STAFF MEETINGS

No matter how large or small they are, most practices will benefit from regular monthly staff meetings. Keep staff informed of protocol changes, insurance changes (i.e., additional insurances accepted), new procedures being performed, etc. Staff meetings help to keep everyone informed on the essential changes within the office and also tend to help staff work together better. Keep records of staff meetings to record changes. Many practices will keep a sheet on which staff can note the issues they think need be discussed at the staff meetings. This is a good time to share compliments that patients have given regarding individual employees, to celebrate office accomplishments, or to note recognition from local media or community groups. Also, some practices prefer to hold a brief morning stand-up meeting to discuss that day's schedule. This can be done at the nursing station or checkout area. If there is no adequate private space available for staff meetings, the waiting room can be used during the lunch period or at some other time when no patients are scheduled.

UNIFORMS

Having staff wear identical uniforms creates a clean, professional look. Some practices prefer all staff to wear scrub tops and pants, while other prefer cotton tops. Consider having different color uniforms for each day of the week. White lab coats can also add to the atmosphere of professionalism (Fig. 4-4).

OFFICE HOURS

Office hours should be convenient for patients, although they must also be reasonable for staff. Consider adding early morning, evening, and even weekend appointments as ways to increase patient load.

Telephone

Some practices may choose to turn off their telephones during lunch and allow an answering machine to pick up the calls. This reduces staff fatigue and burden, although it might miss a potential patient who is shopping around. Another option would be to stagger the staff lunch hours so that the telephones can be monitored throughout the work-

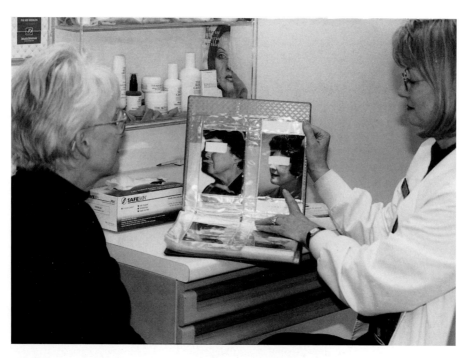

Figure 4-4 Professional-looking staff uniforms and lab coats convey the practice's dedication to patient care during all phases of the patient's visit.

day. Some practices utilize music on hold, while others choose to run practice information while the patient is on hold. One can usually find a local agency to make such a tape or CD; they will be able to provide suggestions and perform the service in a most effective manner.

PHYSICIANS

Physicians must be impeccably dressed and groomed. All physicians should be up to date on all the latest treatments. Physicians should be on time and have a good "bed-side manner," always looking patients in the eye and sitting at their level when possible. It is best always to sit with patients as this tends to make them feel better attended to. The physician's manner should reflect confidence, as most patients will equate confidence with competence. The physician should always treat staff well, especially in front of patients, and never point out their mistakes. The physician's demeanor, in short, is a reflection of the practice.[2–4]

FEES AND FEE COLLECTION

Ensure competitive pricing by periodically having staff check competitors' pricing. For added convenience and to ensure payment, the practice should accept major credit cards. For cosmetic procedures, requiring deposits and prepayment in full will avoid possible future collection problems. For most cosmetic procedures, consider accepting only cash, bank checks, credit cards, and certified checks.

Credit Cards

Most practices today accept major credit cards. In general, fees are lower for Mastercard, Visa, and Discover and highest for American Express. In addition, consider enclosing an authorization for payment by credit card for overdue accounts.

Payment Plans

Some practices will allow patients to pay on a payment plan. It is recommended that patients sign a contractual agreement with stipulations in the event of default. As most practices do not wish to be banks, it is generally not recommended to accept payment plans. In some instances, a patient who is not completely satisfied with his or her outcome may feel that there is no obligation to pay. It may be therefore best to keep the financial aspects of cosmetic surgery apart from the medical. There are some agencies that will provide patients with financing of cosmetic and other surgical procedures at a small fee to the physician. For most practices, this would be a better alternative to accepting payment plans.

Scheduling/Deposits

For all cosmetic procedures, consider taking a 50 percent or greater down payment to reserve the slot for surgery, which will also assure reimbursement for time and materials used by staff to prepare for surgery. This will greatly reduce a practice's no-show rate. If no-shows are a continual problem, consider having patients sign a deposit form, which states the practice's policies (i.e., refund policies). For all cosmetic procedures with set fees, the patient should pay the full amount before the procedure. It is recommended that payment be by credit card, cash, bank check, or certified check to ensure payment in full. For most procedures, consent forms should state that fees are paid for the surgical procedure itself—also that every individual will respond differently and that therefore no guarantees can be made regarding final outcome. In general, it might be wise to have a medical malpractice litigation attorney review all consent forms. Consider sending all consent forms to your malpractice carrier for review.

Fee Quotations

Some practices choose to offer patients written fee estimates. As most practices have set fees for each procedure, this may not be necessary. If patients are to be given written fee estimates, consider adding a disclaimer as to when the estimate will expire, as the practice's fees may eventually change.

Often, prospective patients will call asking for a fee estimate over the phone. Staff offering fees should be well educated. If a practice does not offer fees over the phone, you may lose prospective patients. If one offers a fee that is higher than what the patient is willing to pay, you may lose a prospective patient who, had he or she met the physician, might have chosen to have procedure. On the other hand, quoting reasonable fees over the phone will weed out patients who would not be prepared to spend the amount quoted under any circumstances. Therefore it may be best to quote ranges rather than exact fees. Additionally, inform patients that there may be alternative treatments that they might not have considered. For example, although collagen costs less than autologous fat transplantation or Gore-Tex implantation, the last two might be less expensive over the long run.

Cosmetic Consultations—To Charge or Not to Charge?

Some physicians charge a patient a reasonable fee, such as $100, for a cosmetic consultation. Some physicians will apply this amount later on to any cosmetic procedure they may provide for the patient. Such a fee will help avoid time-wasting consultations with patients who are just "shopping around" and those who are not seriously interested, although it may also turn away some prospective patients. Know what your competition offers. Additionally, how busy are you? If your practice is busy enough that it is reasonable to charge for consultations, then seriously consider charging. Additionally, patients will frequently schedule a "complimentary" cosmetic consultation and inquire about a noncosmetic problem. When this occurs, very diplomatically inform the patient that this time was set aside for cosmetic-related issues only.

Other Services

Know what your competition offers patients—i.e., digital imaging or cosmetic products. Consider adding services that will keep you competitive.

DIGITAL IMAGING

Some patients cannot imagine what they would look like after a cosmetic procedure. Digital imaging with image

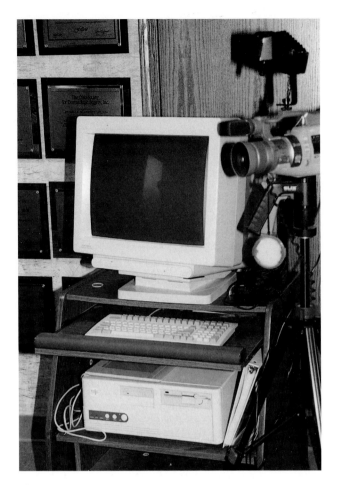

Figure 4-5 The use of digital imaging equipment allows patients to "test drive" their results. Imaging conservative improvement is prudent; it also allows the physician to point out any inherent asymmetries.

manipulation gives patients a true picture of themselves, showing what the results "might" look like. One must, however, be careful to tell patients in writing that such images are for demonstration purposes only and do not guarantee the imaged results. Consider discussing these issues with your malpractice carrier or litigation attorney. Imaging software and hardware now costs between $12,000 and $25,000. Although this is a substantial investment, it allows patients to preview their anticipated result (Fig. 4-5).

PRODUCT SELECTION AND SALES

Most cosmetic practices today sell many products from their offices. One must take extreme care and pay close attention to research products in order to provide patients with the best possible products at a reasonable cost. Spend time researching your patient's needs and desires to contour your product lines to their needs. Often, it is best to start small and grow from there. Private labeling can be of benefit for two reasons: (1) it ensures that you can monitor what the patient is using and (2) encourages patients to return to you

to purchase products they like. Certain staff members should be trained on selecting products for patients, and they must be readily available at all times. In addition, there should be display cases in the waiting and examination rooms (Figs. 4-6 and 4-7). For example, one can purchase a dispenser sim-

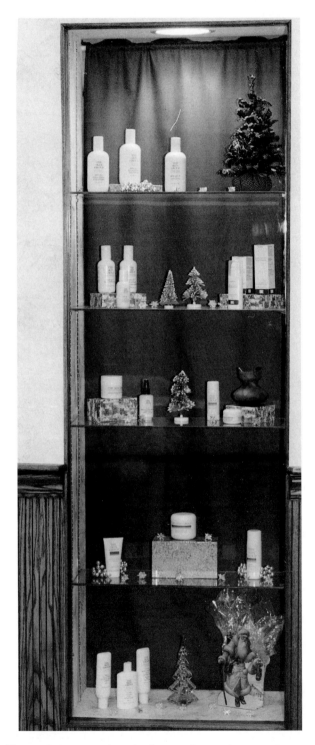

Figure 4-6 A product display window in the reception area can be decorated attractively.

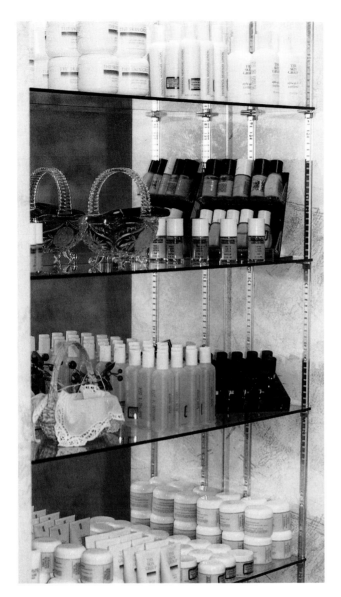

Figure 4-7   Patients can select products from a display area adjacent to the checkout zone, where assistance is available.

ilar to those used in hotels, which could contain a cleanser, a sunscreen, and a moisturizer. This will remove the risk of theft and still offer added convenience to the patient. A sign should be posted above the samples stating that these products are offered for you're the patient's convenience and are available for sale. Some practices choose a more active approach to sales and may even design a small cosmetic consultation room (Fig. 4-8).

PATIENT COMMUNICATION

Communication with patients should strengthen the bond between physician and patient. Considerable time should be spent developing communication aids, which will educate

patients, inform them of the newest procedures, and make them feel welcome and appreciated. Consider developing logo designs and stationery that will present a sophisticated and professional image. Local print shops can assist with development of letterhead stationery, envelopes, mailers, logos, and patient brochures.

Patient Brochure

Every existing and new patient should know about all the services and procedures offered by the practice. This is probably the least expensive marketing you can do and may prove to be the most effective. Existing patients already have trust in you and would probably like to have any cosmetic procedure performed by you rather than another physician. Consider making up a brochure that explains all of the services you offer; it should include some before-and-after photographs. Place these brochures in the waiting and examination rooms and consider distributing them to all new patients before they are seen. The brochure should be well designed, written in layman's terms, and updated regularly. A local print shop can assist with their design. Consider

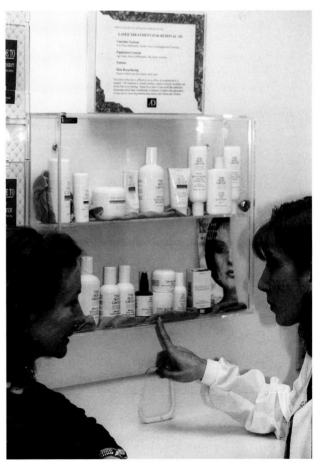

Figure 4-8   Instructions to patients as to the use of daily regimens can be given by staff in an examination or consulting room.

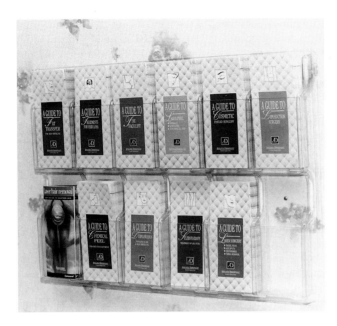

Figure 4-9   A well-organized brochure can familiarize the patient with the physician and the services offered.

adding a page summarizing the physician's credentials and including a photograph (Fig. 4-9).

Welcome Letter

Consider sending all new patients a letter welcoming them to the practice. With it, consider including an orientation packet and the brochure described above. Some physicians prefer to send patient registration and history forms with such letters so that patients may complete them in the comfort of their homes. This helps to keep appointments on time by reducing the time needed for paperwork at the office.

Newsletters and Mailers

Newsletters can be costly, although for some practices they are worthwhile. Monthly, quarterly, or semiannual newsletters can attract referrals from existing patients. If you have recently added a new service, such as microdermabrasion or hair-removal laser, consider sending a mailer to your patients to inform them of this.

Pins for Staff

If you have a new service or wish to promote any particular service or procedure, consider having staff wear a pin. For example, if you have just purchased a new hair-removal laser, consider ordering a pin that reads "Ask Me about Laser Hair Removal."

Patient Recall Cards or Calls

To decrease patient "no-shows," consider calling each patient a day before his or her scheduled appointment or sending a postcard in advance. New automated calling systems

are available that reduce staff time and cost, although are less "personal." Also, the elderly often have trouble using such systems.

Instruction Sheets

All patients should be provided with written pre- and postoperative instructions in addition to verbal communication. Instruction sheets should be professionally printed, not copied, and should include the practice's letterhead. Like everything else, these sheets are a reflection of the practice, and neatness counts.

Fact/Information Sheets

Sheets informing patients about various common treatments—i.e. wrinkle treatment options, hair loss treatments, etc.—should be available. Some physicians may also choose to distribute their recently published articles relevant to a specific procedure.

Postoperative Telephone Calls and Flowers

Consider calling all patients personally the evening after major surgery. This puts patients at ease, also instilling further trust in you and showing your compassion. Nearly every patient will be most appreciative of this gesture. Also, sending a floral arrangement during patient's recovery from cosmetic surgery can help brighten the day and reflects well on you as a caring physician.

Referral-Building Practices

The single most common source of referrals is existing patients, followed by physicians, nurses, and hospital staff. Most physicians neglect to track referral sources and types of referrals.

REFERRAL TRACKING
Patient Questionnaire

All new patients should complete a questionnaire that asks how they found you. Additionally, you may include a list of many of the available services you offer on this questionnaire. This will alert you and nursing staff to what interests the patient. Depending on the physician's preferences, the nurse or physician may address these interests. Additionally, these procedures will inform patients about the services you offer.

What to Track

It is important to track who referred the patient. In addition, it is important to track what type of referrals each nonpatient source is sending. Know you referral sources and treat them well. Take referral sources out for dinner or send their office staff lunch or breakfast.

PATIENT REFERRALS
Thank-You Letters

Send a thank-you letter to patients who refer others to the practice. For patients who have sent several patients to the practice, consider sending a "gift certificate" along with

```
┌─────────────────────────────────┐
│         [letterhead]            │
│                                 │
│ Date                            │
│                                 │
│                                 │
│ Rita Jones                      │
│ 1 Lovely Way                    │
│ Friendship, IL 31000            │
│                                 │
│                                 │
│ Dear Ms. Jones:                 │
│                                 │
│ In the past few months several  │
│ patients have indicated that    │
│ you had recommended me. I would │
│ like to take this opportunity   │
│ to thank you for your           │
│ confidence in me and your       │
│ continued friendship.           │
│                                 │
│                                 │
│ Sincerely,                      │
│ Fred Smith, MD                  │
│ Dr. Smith                       │
│                                 │
└─────────────────────────────────┘
```

Figure 4-10 Sample thank-you letter.

```
┌─────────────────────────────────┐
│         [letterhead]            │
│                                 │
│ Welcome to Advanced Dermatology │
│ Associates!                     │
│                                 │
│ [sample introduction]           │
│ We are pleased that you have    │
│ selected Advanced Dermatology.  │
│ We are committed to providing   │
│ patients with the best possible │
│ care.                           │
│                                 │
│ About Dr. Jones:                │
│ [insert 1–3 paragraphs about    │
│ the doctor, including training  │
│ and areas of special interest.  │
│ Consider underlining notable    │
│ achievements.]                  │
│                                 │
│ [you can use this area to       │
│ insert paragraphs about the     │
│ practice that you feel is       │
│ important for every patient of  │
│ the practice to know, such as:  │
│ Skin Cancer Treatments or       │
│ Cosmetic Surgery. In this       │
│ section, you can discuss        │
│ briefly some of the procedures  │
│ performed in the practice.      │
│ Consider including information  │
│ about the physician in this     │
│ area such as: "Dr. Jones has    │
│ given several lectures on       │
│ advanced facelifing techniques  │
│ at both national and            │
│ international medical           │
│ meetings."]                     │
│                                 │
└─────────────────────────────────┘
```

Figure 4-11 Sample welcome letter.

a letter further thanking them. Patient referrals can be the best source of referrals (Figs. 4-10 and 4-11).

OTHER REFERRAL SOURCES
Rolodex Cards
Send a Rolodex card along with a letter to all prospective and current referral sources (i.e., other physicians). The letter should not be too wordy, only briefly describing what services that prospective referral source may need. Additionally, the Rolodex cards should be simple, noting with a few bulleted points the procedures that you perform.

Other Referral-Building Techniques
Treat your referral sources well. Consider taking your referring physicians out to dinner or lunch on a regular basis. Remember them with a note over the holidays, including a gift of something edible for their staff.

Advertising
All forms of advertising aim at increasing exposure, thus informing current and prospective patients of what you offer and hopefully bringing them to the office. This form of mar-

keting can be expensive and must be monitored for effectiveness. Therefore it is essential that you know how each and every patient found you. A simple and effective way of tracking advertising as well as referrals is via a patient questionnaire. Consider having every new patient fill out a questionnaire that asks how he or she found you (i.e., yellow pages, referred by Dr. Smith, etc.) and lists any services that might be of interest. These questionnaires can be essential as they (1) let all patients know what services you provide, (2) gives timid patients the opportunity to ask about other services/procedures, and (3) allow you to evaluate your advertising and make any necessary changes.

NEWSPAPER
Major-Newspaper Advertising
Advertising in a newspaper can be expensive, although it may be effective. Your newspaper salesperson may work with you in developing the advertisement at no additional cost to you. Do not try to give too much information. Sometimes trying to get more than a few points across will blur the entire message. Consider beginning with a simple idea and then expanding on it. In this medium, as in others, one must rely on trial and error. It will take several revisions to perfect an advertisement. Furthermore, an advertisement

that is not attracting any prospective patients in one section of the paper might work well in another. Consider offering holiday "specials" or a discount in the ad.

Small-Newspaper Advertising

Local papers, which are often free to the public, may be a great medium through which to attract patients. As the area of delivery is usually smaller than that of major newspapers, the cost of advertising may also be less. Furthermore, such advertising may target prospective patients who live closer to the practice. However, as some of these papers are simply given away, a significant percentage of "readers" may not actually read the paper. Again, trial and error is the byword.

TELEVISION ADVERTISING

Although television advertising can be effective, it can also be quite costly. To be effective, such advertising need be well done to make a good impression. Therefore, a good team is needed to ensure good writing, filming, and editing. Unlike other forms of advertising, changes can be quite expensive owing to the costs of production. For such a media, you might consider consulting with a reputable advertising firm.

BUILDING, WINDOW, AND BANNER SIGNS

If you are in an area with any considerable traffic flow, consider creating signs to promote your practice. Any local sign store will be able to discuss your options.

Community Service

Community outreach increases the community's awareness of your practice and can be a good source of patient referrals.

HEALTH FAIRS

Consider offering free skin cancer screenings to major institutions or corporations, depending on your specialty. This can increase public awareness as well as broaden your exposure within the community. Inform local newspapers of the planned skin cancer screening, as they may wish to publicize it. Consider sending nursing staff to other fairs. Always provide brochures to inform people of the services offered by the practice.

BE A GUEST SPEAKER

Many organizations—including businesses, clubs, and other groups—invite speakers. Such organizations may be found through your local chamber or commerce. Organize a clear and concise presentation on subject matter that is easily digested and understood. Find topics that will be of interest for each particular group or organization. For example, a professional women's group may be very interested in leg vein treatments, whereas a local labor union might not. Consider providing the attendees with some of your promotional literature and business cards. Such promotional literature need not be relevant to the information presented. The attendees should know about all the services provided by the practice.

VOLUNTEER WORK

Consider volunteering at a local health care organization. This will increase your exposure to other physicians as well as to patients and keep you in touch with your community.

NEWSPAPER ARTICLES

Consider writing columns for local newspapers as a public service. In addition to educating people, this will increase you exposure at no cost other than your time. Essentially, this becomes free large-scale advertising. Write about subjects that will interest readers. If you are able to write regular columns, your name will become familiar to readers and they will think of you when the need arises.

References

1. Beck LC. Physician's office. In: Beck LC, ed. Princeton, NJ: *Excerpta Medica*, 1977.
2. Tardy ME, Klimsensmith M: Face-lift surgery: Principles and variations. In: Roenigk RK, ed. New York: Dekker, 1989.
3. Stegman SJ, Tromovitch TA, Glogau RG. *General Principles of Office Cosmetic Surgery*, 2d ed. Salem, MA: Year Book; 1990.
4. American Society for Dermatologic Surgery. A Guide to Marketing Your Practice. Schaumburg, IL: ASDS, 1987.

CHAPTER 5

The Consultation Visit

In addition to surgical artistic skill, the art of communication is a key element of dermatologic cosmetic surgery. Thus, the entire surgical process and result are cocreated by surgeon and patient, beginning with the consultation visit. It is important for the cosmetic surgeon to know *how* to operate, but possibly more important is knowing *when* to operate. Cosmetic surgical procedures are elective procedures, and—as with any surgical procedure—the potential for problems and complications exists. The consultation is an extremely important step in the process antedating any procedure. In cosmetic procedures, a special obligation is placed upon the physician to be forthright in describing the procedure, the alternatives, and possible complications. Since the intervention is not therapeutic but is being done as an elective procedure at the patient's will, the physician must be attentive and responsive. The role of proportionality must be respected in the indications for the procedure and the means to obtain the desired objective without compromising patient safety (see Chaps. 6 and 7).

Preconsultation Impressions

The stage is set for the physician/patient relationship long before the first in-person meeting. From word of mouth by former patients or colleagues or other sources of information, patients decide to see the cosmetic surgeon about a particular problem. Patients have preconceived notions of cosmetic surgery and, more specifically, of what their surgeon will be like. At the same time, the patient will often feel a sense of embarrassment or even foolishness about what he or she considers to be an extremely personal issue.

Awareness of these factors will help the surgeon to understand the patient's approach to the consultation. The patient's next impression of the physician comes through contact with the office and is most often made by telephone (see Chap. 4). The office staff, by their telephone manner more than through the information given, convey the tone of the office. Are they friendly and responsive to prospective patients, expressing an interest in helping patients, and being

attuned to their needs? Office staff should be given training in the proper way of handling such telephone conversations as well as specific information (scheduling for appointments, consultation fees, and general areas of cosmetic surgery the physician performs) to be given over the telephone. A general range of costs can be given in some cases, but specific surgical fees and medical advice are inappropriate.

An experienced staff can often spot a difficult patient during this initial phase. More often than not, if the staff suspect that the new patient will be a problem, the physician will find that, at some point, the patient will, in fact, pose a problem. The critical nature of the consultation must be understood. The ability to select appropriate candidates for cosmetic surgery will have a critical impact on the success or lack of success of the practice.

The Initial Consultation

Even before entering the examination room, the physician may review patient history questionnaires to prepare for the meeting. There are two tasks in consultation: the first is to assess the patient's appropriateness for cosmetic surgery and the second is to form a partnership with the patient to plan a cosmetic surgical approach customized to the patient's specific needs.

The consultation frequently begins with the patient outlining his or her cosmetic complaints; frequently the physician asks the patient to rank each complaint in terms of relative importance. It is not uncommon to have a patient initiate a discussion by requesting a surgical procedure such as a blepharoplasty. In evaluating the patient's request, the surgeon must first evaluate the area of concern to the patient—for example, the degree of hooding of the upper lids. After has been done, it is important to evaluate the degree of patient concern with the area. If there is a wide discrepancy between the patient's assessment of the defect and the surgeon's view of it, a red flag immediately shows up in the quality of the patient's expectations. This may therefore, be a poor a poor surgical candidate based on his or her great degree of concern about a small cosmetic problem. It is not uncommon for a patient to ask for a procedure without understanding the true basis of the procedure in relation to the desired effect. It is therefore important to ascertain the level of the patient's knowledge with respect to esthetic surgical procedures as well as his or her expectations and reasons for wanting to have the procedure done.

During the process of gathering this information, relative contraindications to the patient's acceptance for treatments may be revealed. Certain presenting characteristics may be a clue that a patient may have unrealistic expectations. Other basic issues to be considered are the reasons for the procedure—e.g., does a friend or spouse want the procedure performed? Is there a pending divorce or a recent death? The basic rule is to perform the procedure only if the patient is the one who wants the surgery. The patient must be able and willing to share the risk and responsibility of the surgery with the physician, especially in the outpatient setting, where the patient must be actively involved in the postoperative wound care at home.

It is during this visit that impressions are created. Both the surgeon and patient are evaluating each other—based on professional conduct of the surgeon and the office surroundings—while the surgeon is evaluating the characteristics and general makeup of the patient. After this initial discussion, the surgeon will have the patient, with the help of a mirror, detail the exact complaint, ensuring that both the surgeon and patient are clear on the area of patient's dissatisfaction.

Motivation and degree of correction can be discussed, as well as possible approaches. Our initial method is to detail the possible courses of action by first discussing the most conservative approach and then going on through a description of the most aggressive correction (see Chaps. 6 and 7). Discussion of skin quality, relevant sun damage, scars, pigmentary disorders, and asymmetries follows. The corrective procedures are outlined and discussed and appropriate photos are obtained. We usually utilize either previous patient photos and/or digital imaging to present the various approaches. The patient here has the opportunity to better describe his or her expectations, and the surgeon evaluates these as the patient assesses the pictures demonstrating previous results with other patients. For example, if the surgeon feels that a particular patient's photo reveals an excellent result but that the patient sees only marginal improvement, then even an outstanding result may not satisfy this patient because of his or her inappropriate expectations and motivations. It is here that the surgeon must not hesitate to recommend against the surgery. Ultimately, if the initial consultation is acceptable to both parties, a detailed information packet that essentially encapsulates the procedure process is given to the patient to take home and be read carefully at leisure. Included in the packet are pre- and postoperative instructions, photographic examples of the pre- and postoperative results, the consent forms that the patient will have to read in order to see all the risks and benefits in proper prospective, thus guiding the development of realistic expectations as to possible results. The brochure may contain reprints of the surgeon's articles on the procedure, along with his or her credentials and academic accomplishments. A detailed question-and-answer sheet is utilized during the consultation; on it, the patient is asked to review the information and formulate questions, which can be answered later over the phone or in the preoperative visit. It is our policy to obtain a general medical clearance from the family physician prior to any elective cosmetic procedure.

Patient Selection

Patient selection is essentially the hallmark of a successful experience for both the patient and the surgeon. When the surgeon evaluates the patient, many factors must be considered, both medical and psychological. The surgeon must obviously be certain that there are no medical contraindications to the procedure. In addition, the surgeon must review the entire procedure with the patient, stressing the risks and benefits. It is important to assess the patient's expectations to be sure that they are realistic with respect to the anticipated results. The physician must identify the patient's goal and then determine the best way of reaching that goal safely within the limitations of cosmetic surgery. Open-ended questions enable the patient to clarify his or her goals and may reveal personality traits that could affect the physician's view of the patient as a candidate for surgery (Table 5-1).

The patient must be able to understand what cosmetic surgery can realistically accomplish, while the physician must be alert to both physical and psychosocial "caution signals." Some of these may come up in patients' answers to the open-ended questions described previously and may help to identify those individuals who are poor candidates for cosmetic surgery (Tables 5-2 and 5-3).

The importance of this first stage of patient evaluation—the consultation—cannot be overemphasized. It lays the groundwork for all that follows for each patient and is a cornerstone of a successful surgical outcome, translating ultimately to a successful cosmetic surgery practice.

In the next patient visit, the preoperative visit, the procedure, anesthesia, consents, and any questions the patient may have are reviewed. Photographic documentation of the preoperative status is obtained. If the patient is undergoing liposuction, the patient's weight and measurements in

Table 5-1
Open-Ended Questions

How can I help you?

What specific feature do you want corrected?

When you look in the mirror, what is it you don't like?

If you could have only one thing changed, what would it be?

How long have you been thinking about cosmetic surgery?

What caused you to think about it?

What do you think this operation will do for you?

Why do you want the operation at this particular time?

What other cosmetic operations have you had?

Were you happy with the results of those previous operations?

What is the attitude of your family and friends to the proposed operation?

Table 5-2
Caution Signals

Vagueness	Excessive secrecy
Unrealistic expectations	Indecisiveness
Rash decisions	"Very important person" attitude
Great urgency	Failure to establish rapport
Poor motivation	Unsympathetic to physician and staff
Surgery to please others	Hidden infantile motives
Multiple esthetic procedures	Depression (past or present)
Dissatisfaction with previous esthetic operations	Emotional crisis (past or present)
Previous litigation	Psychiatric therapy (past or present)
Disapproval of relatives	Minor or virtually nonexistent defect
Perfectionist attitude	Manipulative behavior

Table 5-3
Common Signs of Unrealistic Patient Expectations

A highly critical attitude toward work done by previous surgeons

A display of antagonistic, angry, or demanding characteristics toward the staff

An overblown concern over subtle defects

Vagueness about the specific change desired

The requirement for perfect symmetry

A personal schedule too tight to allow for adequate recovery time

A hostile personality

inches are obtained. A review of the preoperative clearance and laboratory tests is undertaken and then the patient is given the operative time as well as preoperative medications and is instructed to have a responsible adult available to to drive him or her to and from the ambulatory surgery facility. Finally, the consent forms are signed. The development of informed consent is vigorously guarded as a matter of law. As such, informed consent should not be considered at just one specific point in time but as a continuous process in the management of a patient's treatment, regarding which up-dated information can be provided and the content of the original consultation reviewed. Therefore, informed consent is more than just a consent form. Although many possible problems are presented on the form, not every contingency can be detailed. Again, doctor-patient rapport, built over time, maintains the patient's confidence and faith in the physician. Essentially, whatever time is necessary should be given during each consultation so that both patient and physician have enough time to develop a good rapport.

Complications can occur the patient's recall of these discussions may be less than full; therefore the detailed information packet, along with consents that detail the possible side effects, should be provided several weeks to days prior to the procedure for thorough patient review.

CHAPTER 6

Facial Analysis

Patients who want to look younger often turn to the cosmetic surgeon. This chapter provides the dermatologic surgeon with an overview of the anthropometrics approach to assessment of the condition and quality of skin, soft tissue, and support structures in these patients. The basis for these analyses rests in the proportionality of the youthful face, facial muscle tone, buoyancy of the subcutaneous fatty layer, and quality of young, clear skin. In order to restore youthful features of the face, the cosmetic surgeon must consider the changes in facial shape and proportion produced over time as well as altered quality of skin and substructure associated with aging. Age-related effects present as a spectrum, and each patient needs individual assessment to determine the appropriate rejuvenation strategy and establish realistic expectations and endpoints. Body proportions and morphology are assessed in a similar fashion.

Standards of Beauty

The concept of beauty often appears vague. It can vary with cultural background, ethnicity, and socioeconomic status. The ancient Greeks and Romans demonstrated their idealized forms of beauty in their arts and crafts and attempted to define them metrically. Leonardo da Vinci, however, was the first to clearly establish a metric system for beauty, which is demonstrated in his works and shows his keen sense of esthetics. Throughout the western world, however, ideals of beauty are much the same, given that movie stars and other celebrities are widely regarded as beautiful. It is well known that attractive people are generally more successful. Psychological studies emphasize that higher self-esteem promotes a more optimistic outlook and increases social interaction. This also holds true for elderly people who remain attractive. They appear to be less depressed and lonely and continue to possess higher self-esteem and confidence, making them more successful socially.

The cosmetic surgeon must appreciate the changes associated with aging and have a deeply rooted sense of beauty. Moreover, he or she must be able to define a normal, youthful face. This knowledge will make it possible to offer patients best treatment options.

In general, the telltale signs of aging are viewed very critically in our youth-oriented society. Men and women express frustration with advancing age, in part because they are asked repeatedly about being tired, sad, or angry even though they are not. Their appearance—marked by increasing rhytids, drooping eyebrows, and sagging skin—leads people to draw faulty conclusions. Almost every patient who seeks the attention of the cosmetic surgeon wants to have beautiful skin. The adjectives used by patients to describe beautiful skin most often include *smoothness, radiance,* and *tightness.* These are the characteristics typically associated with youthful skin.

The Skin

Aging is a biological process of tissue involution and evolution resulting in the appearance of sagging skin, rhytids, blotchy discolorations, and subdermal atrophy. There are currently two major theories of aging. One, the programmatic theory, implies that certain "aging" genes are activated by intrinsic and extrinsic stimuli. The stochastic theory, which is also called the oxidative stress and rate-of-living theory, postulates that constant exposure to oxidative stress—in combination with a decline in catalytic enzyme concentrations and activities over time—leads to increasing cell damage due to free radicals. Elements of both theories may help to explain the process of aging.[1,2]

AGING MODELS

The skin ages concurrently with other structures or compartments. These compartments influence each other, possibly via a feedback mechanism. As the skin ages chronologically, the bone mass of the cranium and the entire skeleton is reduced as well. This leads to the perception that the skin envelopes the bony structures only loosely. Facial muscles continue to loose muscle tone, and their muscle mass diminishes further, reducing skin support. Septal structures weaken and give way to gravitational force—i.e., the orbital septum loosens and the underlying fat pads protrude under the skin, forming undesirable bags and bulges. In addition, subcutaneous fatty tissue atrophies throughout the body. As a result, the face comes to appear gaunt and hollow. Epidermal fattening and reduction in the microvasculature makes the skin look pale. In addition, aging increases the vulnerability of the skin to shearing forces, often resulting in ecchymosis. All these phenomena help to explain what happens in aging. This model, like those for other biological systems, emphasizes the interplay of different structures. For the cosmetic surgeon, its implication is that treatment of the aging face requires a multidimensional approach.[3]

Intrinsic Aging

Intrinsic aging is defined as inevitable aging, with changes accumulating over a lifetime. Factors influencing intrinsic aging are genetic features that preprogram subcutaneous tissue atrophy and the resistance to gravity. Examples of changes due to intrinsic aging include sagging skin and dynamic and static rhytids.

Biochemical changes in collagen, elastin, and dermal ground substance occur with aging. Collagen content decreases about 1 percent per year of adult life, with the remaining collagen fibers appearing disorganized and thickened. Elastic fibers are also reduced both in number and diameter. Both collagen and elastin fibers show an increase in calcification and cross-linking in the adult skin. The number of proteoglycans is diminished, contributing to a reduction in skin turgor. In general, the skin appears more rigid and inflexible with aging.

The loss of the epidermal rete ridges leads to a reduction in adhesion forces and makes the skin more prone to injury. The skin appears dry and flaky, perhaps secondary to a proposed reduction in the protein filaggrin. Filaggrin assembles keratin microfibers into keratin filaments and is also reduced in patients with ichthyosis. Moreover, Langerhans cells in the skin are significantly reduced in the aging epidermis, leading to attenuation of the immune response. There is a decrease in blood vessel formation and a reduction in vessel response. Wound healing time is prolonged due to the reduction in nutrition and vascular formation (Table 6-1).

Table 6-1

Signs of Intrinsic Aging

Aging signs	Causes
Sallow skin color	↓ Vascularity and vascular response
Roughened texture	↓ Filaggrin
Fine rhytids	↓ Elastic fibers, ↓ collagen fibers
Subcutaneous and dermal thinning	↑ Genetically programmed atrophy

Table 6-2

Signs of Extrinsic Aging

Aging signs	Causes
Dyschromia, mottled pigmentation	↑ Melanocyte response
Roughened, coarse skin texture	↓ Cell repair, ↓ cell turnover
Rhytid formation	↓ Elastic fibers, ↓ collagen fibers ↑ Dermal and subdermal atrophy

Extrinsic Aging

The skin is the only organ exposed to the harsh external environment, including wind, sun, temperature changes, and chemicals. These environmental factors produce extrinsic aging. Chronic sun exposure correlates with chronic ultraviolet radiation (UV) exposure—both ultraviolet B (UVB) and ultraviolet A (UVA). Both are incriminated in causing photoaging and skin cancer.

Photodamaged skin has a mottled, dyschromic appearance and a tough texture; it appears leathery and thin. Often there are actinic keratoses present as well as ephilids, lentigines, and telangiectasias. In addition, rhytids, from fine lines to deep furrows and creases, can develop. In general, intrinsic aging is accelerated by extrinsic aging, which is superimposed on it. Tobacco smoking contributes to extrinsic aging and exacerbates photodamage (Table 6-2).

There is considerable variation in skin quality among patients seeking rejuvenation treatment. First, fair-skinned people display signs of photoaging at an earlier age than those with darker complexions. Second, patients have varying skin thicknesses. In our experience, patients with thick, relatively "doughy" skin respond better to esthetic treatments than patients with thin, finely wrinkled dry skin. Interestingly, women are better candidates for resurfacing techniques than men, owing to the often highly sebaceous male facial skin. The contractile effect of CO_2 resurfacing is often reduced in men.

AGING TYPES AND REJUVENATION

Our office experience and consultations suggests that there are two dominant forms of aging, involutional and evolutional.

Involutional Aging

Involutional aging involves a marked reduction in subcutaneous tissue over time. The patient usually is of slender to normal build. The skin laxity is progressively visible through jowl formation and increasing accumulation of redundant neck skin. The skin turgor is often lax, without much recoil when the pinch test is performed (Figs. 6-1 to 6-4; Fig. 6-5).

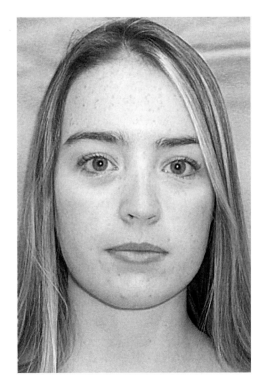

Figure 6-1 Youthful appearance of the face without discernible rhytids.

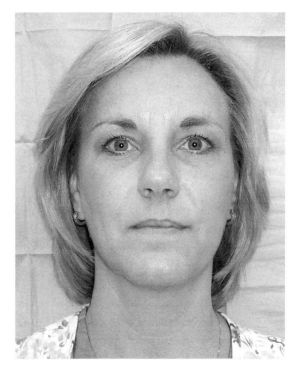

Figure 6-2 Early facial rhytid formation and mild skin laxity (involutional aging).

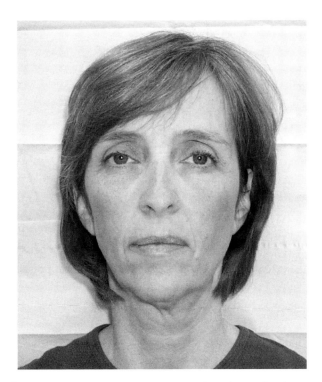

Figure 6-3 Mild rhytid formation and moderate skin laxity (involutional aging).

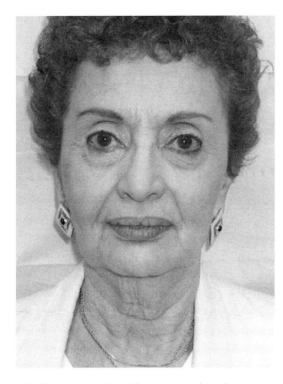

Figure 6-4 Moderate rhytid formation and moderate to severe skin laxity (involutional aging).

1. Early rhytids	2. Dynamic rhytids	3. Deepening rhytids + structural changes
(second and third decades) (Fig. 6-1)	with little static lines (third and fourth decades) (Fig. 6-2)	Improvement fair with makeup (fifth decade) (Fig. 6-3)
Treatment option:		
Topical antiaging products	Botox injection	Botox injection
Superficial chemical peeling	Soft tissue augmentation	Soft tisue augmentation
Microdermabrasion	Collagen	Deep peeling
Botox injection	Fascia lata	Laser resurfacing:
	Micro fat injection	Combination Erb:YAG + Co_2; − CO_2
	Expanded polytetrafluoroethylene	**Surgical intervention**
	Medium-depth peeling	Upper and lower blepharoplasty
	Laser resurfacing: Erb:YAG or CO_2	Facial liposuction
		Full face-lift
	2a. Dynamic rhytids + structural changes surgical intervention:	Combination procedures
	Upper blepharoplasty	**4. Deep rhytids (static/dynamic) and structural changes**
	Facial liposucton	No improvement with makeup (sixth decade and up) (Fig. 6-4)
	Lunch time lift (suture-less facelift)	**Treatment options in addition to 3**
	Mini face-lift	Combination procedures: full face-lift with neck lift, facial liposuction, and CO_2 laser resurfacing

Figure 6-5 Aging and rejuvenation (algorithm).

Evolutional Aging

The second dominant form of aging is the evolutional aging. The patients in this category are of sturdier build. Excess soft tissue deposition is observed in the midface and cheek areas. There is often only minor rhytid formation. The neck appears full and a double chin contour is often visible. The skin turgor is usually good. Gentle pinching and pulling on the skin results mostly in a "snap back," demonstrating elastic recoil. (Figs. 6-6 to 6-9).

AGING AND REJUVENATION

The first noticeable rhytid occurs in patients in their mid- to late twenties. Rejuvenation techniques indicated in this group include the topical antiaging products, microdermabrasion (a physical peeling procedure), superficial peels with hydroxy acid solutions, and botulinus toxin A (Botox) injection. Nonablative laser treatment is also sometimes indicated. These techniques can be used as monotherapy or in combination. The synergistic effect of multiple modalities can increase patient satisfaction (see specific chapters for details).

Dynamic rhytid formation is visible in patients in the fourth decade of life (30 to 39 years). Although relatively little static line formation is detectable in these patients, they may often demonstrate early to moderate photoaging. Procedures to combat the aging effects include medium-deep peels; soft tissue augmentation with collagen, expanded polytetrafluoroethylene, or microlipoinjections; resurfacing with erbium:YAG or ultrapulsed CO_2; botulinus toxin A injections; and adjunct therapies mentioned for the treatment of patients with early photoaging. Although these therapies are effective as monotherapy, combination therapy allows for different approaches toward a youthful-appearing skin. Surgical interventions with upper blepharoplasty, facial liposuction, a lunchtime face-lift or minilift (see Chap. 17) can dramatically restore a youthful appearance. A combination approach is safe and effective.

In their forties, patients display advanced photoaging. Overall wrinkle formation becomes more marked. Dynamic rhytids project prominently and resist improvement with makeup. The nasal structure changes: the nasal tip descends as the columnella relaxes, obscuring the nasolabial angle. The nose may appear elongated, although this is a rare complication. Treatment options for these patients include combinations of CO_2 and erbium:YAG laser resurfacing or solely CO_2 laser treatment, according to the specific patient's needs. Deep peeling and soft tissue augmentation are also indicated, as well as Botox injection. Combination approaches are generally useful. The face-lift procedures to consider include a sutureless face-lift, a mini face-lift, or full face-lift in addition to upper and lower blepharoplasty and facial liposuction.

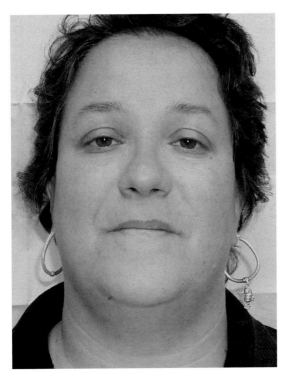

Figure 6-6 Early evolutional aging of the face with minimal rhytid formation.

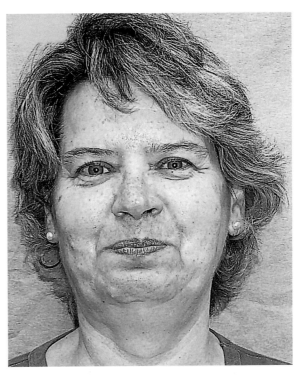

Figure 6-7 Moderately advanced evolutional aging with mild skin laxity and good skin tone.

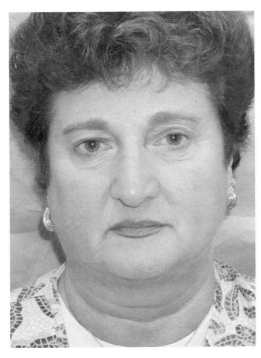

Figure 6-8 Moderate to severe advanced evolutional aging with more pronounced rhytid formation and skin laxity with good skin tone.

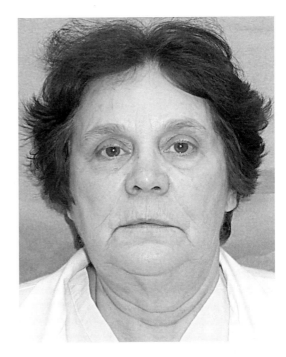

Figure 6-9 More advanced evolutional aging with moderate skin laxity and relatively good skin tone.

In the sixth decade (50 to 59 years), redundancy of neck skin and jowl formation become more noticeable, as do wrinkles and furrows. By the middle of the seventh decade, facial rhytids have become more or less ubiquitous, the brows have descended markedly, and the neck structures have relaxed inferiorly. Toward the eighth decade, there is usually an almost complete loss of facial adipose tissue; the skin is parchment-like and thin, making the bony prominences more visible. This patient group is often characterized as having severe photoaging. In addition to the treatment options outlined for the group of patients with advanced photoaging, these patients benefit most from full face-lift procedure combined with facial liposuction, upper and lower blepharoplasty, and CO_2 resurfacing. Figure 6-5 provides a summary of these rejuvenation options.

The cosmetic surgeon must consider the vectors of aging, which are parallel to the forces of gravity. The vectors of aging for the eyebrows are inferior and for the orbicularis oculi muscle inferolateral. In contrast, in the lower face, the cheek fat and platysma muscle are distorted inferomedially.[4] They are also first noticed at the end of the third decade. The face slowly loses its youthful V shape and takes on a fuller U shape. Blunting of the submandibular angle and subsequent jowl formation result. The effects of these aging vectors are summarized as "the sagging face syndrome." The cosmetic surgeon must combat these processes in order to achieve the best possible result (Figs. 6-10 to 6-13).

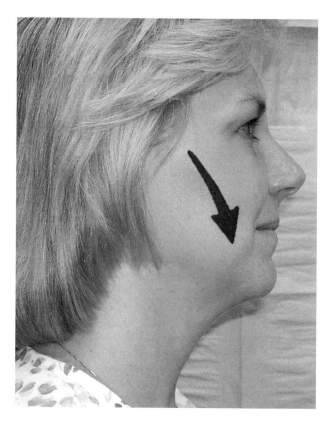

Figure 6-11   Early vector-induced drooping is detectable: the movement is superolateral and inferomedial.

Anthropometrics, Aging, and Rejuvenation Techniques

The cosmetic surgeon must be able to evaluate and improve the esthetic appearance of the patient's face in terms of baseline proportions relating to key anatomic structures. Once these proportions are recognized, each facial region can be analyzed more specifically.

Evaluating each facial area independently and applying the results to the entire face is critically important in facial analysis. The face must be analyzed in different positions and at different angles, from the side view to the oblique view, profile, and en face view, with constant cross-referencing. Facial imaging or multiple photographs should be utilized accordingly on initial consultation. This can help the patient to visualize his or her present appearance, specify present concerns, and outline future expectations.

The Face

Certain generalities apply in describing facial proportions; these are highlighted in each following section. The proportions of the face as compared with the cranium can be assessed simply by using the hand as measure. A hand length is about 80 percent of the cranium, and it can cover half of the face vertically; however, it covers only one-fourth when positioned horizontally. The face is about five eyes across. It can be

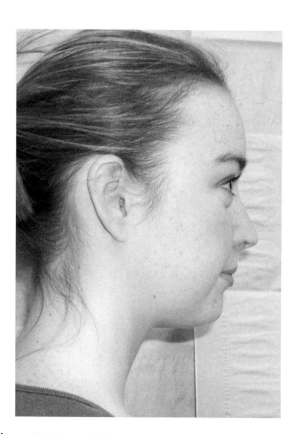

Figure 6-10   Youthful appearance of the face in profile. The effects of aging are not yet detectable.

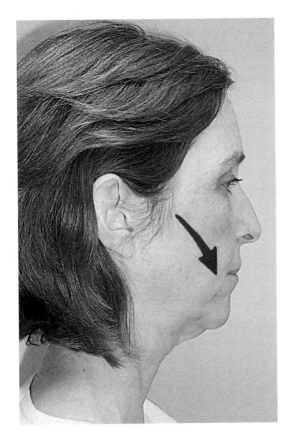

Figure 6-12 More advanced effects of the aging vectors, resulting in pooling of excess skin in the cheek, jowl, and chin area.

factory treatment outcome. Patients with unrealistic expectations should not be treated.

Treatment options vary according to the age and sex of the patient. Because balding patterns progress over time, it is not advisable to perform hair transplantation in men who have not established a clear hair-loss pattern (Figs. 6-16 to 6-19). The hairline in these young men is naturally low, and they often have unrealistic expectations during consultation. Topical application of a minoxidil solution in a concentration of 2 or 5 percent is a first-line option. All-*trans*-retinoic acid (tretinoin) 5% solution, also used topically in conjunction with minoxidil, has been reported to improve hair loss.[5] The minoxidil 5% solution is officially not indicated for women.

Finasteride, a specific 5-alpha reductase receptor blocker, is available only for men and currently is the sole systemic treatment option for hair loss. Prior to the initiation of finasteride therapy, the prostate-specific antigen (PSA) level, free and bound testosterone levels, and dihydroepiandrostenedione level should be obtained as a baseline. Women of childbearing age should not touch or handle finasteride. Recent studies in postmenopausal women did not show any improvement compared with placebo. Progesterone—either administered topically or injected intradermally—is advocated anecdotally as a 5-alpha reductase blocker.[6] Hair transplantation is indicated when the hair-loss pattern is established, mostly in patients in their mid-thirties or beyond. Placement of the new hairline in the balding patient must be considered carefully and should

divided into equals of three horizontally—the upper face extending from the hairline to the glabella, the midface from the glabella to the subnasal region, and the lower face from the subnasal region to the menton. In the following discussion, the contained structures are considered within this context.

Upper Face

Hair and Hairline The frontal hairline marks the superior margin of the upper third of the face. The hair frames the face, and full hair is a desirable feature. It is associated with power and success in men and with attractiveness in women. Hair loss is a frequently encountered problem among both sexes. The focus of the following discussion is androgenic alopecia.

In men, the low youthful hairline recedes with time, initially in the temporal areas, followed by thinning in the crown region. This process is continuously progressive, as demonstrated by the Hamilton classification (Fig. 6-14). In women, the androgenic hair loss is characterized by persistent thinning of the frontoparietal scalp hair while the frontal hairline often remains intact (Ludwig classification) (Fig. 6-15).

The evaluation of androgenic alopecia requires a sympathetic and sensitive cosmetic surgeon, because this problem is frequently associated with a social stigma resulting in reduced self-esteem and self-confidence. On the other hand, proper patient selection is critical for a successful and satis-

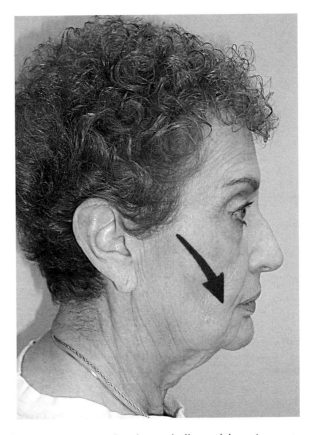

Figure 6-13 Severely advanced effects of the aging vectors, with skin drooping clearly observed.

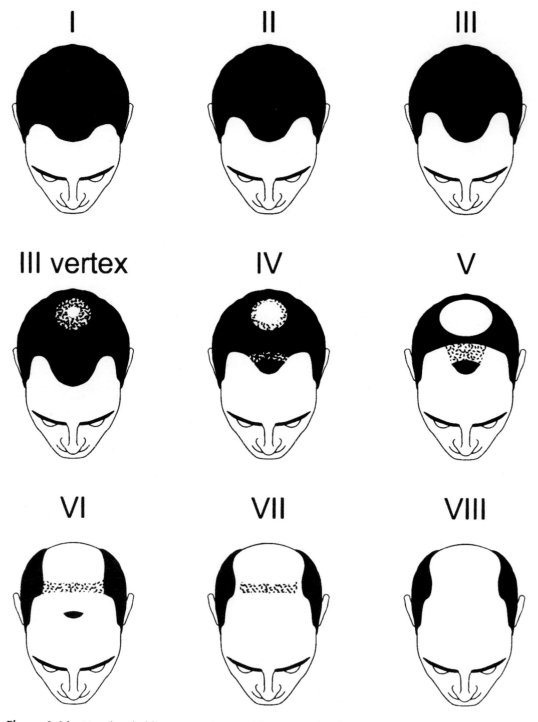

Figure 6-14 Hamilton balding pattern in men. (© 2001 Mark Palangio.)

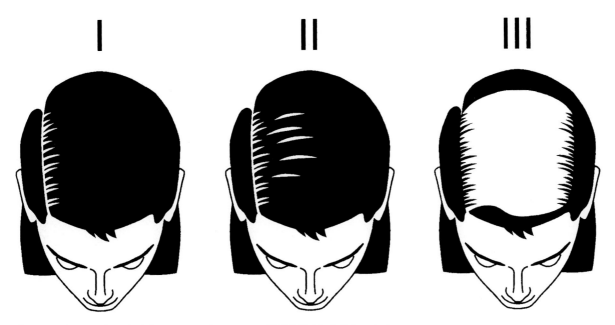

Figure 6-15 Ludwig balding pattern in women. (© 2001 Mark Palangio.)

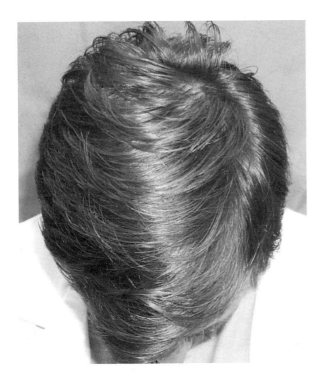

Figure 6-16 Youthful "full head of hair."

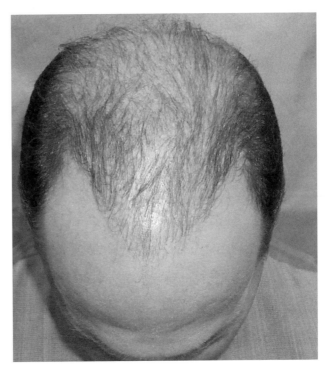

Figure 6-17 Moderate androgenic alopecia, with recession at the temples and overall thinning.

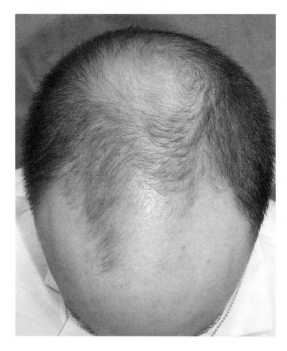

Figure 6-18   Severe androgenic alopecia, with the majority of the hair transformed into vellous hair.

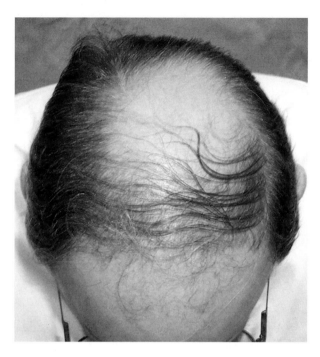

Figure 6-19   Severe androgenic alopecia, with almost complete balding of the frontal and parietal scalp with vertex.

never be too low. Often a strong central forelock is all that is required for esthetic definition of the hairline. Mini- and micro-grafts are used currently in hair transplantation to achieve the desired natural look (Table 6-3).

The Forehead   The forehead, from glabella to hairline, encompasses the upper third of the face. It arches slightly backward with an angle of 7 degrees in men and 10 degrees in women. In children, dynamic forehead lines can serve to express surprise, anger, or questioning. Naturally, these lines disappear in children without a trace. In adults, facial gestures made as continuous responses to certain emotional states lead to the formation of furrows and creases. Patients in the third decade of life (20 to 29 years) may

notice deepening of forehead and frown lines on the glabella. Minor rhytid formation is detectable. Patients in their forties seek attention for more noticeable dynamic lines. In them, photoaging is more advanced. Individual patient assessment is required to select the most appropriate therapy.

Between the ages of 40 and 50, dynamic rhytids become permanent even at rest. These lines on the glabella and forehead cannot be covered with makeup. Some patients try to hide them behind long bangs. Patients in their sixties experience continued line and rhytid formation due to severe photodamage. These prominent lines can sometimes produce bizarre frown patterns that may mistakenly convey sterness, anger, and disgust (Fig. 6-20*A* through *D*; Fig. 6-21).

Table 6-3
Summary of Treatment Options for Androgenic Alopecia

	Treatment Options		
Patient Group	Topical—Minoxidil	Systemic—Finasteride	Surgical—Hair Transplantation, Scalp Reduction
Men Hair loss pattern not established	✓	✓	—
Men Established hair loss pattern	✓	✓	✓
Women	✓	—	✓

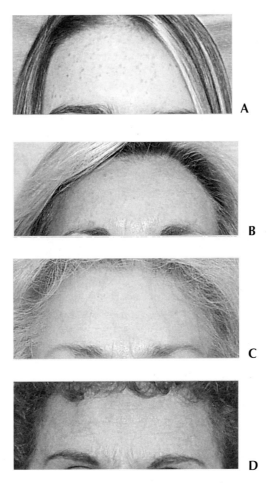

Figure 6-20   Aging of the forehead: (**A**) youthful forehead (early photoaging), (**B**) early rhytid formation (mild photoaging), (**C**) moderate rhytid formation (moderate photoaging), (**D**) prominent line formation (severe photoaging).

Photoaging			
1. Early	**2. Mild**	**3. Moderate**	**4. Severe**
Superficial rhytids with movement only (second decade) (Fig. 6-20A)	Superficial rhytids at rest (third to fourth decades) (Fig. 6-20B)	Deepening lines (fifth decade) (Fig. 6-20C)	Prominent lines/grooves (sixth decade + up) (Fig. 6-20D)
Treatment options:			
Topical antiaging	Microdermabrasion Superficial peels Botox injection	Botox injection Medium-depth peels Soft tissue augmentation Laser resurfacing: Erb:YAG, or CO_2 laser Combination procedures	Botox injection Deep peels Soft tissue augmentation CO_2 laser resurfacing Forehead lift Combination procedures

Figure 6-21   Forehead and glabella—aging and rejuvenation (algorithm).

REJUVENATION Microdermabrasion and superficial resurfacing agents are the treatment of choice for superficial lines on the forehead and glabella. In patients who present with moderage photoaging, the rejuvenation techniques include medium-depth peels or laser resurfacing in combination with Botox injection, because superficial peeling agents will not provide the outcome desired. Moderate to severe photoaging indicates laser resurfacing, either with the erbium: YAG laser or with the ultrapulsed CO_2 to improve skin quality and to diminish static rhytids. To fill deep furrows and creases, soft tissue implants offer another line of treatment. Expanded polytetrafluoroethylene provides permanent improvement with low risk.

Botox injection can eliminate dynamic lines very effectively and helps to preserve the improvement achieved through resurfacing techniques. In the pre-Botox area, forehead lifts were a mainstay of cosmetic treatment. Forehead lifts are no longer performed as frequently because Botox can provide the same effect in patients with mild to moderate forehead droop without the morbidity inherent in the forehead lift. However, the forehead lift is still indicated in selected patients with severe forehead droop.

The Midface

In the transverse or en face view, the midface makes up the widest point at the junction of the zygomatic arch and the zygoma, while the upper and the lower parts of the face are of equal width when measured in the temporal and gonion area respectively.[7,8]

The superficial musculoaponeurotic system (SMAS), which is attached to the dermis via small fibrous septa, is divided at the zygomatic arch into the upper face-and-scalp plane and the lower face-and-neck plane. The forehead and the scalp are freely movable above the arch, while pulling of the SMAS below the arch lifts the lateral cheeks, jowl, and neck areas only. The reason for this subdivision is explained by its embryonic development. The helm-like muscle arrangement of the forehead and scalp area is derived from sphincter colli profundus muscles, which are still found in lower animals, whereas the primitive platysma muscle is the origin of the lower face-and-neck SMAS plane.

The lower face-and-neck plane components of the SMAS include the parotid fascia, a fibrotic degeneration of the platysma muscle and the platysma muscle itself; the rhisorius muscle; and the depressor anguli oris muscles. There is no connection to the subgaleal plane. The platysma muscle extends down to cover the neck anteriorly. The parotid gland rests on the masseteric fascia, which creates the deeper plane of the lower face. Together, these two fascial planes ensheath Stenson's duct and facial nerve branches in addition to the parotid gland. On the neck, the cervical fascia creates the deep plane.

Above the zygomatic arch are the superficial temporal fascia and the underlying galea aponeurotica. Between them, they ensheath the frontalis, occipital, superior, and anterior auricular muscles and the procerus muscle. The superior temporal fascia and galea aponeurotica are connected through the subgaleal space. Their attachment is, anteriorly, the superior orbital rim under the eyebrow; later-

ally, the zygomatic arch and mastoid; and posteriorly, the nuchal line. Knowledge of the SMAS division is important to reverse the vectors of aging and especially when lifting procedures are performed.

The midface includes the eyebrows and eyes, the cheeks, and the nose. The nose together with the lips, the nasolabial crease, and the chin form the "muzzle region." Each region is explained below.

The Eyebrows and Eyes The eyebrows mark the line where the upper face ends and the midface begins. The eyebrows are usually located prominently along the superior orbital rim. They reach their highest point at the juncture of the medial two-thirds and lateral one-third superior orbital rim. From there they slope down gradually toward the temporal crest. The arc of the eyebrows is higher in women than in men, where often little or no arching is detected. The preferred eyebrow arch varies among different cultures and with changing trends in fashion.

The exact resting location of the eyebrows is determined by having the patient relax the forehead muscle and then following the eyebrow slope with mild pressure. It is easily detectable if the eyebrows follow the superior orbital rim or if they are located beneath it. An eyebrow lift is indicated only if the eyebrows are located below the superior orbital rim at rest. Because of gravity, the vectors of aging cause a downward droop of the eyebrows, sometimes in association with the increased forehead laxity. Early evidence of such a droop includes the loss of brow symmetry and the accumulation of excess skin on the upper eyelid. Eyebrow drooping is initially more noticeable in men than in women. To camouflage the eyebrow drooping, women may pluck this region to make the eyebrow appear higher and symmetrical. The eyebrows may also be made to appear higher by constantly raising them with a contraction of the frontalis muscle, but this compensatory maneuver usually fosters forehead creases and furrows. If this compensatory behavior is not recognized, leading to the injection of Botox to alleviate forehead lines, a significant and troubling drop in eyebrow height will result. On the other hand, when placed correctly, Botox injection can induce an upward lifting of the eyebrows, comparable to a temporary eyebrow lift (Fig. 6-22A through D, Fig. 6-23).

The relationship between the bony structures of the orbit and the cornea is such that the superior orbital ridge protrudes 8 to 10 mm anterior to the cornea, while the lateral orbital ridge is located 12 to 16 mm posterior to the cornea.[7] The upper eyelid's most superior point is located at the border between the medial and the middle thirds of the eyelid at the superior orbital rim. The slope of the lateral upper lid margins is parallel to the slope of the vermilion border of the upper lip. The most inferior aspect of the lower lid is found at the border of the medial to lateral thirds. From this inferior point, the lower eyelid slants slightly upward. The lateral canthus is generally 2.1 mm higher than the medial canthus in men and 4.1 mm higher in women. A slight upward slant is often considered a glamorous feature.

AGING Early in the third decade, skin redundancies develop at the upper eyelids, and the crisp definition of the palpebral line is lost. The lower eyelid folds as well as

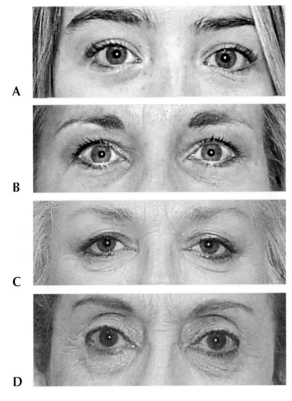

A

B

C

D

Figure 6-22 Aging of eyes and eyebrows: (**A**) youthful appearance without dermatochalasis, or discernible rhytids; (**B**) moderate dermatochalasis, mild blepharochalasis, and mild dynamic rhytid formation; (**C**) moderate to severe dermatochalasis with moderate blepharochalasis and smile lines at rest; (**D**) severe dermatochalasis with severe blepharochalasis and deep periorbital lines.

Eyebrow position along superior orbital rim

1. Droop after forehead relaxation, loss of symmetry

a. Mild excess upper eyelid skin: b. Moderate to severe dermatochalasis:
   Botox injection   Eyebrow lift and forehead lift combination
   Eyebrow lift

2. No droop after forehead relaxation, no loss of symmetry

Upper- and lower-eyelid dermatochalasis and blepharochalasis, periorbital rhytids

| a. No dermatochalasis (second decade) (Fig. 6-22A) | b. Moderate dematochalasis Mild blepharochalasis Mild dynamic rhytids (third to fourth decades) (Fig. 6-22B) | c. Moderate to severe dermatochalasis Moderate blepharochalasis Smile lines at rest (fifth decade) (Fig. 6-22C) | d. Severe dermatochalasis Severe blepharochalasis Deep periorbial lines (sixth decade and up) (Fig. 6-22D) |

Treatment options

| Topical antiaging products | Botox injection periorbital Superfical peels (lower eye lid) Laser resurfacing: Erb:YAG CO_2 laser Upper lid blepharoplasty | Botox injection periorbital Medium depth peels (lower eyelid) Laser resurfacing: CO_2 laser Upper/lower lid blepharoplasty Blepharoplasty/CO_2 laser/ Botox combination | Botox periorbital Upper/lower lid blepharoplasty CO_2 laser/Botox combination |

Figure 6-23 Eyebrows and eyes—aging and rejuvenation (algorithm).

the nasolabial and the buccolabial folds are more pronounced. In the fourth decade (30 to 39 years), glabellar rhytids and wrinkles in the lateral canthi are apparent at rest. Eyelid redundancy is more evident on the upper than the lower eyelids.

There are five septate compartments periorbitally; these contain the majority of the periorbital adipose tissue. Over the decades, an increased fullness can develop that is especially noticeable in the medial canthus of the upper lid and the inner, middle, and outer regions infraorbitally. The prominence of these bulges increases continuously; they have been described as "herniated fat pads." The periorbital septa relax with age, and gravity allows the fat pads to protrude in the lid space. The amount of herniated fat is not related to body weight; however, it is assumed that hereditary factors play a major role.

In the fifth decade (40 to 49 years) and the sixth (50 to 59 years) the excess upper-lid skin may rest on the eyelashes and extend to the lateral canthus. Subsequently, the lateral canthi develop a downward slope. Protrusion of the fat pad can be so prominent as to obscure the individual's vision; that is, the upper eyelid may obstruct the line of sight or may cause excessive scleral show by creating lower lid rounding, ectropion, or even festoons in more advanced age. (Fig. 6-22A through D)

REJUVENATION Treatment options for patients in their third decade (20 to 29 years) with mild fullness periobitally and a small amount of redundant skin include laser resurfacing, depending on the severity, either with erbium:YAG laser in very mild cases or the ultrapulsed CO_2 laser when there is a greater amount of excess skin or fullness periorbitally. Because of a contractile effect, CO_2 laser resurfacing in this area can, in selected patients, replace a upper-lid blepharoplasty. It is a valuable tool for the treatment of patients in their fourth decade (30 to 39 years) and those in their fifth (40 to 49 years) who usually present with early fat pad herniation and an increased amount of redundant skin.

Upper and lower blepharoplasty is indicated in patients with moderate to severe blepharochalasia and infraorbital fullness. Intraoperatively, the surgeon must take exquisite care not to damage the lacrimal gland, which is normally located in the lateral upper canthus. Occasionally, this gland relocates medially because of the repositioning of the adipose tissue. The cosmetic surgeon must be aware that the inferior oblique muscle extends between the medial and central fat pad and that it must be protected during a lower blepharoplasty with extensive fat removal.[8]

Periorbital rhytids can be treated with superficial peels in early photoaging. Microdermabrasion is another treatment option. Medium to deep peels are effective for moderate to severe photoaging. The formation of periorbital rhytids is dynamic in that they will most likely reappear owing to muscle contraction. Botox injections are very effective in this area, especially for the squint lines. This rejuvenation technique can be applied to patients in their twenties and thirties with early rhytids. It can again be used as adjunctive therapy after blepharoplasty or laser resurfacing in patients with deep lines and advanced photodamage. (Fig. 6-23)

Malar Prominence This area is generally highly variable. The malar complex is made up of a medial or paranasal part, a middle or malar part, and an outer part comprising the zygomatic arc. The malar eminences are situated medially and anteriorly to the widest point of the face, the junction of the zygomatic arc and the zygoma. Measuring the inclination of the malar complex vertically from the lateral orbit to the alar lobule results in an angle of 45 degrees when the face is in neutral position.[7]

AGING In the aging face there is often a prominent protrusion of fat, frequently with festooning noticed inferiorly to the lateral lower eyelid. This "sad bag" produces an appearance of constant worry and fatigue and is due to the influence of the aging vectors. As previously mentioned, the orbicularis oculi muscle, which is a tight muscle sphincter in youth, relaxes with age, and its inferior part forms the malar cresent. Thus, influenced by gravitational force, the muscle component moves inferolaterally and extends below the bony malar prominence. This inferior part of the orbicularis oculi muscle can be compared to a drawn curtain, the gathers of which are visible as festoons.[4] In response, the overlying fat pads reposition themselves anteroinferiorly, creating the sad bag and the formation of a prominent nasojugal line. The abnormal position of the malar fat pad is stressed by the relocation of the buccal fat pad medially and inferiorly (Fig. 6-24A through D).

REJUVENATION Rejuvenation options include liposuction of the malar fat pads. This procedure is usually very satisfying, although it can take several months for the postoperative edema to subside. Another therapeutic approach is to reposition and excise part of the inferior orbicularis oculis muscle. Both procedures can restore the youthful proportions of the midface (Fig. 6-25).

The Nose Lengthwise, the nose encompasses the middle third of the face. In the frontal view it can be divided into two planes. In the vertical view the ideal width of the nose is equal to the width of an eye. A vertical line drawn straight from the medial canthus to the lower face should meet the lateral aspects of the alae nasi and document the nose's width. A line drawn from the lateral canthus toward the nose should connect to the lateral alar base. Another way to elevate the width of the nose is to measure the distance between the lower lateral cartilages and the width of the nasal root.[9]

On the lateral view, the projection of the nose from the face is assessed by the Frankfort line, which is a line extending from the external auditory meatus through the inferior orbital rim to the nose. Dropping a perpendicular line straight from the nasal root and adding another line from the rhinion to the nasal tip defines the angle of protrusion, which is generally between 30 and 36 degrees. A greater angle suggests a possible hump deformity; a smaller angle defines a small nose, which may require augmentation.[7] In the profile view, 2 to 3 mm of the columella should be visible below the ala. To evaluate the projection of the nose to the face, a line is drawn from the nose tip to the base of the columella and extended to the vermilion border of the upper lip. This angle is called the nasolabial angle and is usually 95 to 110 degrees in men and 90 to 95 degrees in women.[8,9]

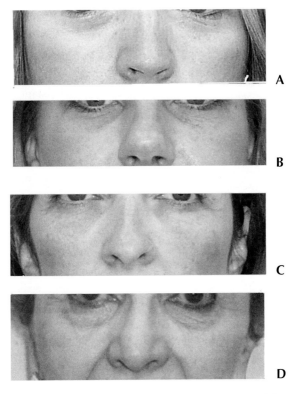

Figure 6-24   Aging of malar prominence: (**A**) youthful appearance; (**B**) mild drooping of the malar prominence; (**C**) and (**D**) increasing distance to infraorbital area.

Position of malar prominence

1. On bony prominence
   (second decade) (Fig. 6-24*A*)
   Youthful appearance

2. Below bony prominence
   (development from third to sixth
   decades and up) (Fig. 6-24*B* to *D*)

   a. Increasing distance to infraorbital area   b. With or without "sad bag" formation

   Treatment options
   a. Discrete liposuction
   b. Partial removal and redraping of relaxed orbicularis oculi muscle
   c. Combination therapy

Figure 6-25   Malar prominence—aging and rejuvenation (algorithm).

The basal view allows an analysis of the size, shape, and possible asymmetry of the nares and nose tip. Every preoperative evaluation for any nasal procedure that can possibly affect the nares (including cosmetic surgery and Mohs' micrographic surgery) requires a basal-view photograph of both nares and an en face view to document possible preexisting asymmetries. Often patients will notice their inherited asymmetries only postoperatively, upon critical inspection of the closure. They will appreciate the care of the attentive surgeon who discreetly pointed out these asymmetries during the consultation.

The nose is the site most frequently affected by nonmelanoma skin cancer. The dermatologic surgeon has to have a solid base of knowledge of the nasal proportions if the most favorable surgical outcome—customized to each individual patient—is to be achieved. Mohs' closures on the nose depend on the exact size and the location of the defect. Examples of these include straight-line closures on the lateral and middle dorsum and lateral advancement flaps in different shapes and often ala-based, pedunculated transposition flaps used for defects on the nose tip, grafting procedures, and more. Aging of the nose results in relaxation of the columella, causing a protrusion of the nose tip and making the nose appear longer. The nose—together with the lips, the nasolabial folds, and the chin—is part of the "muzzle region." The maxilla and mandible are the bony parts of this area (Fig. 6-26A through D).

Proportion of Maxilla and Mandible The lip-tooth relationship is a key factor in determining the relationship between the maxilla and the mandible. While lips are at rest, slight touching or a small gap of 3 to 4 mm is favorable. The smiling lip should expose about 2 mm of the maxillary incisors, while the lip edges are parallel. A "toothy smile" with more than 2 mm incisor show suggests vertical maxillary excess. In a case with hardly any upper tooth exposure, a vertical maxillary deficit is assumed.

Little or no lower tooth exposure at rest or during animation is associated with the mandible. Lip incompetence or lower incisor exposure is most likely a sign of vertical excess of the mandible. Flattening of the labionasal fold with straining of the mentalis muscle, followed by upward displacement of the chin soft tissue, is a consequence of forced lip closure and also a sign of mandibular excess. Mandibular deficiency is suspected when the distance between the lip and the chin decreases and the lower lip protrudes over the dependent labiomental fold. This appearance is termed the *overclosed look.*[7]

There is evidence that relative changes in the bony structure of the maxilla in the aging face contribute to the depth of the nasolabial folds. A recent imaging study demonstrated that the relative distance between the medial canthus and the nasolabial crease is equal to the distance from the nasolabial crease to the mouth in the aged face. However, the youthful proportions display a ratio of 1.5 to 1 respectively. Surprisingly, the ratio of these distances measured in infants showed a ratio of 1 to 1, similar to that of the aging face. It appears that the maxilla is relatively hypoplastic in infancy and advanced age, whereas there is a relative hyperplasia during early adulthood. These findings suggest that there is selective bony remodeling throughout life, thus changing the ratios between key structures.[3]

THE LOWER FACE

The lower face extends from below the columella to the chin. It encompasses the major part of the muzzle region, including the nasolabial crease, lips, and chin.

The Nasolabial Crease

In the youthful face, only a superficial fine line separating the cheeks from the periorbital region is visible. With aging, this crease continues to deepen and is often cause of concern for patients in their forties. Maxillary retrusion, medial-inferior movement of the buccal fat pat due to gravitational forces, and atrophy of subcutaneous adipose tissue are the main factors underlying the prominence of the nasolabial crease.

Aging In the fifth decade (40 to 49 years), as the laxity of the lateral cheek increases, the septate attachments to the SMAS loosen and the lax skin moves medially along the jaw, deepening the nasolabial fold even further, while at the same time creating a soft tissue prominence, the jowls, in the middle of the jawline. In the sixth decade (50 to 59 years) and beyond, both the nasolabial crease and the jowl formation are more accentuated (Fig. 6-26A through D).

Rejuvenation Treatment of the nasolabial crease can be achieved temporarily through soft tissue augmentation with collagen, fascia lata, and fat injection. The implantation of extended polytetrafluoroethyl is well tolerated and results in a permanent improvement. Surgical techniques, including face-lifts and excision of the nasolabial fold, contribute only marginally to the rejuvenation of the nasolabial crease. Fold excisions often result in prominent scarring, which is difficult to camouflage. Improvements seen with deep-plane middle face-lifts are transient at best.

The Jaw Line

The youthful jaw line at the inferior margin of the lower face is sharp and uninterrupted. It forms the desirable V shape of the youthful face. With the sagging of the cheek skin, the U configuration of the aging face is noted, sometimes as early as in the fourth decade (30 to 39 years). Initially the jowl is discreetly located superior to the mandible. However, continued vector force directs the jowl downward medially, finally disrupting the sharp contour of the jaw. Patients often notice it in their forties or shortly thereafter. The angle between the mandible and the neck loses its acuity and becomes blunted. From the seventy decade (60 to 69 years) onward the jowls may come to protrude even more. At this point the skin laxity is severe, allowing the jowls to extend into the neck area below the mandible.

Rejuvenation Treatment options consist of facial liposuction of the jowl and submandibular area alone, which is indicated in early jowl formation. A combination of facial liposuction with various lifting procedures is indicated for more advanced skin laxity. The lifting procedures range from the sutureless face-lift in early skin redundancy, to the

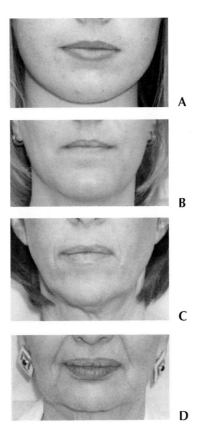

Figure 6-26   Aging of the "muzzle region": (**A**) youthful V-shape of jaw line, (**B**) blunting contour with deepening nasolabial folds (NLF); (**C**) U-shape appearance of jaw line; (**D**) square U-shape of jaw line. See change in lip contour.

Shape of jaw line			
1. Youthful **V-shape** (second decade) (Figs. 6-26A and 6-28A)	2. Blunting contour with mild cheek laxity, deepening nasolabial folds (NLF) (third to fourth decades) (Figs. 6-26B and 6-28B)	3. Change to **U-shape** jowl formation, deep NLF (fifth decade) (Figs. 6-26C and 6-28C)	4. **Square U-shape**, jowls below mandible Prominent NLF (sixth decade and up) (Figs. 6-26D and 6-28D)
Treatment options			
	Facial liposuction Combination with sutureless face-lift	If skin snap test +/ evolutional aging Facial liposuction	Facial liposuction with full face-lift Combination facial liposuction/full face-lift/ neck lift
		If snap test −/ involutional aging Combination facial liposuction/ mini face-lift or full face-lift	

Figure 6-27   Jaw line—aging and rejuvenation (algorithm).

mini face-lift indicated in moderate to severe jowl formation and skin laxity, and to the full face-lift, which is performed in patients with severe skin laxity and jowl formation. The vector of the lifting procedure is always directed opposite to the direction of the aging vector. Laser resurfacing as an adjunctive treatment modality, preferably with the ultra-pulsed CO_2 laser, improves skin quality and helps firm the underlying skin structures (Fig. 6-27).

Mouth and Lips

The lower face can be divided into thirds: the distance from the base of the nose to the upper lip is one-third, and the remaining distance comprises the lower lip and the chin. The lower face is usually highly variable due to variations in the bony structure, the muscles, and the soft tissue structures. The diagonal distance parallels the bitemporal distance of the upper face, both being smaller than the widest facial point. The mouth is, of course, the most prominent feature of the lower face.[8]

Ideally the upper lateral lip margins should align with a vertical line projected from the medial irides. The medial slope of the upper lip is parallel to the slope of the supero-lateral eyelid. Though the configuration of the lip is often variable, the upper lip should resemble a minimally slanting M; it should be flatter and wider than the lower lip. The lower lip ideally has a W configuration.

Dynamic Perioral Rhytids At the end of the fourth decade (around age 39), the aging of the lips is first visible by the appearance of perioral radial lines. These lines are dynamic in origin and result from the contraction of the perioral muscle sphincter. Initially these lines are superficial, mostly seen on the upper lip. Mild resurfacing methods, such as microdermabrasion and superficial to medium peels, are indicated. Medium-depth peeling agents and laser resurfacing can even eliminate deeper perioral lines temporarily. However, because these lines are due to contraction of the perioral orbicularis oris muscle, they will recur. Dynamic lines like these may respond to Botox injections. Botox inactivates injected muscles temporarily. The patient should be warned, however, that movements of the lips, as during smiling and talking, might feel unusual even though no obvious distortion is detectable. Most likely the patient will experience muscle interplay during these movements, which will feel unfamiliar.

Patients in their forties and fifties will often seek the attention of the cosmetic surgeon due to the continued increase in the number and depth of these perioral creases. The patient will complain of "bleeding lipstick" from the lip to the surrounding skin into these rhytids. When patients purse their lips, a concertina effect is produced by the radial arrangement of these rhytids (Fig 6-26A through D).

REJUVENATION Filler materials such as fascia lata, collagen, and autologous fat can be injected and provide a temporary improvement. Soft tissue augmentation can be combined with resurfacing techniques to improve the skin quality periorally even further. Medium to deep peels as well as laser resurfacing—either with the long-pulsed erbium: YAG laser of the ultrapulsed CO_2 laser—is the treatment of choice (Fig 6-29).

Lip Volume, Vermilion Prominence, Philthrum In the fifth decade (40 to 49 years) a noticeable loss of the upper lip's volume and reduction of the vermilion prominence are observed, together with flattening of the upper lip. At the same time the distance from the columella base to the vermilion enlarges, making the upper lip appear even thinner (Fig. 6-26A through D).

REJUVENATION Soft tissue augmentation is a valuable tool in augmenting the lip volume and contour, with recreation of the vermilion border. Temporary improvement is achieved with collagen and fascia lata, often in conjunction with laser resurfacing and Botox injection. Expanded polytetrafluoroethylene can permanently recreate the vermilion border and augment the lip volume. Shortening of the distance between the columella and the vermilion border surgically reestablishes the youthful proportion (Fig. 6-29).

Marionette lines Continued facial drooping and progressive atrophy of the subcutaneous tissue lead to the downward formation of both lip angles. This creates two bilateral creases extending down lateral to the chin. These lines give the face a marionette-like appearance, thus the name *marionette lines.* They can be seen in patients in their sixties and beyond. (Fig. 6-26A to D).

REJUVENATION A variety of surgical techniques can reverse the downward turn of the lip angles. These interventions are technically demanding and pose an increase risk of scarring. Face-lifting procedures can aid in reversing skin ptosis, but for the perioral region, including the nasolabial creases, they are not the ideal option. The results might be disappointing for both the patient and the surgeon (Fig. 6-29).

The Chin

The chin is commonly associated with adjectives connoting certain character traits: a "chiseled" chin attests to virility and strength in a man, while a weak chin implies a lack of discipline and lack of control.

Ideally, the chin in profile touches a line drawn vertically from the medial eyebrows to upper lip and advanced to the chin. The line should touch the most prominent part of the chin in men; in women, the chin is slightly posterior to this line.

Hypoplasia of the chin, sometimes referred to as the "bird face" or fleeting chin, can be treated with several different approaches. The creation of a sharp submandibular angle via liposuction helps to improve a weak chin. Fat injection is another option to augment the chin temporarily. Finally, a chin implant made of expanded polytetrafluoroethylene or other inert material can provide permanent improvement. Occasionally these implants can dislocate. Careful placement of an appropriately sized implant can help to prevent this complication. In chin hyperplasia, a reduction of the bony chin prominence is indicated, with occasional reduction of the mandible as well, to achieve the most satisfying results.

Aging Three vectors of aging influence the aging appearance of the chin: (1) the chin pad becomes ptotic and often moves forward while deepening the sublabial sulcus,

(2) the lateral neck loses its sharp angle and becomes blunted, and (3) the submental triangle stays intact or projects a rounded contour. These signs of aging are apparent in the late forties and early fifties; they become more obvious during the sixties. A configuration known as the "witch chin" is the end result (Fig. 6-26A through D and Fig. 6-28A through D).

Rejuvenation Rejuvenation can be expected after submental and jowl liposuction moderates the prominence of the abnormal chin pad. Lifting procedures, including neck and face-lifts, will reverse the aging vectors and reestablish a youthful contour, with an improved mandibular-neck angle (Fig. 6-30).

The Neck

The shape, contour, and proportion of the neck in reference to the face play an essential role in rejuvenation strategies for the aging face.

The neck extends superiorly to the chin and inferiorly to the sternal notch. The thyroid cartilage and hyoid bone are two of its landmarks. The most important structure responsible for the appearance of the aging neck is the platysma muscle. It originates from the pectoralis fascia and extends like a sheet upward, where it inserts medially at the mandible. It forms the lower face-and-neck SMAS plane in conjunction with the superficial parotid gland fascia, the risorius muscle, and the depressor anguli oris muscle inserting below the zygomatic arch. There are a variety of platysma muscle variants which directly affect the aging neck. If the platysma muscle divides in the midline, early "turkey gobbler" formation is expected. If, on the other hand, the platysma muscle is interlaced in the midline, aging effects are seen later in life.

The cervicomental angle is created through the attachment of the platysma muscle to the hyoid bone. A youthful angle measures between 105 and 120 degrees. The other criterion for a youthful neck is a submental-sternocleidomastoid angle of 90 degrees (Fig. 6-28A).

Aging The neck ages slowly and gradually, following the vectors of aging medial to inferior and the gravitational force from superior to inferior. During the twenties, fine horizontal lines appear; however, the youthful contour of the neck is maintained. During the thirties, mild skin laxity begins to appear, leading to progressive blunting of both the cervicomental and submandibular-sternocleidomastoid angle. Fine platysmal bands begin to show and the horizontal lines increase in depth and number. The submental triangle loses its firmness and appears rounded rather than flat. Thick platysmal bands, subplatysmal and submental fad pads, and moderate jowl formation are seen during the forties. The skin laxity is now moderate. Dyschromia and poikiloderma of Civatte are signs of advanced photodamage to the neck skin. The chin pad descends. From the fifties onward, the neck loses its contour. Thick, hypertrophied platysmal bands and severe skin laxity with deep horizontal folds as well as complete chin ptosis dominate the appearance of the neck (Fig. 6-26A through D and Fig. 6-28A through D)

Rejuvenation Treatment techniques vary according to the extent of aging in each individual. In the early stage,

horizontal lines can be treated with superficial resurfacing approaches, microdermabrasion, and superficial peels. Because the neck skin is structurally thinner with a smaller amount of sebaceous structures for reepithelization, more aggressive resurfacing of the neck carries an increased risk of complications, especially scarring.

Liposuction of the submental and subplatysmal fat pad and jowls can be performed alone in patients with mild to moderate signs of aging who are in their late fourth decade (30 to 39 years) and early fifth decade (40 to 49 years). Skin elasticity can be assessed with the snap test. The more the skin snaps back after a mild pull in the submental area, the higher the success rate with redraping after liposuction. Liposuction can be performed in combination with a neck-lift, or a face-lift procedure without increased morbidity. Laser resurfacing improves the skin quality and creates a more youthful epidermis. However, a conservative approach is recommended, with keeping in mind the potential for scarring.

Elimination of platysmal bands and horizontal lines is often successfully achieved with Botox injections, because the bands and lines are due to dynamic muscle contraction. The finer the bands and lines, the better the response. Platysmal banding has been especially advocated in patients with "turkey gobbler" deformity (Fig. 6-26A through D, Fig. 6-28A through D, and Fig. 6-31).

Neck structures influence the appearance and function of facial structures and vice versa, consistent with the integral model of aging. Rejuvenation of the aging neck in concert with treatment of the aging face provides the balance seen in the youthful face and neck.

The Ears

The external auditory canal is situated halfway between the alar facial junction and the outer canthus of the eye. The Frankfort line, as defined previously, aids in the alignment of profile photos and is used in facial reconstruction. The width of the ear is half the ear's length. The ear's long axis runs parallel to the long axis of the dorsal nose. Normally, the ear protrudes about 20 degrees from the skull.

Congenital deformities often require reconstruction or augmentation of the auricle. The use of muscle-and-cartilage grafts from ribs as donor sites is common. Protuberant ears must be corrected early because of the psychological burden carried by children with this condition.

Aging The aging of the ear can increase the length of the auricle by as much as 1 cm, often starting in the fourth decade (30 to 39 years). As a result of the overall decrease in skin elasticity, the auricular shape flattens and the earlobe becomes elongated. Photodamage leads to a wrinkled appearance of the lobular skin surface.

Rejuvenation Laser resurfacing eliminates these static wrinkles. When it is performed with the CO_2 laser, it can, through the shrinkage effect, reduce the size of the lobule. This resurfacing procedure can be performed as part of a facial resurfacing.

The most frequently encountered ear-related cosmetic procedure is the repair of a torn earlobe. After surgery, the patient is advised against wearing earrings for about 6 weeks.

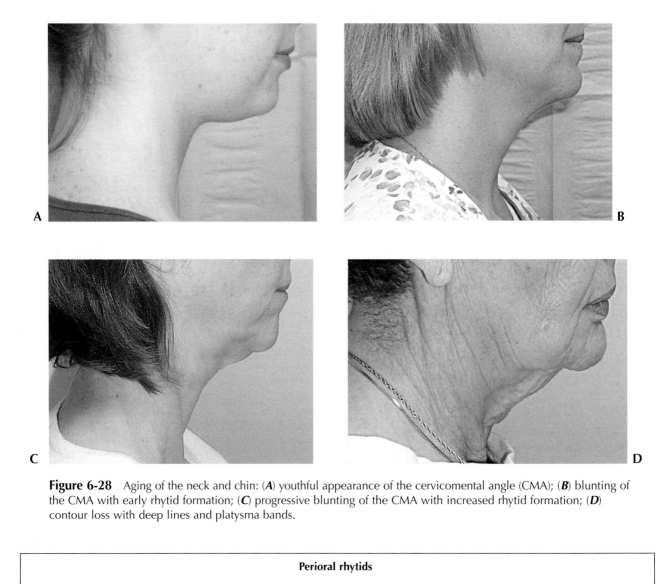

Figure 6-28 Aging of the neck and chin: (**A**) youthful appearance of the cervicomental angle (CMA); (**B**) blunting of the CMA with early rhytid formation; (**C**) progressive blunting of the CMA with increased rhytid formation; (**D**) contour loss with deep lines and platysma bands.

Perioral rhytids			
1. Upper lip: minimally slanted M lower lip: slight W configuration (second decade) (Fig. 6-26A)	2. Dynamic rhytids, mild at rest (third to fourth decades) (Fig. 6-26B)	3. Deeper lines, increased number (fifth decade) (Fig. 6-26C)	4. "Bleeding" of lipstick, "concertina" effect (sixth decade + and up) (Fig. 6-26D)
Treatment options			
	Botox injection Microdermabrasion Superficial peels Soft tissue augmentation	Botox injection Soft tissue augmentation Medium-depth peels Dermabrasion Laser resurfacing: CO_2	Botox injection Deep peels Dermabrasion Laser resurfacing CO_2 Combination procedures and soft tissue augmentation
Lip volume, vermilion			
1. Slope-like vermilion border full upper and lower lips (second decade) Figs. 6-26A and 6-28A	2. Early blunting of vermilion prominence (third to fourth decades) Figs. 6-26B and 6-28B	3. Reduction of vermilion, thinning of upper lip (fifth decade) (Figs. 6-26B and 6-28B)	4. Loss of vermilion prominence, elongation of philtrum, thinning of lips (sixth decade and up) (Figs. 6-26D and 6-28D)

Figure 6-29 Lips—aging and rejuvenation (algorithm).

Treatment options			
	Microdermabrasion Soft tissue augmentation	Soft tissue augmentation CO_2 laser resurfacing	In addition to (3), surgical intervention: Augmentation cheiloplasty Advancement of vermilion Resection of nose base
	Marionette lines, downturn of lip angles		
1. Lip angle upwards, no marionette lines (second decade) (Fig. 6-26A)	2. Lip angle flat no marionette lines (third to fourth decades (Fig. 6-26B)	3. Early downturn of lip angles early marionette lines (fifth decade) (Fig. 6-26C)	4. Downturn of lip angles prominent marionette lines (sixth decade and up) (Fig. 6-26D)
Treatment options			
	Botox injection	Botox injection Soft tissue augmentation	Soft tissue augmentation Surgical intervention: corner lift

Figure 6-29   *(Continued)*

Chin			
1. Well defined, in line with submandibular angle (second decade) (Figs 6-26A and 6-28A)	2. Contour maintained, but mild skin laxity (third to fourth decade) (Figs. 6-26B and 6-28B)	3. Early ptosis of chin pad (fifth decade) (Figs. 6-26C and 6-28C)	4. Ptotic chin, increased sublabial sulcus (Figs. 6-26D and 6-28D)
Treatment options			
	Submental/jowl liposuction Sutureless face-lift	Liposuction in combination with minilift or full face-lift	Liposuction with full face- lift/neck lift combination

Figure 6-30   Chin—aging and rejuvenation (algorithm).

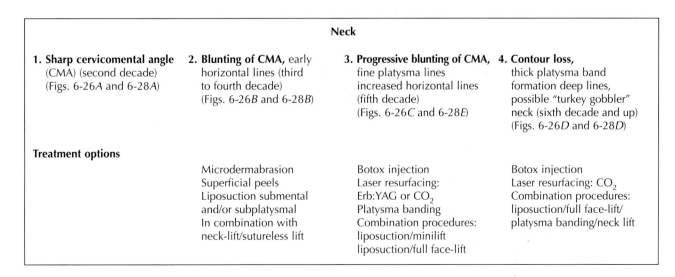

Neck			
1. Sharp cervicomental angle (CMA) (second decade) (Figs. 6-26A and 6-28A)	**2. Blunting of CMA,** early horizontal lines (third to fourth decade) (Figs. 6-26B and 6-28B)	**3. Progressive blunting of CMA,** fine platysma lines increased horizontal lines (fifth decade) (Figs. 6-26C and 6-28E)	**4. Contour loss,** thick platysma band formation deep lines, possible "turkey gobbler" neck (sixth decade and up) (Figs. 6-26D and 6-28D)
Treatment options			
	Microdermabrasion Superficial peels Liposuction submental and/or subplatysmal In combination with neck-lift/sutureless lift	Botox injection Laser resurfacing: Erb:YAG or CO_2 Platysma banding Combination procedures: liposuction/minilift liposuction/full face-lift	Botox injection Laser resurfacing: CO_2 Combination procedures: liposuction/full face-lift/ platysma banding/neck lift

Figure 6-31   Neck—aging and rejuvenation (algorithm).

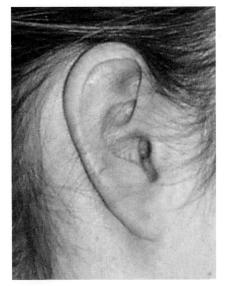

A

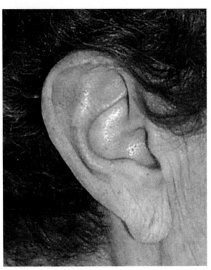

Figure 6-32 Aging of the ear: (**A**) youthful ear; (**B**) aged ear with flattening of cartilage structure and earlobe elongation.

B

Ears

1. Firm earlobe, firm helix youthful ear (second decade) (Fig. 6-32A)

2. Increased lengthening of the ear
   Ear shape flattened
   Increased wrinkling of earlobe
   Stretching and thinning of earlobe (sixth decade and up) (Fig. 6-32B)

Treatment options

Resurfacing procedures: Microdermabrasion
Superficial peels
Laser: Erb:YAG or CO_2
Soft tissue augmentation of the earlobe
Surgical reshaping of the earlobe
Combination procedures

Figure 6-33 Ears—aging and rejuvenation (algorithm).

Table 6-4
Rejuvenation Techniques for Chronological Aging

Treatment Options	Chronological Age, Years			
	20–30	*30–40*	*40–50*	*50 and up*
Topical antiaging products	✓	✓	✓	✓
Superficial peels	✓	✓		
Botox injections	✓	✓	✓	✓
Microdermabrasion	✓	✓	✓	✓
Medium-depth peels		✓	✓	
Microlipoinjection		✓	✓	✓
Expanded polytetrafluoroethylene		✓	✓	✓
Collagen		✓	✓	✓
Erbium:YAG laser		✓		
Combination Erbium:YAG/CO_2 laser		✓	✓	
CO_2 laser ultrapulsed		✓	✓	✓
Face-lift: sutureless		✓	✓	
Face-life: minilift			✓	✓
Face-lift: full facelift				✓
Forehead lift		✓	✓	✓
Brow lift		✓	✓	✓

References

1. Gilchrest BA, Yaar M. Aging of skin. In: Fitzpatrick TB, Eisen AZ, Wolff K, et al. eds. *Dermatology in General Medicine*, 5th ed. New York: McGraw-Hill; 1998:1697–1706.

2. Kohen R. Skin antioxidants: Their role in aging and oxidative stress—New approaches for their evaluation. *Biomed Pharmacother* 1999; 53:181–192.

3. Pessa JE, Zadoo VP, Yuan Ch, et al. Concertina effect and facial aging. *Plast Reconstr Surg* 1999;103(2):635–644.

4. Hamra ST. Basics. In: Hamra St, ed. *Composite Rhytidectomy*. St. Louis: Quality Medical Publishing; 1993:28–78.

5. Bergfeld WP. Retinoids and hair growth. *J Am Acad Dermatol* 1998; 39:586–589.

6. Samule Ayres III. Hair transplantation. In: Epstein E, Epstein E Jr, eds. *Skin Surgery*, 5th ed. Springfield, IL: Charles C Thomas; 1982:437–529.

7. Bartle S, Wornom I III, Whitaker I. Evaluation of facial skeletal esthetics and surgical planning. *Clin Plast Surg* 1991; 18(1):1–9.

8. Beeson WH. Facial analysis. In: Beeson WH, McCollough EG, eds. *Aesthetic Surgery of the Aging Face*. St. Louis: Mosby; 1986:1–9.

9. Willett JM. How to assess the nose for rhinoplasty. In: Willett JM, ed. *Facial Plastic Surgery*. Stamford, CT: Appleton & Lange; 1997:33–35.

In general, the patient is discouraged from wearing heavy ear jewelry and loops, as they seem to contribute directly to the stretching and tearing of the earlobe (Fig. 6-32*A* and *B*, Fig. 6-33).

In summary, it is important for the cosmetic surgeon to understand the value and application of facial analysis. Through an integrated model of aging, the cosmetic surgeon can interpret age-related changes in the context of a patient's unique facial features and propose a treatment plan that can promote beauty and confidence (Table 6-4).

CHAPTER 7

Body Analysis

This chapter is a continuation of Chap. 6 ("Facial Analysis") in the sense that the same principles of symmetry, proportion, and dimension, paired with functionality, define a beautiful body. We know that there are cross-cultural differences in what such a body—for example, the female figure—should look like. However, in western society, android body types are favored for both men and women. Patients who present for esthetic body improvements often have very concrete concerns, and it is the cosmetic surgeon's obligation to develop a rejuvenation plan tailored to each individual patient.

Factors Influencing Body Shape

Next to fashion, there are several other factors influencing and contributing to the body's shape. They encompass hormones, genetics and gender, diet and exercise, diseases and medication, and advancing age. Psychological factors can influence the patient's body image negatively. The cosmetic surgeon has to assess what the patient's motivation is and whether he or she is able to focus on a realistic endpoint. If, during a thorough clinical evaluation and consultation, an obvious body image problem exists, as in the case of anorexia nervosa, the patient will not benefit from a cosmetic procedure but requires a psychiatric evaluation.

Physiognomic factors, such as lordosis, can simulate a protruding, round abdomen, suggesting a cosmetic problem. However, physical therapy is the treatment of choice in this case, not cosmetic surgery. A number of practical criteria can help the experienced surgeon to detect those patients who would actually benefit from a rejuvenation procedure. Anthropometrics is another method used to assess body shape by taking height, body mass, and fat percentage into account. However, the formula to determine the body's proportions is rather complicated; therefore a simpler practical approach is often more helpful.

A "normal" body type is usually associated with symmetrical proportions, with equal muscle tone on the right and left sides of the body, the absence of localized or even generalized obesity, and good skin turgor in an alert, communicative patient.[1] Even if the portions are symmetrical, patients of the same height can have very different body shapes. The obese and the emaciated body are the extremes, in contrast with the normal body shape. Moreover, a patient's bone structure can range from petite to regular to large. The proportion of the trunk to the legs can vary, meaning that the torso can be relatively long compared to the legs or that the legs may be long relative to a short trunk.[1] The latter is favored.

HORMONES

Hormones and hormone imbalances have a direct effect on the body's morphology. For example, an imbalance of thyroid hormones has devastating effects. If thyroid function is depressed, the patient's skin yellows over time, the patient may appear mentally slow, the metabolism is decreased, and the patient gains weight. He or she appears "pudgy." In contrast, if thyroid function is excessive, the opposite happens: the body's metabolism is geared up and the patient can lose weight despite increased food intake. The skin is warm and moist and the eyes may protrude. With treatment, homeostasis will be established and the body will regain its normal shape.

Gynecoid and Android Body Shapes

Body shapes are also determined by genetics and gender. It is not uncommon for both a mother and daughter to present for the correction of the same cosmetic problem. Localized fat deposits on the lateral thigh, colloquially called "riding breeches" or "saddlebags," are seen often in women within the same family.

Obviously hormones play an important role in creating a characteristic body shape, according to the patient's gender. The gynecoid or female shape embodies the ideal seen in paintings of the old masters, with voluptuous curves and round hips and bellies. The android body shape, with straight flanks and hips and relatively broad shoulders, is commonly associated with the male body image.[2] In our culture today, the android body type is also favored for women. Some people do not fit this classification. They may be somewhere in between, showing features of both the gynecoid and the android body types. Also, there are a significant number of men with a gynecoid body type and women with an android body shape. Body fat topography has been shown to correlate with certain adverse health consequences. In general, excessive abdominal girth is associated with an increase in hypertension, diabetes mellitus, and cardiac morbidity and mortality (Figs. 7-1 and 7-2)[3,4]

Disease and Medication

Overall health contributes to one's body shape and figure. Imbalance of hormones in certain diseases may have marked effects, as in Cushing's syndrome, which is associated with moon facies, "buffalo hump," and central obesity. Postural problems such as slumped shoulders can present with fullness in the superior and lateral pectoral areas. Lordosis leads to protrusion of the abdomen—a problem that is not solved with liposuction but rather calls for physical therapy.

Drug intake can also change the body's morphology. The latest example is the "Crix belly," an unusual fat distribution due to protease inhibitors, a well-known result of HIV drug therapy. The typical features are loss of subcutaneous facial fat and a gain in visceral fat. This excess visceral fat gives the abdomen the appearance of a pouch. Liposuction cannot reduce the visceral fat deposits, and only mildly alleviates the symptoms of dyslipomorphia in these patients. Correcting the hormonal imbalance or a change to medications without this side effect is the proper treatment.

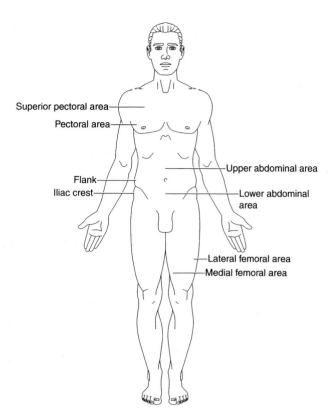

Figure 7-2 Android or male body shape with areas of importance, anterior view. (© 2001 Mark Palangio.)

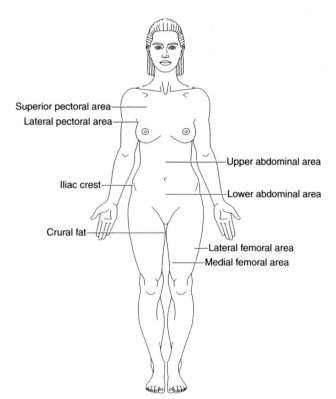

Figure 7-1 Gynecoid or female body shape with areas of importance, anterior view. (© 2001 Mark Palangio.)

Age

The aging body undergoes changes similar to those described for the face in Chap. 6 ("Facial Analysis"). In general there is progressive loss of skin tone and elasticity. The aging vectors in association with gravity promote a downward draping of the skin, which can be observed by patients particularly when a tattoo "moves" with age. Loss of subcutaneous tissue in addition to the continuous loss of muscle mass and bone substance over the years increases the prominence of skin folds and rhytids. A recent study observed a relative reduction in skeletal muscle mass (SMM) in the third decade of life in both men and women. However, significant loss of SMM was not observed till the end of the fifth decade. Additional findings indicate that men have more SMM than women, especially in the upper body, where the gender difference is the greatest in this regard. Independent of gender, however, aging is associated with a decrease in SMM in the lower body in the fifth decade.[5] There is also a loss in height. The posture changes as well, often becoming kyphotic. Aging in our society is generally associated with weight gain. One study suggests that continuous weight gain of an average of 1 lb over the holiday season per year helps to explain the considerable weight increase in the aging population.[6]

These examples illustrate the need for a thorough evaluation of each patient in order to rule out underlying factors other than genetics, gender, and aging that may be deforming the body shape. Realistic goals and good communication are also important.

Body Regions

The various body regions may be discussed individually with regard to their changes over time and in relation to the rejuvenation methods used to correct them. However, although the focus is on relatively small areas, it is important for the cosmetic surgeon to see these regions as parts of a whole. Below, individual body regions are discussed in terms of cosmetic units.

COSMETIC UNITS

In contrast to the facial cosmetic units, those of the body are not firmly standardized. Our pragmatic definition of cosmetic units involves several subunits that are often continuous with each other in terms of fat deposition and treatment. Accumulation of fat deposits can occur in localized, individual regions or in a certain grouping of regions. For example, submammary rolls of adipose tissue can extend laterally and dorsally to become thoracic rolls connecting with rolls of the iliac crest. These areas are a cosmetic unit, because treatment of only an isolated region in this setting leads to a suboptimal result. Lipid deposits of the posterior upper arms are one such subunit, which can be continuous with the lateral and even superior pectoral areas. The lateral pectoral areas, in turn, can merge with thoracic fat rolls. The thoracic rolls connect the upper back as a cosmetic subunit with the flanks and waist, which, in turn, unite with the abdomen and the iliac crest rolls. The flanks and iliac crest rolls can extend into the buttocks caudally and the outer thighs laterally. The crural fat and the medial thigh fat deposit extend toward the anterior thigh when these are seen as three-dimensional fat deposits. The suprapatellar region of the lower anterior thigh can merge with the medial knee fat deposit. Calf and ankle fat deposits can be continuous and give the lower legs a stovepipe-like appearance. These band-like connections, within our definition of cosmetic units of the body, should be treated together in order to achieve the most esthetically pleasing results (Figs. 7-3, 7-4A and B, and 7-5A and B).

On the body, the most frequently employed rejuvenation technique is liposuction. This, in concert with diet and exercise, will achieve the best cosmetic outcome. However, liposuction will not change a person's basic somatotype, and it is not indicated as primary treatment for obesity.[2] In our experience, the adipose tissue in men is generally more fibrous than that in women. Darker-skinned individuals may also have a more fibrous adipose tissue than those with lighter skins.

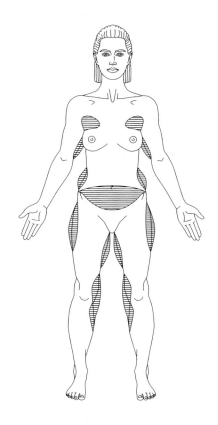

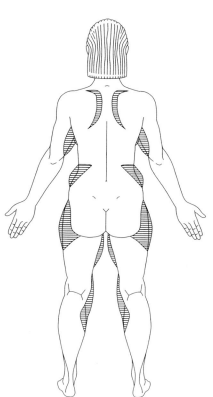

Figure 7-4   (**A**) Areas of frequent fat deposition in women, anterior view. (**B**) Areas of frequent fat deposition in women, posterior view. (© 2001 Mark Palangio.)

---

1. Posterior upper arms → lateral/superior pectoral bulges → thoracic rolls
2. Thoracic rolls → flanks/waist → outer thighs (trochanteric bulges)
3. Thoracic rolls → iliac crest rolls → abdomen → pubis
4. Crural fat → medial thigh bulge → anterior thigh/ suprapatella region → medial knee
5. Calves and ankles

Figure 7-3   Band-like grouping of cosmetic units (algorithm).

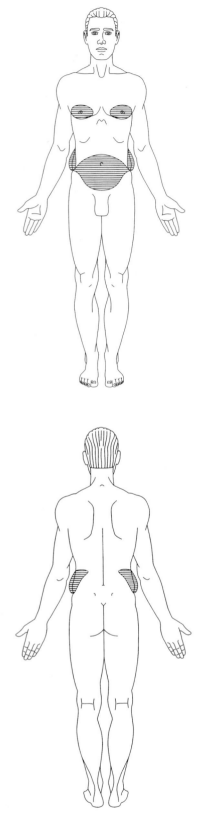

Figure 7-5 (**A**) Areas of frequent fat deposition in men, anterior view. (**B**) Areas of frequent fat deposition in men, posterior view. (© 2001 Mark Palangio.)

The Posterior Upper Arms

The ideal upper arm is well formed, with an even increase of its circumference from the elbow to the shoulder. This circumferential increase is more dramatic in the male. In women, the ideal arm profile tends to be more linear than in men. Ideally the arm circumference should be 0.18 to 0.19 times the patient's height.[1] The ideal arm is firm, with definition of the underlying muscles. There is no excess fat deposit. When the upper arms are held abducted, with bent elbows, only minimal skin laxity in the posterior triceps area should be visible, especially in women (Figs. 7-6 and 7-7).

Aging   With time, a loss of muscle tone, especially in the posterior triceps area, is often noted during the abduction maneuver. At the same time, subcutaneous adipose tissue accumulates. Thus disproportionately full upper arms develop. With the loss in skin tone, the abduction maneuver finally demonstrates floppy posterior upper arms, most notably in women. The excess skin above the elbow drapes towards the elbow like a pleated towel (Figs. 7-4*A* and *B*, and Fig. 7-5*A*).

Rejuvenation   If the upper arms are just full but not yet floppy, liposuction achieves good skin retraction and is the rejuvenation technique of choice even for obese arms. The cosmetic surgeon must, however, discuss the problem of possible skin "dimpling." This is especially important in the case of floppy upper arms, where there is an excess amount of redundant skin. The improvement in contour will still be very favorable, especially in clothes. Another surgical procedure, brachyplasty, achieves a lipectomy with excision of redundant skin. This procedure often leaves the patient with a very obvious scar, which may be hidden under long sleeves. A thorough discussion of both procedures and their indications is recommended to ensure realistic expectations of improvement.

The entry point for the liposuction cannula is a fine skin fold just above the elbow. The surgeon must be careful to avoid injury to the brachial plexus in the axillary region—a danger zone.

Superior and Lateral Pectoral Areas— Superior and Lateral Bulges

These isolated fat deposits are not usually seen in the youthful body. The lateral rib cage is sharply outlined and there are no localized fat deposits in the suprapectoral areas (Figs. 7-1 and 7-2).[2]

Aging   These isolated fat deposits build up over time and, in most patients, are a result of weight increase and lack of upper-body exercise. They are easily noticeable when women wear tops or gowns with thin straps because they disrupt the otherwise smooth contour of the upper chest. These bulges can protrude beneath the bra straps and are not appealing. Lateral bulges and inframammary extensions of these fat pads are more obvious than medial ones. In the side view, an indentation is seen between these areas and the breasts (Fig. 7-4*A*).

Rejuvenation   In our experience, fat deposits in these areas are more often found in obese women or women with lack of upper-body exercise as well as in some women

other areas, such as the flanks and iliac crest rolls, the thoracic rolls can often be treated through the same incision. Often the subcutaneous adipose tissue presents as firm and fibrous, and some strength is required to perform the procedure. The risk is that the liposuction cannula might accidentally pierce the ribs and cause internal injury. This is especially true of cannulas smaller than 4 mm. If the thoracic fat deposit is treated too aggressively, there is also a risk of injuring the brachial plexus, as it abuts the axillary fold.

The Female Breasts

Youthful female breasts are firm, well rounded, and framed by the lateral part of the pectoralis muscle, which creates a soft slope toward the inner upper arm. This is appreciated when the arm is held up with the hand behind the head. The breast ideally extends from the widest part of the shoulder/axilla to the widest part of the upper arm (Fig. 7-1).[1]

Aging   Over time, the force of gravity together with the vectors of aging promote a downward positioning of the breast. The breasts lose their firmness and become pendulous. Pregnancy and nursing contribute to these changes. The nipples begin to point downward rather than upward. With age, the breasts appear flat and their gland tissue involutes.

Rejuvenation   Although there are a variety of rejuvenation techniques available, the surgeon must be able to find

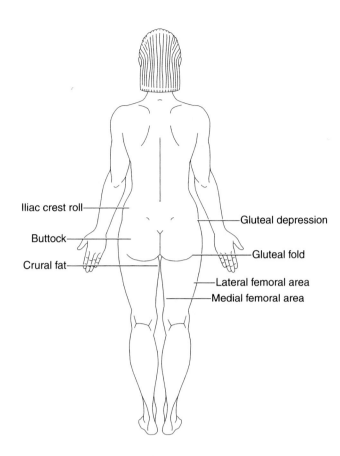

Figure 7-6 Gynecoid or female body shape with areas of importance, posterior view. (© 2001 Mark Palangio.)

with breast hypertrophy. Although liposuction is a viable rejuvenation method, we find that most patients improve with exercise and a healthy diet regimen.

Upper to Midlateral Back—Thoracic Rolls

These bulges are often detected as lateral and posterior extensions of the superior and lateral pectoral fat deposits. Caudally, these rolls can extend to the waist. The patient usually seeks esthetic improvement because these bulges can be seen through clothing, often protruding around the bra straps.

Aging   Ideally, the upper to midlateral back is sharply defined. The skin tone is firm and no localized fat rolls are seen. The development of initially small local fat deposits, often around the bra straps, is barely noted by the patient. Over the years, these small lipid deposits can enlarge and develop into bulges connecting with the fat deposits of the superior and lateral pectoral areas. Over the fourth to sixth decades, a relaxation in skin tone is noted, with mild drooping of the skin, which can form shelf-like arrangements (Fig. 7-4B).

Rejuvenation   The cosmetic surgeon knows that, without liposuction, it is very difficult for a patient to eliminate these bulges with diet and exercise alone. Liposuction is the procedure of choice. The access point for the cannula is on the lateral torso. When the liposuction procedure includes

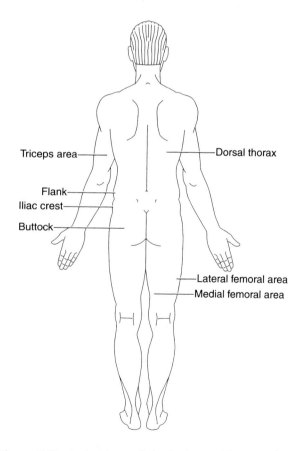

Figure 7-7 Android or male body shape with areas of importance, posterior view. (© 2001 Mark Palangio.)

the least invasive but most appropriate method for each given patient. Micro fat transfer has been shown to provide good cosmetic results but has only temporary effects. Possible side effects include microcalcification of the breast tissue, which can be indistinguishable from that due to breast cancer. Breast implants, though once controversial, are another treatment alternative. While the concept of breast lifting may be appealing, it can be associated with considerable scarring.

The Male Breasts—Gynecomastia

In men, the ideal breast appears flat—not rounded—with strong, well-defined pectoralis muscles creating a rectangular outline (Fig. 7-2). In young men, a small breast bud often develops before the pectoralis muscles become prominent. The result is that the breasts appear rounded and feminine. A majority of these young men attempt to resolve this problem by lifting weights in order to develop the pectoralis muscles. However, they achieve just the opposite result. A strong, thick pectoralis muscle makes the overlying breast bud protrude even more. In consultation with these patients, the cosmetic surgeon must be very tactful, because these patients are often psychologically traumatized. The surgeon must also make sure that they have realistic expectations.

Aging   A fullness of the male breast with aging is very common, and at least mild gynecomastia develops in most men over time. However, the patients who seek surgical correction often have a moderate to severe degree of gynecomastia. These patients are often obese (Fig. 7-5A).

Rejuvenation   The first-line treatment for gynecomastia is liposuction under tumescent anesthesia, which avoids the serious morbidity of open reduction. Pretumescent-era complications, such as subcutaneous hematoma, frequently resulted in increased scarring and deformed anatomic landmarks. Since this patient group is very critical, sometimes a second intervention is required, which may include excision of the breast bud. This directly improves the contour of the male breast, especially in the younger patient group described above. The cannula's access point is via an incision from the lateral sternum in the inframammary crease.

The Abdomen

As a cosmetic unit, the abdomen can be divided into upper and lower regions. The upper abdomen extends from the xyphoid to the umbilicus while the lower abdomen extends from the umbilicus to the mons pubis. These two areas are cosmetic subunits and connect with the flanks laterally and the iliac crest rolls inferiorly and laterally, forming a continuous cosmetic unit with several subunits (Figs. 7-4A and 7-5A).

Aging   The youthful abdomen is firm and flat. It does not demonstrate localized fat deposits and the skin turgor is good. There are no striae distensae. The abdominal wall's muscle system is well developed and no periumbilical hernia or rectus diastasis is found. Because of the specific anatomy, the upper abdomen is generally firmer and has less localized deposits of fat than the lower abdomen (Figs. 7-1 and 7-2).

In women, the lower abdomen often contains either localized fat deposits or is actually transformed into a large bulge in those who are overweight. Not only the excess fat but also weak abdominal muscles can make the abdomen appear large and protruding. Pregnancies can weaken the muscles of the abdominal wall. Pregnancy is a big influence on the appearance of a woman's body. The stress it places on the body is better tolerated if the woman is in her twenties rather than her forties during her pregnancy. On the other hand, many women nowadays decide to delay childbirth until their middle to late thirties. These women will most likely have more trouble getting "back into shape." They will often have developed lax and/or elongated, stretched abdominal muscles with excess skin overlying the abdomen. The appearance of striae distensae, commonly called stretch marks, is common. These changes are more pronounced in the lower abdomen. Weight loss and exercise may help to improve the body shape, but only to a degree (Figs. 7-4A and 7-8).

In our experience, as they age, women will accumulate fatty deposits in the lower abdomen. Interestingly, these kinds of localized lipid deposits are usually not seen in men, suggesting that female hormones contribute to a rounding of the lower abdomen. Men develop a "pot belly" configuration with age, which usually means an even increase in the subcutaneous tissue[7] throughout the abdomen. For both men and women, it is well established that an increase in abdominal girth is associated with increased cardiac morbidity, although it is the increase in visceral fat that is most implicated (Fig. 7-5A).[3,4]

Because of the vectors of aging as well as the force of gravity, the abdominal skin relaxes over time, the umbilicus appears to move caudally, and muscles of the abdominal wall often increase in length while their strength decreases. The excess abdominal tissue can appear to be lying on the mons pubis, either just as excess skin or protruding in the form of a pannus, which can cover the groin area like an apron.

Rejuvenation   In choosing the best rejuvenation procedure for a given patient, it is vital to assess his or her needs. On clinical examination, the centripedal adiposity is assessed with the pinch test, whereby the tissue is pinched between the thumb and the index finger. The patient then assumes the diving position (bent form just prior to a dive) to assess the laxity of the abdominal wall musculature. Finally, the patient lies in the supine position and contracts the abdominal muscles by elevating both head and legs. This maneuver is used to detect possible periumbilical hernias

---

1. Lower abdominal adiposity only → liposuction alone treatment of choice
2. Abdominal adiposity combined with discrete skin laxity → combination liposuction with miniabdominoplasty
3. Abdominal adiposity combined with skin laxity and abdominal muscle flaccidity → combination of liposuction, with rectus muscle plication and miniabdominoplasty
4. Mild to moderate pannus formation → two-stage liposuction procedure

Figure 7-8   Treatment algorithm for various cosmetic problems of the abdomen (algorithm).

and rectus diastasis. A thorough preoperative physical examination helps to avoid intraoperative complications.

Miniabdominoplasty and its variations are indicated if the patient has a partially lax abdominal muscle system, either due to multiple pregnancies or constitutionally. A direct tightening of the rectus muscle by means of plication sutures helps to eliminate this problem. On the other hand, if the patient's abdominal wall shows good muscle tone and only localized skin laxity associated with mild to moderate adiposity, the removal of the excess skin in conjunction with liposuction leads to cosmetically superior results. A prerequisite for the performance of these procedures is that the cosmetic surgeon be appropriately trained and experienced (Fig. 7-8).[8]

In the case of a pannus formation, we recommend liposuction as a two-stage procedure, starting with the lower abdomen. A prolonged healing period of 3 to 6 months allows for the ensuing fibrosis to elevate and contract the lower part of the pannus so that it appears lifted above the groin area. The skin is tightened to the abdomen. The second liposuction procedure then corrects the superior portion of the pannus. This two-stage method leads to esthetically superior results, often without excision of excess skin (Fig. 7-8).[9]

Flanks—Love Handles

The flanks are the area lateral between ribs and iliac crest, extending posteriorly to near the midline. The flanks are ideally trim and either straight, connecting to the iliac crest in men, or narrow, to create an hourglass waistline in women. The waist circumference should ideally be up to two-fifths of the height of patients (Figs. 7-1 and 7-2).[1]

Aging   Over time, the sharp contour of the flanks is broken by slowly developing bulges. In men, fat is deposited in this area, often to a point where the fat accumulations are colloquially called "love handles." The main complaint is that these bulges protrude above the belt line. Men then tend to wear their trousers lower on the hips instead of at the waist area so that their clothes will still fit. In women, the waist gradually fills in, so that the narrow hourglass shape is replaced by a straighter, more masculine outline. Women then tend to wear their skirts and slacks higher up in an attempt to make their cutomary clothing still fit this new shape. In general, these fat deposits occur as isolated pockets; often, however, they are continuous with the lower abdominal fat deposits and/or with the posterior back as thoracic rolls and the iliac crest rolls (Figs. 7-4A and B and 7-5A and B).

Rejuvenation   Liposuction is the ideal technique for reducing the flank bulges in men and creating a new waistline in women. The surgeon must begin by evaluating the patient's overall body proportions. Especially in the flank and waist regions, it is important to determine whether adjacent cosmetic subunits—like the lower abdomen, the iliac crest areas, or the buttocks—are also involved. This is easily done by the pinch test, which can demonstrate excess adipose tissue in these areas. Rarely, the flank and waist truly contain only isolated fat deposits. The patient may be aware of only one particular area, but in order to achieve the most esthetically pleasing result, the surgeon should point out contiguous zones in need of treatment. Future treatments can also be planned accordingly. The patient will soon begin to appreci-

ate that after liposuction in one specific area, neighboring areas will appear far more prominent. The patient will accept this fact far better if the cosmetic surgeon has already made him or her aware of it during the initial consultation.

Iliac Crest—Iliac Crest Rolls

This is the area overlying the ileum and the upper part of the sacrum; fat deposits here are colloquially called "high hips," which extend forward to just below the iliac crest. In both sexes, adipose bulges (called iliac crest rolls) are frequently encountered here. Often, they are associated with an excess bulge in the lower abdomen anteriorly, flank bulges superiorly, buttocks posteriorly and inferiorly, and outer thighs laterally. The combination of iliac crest rolls with abdominal fat results in a "lifesaver" appearance by creating a ring of excess fat in the lower torso. When the iliac crest rolls associate posterior with thoracic rolls, a butterfly deformity is created. The iliac crest rolls may be depicted as the lower wing pair, which is wider than the upper wing pair, the thoracic rolls. The term *violin deformity* is used when the iliac crest rolls continue into bulges of the outer thighs. When such a torso is viewed posteriorly, the shape of a violin is outlined (Figs. 7-4A and B and 7-5A and B).[2]

Aging   The youthful iliac crest area is free of fatty deposits. The bony crest is visible as a landmark. The sacral areas have a "ski slope" appearance where they connect with the buttocks (Figs. 7-1, 7-2, 7-6, and 7-7). With aging, the sacral part develops a more rounded contour, starting usually in the late thirties and early forties. This results in loss of the ski slope appearance. The anatomic landmarks of the iliac crest become obliterated by fat accumulations, as is commonly seen with an average weight gain of 1 lb per holiday season.[6]

Rejuvenation   Liposuction is the treatment of choice. Even when several cosmetic subunits are involved—as mentioned in discussing the butterfly deformity, the lifesaver deformity and the violin deformity—marked improvement with re-creation of a youthful contour leads to high patient's satisfaction. The cosmetic surgeon must once again take care not to injure any viscera during the procedure.

The Buttocks

The ideal buttock is well rounded—apple-shaped. It is uplifted and firm, with minimal surface irregularities or dimples due to cellulite. Since the gluteal musculature is often neglected in everyday life owing to sedentary lifestyles, improvement of the buttocks is an important rejuvenation procedure in the dermatologic surgeon's practice.

Aging   Some buttocks never droop until late in life; however, others are droopy and square-shaped at an early age. As an explanation, it was proposed that, in the cosmetically pleasing buttock, there is a connection of the superficial layers with the deeper structures. This ultimately reduces the buttocks' mobility. Combined with good skin turgor, such buttocks can resist the force of gravity longer (Figs. 7-6 and 7-7).

On the other hand, buttocks with superficial hypertrophy and no connection to deeper muscular structures are increasingly involved in body movement and unsupported against the forces of gravity. With the additional combination of a lax skin tone and excessive weight, the fat is not held in place and starts to sag, with the fat accumulating most often caudally in the sagged, drooping part. The frequently seen surface irregularities, in the form of dimpling and cellulite in the ischiocrural part, might be due to increased compression to the tissue when sitting and in general a sedentary lifestyle. In the forties and fifties, the decrease in muscular tissue and bone mass results in excess skin, especially in the caudal part. The skin folds appear like the folds of a drawn curtain. The natural convexity of the buttock flattens with age, resulting in a squared, flattened appearance. Individuals with more fibrous tissue have a relative advantage. For them, the signs of aging in this area are delayed, as the fibrous structure can better withstand the force of gravity.

Gluteal Depression Patients often seek the attention of a cosmetic surgeon for evaluation and improvement of what they perceive as an unsightly indentation in the buttock region. The gluteal depression is the area overlying the gluteal muscle laterally and often lacks fat. In combination with trochanteric fat deposits and iliac crest fat accumulations, this depression is partially responsible for a violin deformation. The cure is elimination of surrounding bulges via liposculpture and possibly also fat transfer (Fig. 7-6).[2]

Gluteal Fold The gluteal fold outlines the buttock shape inferiorly and separates it from the posterior thigh. The gluteal fold is an important anatomic landmark contributing directly to the buttock shape. Nowadays, with the trend toward activities like jogging and roller blading, a more athletic look does not require a very pronounced gluteal fold. The ideal buttock nowadays is a continuum of the thighs, with only the medial buttock crease being seen while the remaining part is eliminated by the uplifted buttock cheeks. It is clear that the length or shape of the gluteal fold is not necessarily identical with the border of the underlying gluteal muscle; rather, this structure is variable (Fig. 7-6).

Interestingly, an anatomic fixed point of the medial part of the gluteal fold can be identified. The ligament of Luschka originates from the ischeal tuberosity and connects posteriorly and laterally with the deep dermis, determining the medial portion of the gluteal fold. This fixed point can function as a hinge point. It can end up being positioned very close, medially and caudally, to the buttock crease, and as such predispose the patient to develop a double gluteal fold, colloquially called a "banana fold," due to variations in the ligamentous insertion points. The lateral part of the gluteal fold is extremely variable and depends on the buttock's weight, skin and muscle tone, and fat accumulations in the neighboring areas. A concave fold is esthetically more pleasing than a straight or even inverted fold, as commonly detected in heavy, drooping buttocks with loose skin tone.[2,7]

Rejuvenation To achieve firmer, fuller buttocks, buttock implants can be placed. These are becoming increasingly popular among South American patients. As with all implants, there are possible side effects associated with them, including displacement, tissue reactions, and infection. The patient must be reminded to avoid intramuscular injections in the buttock.

Liposculpture and fat injections are more pliable rejuvenation techniques. An enlarged buttock can be reduced and an irregular, asymmetrical silhouette improved by fat removal in the cephalic buttock area. The resulting fibrosis also helps to lift a drooping buttock. Surface changes like depressions and cellulite dimples cannot be improved by liposuction, but fat injection might be indicated here. The region of the gluteal fold is a danger zone. Compromising the fibrous attachments with aggressive liposuction will destroy this attachment system and remove the buttocks' caudal support. The weight of the cephalic part in conjunction with the force of gravity leads to a drooping buttock and gluteal fold deformities. These deformities are very difficult to correct. Dermatolipectomy will result in permanent scarring. Fat transfer might provide some improvement.[10] The cosmetic surgeon must respect this potentially troublesome zone in order to avoid possible pitfalls.

Access by liposuction cannula is from the midsacrum to treat the cephalic part, from the trochanteric region to treat the lateral inferior part, and just inferior to the gluteal fold to treat the banana-fold area. The cosmetic results achieved are generally very satisfying.

The Thighs

The thighs are frequent sites of rejuvenation. Ideally, they are slender and firm and the skin surface is smooth. The trochanteric region of the outer thighs does not extend beyond the line shaped by the buttocks and the inferior lateral thighs. In the youthful patient, the crural fat is located at the superior inner thigh, close to the vulva. The overlying skin is thin, and a smooth surface here is desirable. The medial thighs should not touch when the feet are placed close together; they should taper gradually to join the midthigh. A natural mild depression in the midthigh region may produce a bow-legged appearance if it is accentuated. Ideally, the thighs encompass about one-quarter of the body's height (Fig. 7-1).[1]

The Outer Thighs—Trochanteric Bulges, "Riding Breeches" In general, women have a tendency to deposit fat in the trochanteric region of the outer thighs as part of the gynecoid body morphology. Like those of the lower abdomen, these fat reserves do not resolve with exercise and dieting. Frequently a genetic disposition in female members of a family is brought to light during the initial consultation, when the patient states that all the women in her family have the same body shape, characterized by exuberant outer thighs. On clinical examination the outer thigh region assumes the appearance of riding breeches or saddlebags. Often there is additional excess fat in the superior iliac crest region and the inner thigh areas medially. These fatty deposits can be so extensive that they create a morphologic discrepancy between the disproportionately small upper body and the lower body, which may be more than one clothing size larger (Fig. 7-4*A* and *B*).

Rejuvenation Liposuction of the excess fat accompanied by liposculpture of the neighboring regions—such as buttocks, iliac crest rolls, and inner thighs—improves the body silhouette of the patient dramatically and can literally change a patient's life.

The surgeon must be familiar with the fascia lata zone. The fascia lata is a large tendinous structure along the outer thigh. Removal of too much adipose tissue and/or injury to subdermal fat overlying this fascial structure results in surface irregularities that are difficult to repair. Sometimes the adipose layer is accidentally so thinned that the movement of the fascial structure can be seen with the naked eye. The patient will be very disappointed with this kind of result.

The Medial Thigh with Crural Fat, the Anterior Thigh
The superior medial aspect of the thigh contains a mild fatty deposit called crural fat. The crural fat of both thighs may slightly touch when both knees meet (Figs. 7-1 and 7-6). The hypothetical function of this compartment is protection of the vulva. Additional fat deposits in the mid-medial thigh frequently accompany fat accumulations in this region. The shape of the mid-medial thigh then changes from a mild natural depression to fullness, sometimes in such excess that the medial thighs rub and patients develop an elephant-like way of walking, trying to avoid this abrasion.

The fat deposits must be seen three-dimensionally, since the anterior thigh can have a continuation of excess fat accumulations as well. Frequently there is a localized deposit in the suprapatellar region, which gives the impression of a skin ptosis overhanging the patella.[7]

Aging   The crural fat region changes in the mid-thirties and early forties. The smooth surface becomes irregular and wavy owing to the loss of skin turgor and elasticity. In the fifties and sixties, the crural fat atrophies and a widening gap in the upper thigh closure may result when both knees meet. In the late thirties and early forties, the mid-medial thigh region undergoes similar changes. The inner thigh region appears flabby from the seventh decade onward. An increase in skin rhytids accompanies these changes (Figs. 7-4A and B).[2]

Rejuvenation   The fatty deposits of the thigh can be removed via liposuction. We usually start with the upper inner thigh first, while the patient's leg is in the frog-leg position. The liposuction is initially confined to the triangle marked as the crural fat region. After removal of excess fat in this area, the cannula is directed caudally, performing liposuction in a marked triangle pointing toward the medial knee. The patient's leg is straight. If liposuction of the anterior thigh is included, this area is treated last. Special care must be taken not to remove too much deep adipose tissue in order to avoid a step in the anterior thigh contour. Removal of the suprapatellar fat deposit is difficult because that area is very localized and liposuction should not include the patella. The patella is one of the fixed points, and if this region is not respected, deformity of the anatomic landmarks can result. There is, in addition, the danger of creating a step with an indentation in the suprapatella area.

The suggested sequence of liposuction is very important. If the fat of the medial thigh is removed prior to the excess crural fat, the sense of proportion is lost and it is technically more difficult to remove this fat deposit. The removal of an exaggerated amount of fat causes a gap to form in the crural fat region; this is generally undesirable.[7]

The cosmetic surgeon must be gentle in this region, because aggressive rasping of the dermis can induce scar-ring, even keloid formation. Superficial liposuction should be avoided; otherwise skin irregularities and dimple formation can develop. Further, excessive fat removal in the medial thigh can overemphasize the natural depression and lead to a bowlegged appearance or an "O" formation when both knees meet. In addition the patient must be instructed to keep the compression garment in place so that folds and depressions, which can persist permanently, are not created.

The Knees
A very important aspect of a beautiful leg is the knee. It should be shapely, with a condylar prominence and no localized fat deposits. The bony patella should be outlined when the knee is bent.

Aging   With aging, the knees become rounded and encased medially; less frequently, lateral fat deposits may appear. Excess fat can extend from the lower medial thigh to the superior aspect of the lower medial leg, in the sense of a cosmetic unit composed of several subunits. Sometimes these fatty deposits include the anterior thigh in the suprapatellar region, as described earlier. These changes usually start in the late twenties and early thirties. In women in their sixties and beyond, these changes are often compounded by osteoporosis, creating an "O" shape of the legs when the feet are placed together.

Rejuvenation   The knees are difficult areas to treat. Liposuction is usually performed with small cannulas only. The surgeon must be careful not to injure joint structures or damage the saphenous vein and nerve medially. The popliteal area is a fixed point and should not be disturbed.[7] Treatment of the fat deposit in the suprapatellar region was discussed earlier. In addition, an increase in wrinkles and folds after liposuction can occur. Excision of the excess skin is not advised, since the remaining scar can be very disfiguring. Last but not least, the final result of the liposuction procedure is demonstrated only after a prolonged healing phase, since it takes time for the postoperative edema to resolve.[10]

Calves and Ankles
The ideal calf for men and women is well shaped by a trained gastrocnemius muscle, with no excess adipose tissue obscuring this anatomic landmark. The normal gastrocnemius muscle mass projects a shadow towards the ankle, defining the desirable shape laterally and dorsally. In women who prefer to wear high heels, the calf profile is often flat and appears skinny. This is the result of gastrocnemius hypotrophy. Patients with lower calf fat deposits, which obliterate the gastrocnemius's silhouette, present with the complaint of "shapeless calves"; their calves appear pipe-like, with a pursestring cutoff just above the mallelolei, where these fat accumulations abruptly end. This kind of calf deformity is hereditary.[2]

The ankles are ideally defined with the Achilles' tendon projecting at the most posterior point of the ankle. At both sides of it, there should be a hollow, with prominent malleoli anteriorly.

Aging   Over time the gastrocnemic muscle mass will atrophy and the pleasing shape of the calf slowly diminishes.

The reduction with aging of the lower body skeletal muscle mass occurs after the forties.[5] The calf profile changes from well rounded to flat. The skin of the lower legs becomes roughened and often discolored with rust to brownish macules. These changes are starting to occur in patients in their forties. Varicosities develop and trophic changes can lead to skin edema and even sclerosis. Skin rhytid formation is noticeable in patients in their fifties and sixties.

The ankles often start to appear plump and edematous in the thirties and early forties. Age conditions like hypertension, cardiac problems, and diabetes lead to fluid accumulation, with edema of the ankles. If these conditions are left untreated, the lower legs and ankles become indurated and even sclerous, making both areas unforgiving rejuvenation treatment zones.

Rejuvenation   The cosmetic surgeon must assess the cause of calf and ankle deformity. If a medical condition is most likely to blame, rejuvenation therapy is contraindicated. However, if inherited excess fat accumulation is the cause, liposuction can be used to reshape the calf and redefine the ankles. Thorough and gentle liposuction with attention to the danger zones in the gastrocnemius and Achilles' tendon areas should be performed. The fat layer is often firm in those regions, and a pinch test to examine the amount of remaining adipose tissue is often impossible to perform.[7] The surgeon must use small cannulas and be careful not to injure any vital structures in this region. The postoperative recovery is prolonged, since the liposuction procedure disrupts the lymphatic vessels, thus prolonging edema and dysesthesia. This must be discussed with the patient preoperatively in order to set realistic goals. The postoperative edema can take 6 or more months to subside. A high incidence of pigmentary changes is reported. Despite all these difficulties, there is noticeable improvement and, as a rule, the patient is finally satisfied.

Calf implants help to improve the contour of the hypothrophied gastrocnemic muscle. There is a preference for these in California. As with all implants, potential side effects must be thoroughly discussed with the patient, and the discussion points should be clearly documented.

DANGER-ZONE SUMMARY

The liposuction technique is reviewed in greater detail in Chap. 16. In general, the harvesting part of the liposuction cannula should always be directed toward the adipose tissue and away from the dermis. This helps to avoid dermal injury and subsequent surface irregularities. There are collision zones where cannulas can become too superficial, by abutting either a bone, a tendon, or fascial structures.

The Collision Zones

In general, a definition of such a zone is any anatomic structure that can induce a change in direction of the cannula. Natural flexion creases—as at the elbows, the popliteal area, and the inframammary region—are included. Some authors suggest that the lower abdomen and the umbilicus each embodies such a zone. The fascia lata zone has been defined above. The three colliding zones of the lower leg—which include the gastrocnemius muscle, Achilles' tendon, and

malleolei—have also been discussed above. It is obvious that trophic changes make the calf and ankle area unforgiving regions for liposuction. Adverse sequelae are dysesthesia, pigmentary alterations, and dimpling. Trauma to the Achilles' tendon during lipoaspiration should be avoided, as it can lead to noticeable fibrous adhesions.[7]

The Fixed Points

Fixed points are either variable, meaning they adapt to body movement and skin tension, or invariable. These points cannot be changed regardless of the rejuvenation techniques employed. They have been discussed previously and are briefly summarized here. They are the inguinal crease, the area of the fascia lata, the gluteal fold with medial hinge point, a double or banana fold if present, the popliteal area, and the region overlying the patella. These fixed points direct and influence body shape and fat distribution. In order to perform a natural-appearing, dynamic liposculpture, the surgeon must take these pivotal points into consideration.[7]

In summary, the aging body allows for a variety of rejuvenation methods. Those most often employed are liposuction and liposculpture. Dramatic results can be achieved in the "right" patient. This again emphasizes the value and importance of patient selection and physical examination of the problem area as well as awareness of the body proportions. This will allow the dermatologic surgeon to customize each treatment for the individual patient, thus achieving superior cosmetic results.

References

1. Toledo LS. The preoperative examination. In: Knopp D, Donnellan K, Palumbo R, eds. *Refinement in Facial and Body Contouring*. Lippincott-Raven; Philadelphia: 1999:29–41.

2. Hetter GP, Lewis CM, Arner P. Nomenclature. In: Hetter GP, ed. *Lipoplasty*. Boston/Toronto/London: Little, Brown; 1990:65–75.

3. Kahn HS, Simoes EJ, Koponen M, et al. The abdominal diameter index and sudden coronary death in men. *Am J Cardiol* 1996; 78(8)961–964.

4. Rexrode KM, Carey VJ, Hennekens CH, et al. Abdominal adiposity and coronary heart disease in women. *JAMA* 1998; 280(2)1843–1848.

5. Janssen I, Heymsfield SB, Wang ZM, et al. Skeletal muscle mass distribution in 468 men and women aged 18–88 years. *J Appl Physiol* 200; 89(1):81–88.

6. Yanovski JA, Yanoski SZ, Sovik KN, et al. A prospective study of holiday weight gain. *N Engl J Med* 1998; 342(12):861–867.

7. Illouz YG. The study of the subcutaneous fat. In: Hetter, GP, ed. *Lipoplasty*. Boston/Toronto/London: Little, Brown; 1990:77–98.

8. Bisaccia E, Scarborough DS. Miniabdominoplasty using combination liposuction and limited skin resection. *Cosmet Dermatol* 1997; 7(10):10–12.

9. Bisaccia E, Scarborough DS. Liposuction for the pendulous lower abdominal panniculus. *Cosmet Dermatol* 1997; 12(10):12–14.

10. Toledo LS. The buttocks. In: Knopp D, Donnellan K, Palumbo, R, eds. *Refinement in Facial and Body Contouring*. Philadelphia: Lippincott-Raven; 1999:135–163.

CHAPTER 8

Anesthesia

Successful cosmetic surgery depends highly on effective anesthesia. Most importantly, anesthesia involves the patient's safety and comfort, physical and mental. Studies have shown that patients are more apt to return for a second procedure if adequate anesthesia was given during the initial procedure. Since ancient times, local anesthesia has been used. For instance, the Incas chewed coca leaves, allowing their saliva to drip into wounds to minimize pain.[1]

Anesthesia for dermatologic surgery has progressed from local anesthesia to sedation with monitored anesthesia. Newer agents—topical and parenteral—have become available, making ambulatory surgery an affordable, less stressful option. Regional anesthesia can be categorized according to means of application: (1) topical, (2) infiltration, (3) peripheral nerve block, and (4) central neural block—i.e., epidural.[2] Central neural blocks are not be discussed in this text.

Topical Anesthesia

Topical anesthesia has revolutionized invasive procedures. Traditional local anesthesia, most commonly the injection of lidocaine, involves two painful experiences. First "the needle stick" and then the burning sensation resulting from infiltration.[3] In fact, 14 percent of 20-year-old adults are "needle phobic."[3]

One of the skin's main functions is to protect the body from harmful penetrating agents. Thus, it is easy to understand the difficulty in developing the perfect topical anesthetic. The main barrier in the diffusion of all substances is the stratum corneum.[3] Topical anesthesia has been prevalent in oral, genital, and tracheal procedures for many years. These preparations include 2% xylocaine jelly, benzocaine, and TAC (a mixture of tetracaine, adrenaline, and cocaine), but these agents are not effective on nonmucosal intact skin.

Topical anesthetics fall into two groups—chemical and physical.[3] The chemical methods include a variety of agents. Of these, EMLA, or "eutectic mixture of local anesthetics," is by far the most commonly used. It is a one-to-one mixture of 25 mg/mL lidocaine and 25 mg/mL prilocaine in an oil-in-water emulsion. The melting points of the two crystalline anesthetic salts is lowered in the mixture. This defines a eutectic mixture, which allows for a higher concentration of active ingredient per droplet of emulsion.[3] It is excellent for dermal analgesia up to 3 mm in depth, requiring 60 to 90 min under occlusion to take effect. Anesthesia continues for 30 to 60 min after the cream is removed.[4] It is not recommended for use in infants less than 3 months of age because of the risk of methemoglobinemia.[4]

Liposomal agents are new forms for drug delivery. One of these, ELA-Max cream, uses lipid bilayers encapsulating 4% lidocaine to deliver the anesthetic to the dermal target. Unlike EMLA, it does not require occlusion and needs to be applied only 15 to 45 minutes preoperatively.[5]

Other newly formulated, proprietary, patented topical agents include Betacaine-LA ointment (lidocaine, prilocaine, and a vasoconstrictor) and tetracaine gel (containing 4% tetracaine in a lecithin gel base). Neither is approved by the U.S. Food and Drug Administration (FDA).[5] Pramoxine hydrochloride (Tronothane) is a surface anesthetic agent; it is not used for injections but mainly as an antipruritic in dermatology.

Anesthetic patches have been developed to simplify administration and quantify the dose to an area of skin. One preparation, 30% lidocaine mixed in an acid mantle cream, requires mixing 9 g of lidocaine powder with 30 g of the acid mantle cream; the mixture is applied to various sizes of gauze and occlusively sealed. The patch has fallen out of favor because of the high concentration of lidocaine necessary for anesthesia and the onerous task of compounding each prescription.[3] Amethocaine (4% amethocaine) and Lidogel patch (10% lidocaine gel with an absorption promoter) are other available patch systems.

Physical methods utilize electric current or ultrasound, in iontophoresis and phonopheresis, respectively, to drive topical agents via percutaneous absorption. Iontophoresis has been most notably used in hyperhidrosis. A number of dermatologic procedures have been performed under acceptable iontophoretic anesthesia, including pulsed dye laser for port wine stains; shave biopsies of the nose; and injection, dermabrasion, cautery, and electrocoagulation of spider veins.[3,6] The greatest advantages are avoidance of injection pain and quick onset of action (less than 10 min). The main disadvantage is the bulkiness of the apparatus, making it difficult to treat the face and fingers. Large areas are tedious to treat. The major potential side effect is burning of the exposed skin due to the direct current.[3]

The effectiveness of phonopheresis in anesthetic delivery has been debated in the literature. Further research in this area is necessary. It has been shown to be very successful in the treatment of musculoskeletal disorders—sprains, strains, arthritis, and bursitis.[6] Phonopheresis has been shown to be particularly useful in driving hydrocortisone ointment into muscle (100 percent) and neural tissue (145 percent).[6]

SPECIAL SITES

Proparacaine and tetracaine are benzoic acid esters that are useful as ophthalmic anesthetics for eyelid surgery and the placement of eyeshields prior to facial resurfacing. Proparacaine eyedrops have been shown to cause less pain than tetracaine and the anesthesia lasts slightly longer (10.7 versus 9.2 min.).[7] Topical lidocaine, benzocaine, and cocaine preparations have been used for mucosal surfaces. Topical anesthetics may impair swallowing and cause aspiration. Unintentional biting can occur.[7]

OTHERS

Other modes of anesthesia have been employed. Saturated phenol (88%) has been used to achieve temporary anesthesia in small, manually dermabrated areas.[8] Since the applied phenol is removed by dermabrasion, further inflammation and penetration is not a problem.[8] Potential cardiac and renal toxicity is the main concern with the use of phenol. Contact skin cooling with ice or chilled gels and spray coolants has been used for anesthesia for many years. In recent times, with the development of visible and infrared lasers, heat targets below the skin have been of interest. Cold sapphire contact handpieces that are held against the skin surface with compression allow for deeper penetration of the light beam to the dermal targets and are also beneficial for topical anesthesia.[9]

Infiltrative

The conventional technique of injecting an anesthetic is via infiltration. All local anesthetics block sodium influx through sodium channels in local nerve endings.[10] Smaller, non-myelinated C fibers carrying pain are blocked first.

Derivatives of paraaminobenzoic acid (e.g., procaine) or aniline (e.g., lidocaine), esters, and amides, respectively, make up the two groups of local anesthetics. Each group is characterized by a principal site of biotransformation and allergic profile. The ester anesthetics are primarily metabolized by plasma cholinesterase and much less by hepatic cholinesterase. The amide anesthetics are degraded in the liver via microsomal enzymes. Thus, after multiple dosings, notable amounts of amides may accumulate in the serum—as opposed to esters excluding cocaine, which are rapidly metabolized.[2] Patients with severe hepatic disease may have reduced metabolism of amides and esters. Genetic or sup-

pressed esterase activity may decrease ester metabolism.[2] Over 90 percent protein-bound, the amides may be markedly elevated in situations of decreased protein binding. Due to the decreased volume of distribution, plasma concentrations may be elevated in patients with congestive heart failure (CHF).

AGENTS

Procaine, a representative ester, is an aromatic compound with an ester bond linking either an amino or piperidine group (Table 8-1).[11] Other esters include cocaine (for topical use only) and tetracaine. The ester-linked anesthetics (e.g., procaine) have fallen out of favor with dermatologic surgeons due to allergic and cross-reactions with benzocaine, PABA, paraphenylenediamine, and sulfonamides.[11]

Lidocaine, a representative amide, is the most popular local anesthetic because of its rapid onset of action, long duration (45 min to 3 h without epinephrine), and low toxicity.[1] The amide anesthetics are preserved with methylparabens and should be avoided in patients with a history of paraben allergy.[11] The maximum recommended dose of lidocaine for topical and injection anesthesia is 300 mg (4 to 5 mg/kg up to 30 mL of a 1% solution or 25 to 35 mL of a 2% solution) without epinephine or 500 mg (7 mg/kg up to 50 mL of a 1% solution or 25 mL of a 2% solution) with epinephrine 1:200,000, every 2 h.[2] Higher doses may be given in tumescent anesthesia (see "Tumescent Anesthesia," below). Other amides include bupivacaine, prilocaine, and etidocaine.

If the amide and ester anesthetics are contraindicated, diphenhydramine or normal saline are options. A 1% solution of diphenhydramine, an antihistamine, produces the equivalent anesthetic effect of 1% lidocaine.[12] The pain resulting from the injection of diphenhydramine injection is worse and the duration of action is shorter than with lidocaine.[12]

ADDITIVES

Excluding cocaine and prilocaine, local anesthetics directly relax vascular smooth muscle, resulting in vasodilation. By adding epinephrine, a vasoconstrictor, to the local anes-

Table 8-1
Representative Chemical Structures

	Chemical Structure	
Aromatic Terminal	Intermediate Chain	Amine Terminal
Esters Procaine H_2N-*	$COOCH_2CH_2$	$N\begin{cases} C_2H_5 \\ C_2H_5 \end{cases}$
Amides Lidocaine $\begin{cases} CH_3 \\ *-NH \\ CH_3 \end{cases}$	$COCH_2$	$N\begin{cases} C_2H_5 \\ C_2H_5 \end{cases}$

thetic, bleeding is decreased, larger total anesthetic doses are possible, and the duration of action is prolonged.[1] Maximal vasoconstriction from epinephrine takes approximately 7 to 15 min and lasts approximately 40 min in lidocaine mixtures of 1:100,000 to 200,000.[1]

Epinephrine is to be avoided in labor, thyrotoxicosis, and severe cardiovascular disease.[2] Tricyclic antidepressants or monoamine oxidase inhibitors may enhance epinephrine's systemic effects.[2] Epinephrine-induced vasoconstriction may predispose contaminated wounds to infection secondary to tissue ischemia[12] and should be avoided in tissues supplied by an end artery (digits, pinna, nasal ala, penis, and skin flap). Premixed commercial local anesthetics with epinephrine contain various acids that lower the pH to decrease epinephrine degradation over time.[1] Since these solutions are acidic, more pain is produced on injection.

To decrease injection pain, a mixture of 8.4% sodium bicarbonate per 10 mL of local anesthetic may be used; more postoperative edema may result.[1] The addition of 1 mL of sodium bicarbonate (1 meq/mL) to each 10 mL of local anesthetic results in 0.1 meq/mL.[11] The solution is prepared fresh daily. Hyaluronidase added to the anesthetic solution enhances anesthetic spread.[13]

METHOD OF INJECTION

To decrease the pain of injection, several injection methods have been employed. Warming the local anesthetic to 40°C prior to subcutaneous injection has been shown to reduce local pain.[14] The "two-finger confusion technique" involves distracting the patient with a series of questions throughout the injection maneuver while the patient is concentrating on two fingers placed on either side of the wound.[12] There is also less pain with slower injection rates, placing pressure on the injection site, and injecting proximally on extremity sites.[12] Also, the patient experiences less pain when the injection is made on the way out of the surgical site.[13]

Nerve Blocks of the Face

Dentists have long used nerve blocks for regional anesthesia in order to minimize discomfort. With the advent of full-face laser resurfacing and dermabrasion, cosmetic surgeons have incorporated nerve blocks for these outpatient procedures, thus reducing the need for sedation. A lidocaine solution ranging from 0.5%[15] to 2% with 1:100,000 epinephrine[16] or bupivicaine 0.5% with 1:200,000[16] have been shown to provide excellent results. Facial anatomy is crucial to the successful anesthesia of facial units. In a vertical plane 2.5 cm from a line drawn through the length of the nasal midline lie the supraorbital notch, infraorbital foramina, and mental foramen[17] (Fig. 8-1).

The supraorbital notch, which contains the supraorbital foramina, is palpable in the middle portion of the supraorbital rim. Exiting cephalad from the supraorbital foramina 2.5 cm from the midsagittal plane of the head are the supraorbital and supratrochlear nerves, which are divisions of the frontal nerve.[17] The supratrochlear nerve, which is medial to the supraorbital nerve, innervates the upper medial orbit

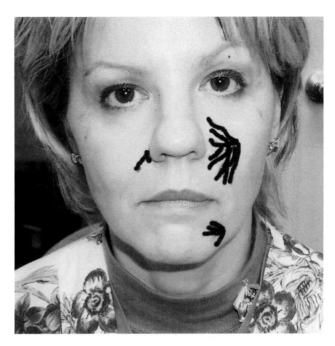

Figure 8-1   In a sagittal plane 2.5 cm from the midline, one will find the supraorbital notch and exiting nerves proximally, the infraorbital foramina and nerve centrally, and the mental foramina and nerve distally.

and the lower medial forehead; the supraorbital nerve innervates the upper eyelid, forehead, anterior scalp, and vertex of the scalp. The medial eyelids and the side of the nose above the medial canthus is supplied by the infratrochlear nerve, a branch of the nasociliary nerve.[13] For a supratrochlear/supratrochlear/infratrochlear block, the needle is inserted at the lateral middle third of the eyebrow while aiming at the suprorbital notch (Fig. 8-2). A sensation of "heaviness" of the upper eyelid is a sign of a successful nerve block, since the supraorbital nerve innervates the upper eyelids.[15] Periorbital ecchymosis may occur with this block.

The infraorbital foramen is about 5 to 7 mm below the infraorbital rim; it is in line with the medial limbus and contains the infraorbital nerve, which exits inferiorly and medially. An infraorbital block can be used to anesthetize the nose, upper lip, and lower eyelid. Injection occurs lateral to the alar rim and medial to the nasolabial fold (Fig. 8-3).[13] While the patient is supine and looking directly at the ceiling, the needle is advanced upward in line with the medial limbus and laterally to a point 5 to 7 mm below the infraorbital rim; then 1 to 2 mL is injected.

To avoid painful injections at the nasal tip, a dorsal nasal block should be used. The dorsal (external) nasal nerve is a branch of the nasociliary nerve. On both sides of the nose 6 to 10 mm from the midline, where the nerve exits from a small groove in the nasal bones, 1 to 2 mL of anesthetic is injected.[13]

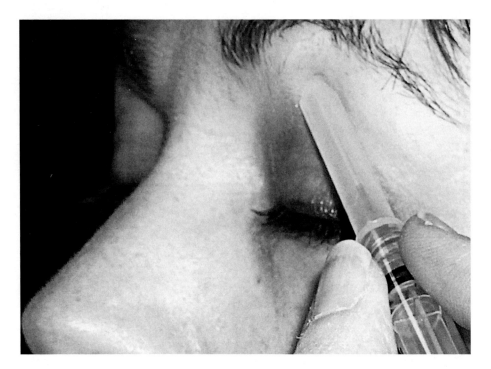

Figure 8-2 The supraorbital and supratrochlear nerves are approached laterally from the middle third of the eyebrow. With his or her free hand on the supraorbital rim, the operator injects 1 to 2 mL of the anesthetic prior to the notch and then moves medially, depositing 1 mL along the rim and another 1 mL at the nasal bones.[13]

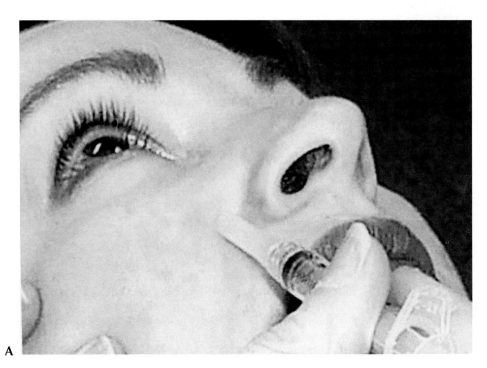

A

Figure 8-3 (**A**) and (**B**). In the infraorbital nerve block, the needle is held like a pen and directed upward and laterally to the infraorbital foramina in the center of an imaginary inverted "V" defined by the nasolabial fold and the alar base, while the index finger of the opposite hand is placed on the infraorbital rim.[13]

The zygomatic nerve, a terminal branch of the maxillary trigeminal nerve, V_2, splits into the zygomaticotemporal and the zygomaticofacial nerves. The zygomaticotemporal block allows one to anesthetize an area spanning a fan-like distribution from the lateral canthus into the temporal scalp abutting the forehead (supraorbital) block.[13] The zygomaticofacial block desensitizes the lateral face in the distribution of an inverted isosceles triangle with the apex just anterior to the palpable portion of the anterior ramus of the mandible and the base starting along the outer third of the orbit, ending at midcheek (Fig. 8-4).[13] The zygomaticotemporal block calls for an approach from above the patient, so that a 1.5-in. needle can be inserted 10 to 12 mm behind and just below the zygomaticofrontal suture and behind the lateral orbital rim as far as 1 cm below the canthal level. Injection occurs on the way out.[13]

To anesthetize the lower third of the ear and the lower postauricular skin, block of the great auricular nerve is incorporated. Some skin over the mandibular angle from the tragus may be desensitized. The largest ascending branch of the cervical plexus C2 and C3, the great auricular nerve, passes almost straight upward on the fascial surface of the sternocleidomastoid muscle after it rounds the posterior border of this muscle. This nerve lies approximately 6.5 cm inferior to the lower external ear canal (Fig. 8-5).[13]

To anesthetize the bulk of the cheek, upper preauricular, and auriculotemporal regions, the V_3 nerve block is employed. The mandibular branch of cranial nerve V includes the auriculotemporal, buccal, and mental nerves (Fig. 8-6); it

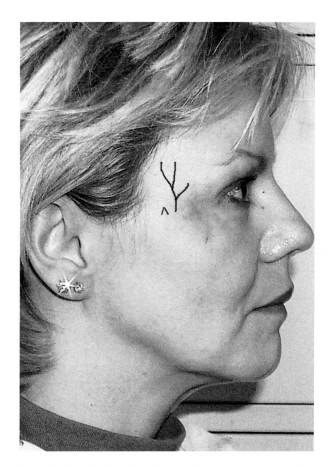

Figure 8-4   The boundary limits of zygomaticotemporal block anesthesia (||) and zygomaticofacial block anesthesia (—) are illustrated.[13]

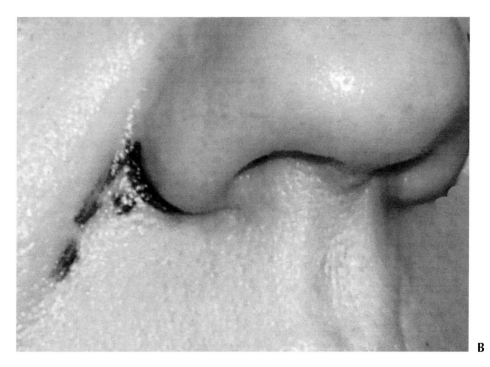

B

Figure 8-3   *(continued)*

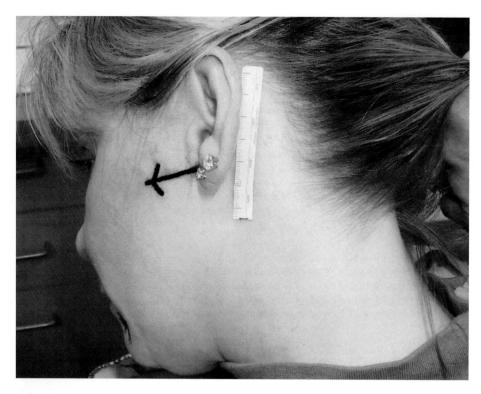

Figure 8-5 For anesthesia of the greater auricular nerve, the nerve is approached by injecting a nickel-sized circle of anesthetic into the sternocleidomastoid (SCM) fascia at the intersection of an imaginary 6.5-cm line drawn from the lower border of the external acoustic canal to the middle of the SCM muscle belly.[13]

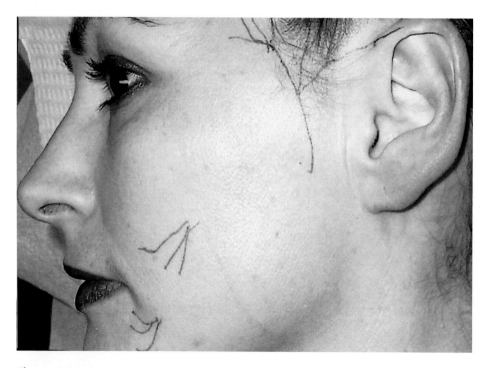

Figure 8-6 The auriculotemporal nerve superiorly, the buccal nerve centrally, and the mental nerve inferiorly are shown.

travels 1 cm posterior to the pterygoid plate behind the pterygoid muscles.[18] The V$_3$ block is approached by injecting a local anesthetic in the center of the sigmoid notch, which, with the patient's mouth slightly open, can be palpated 2.5 cm anterior to the tragus. Then, a 22-gauge spinal needle is advanced until it hits the pterygoid plate. The needle is retracted and redirected 1 cm posterior to the original direction with injection (approximately 3 to 4 mL) occurring at the same depth as the original pterygoid plate bump. Since the maxillary artery is directly behind the pterygoid muscles, it is important to aspirate before injecting the anesthetic.

Nerve damage from blocks is possible, although careful technique and knowledge of anatomy should decrease this risk. Burning or tingling sensations should be avoided; they indicate direct contact with a nerve trunk. Normal sensation generally returns; the block is rarely permanent.[15] Injury of the orbital nerve and blindness is a major complication of the V$_3$ block.[17] Other rare complications include infection and central nervous system (CNS) or systemic cardiovascular toxicity.[15] Areas around the ear and lateral temporal region may fail to become anesthetized even with perfect technique.[19]

INTRAORAL NERVE BLOCKS

Both the infraorbital and the mental nerves may be approached via intraoral nerve blocks. Pain from needle introduction is eliminated by applying a topical benzocaine agent to the mucosa, which has been cleaned with alcohol and wiped with sterile gauze. At approximately a 10-degree angle, a 1-in. 30-gauge needle is directed proximally into the sulcus of the upper lip over the maxillary canine (Fig. 8-7)

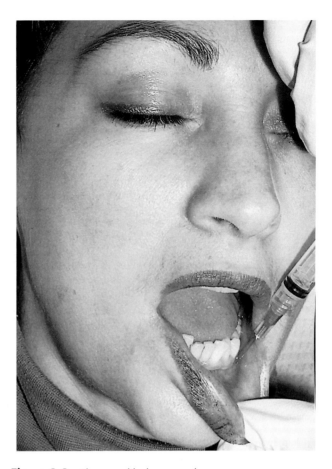

Figure 8-8   The mandibular premolars.

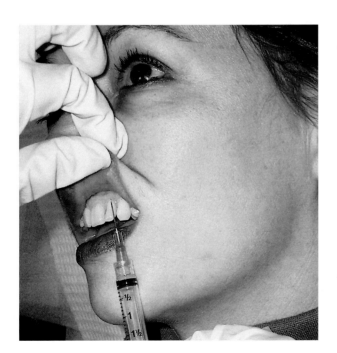

Figure 8-7   The maxillary canine teeth.

and 0.3 mL of anesthetic is deposited into the mucosa. The noninjecting hand is retracting the lip with the pad of the index finger placed on the inferior orbital rim just superior to the foramen. The needle is redirected toward the infraorbital foramen and 0.5 mL of anesthetic is injected.[16]

The mental nerve, which innervating the lower lip and chin, may be anesthesized via an intraoral block as well. The mental foramen is found between the mandibular premolars or beneath the second premolar and about 10 to 12 mm above the inferior border of the mandible.[16] With the lower lip retracted, the mucosa is cleansed and anesthesized as above; the 1-in., 30-gauge needle is then directed inferiorly and 0.3 mL of anesthetic is injected. The mental foramen is then palpated with the noninjecting hand and 0.5 mL of anesthesic is injected into the mental foramen (Fig. 8-8).[16]

TUMESCENT ANESTHESIA

The tumescent technique was introduced by Dr. Jeffrey Klein in 1987, originally for liposuction.[20] It has been a standard for local anesthesia in liposuction and more recently has been incorporated into scalp surgery, dermabrasion,[21] ambulatory phlebectomy,[22] and skin cancer[23] and soft tissue reconstruction.[24] This technique is increasingly popular because it eliminates the need for general anesthesia and intravascular fluid replacement. Patients recover quickly yet have long-lasting analgesia, up to 16 h.[25] In tumescent anesthesia, more dilute and larger volumes of anesthetic—usually lidocaine—are used, allowing for a greater total mass of anesthetic to be administered with fewer systemic effects.[24] Different for-mulas for tumescent anesthetic solutions have been used depending on the body area being treated. Typically, for body contouring, the lidocaine concentration is more dilute, ranging from 0.05 to 0.1%, depending on the size of the area, while facial procedures require a more concentrated lido-caine solution containing 0.05% lidocaine and 1:100,000 epi-nephrine (Table 8-2).[26]

Table 8-2
Tumescent Anesthetic Solution Formulas

Procedure	Volume/Mass	Ingredient
1. Klein-body liposuction[20]	1 L	0.9% NaCl
0.091% lidocaine	100 mL/1 g	1% Plain lidocaine
1:1,000,000 epinephrine	1 mL/1mg	1:1000 Epinephrine
2. Hair transplant/Scalp reduction[24]	30 mL	0.9% NaCl
0.1% lidocaine	2 mL	2% Plain lidocaine
1:320,000 epinephrine	0.1 mL	1:1000 Epinephrine
	0.2 meq	Sodium bicarbonate
3. Localized dermabrasion[24]	30 mL	0.9 % NaCl
0.5% lidocaine	11 mL	2% Plain lidocaine
1:420,000	0.1 mL	1:1000 Epinephrine
	1.1 meq	Sodium bicarbonate
4. Full face dermabrasion/face lift[24]	500 mL	0.9% NaCl
0.1 % lidocaine	25 mL	2% Plain lidocaine
1:500,000	1 mL	1:1000 Epinephrine
	2.5 meq	Sodium bicarbonate
5. Body liposuction[25]	1 L	0.9% NaCl
0.05–0.1% lidocaine	500–1000 mg	Lidocaine
1:2,000,000	0.5 mg	Epinephrine
	10 mEq	Sodium bicarbonate
	10 mg	Triamcinolone
6. Facial tumescence[26]	500 mL	0.9% NaCl
0.08% Lidocaine	400 mg	Lidocaine
	0.4 mg	Epinephrine
	6 mL	Sodium bicarbonate, 8.4 %
7. Scalp surgery[15]	237.5 mL	0.9% NaCl
0.1% lidocaine	12.5 mL	2% Lidocaine
1:250,000	1 mL	1:1000 Epinephrine
8. Dermabrasion[21]	500 mL	0.9% NaCl
	25 mL	2% Lidocaine
	1 mL	1:1000 Epinephrine
	12 meq	8.4% Sodium bicarbonate
9. Ambulatory phlebectomy[22]		0.9% NaCl
0.2% Lidocaine	——	Lidocaine
1:100,000 Epinephrine	——	Epinephrine
	1 meq/100 mL of solution	Sodium bicarbonate

Studies have shown that 55 mg/kg of lidocaine in tumescent anesthesia is a safe upper limit for liposuction of the abdomen, flanks, and/or thighs.[25] In more vascular procedures of the head and neck, such as hair transplantation and face lifts, the 500-mg lidocaine maximum should be adhered to until further studies are completed.[24] In the head and neck areas, the volume needed for anesthesia is not as great; the upper-limit lidocaine dose is rarely reached. Although tumescent anesthesia has eliminated the need for general anesthesia, patients may experience a burning or stinging sensation during infiltration of the tumescence fluid. In a double-blinded randomized study, warming the tumescence fluid to 40°C significantly reduced infiltration pain.[27] The same has been noted in local infiltration.[14]

The equipment and methods of infiltration are discussed in the respective chapters detailing procedures utilizing tumescence.

ADVERSE REACTIONS

The use of local anesthetics may be associated with three types of adverse reactions, including those unrelated to the drug used, toxic reactions, and allergic reactions. The most common is a vasovagal reaction unrelated to the drug; it is resolved by placing the patient in the Trendelenburg position. A bolus infusion to resolve the hypotension is rarely needed.[12]

Lidocaine and other amide anesthetics are metabolized by the hepatic microsomal enzymes. As a result, increased plasma levels may occur in patients with hepatic insufficiency or those on medications that impair microsomal enzyme function, such as propanolol, cimetidine, and halothane. At toxic plasma levels of lidocaine, there are well-recognized signs and symptoms. At plasma levels of 3 to 5 μg/mL, light-headedness and drowsiness may be apparent. At plasma levels of 5 μg/mL, signs include tinnitus, shivering, and paresthesias.[25] Above plasma levels of 10 μg/mL, seizures and coma may occur.[25] Beyond 20 μg/mL, bradycardia, hypotension, heart block, and cardiac arrest occur.[25] Ester-type anesthetics are metabolized by plasma cholinesterase; patients with pseudocholinesterase deficiency will have impaired metabolism of ester anesthetics.[28]

Less than 1% of adverse reactions to local anesthetics are allergic in nature.[28] There are two types of allergic reactions to local anesthetics: IgE-mediated reactions and allergic contact dermatitis. IgE-mediated reactions occur secondary to ester and amide anesthetics. Rare cases of allergy to parabens—antibacterial preservatives found in the anesthetic solutions—have been reported.[28] IgE-mediated symptoms begin within seconds to minutes and are sometimes delayed up to an hour.[29] These symptoms are characterized by erythema, pruritus, feelings of impending doom or oppression, hives, angioedema, faintness, crampy abdominal pain, laryngeal edema, bronchospasm, rhinorrhea, sneezing, diaphoresis, disorientation, fecal/urinary incontinence, and/or shock.[28,29] In shock, usually the above signs precede hypotension. Sometimes the accompanying signs in shock are absent—excluding sinus tachycardia, which is always present. In vasovagal and cardiac syncope, bradycardia and rhythm disturbances are common. Contact hypersensitivity accounts for 80 percent of the allergic responses reported

with local anesthetics[30] and is most notorious with benzocaine, an ester. Contact cross-reactivity has been postulated among the esters but is less definite among the amide anesthetics. Injection of other ester anesthetic agents and the use of sulfonamides and paraphenylenediamine (in hair and fur dyes)[31] should be avoided in patients with an ester contact hypersensitivity. Amide-sensitive patients, though rare, should be patch tested to other amides and esters as well.

The approach to the -caine-sensitive patient is a thorough history with precise details of the reaction symptomatology. Patients with a presumed history of local anesthetic-induced anaphylaxis, borderline history (symptoms within 2 h of the local injection), or an incomplete history should be referred to an allergist and undergo local anesthetic skin testing and incremental challenge.[28,30] Malignant hyperthermia (MH) is a relatively rare autosomal dominant skeletal muscle disorder triggered by volatile inhalational anesthetics (halothane, isoflurane, enflurane, sevoflurane, desflurane) and depolarizing muscle relaxants (succinylcholine, decamethonium). Major clinical signs of MH include tachycardia, tachypnea, lacy cyanosis, muscle rigidity, elevated temperature, coagulopathy, and myoglobinuria.[32] Local anesthesia is considered safe in MH patients. More invasive or longer procedures—such as hair transplantation, laser resurfacing, or extensive Mohs' surgery—in susceptible patients may require an anesthesiology consultation.[32] Dantrolene IV (1 to2 mg/kg maximum) is the key to effective treatment. Dantrolene directly interferes with skeletal muscle contraction by interfering with the release of calcium from the sarcoplasmic reticulum.

Sedation and Analgesia

Patients are reluctant to undergo painful procedures with only local or regional anesthesia, and operating rooms can be anxiety-provoking. Moreover, long periods of immobility may be uncomfortable for patients. Intravenous sedation and analgesia alleviate patients' concerns about experiencing pain during surgical procedures and aid the surgical team, as the patient is more likely to cooperate fully. Since there is no ideal anesthetic agent, a cocktail of agents are used to closely approximate ideal sedation and anesthesia. The use of newer agents has led to greater patient satisfaction.

As with general anesthesia, the patient must undergo a complete preoperative evaluation and obtain clearance from his or her primary physician. An anesthesia practitioner must monitor the patient receiving IV sedation. Since cosmetic procedures are elective, patients should be fasting for an appropriate period because there is always the potential for loss of airway reflexes if the patient becomes deeply sedated.

MONITORING

Patients receiving more than local anesthesia are monitored during the procedure with a transcutaneous pulse oximeter, an automated noninvasive sphygmomanometer, and real-time electrocardiography (Fig. 8-9). Pulse oximeters estimate the arterial saturation of oxygen (SaO_2), and readings are recorded as oxygen saturation pulse (SpO_2) values. In the SaO_2 range of 70 to 100%, pulse oximeters are quite accurate.[33]

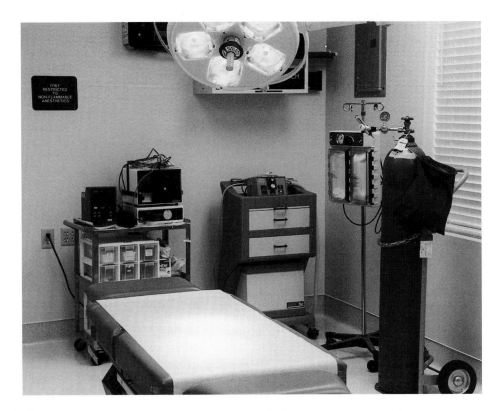

Figure 8-9 Standard monitoring equipment includes a transcutaneous pulse oximeter, blood pressure monitor, pulse monitor, and ECG monitor.

Conditions that may affect or distort SpO_2 readings include some arrhythmias and cardiac arrest, hypovolemia, hypothermia, vasoconstriction, anemia (underestimation of SaO_2 readings), injection of dyes (methylene blue, indocyanine green, indigo carmine), and dyshemoglobin.[33] External factors that may affect SpO_2 readings include an inflated blood pressure cuff and tourniquet, ambient light, electrocautery, motion, fingernail polish, and/or synthetic nails.[33] Actual cardiac performance must be monitored, since adequate saturation in the skin circulation does not always parallel oxygen delivery to the myocardium.

Desaturation after sedation is a late event; corrective measures should be instituted when the oxygen saturation falls below 90%. Several methods have been used to monitor the level of sedation. The Ramsay scale is an objective scoring system that quantitates drug-induced sedation by the patient's responsiveness. Other methods have been described. The electroencephalogram (EEG) is the most common neurophysiologic technique for determining depth of sedation. A computerized EEG analysis, the EEG-BIS index, has simplified EEG interpretation. As depth of sedation increases with sedative drugs, there are consistent decreases in the EEG-BIS index. This tool may help anesthesia personnel improve on the titration of sedative-hypnotic drugs.[34]

SEDATIVE/ANXIOLYTICS
Benzodiazepines

Benzodiazepines are widely used during MAC because they provide anxiolysis, amnesia, and sedation.[34] Diazepam, the prototype benzodiazepine, is not desirable for parenteral use because of the high incidence of pain on injection, venoirritation, and phlebitis.[34] It is helpful as an adjunct if taken orally the night before and the morning before surgery. Midazolam is more widely used in monitored anesthesia than diazepam. Midazolam's advantages include its rapid onset and short onset of action; it also causes less pain and less venous irritation upon injection. It is often bolused and may be followed by an infusion.

Barbiturates

Methohexital has shown good sedative effects and rapid recovery with bolus or infusion. A sedative dose produces pain on injection (less than propofol), paradoxical excitement, antianalgesic effects, nausea and vomiting, hiccupping, and excessive postoperative drowsiness (more than propofol).[34] Pentobarbital IV or IM, when used in combination with other sedative or opoid hypnotics, has caused marked hypoxemia and an increase in airway obstruction.

Ketamine

Ketamine, a phencyclidine derivative, produces excellent analgesia but also a "dissociative" sedative state. Because of such psychic disturbances, ketamine is used in small doses with other medications, mostly benzodiazepines.

Propofol

Propofol is the newest parenteral medication. It is short-acting and has a rapid onset of action. Its advantages over midazolam include a more rapid recovery of cognitive function and less postoperative sedation, drowsiness, confusion, and amnesia. Side effects include pain on injection, excitatory phenomena, and involuntary movements. Also, supplemental oxygen should be available, since propofol can depress the hypoxic ventilatory response and cause more frequent and longer apnea.[34]

ANALGESICS

Fentanyl is the most commonly used of the opioids for analgesia. The biggest concern with fentanyl in combination with other sedatives is respiratory depression. Typical opiod- related side effects include emesis, pruritus, and, as already stated, respiratory depression. Alfentanil, a short-acting analog of fentanyl, is asociated with a shorter duration of respiratory depression than fentanyl and fewer perioperative side effects.[34] Remifentanil is another opioid analgesic with an extremely short half-life (3 to 5 min), therefore minimizing opioid-related side effects. Excessive respiratory depression can result with infusion when remifentanil is used alone.

Ketorolac, a potent nonsteroidal anti-inflammatory drug (NSAID) in a parenteral formulation, has been used for analgesia to avoid the opioid-related side effects of pruritus, nausea, and vomiting. Some studies have shown that larger intraoperative doses of propofol were necessary with ketorolac-treated patients.[34]

ANTAGONISTS

Flumazenil

Flumazenil reverses sedation and amnesia better than it does respiratory depression caused by benzodiazepines. Some authors routinely use flumazenil at the end of a surgery to reverse the effect of midazolam. The increased cost of using two agents and the secondary sedative effect due to the brief reversal effect (<90 min) has deterred practioners from using flumazenil routinely. It is helpful for patients who experience persistent excessive sedation after MAC.

Naloxone and Nalmefene

Naloxone (elimination half-life 1 to 1.5 h) and nalmefene (elimination half life 8 to 10 h.) are opioid antagonists that rapidly reverse opiate-induced respiratory depression but may also reverse analgesia. Respiratory depression can recur, and side effects have been associated with nalmefene: light-headedness, drowsiness, dizziness, mental fatigue, hypertension, tachycardia, and pulmonary edema.

DRUG COMBINATIONS

In the dermatologic literature, several combinations have been described for MAC.[35–38] Glycopyrrolate (0.2 mg IV), metoclopramide (10 mg IV), midazolam (1 to 3 mg IV) followed by a propofol bolus and infusion (10 to 100 µg/kg per minute) produces effective sedation, anxiolysis, and amnesia. Several 10-mg boluses of ketamine are given for analgesia throughout the procedure. Boluses of fentanyl may be administered as needed. Increased risk of drug reactions occurs with combinations of sedatives, analgesics, and local anesthesia. The respiratory system is at risk of depressed esophageal and laryngeal reflexes, upper airway obstruction, and depression of central hypercarbic and hypoxic ventilatory responses. Respiratory depression has been shown to be minimized by carefully titrated sedative infusions. Hypoventilation is still a risk despite the use of supplemental oxygen. Postoperative nausea and vomiting are increased when multiple agents are used.

Inhalation Anesthesia

LARYNGEAL MASK AIRWAY

The laryngeal mask airway (LMA) is helpful in deep sedation or general anesthesia.[19] It does not require endotracheal intubation or an anesthesia machine. Coughing, vomiting, or laryngospasm may occur if anesthesia is not deep enough. All or part of the esophagus may be contained within the bowl of the LMA; its use is contraindicated in patients with a full stomach, gastroesophageal reflux, obesity, an airway known to be difficult, trauma, prone or lateral patient positioning, or surgery of the upper abdomen.[33]

NITROUS OXIDE

Studies have shown that inhalation of nitrous oxide, which has a low anesthetic potency, and at least 30% oxygen prior to infiltration of local anesthesia reduces anxiety and pain.[39] Nitrous oxide concentrations above 40% may make some patients anxious. Since the patient's protective reflexes are intact, cardiovascular and respiratory monitoring is not necessary. N_2O_2 and O_2 are usually given at an initial flow rate of 6 L/min each; after approximately 1 min, the flow rates are reduced to 3 L/min for both gases.[40] Since nitrous oxide is 35 times more soluble in blood than oxygen, the patient is ventilated for 1 min on 100% oxygen after N_2O_2 flow has been discontinued.[40] Patients recover within minutes of stopping N_2O_2 gas administration, but they may experience light-headedness and paresthesias of the distal extremities for several minutes.[40] Some 15 percent of patients develop nausea and vomiting postoperatively. Fire is another risk; thus, wetting the hair and covering the exit ports of the nasal piece with saline-soaked gauze is advised.[40] Conscious sedation, pre- and postoperative instructions, consent forms, and a discharge protocol are given in Tables 8-3 to 8-4.

Table 8-3
Conscious Sedation—Pre-Operative Instructions

For all surgical patients receiving presedation, the instructions listed below should be strictly followed regarding certain medications that should be taken upon rising, with just enough water to swallow the medication.

Intravenous sedation (similar to "twilight sleep") will be given by our anesthetist to eliminate any potential discomfort during the procedure. Discuss this with the doctor prior to surgery, and please be aware that it will necessitate having your doctor sign our medical clearance letter and arranging for you to have an ECG and chest x-ray.

If you routinely take specific medicines daily, on the day of your surgery you should plan to take:

Hypertension (high blood pressure) medications	Angina (heart-chest pain) medications
Asthma medications	Convulsion-prevention medications
Cardiac dysrhythmias (irregular heartbeat) medications	Parkinson's medications
Any other heart medication that you take on a regular basis	Discuss with the doctor any diabetic medications

DO NOT TAKE:
Anticoagulants (blood-thinners or any form of aspirin). If you take an anticoagulant on a regular basis, please check with your doctor. It may be necessary to change your medication to a shorter-acting type several days in advance of your surgery.

Despite the many benefits, some vitamins and herbal remedies can have detrimental effects on a person undergoing surgery.

Herbal and Other Remedies Possible Complications

Aspirin	Increases bleeding and bruising.
Ibuprofen	Increases bleeding and bruising.
Nonsteroidal anti-inflammatory drugs (NSAIDS)	Increases bleeding and bruising.
Selenium, chromium, vitamin E	Antiplatelet activity and induces bleeding.
Ginger, garlic, cayenne and bilberry	Antiplatelet activity and inhibit clot formation.
Ginkgo biloba	Powerful anticoagulant and induces bleeding.
Aloe	Topical can cause dermatitis.
Vitamin A	Liver toxicity in high amounts.
St. John's wort, yohimbine, and licorice root	May intensify effects and potency of anesthesia.
Ginseng and Ma-huang extract (6% ephedrine)	May induce high blood pressure and rapid heart rate.

Except for the sips of clear liquids needed to take any of the above medications, it is very important that each patient not eat solid food or drink milk for eight (8) hours prior to the scheduled surgery.

No food or drink after midnight if twilight sleep or presedation is to be administered. Please refer to the following diet guidelines:
1. No solid food or milk after midnight on the day of surgery.
2. Unlimited clear liquid from the list below may be taken up to 3 hours before the scheduled time of surgery. After this time, only oral medications may be taken. Oral medications should be taken with no more than 1 ounce of water up to 1 hour before surgery.

ONLY CLEAR LIQUIDS ARE ACCEPTABLE
Water, black coffee or tea (no milk, cream, or non-dairy creamer), apple juice (clear), club soda, ginger ale, Seven-Up, cola

If there are any questions as to whether a medication should be taken on the day of your surgery, please contact us at
(   ) _____.

These instructions concern only medicines you take at home before coming to our office. Your anesthetic and any medications that you will receive here will be discussed with you on your surgery day.

Table 8-4
Conscious Sedation—Outpatient Discharge Instructions

For patients who have had: _____ Spinal epidural

_____ Local anesthesia with sedation

_____ Nerve block

_____ General anesthesia

_____ Conscious sedation

The medicine that was used to sedate you will be acting in your body for the next 24 hours. As a result, you might feel a little sleepy or dizzy when you get home. This feeling will slowly wear off.

For the next 24 hours you should not:
- Drive a car, operate machinery or power tools, etc.
- Drink any alcoholic beverages, even beer
- Take any medication not prescribed by your physician
- Make any important decisions, such as to sign important papers

You may eat anything, but it is better to start with liquids such as soft drinks (soda), then go on to soup and crackers and gradually work up to more solid foods. It is not uncommon to be a little nauseated after surgery.

We strongly suggest that a responsible adult be with you for the rest of the day and also during the night for your protection and safety. After 24 hours, you may resume your daily activities within the limits set by the surgeon.

You may experience a slight sore throat and/or some degree of muscle soreness after the anesthetic. This is not uncommon and should clear up quickly. It is due to breathing through your mouth while you were lightly sedated, not unlike snoring.

If you receive a nerve block, the anesthetized body part may not have the normal sensations that usually protect it from injury. Care must be taken to protect the anesthetized area until full sensation returns.

If any questions should arise, call the office immediately at (   ) _____.

References

1. Seager DJ. Local anesthesia in hair transplantation. In: Stough DB, Haber R, eds. *Hair Replacement*. St. Louis: Mosby; 1996:81–89.

2. American Medical Association. Local anesthetics. In: *Drug Evaluation Annual 1995*. Chicago: American Medical Association; 1995;157–171.

3. Lener EV, Bucalo BD, Kist DA, Moy RL. Topical anesthetic agents in dermatologic surgery. *Dermatol Surg* 1997; 23:673–683.

4. Juhlin L. Evers H. EMLA: A new topical anesthetic. *Adv Dermatol* 1990; 5:75–92.

5. Friedman PM, Fogelman JP, Nouri K, et al. Comparative study of the efficacy of four topical anesthetics. *Dermatol Surg* 1999; 25:950–954.

6. Kassan DG, Lynch AM, Stiller MJ. Physical enhancement of dermatologic drug delivery: Iontophoresis and phonpheresis. *J Am Acad Dermatol* 1996; 34:657–656.

7. Huang W, Vidimos A. Topical anesthetics in dermatology. *J Am Acad Dermatol* 2000; 43:286–298.

8. Ruiz-Maldonado R. Saturated phenol as a local anesthetic for manual dermabrasion. *Dermatol Surg* 1997; 23:187–190.

9. Alora MB, Anderson RR. Recent developments in cutaneous lasers. *Lasers Surgery Med* 2000; 26:108–118.

10. Graham HD, Duplechain G. Anesthesia in facial plastic surgery. In: Willet JM, ed. *Facial Plastic Surgery*. Stamford, CT: Appleton & Lange; 1997:5–26.

11. Scarborough D, Bisaccia E. Choosing the appropriate anesthesia for dermatologic anesthesia. *Cosmet Dermatol* 1991; 8:8–11.

12. Emslander HC. Local and topical anesthesia for pediatric wound repair: A review of selected aspects. *Pediatr Emerg Care* 1998; 14(2):123–129.

13. Zide BM, Swift R. How to block and tackle the face. *Plast Reconstr Surg* 1998; 101:840–851.

14. Fialkov JA, McDougall EP. Warmed local anesthetic reduces pain of infiltration. *Ann Plast Surg* 1996; 36:11–13.

15. Haber RS, Khan S, Stough DB. Nerve block anesthesia of the scalp. In: Stough DB, Haber R, eds. *Hair Replacement*. St. Louis: Mosby; 1996:89–93.

16. Bisaccia E, Scarborough DA. Intraoral nerve blocks. *Cosmet Dermatol* 1989; 2 8:629–637.

17. Scarborough DA, Bisaccia E, Schuen W, Swensen R. Anesthesia for the dermatologic surgeon. *Int J Dermatol* 1989; 28:629–637.

18. Salasche SJ, Bernstein G, Senkarik M. *Surgical Anatomy for Surgery*. East Norwalk, CT: Appleton & Lange; 1988.

19. Fitzpatrick, RE, Williams B, Goldman MP. Preoperative anesthesia and postoperative complications in laser resurfacing. *Semin Cutan Med Surg* 1996; 15:170–176.

20. Klein JA. The tumescent technique for liposuction surgery. *Am J Cosmet Surg* 1987; 4:263–267.

21. Goodman G. Dermabrasion using tumescent anesthesia. *J Dermatol Surg Onco* 1994;20:802–807.

22. Keel D, Goldman MP. Tumescent anesthesia in ambulatory phlebectomy: Addition of epinephrine. *Dermatol Surg* 1999; 25:371–372.

23. Acosta AE. Clinical parameters of tumescent anesthesia in skin cancer reconstructive surgery with a review of 86 patients. *Arch Dermatol* 1997; 133:451–454.

24. Coleman WP, Klein JA. Use of tumescent techniques for scalp surgery, dermabrasion, and soft tissue reconstruction. *J Dermatol Surg Oncol* 1992; 18:130–135.

25. Ostad A, Kageyama N, Moy RL. Tumescent anesthesia with a lidocaine dose of 55 mg/kg is safe for liposuction. *Dermatol Surg* 1996; 22:921–927.

26. Namias A, Kaplan B. Tumescent anesthesia for dermatologic surgery: Cosmetic and non-cosmetic procedures. *Dermatol Surg* 1998;24:755–758.

27. Kaplan B, Moy RL. Comparison of room temperature and warmed local anesthetic solution for tumescent liposuction. *Dermatol Surg* 1996; 22:707–709.

28. Glinert RJ, Zachary CB. Local anesthetic allergy—Its recognition and avoidance. *J Dermatol Surg Oncol* 1991; 17:491–461.

29. Kennedy KS, Cave RH. Anaphylactic reaction to lidocaine. *Arch Otolaryngol Head Neck Surg* 1986; 112:671–673.

30. Assem ESK, Punnia-Moortly A. Allergy to local anesthetics: An approach to definitive diagnosis. *Br Dent J* 1988; 164:44–47.

31. Fisher AA. Local anesthetics. In Fisher AA, ed. *Contact Dermatitis*, 3rd ed. Philadelphia: Lea & Feibiger; 1986,220.

32. Murray C, Sasaki SS, Berg D. Local anesthesia and malignant hyperthermia. *Dermatol Surg* 1999; 25:626–630.

33. Burns LS. Advances in pediatric anesthesia. *Nurs Clin North Am* 1997; 32:45–71.

34. Sa Rêgo MM, Watcha MF, White PF. The changing role of monitored anesthesia care in the ambulatory setting. *Anesth Analg* 1997; 85:1020–1036.

35. Scarborough DA, Bisaccia E, Swensen RD. Anesthesia for outpatient dermatologic cosmetic surgery: Midazolam-low-dosage ketamine anesthesia. *J Dermatol Surg Oncol* 1989; 15:658–663.

36. Abeles G, Sequeira M, Swensen RD, et al. The combined use of propofol and fentanyl for outpatient intravenous conscious sedation. *Dermatol Surg* 1999; 25:559–562.

37. Friedberg BL. Facial laser resurfacing with the propofol-ketamine technique: Room air, spontaneous ventilation (RASV) anesthesia. *Dermatol Surg* 1999; 25:569–572.

38. Abeles G, Warmuth IP, Sequeira M, et al. The use of conscious sedation for outpatient dermatologic surgical procedures. *Dermatol Surg* 2000; 26:125–126.

39. Maloney JM, Coleman WP, Mora R. Analgesia induced by nitrous oxide and oxygen as an adjunct to local anesthesia in dermatologic surgery—Results of clinical trials. *J Dermatol Surg Oncol* 1980; 6:939–943.

40. Fitzpatrick RE, et al. Anesthesia for cutaneous laser surgery, In: Goldman MP, Fitzpatrick RE, eds. *Cutaneous Laser Surgery: The Art and Science of Selective Photothermolysis.* St. Louis; Mosby; 1994:269–282.

CHAPTER 9

Soft Tissue Augmentation

Dermal Fillers

The wish to maintain a youthful and attractive appearance is a primary motive of patients who choose to consult a cosmetic dermatologist. Soft tissue augmentation is a modality that is often used to enhance or improve a patient's appearance. This procedure has the unique benefit of limited "down time." In fact, soft tissue augmentation has been performed for several decades because it performs this valuable function so well. Driven by public demand, augmentation procedures have been done throughout history. Before modern procedures were established, soft tissue augmentation was performed utilizing candle wax, beeswax, paraffin, and various other oils. These methodologies were discarded owing to various undesirable reactions to these substances, movement of the material, chronic edema, scarring, and granulomata.

Filling Agents

These can be divided into autologous and heterologous fillers. The risk of inducing immunologic reactions is not present with autologous fillers. The autologous group for lip augmentation encompasses fat microinjections, which are also used in flattening of radial rhytids; autologous collagen (autologen); temporal fascia, galea and subgalea, superficial musculoaponeurotic system (SMAS) strips, and breast implant capsules.[1–5] The use of fat as a filling agent has increased dramatically. Autologous fat implantation is utilized for lip augmentation, leveling of radial rhytids, and to modify the nasolabial fold. Fat injection is combined with a variety of other procedures that have been performed in combination with laser resurfacing and facial liposuction without negative outcome. In our experience, microlipoinjection shows persistently good results. We consider it a very safe procedure for the rejuvenation of the aging mouth. In addition, this filling material is often readily available, and hypersensitivity reactions do not occur. It is our observation that, although the filling effects diminish over time, there remains a persistent benefit, most likely due to a survival and growth of intact lipocytes from the fat implant. For this procedure, the patient must undergo a minor harvesting procedure.[3–6]

Autologous fascia and SMAS implants seem to have persistent long-term effects. However, a donor-site scar is usually the trade-off for harvesting. Subsequently, these procedures are often combined with face-lifts. Patients commonly complain postoperatively about firm lips with disturbances of sensation.[1,5] There are rare reports of lip augmentation using autologous breast implant capsules. Candidates for this procedure are patients who undergo a breast augmentation revision or repeated augmentation enhancement. The graft can be harvested then without creating an additional donor scar. The small series of patients we have studied demonstrated a long-term effect. It is advised not to use graft material from a silicon implant capsule or breast implant capsules developed by an infectious process.[4]

Heterologous Filling Agents

Heterologous fillers are used very frequently and have a good profile. There is, however, a potential for allergic reactions (with collagen injection other than autologous collagen) and risk of infection and/or extrusion of these materials. These substances are made up of expanded polytetrafluoroethylene and different variants of collagen.

EXPANDED POLYTETRAFLUOROETHYLENE

Expanded polytetrafluoroethylene, in our hands, is a pliable, inert material implanted into lips and folds and several other areas. In our experience, it provides consistently good results. The insertion technique is made easier by the newly developed tunnel structures and multistripe lengths. These allow for custom-molding according to the patient's need. As the aging process continues, further touch-ups may be required. The insertion techniques can vary, depending on whether swaged materials are used. Cutting the implant to an appropriate length and width and customizing it to the nasolabial, lip, or glabellar areas will help to avoid inflammation and pouching. Theoretically, there can be displacement and rarely extrusion of the implant, but appropriate placement helps to minimize these complications.

Autologous Fat Transplantation

HISTORY

Fat-transplant surgery dates back over 100 years to when, in 1893, the German physician Neuber[7] reported on the clinical use of free fat transplants to the 23rd Congress of the German Surgical Society. Using bean-sized pieces of free fat taken from the upper arm, Neuber successfully reconstructed a depressed facial defect secondary to tuberculous osteitis. In 1911, Brunings[8] reported the earliest use of the technique of fat injection. He placed small pieces of fat into a syringe and used fat transfer to correct postrhinoplasty deformities. During the second third of the twentieth century, free fat transplants were neglected. Most surgeons preferred the use of pedicle flaps, which conserved blood supply, making the outcome more predictable. Artificial substances (e.g., paraffin and silicone) became available during this period. However, in 1950, fat transplantation was rediscovered and Peer[9] reported his classic studies involving autologous fat transplants. He demonstrated that over 50 percent of the fat remained as a viable transplant 1 year after grafting.

The contemporary phase of fat transplantation began with the introduction of a new method of fat extraction. In the late 1970s, Illouz[10] and others introduced the method known today as liposuction. Liposuction gave the cosmetic surgeon access to an abundant supply of viable adipose tissue. Initially, this adipose tissue was discarded, but soon reports appeared in the literature describing the successful use of the fat as a soft tissue substitute to fill in defects in the face and body. Thus, very recently, the technique of fat transfer by injection has received a great deal of attention and has found ever-widening clinical applications.[11]

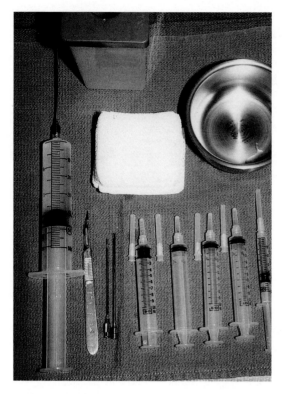

Figure 9-1 The fat-transfer/microlipoinjection setup contains a #11 blade, an infusion cannula attached to a syringe containing tumescent solution, two types of fat harvesting cannulae, a container in which to store the syringes and in which to drain serosanguineous fluid, several 10-mL syringes, and an 18-gauge needle.

Fat-Transfer Technique

The technique of fat transfer involves very basic equipment and instrumentation (Fig. 9-1). The setup includes an infusion catheter attached to a 60-mL syringe holding 0.25% lidocaine (Xylocaine) with 1:400,000 epinephrine. This is made up by diluting 10 mL of 1% lidocaine with 1:100,000 epinephrine and 30 mL of normal saline. A no. 11 blade is used to make an opening 1 mm in diameter in the corium, which gives access to the subcutaneous plane.

The donor site is often chosen on the basis of patient preference. Ideally, it would involve an area that is metabolically more or less resistant to weight fluctuations (i.e., the areas of the body in which the patient notices a persistent collection of fat even after losing weight). The hip, buttock region, lateral thigh, and lower abdomen are all acceptable. Our favorite site is the medial knee when adequate fat is available there. There the fat tissue is "smoother"—that is, it has a less fibrous consistency. In males, the donor region is often limited to the lateral flanks or "love handles."

A wide area of skin overlying the donor site is prepped with povidone/iodine (Betadine). The center of the area is grasped in a pinching fashion and a puncture is made with a no. 11 blade. The dilute lidocaine mixture is injected in a radial fashion into the subcutaneous plane via an infusion

cannula. The tip of the infusion cannula is constantly palpated and is then carried out. This process is virtually painless and produces tumescence of the donor site. The patient's comfort can be enhanced by appropriate "vocal" anesthesia. A sterile ice pack is then applied to the region for 20 min, adding to the firmness of the tissue. After adequate chilling, a 14-gauge accelerator extraction cannula attached to a 10-mL syringe is inserted into the donor area (Fig. 9-2). The cannula is advanced along the subcutaneous plane parallel to the overlying skin. The syringe's plunger is then withdrawn and stabilized in the grasp of the "working" hand. With a gentle in-and-out motion directed in a radial, fan-shaped pattern, the syringe quickly fills with adipose tissue. This is in essence a blunt lateral punch extraction of subcutaneous tissue.

Normally, only 15 to 20 mL of material is needed. After the required syringes have been filled, they are capped and placed in the upright position (tip downward) for 10 min. This allows the serosanguineous fluid to separate from the fat. The fluid is mostly local anesthetic with small amounts of blood. This admixture, which drains to the base of the syringe by gravitational pooling, is discarded. In effect, this fluid washes the fat. One can see the intact fat globules that make up the final donor material. In our experience, no additional washing or manipulation of the fat is needed and may even be detrimental to the survival of the intact fat globules.

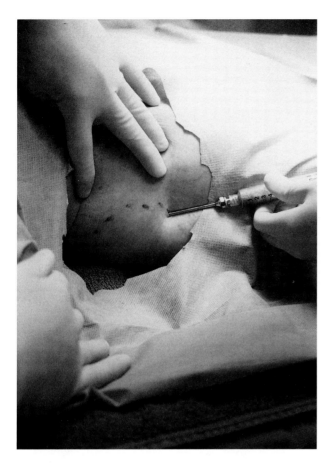

Figure 9-2 As the fat harvesting gets under way, the marked site has been infused with anesthesia. The plunger of the syringe is withdrawn and the to-and-fro motion in a spoke-wheel pattern obtains the transfer harvest.

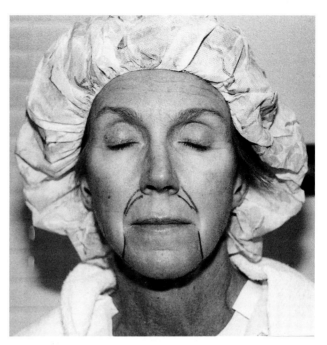

Figure 9-3 The patient is marked in the seated position. The area to be filled is outlined with gentian violet.

The patient is generally marked in the seated position (Fig. 9-3). We typically place a small wheal of local anesthetic at each injection point of the face. The fat graft is then placed by injection through a 1½-in. 18-gauge needle, using the same syringe. The 18-gauge needle is directed into and parallel with the surface of the skin, sliding just along the dermal-subcutaneous junction, analogous to the linear threading technique used for bovine collagen injection. If the grooves are quite deep, we will often create a small tubular pocket in which to place the fat by making minute 1-mm side-to-side "windshield" wiper–like motions. This not only creates the tubular pocket for the placement of fat, but also lyses the bound-down connective tissue. We have found that the key to accurate placement is using a "lateral pinch technique," where manual pressure is applied bilaterally along the edges of the defect to be filled (Fig. 9-4). The linear or curvilinear placement of the operator's first two to three fingers on one side of the defect, mirrored by the placement of the assistant's fingers, creates a walled chamber for the infused donor fat. This simple maneuver allows total control of fat deposition and has been free of complications. If additional injection pressure on the syringe is required, the described

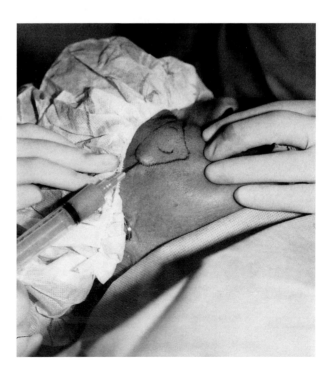

Figure 9-4 Fat transfer to the malar area is under way. The fat is injected via an 18-gauge needle as manual pressure outlines the area to be enhanced.

technique prevents an overspill of the fat into unwanted areas. Occasionally, a fibrous globule of fat will block the entrance to the needle; then simply changing the needle is all that is required. We have found the use of "injection guns" cumbersome and totally unnecessary.

Once the donor tissue is in place, it can be smoothed or worked into exact position, if necessary, although linear threading using the lateral pinch technique rarely necessitates this.

The complications have included only mild bruising and slight edema, which may persist from 12 to 24 h, rarely up to 72 h. Applying ice for 15 to 20 min three times during the first 12 h after the procedure is beneficial. The patient can bathe normally and clean the face gently the same day. Exercise and exertion is avoided for the first 24 h. Makeup can be applied after the first 24 h. The donor site is bandaged with a compression dressing and patients are instructed to leave it in place for 48 h.

Discussion

Conceptually, it seems beneficial to limit the diameter of the volume of fat injected at any one point to 4 mm or less. We feel that this is analogous to the optimal size for hair transplant graft survival, allowing for the necessary vascularization and metabolic influx to sustain the donor material. We are cautiously optimistic regarding the duration of correction. At 6 months, the degree of correction is quite substantial in the majority of patients. Clinical experience has shown 20 to 80 percent of the graft tissue surviving in excess of 3 years, with good correction. It is reasonable to anticipate that some future touch-ups will be needed due to "tissue fatigue" from the constant flexion and because of the ongoing aging process.

The clinical applications for treating the aging face are numerous. This technique is often the treatment of choice for deepened nasolabial folds, oral commissures, and glabellar furrows. Fat transfer is commonly a very satisfactory treatment for the fallen and receding upper lip with radial perioral lines, sunken cheeks, and transverse forehead creases. There is also a widening application for congenital and acquired facial malformations and certain types of depressed scars. Using the body's own living tissues to augment involuted and weakened facial tissues as we have done represents a reawakening of a century-old science and is ideally suited for facial restoration in the outpatient setting (Fig. 9-5A and B).

Autologous Collagen

Autologous injectable collagen (Autologen)[12] is another viable option for soft tissue augmentation. As with autologous fat transfer, the main advantage is the low risk of an allergic reaction[13] due to autologous tissue. In this procedure, donor skin is removed during various procedures (abdominoplasty, face-lift, breast reductions, or skin biopsy) and sent to Collagenesis Inc., Beverly, MA, for tissue processing. This requires freezing before the tissue is sent. Collagen is then grown in culture and processed. The

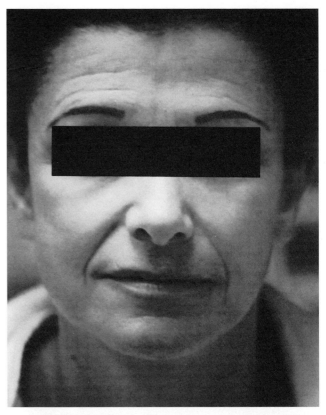

A

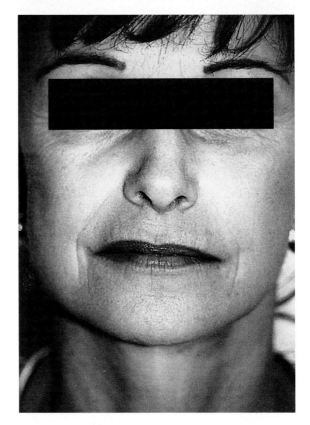

B

Figure 9-5 (*A*) Before fat transfer. (*B*) 6 months after fat transfer.

patient's own material (collagen) is placed in a syringe and returned to the physician for appropriate use. This "natural" technique avoids the possibility of allergic reaction; however, the logistics for transport and transfer of the biopsy to be cultured in the laboratory within 48 h can be daunting. Patients' expectations might not be met, and the procedure is currently very costly. Collagen injections must be repeated in intervals ranging from 6 weeks to 3 to 6 months, as the material is often readily degraded[14,15] (Fig. 9-6A). In addition, homologous tissue (Alloderm) and fascia lata have become popular products because of their relative lack of allergic reaction.

COLLAGEN

Bovine collagen has a long-standing history of being used as a filling substance in cosmetic surgery for facial lines and wrinkles.[15] There are currently several variants available: Zyoderm I and II are injectable suspensions of bovine collagen types I and III, which are placed into the papillary dermis and commonly used for lip augmentation as well as in concert with Zyplast for the leveling of perioral rhytids. Zyplast is processed with glutaraldehyde, thereby increasing the collagen cross-linking and prolonging the effect (for an average 3 to 6 months). It is injected into the deeper dermis. Hypersensitivity develops in about 3 percent of patients with a positive skin test, and the 1 percent rate of hypersensitivity is relatively low.[13] It is nevertheless a concern. Serum sickness has been reported after bovine collagen injections in single cases.

We recognize a definite trend in cosmetic surgery toward the use of autologous substances like fat and autologous collagen for implantation over foreign and potentially harmful materials. We currently prefer microfat injection over the collagen implant procedures, although all of these procedures are available to our patients. Again, correct implantation technique in our office minimizes effects such as mild erythema and edema at the injection site.

Human fascia can function as a filling substance (Fig. 9-6A and B). Typically the product is obtained from a cadaver, processed, screened, and preserved by freeze-drying. For implantation, it is reconstructed and injected via an 18- to 22-gauge needle. Although the ideal filler substance has not yet been developed, we prefer methods of augmentation that pose the least potential for morbidity and an adverse outcome. Therefore we commonly use autologous implants such as microfat injection, autologous collagen, and Zyderm products.

Fibrel

Fibrel was approved by the U.S. Food and Drug Administration for the treatment of scarring in 1988 and for the treatment of age-related lines (wrinkles) in 1990. Owing to the need for handling blood products in the office, Fibrel's popularity declined, and it ultimately went off the market. It is no longer available in the United States. Historically, Spangler performed the initial studies on this collagen-based product by mixing fibrin foam (Gelfoam) with human plasma and thrombin for the treatment of persistent scars. Later this

was modified by Gottlieb to involve gelatin foam (G), epsilon-aminocaproic acid (A), and human plasma (P). This was available as a kit, which required obtaining the patient's plasma mixed in a 1:1 ratio with the porcine gelatin powder and epsilon-aminocaproic acid (a 0.9% sodium choride solution) and then placed in syringes. It was found that the gelatin matrix implant was most effective when placed in the mid-to-deep dermis. If it was placed superficially, there were often frequent skin irregularities.

Of interest, in a 2-year clinical trial performed by Millikan,[16] no allergic reactions were reported at the treatment site. Additionally, Gottlieb reported no treatment site reactions after 11 years and Spangler reported none after 17 years. Fortunately, the introduction of autologous filler materials made the disappearance of Fibrel less problematic.

Polytetrafluoroethylene (Soft Form or Gore-Tex) Augmentation

State-of-the-art dermatologic cosmetic surgery employs a wide array of interventions now available to enhance appearance and correct facial aging changes; these techniques are adapted specifically to the patient's requirements. One such option is the use of expanded polytetrafluoroethylene (ePTFE) as a permanent filler for deep lines and rhytids; it has been gaining in popularity in recent years. ePTFE has been used for more than 4 million clinical implants since the 1970s as a vascular graft and patch for soft tissue reconstruction, and it is one of the most inert biomaterials available. This material has now begun to be used extensively in cosmetic surgery.[17–25]

MATERIAL

The inert biomaterial PTFE is expanded to provide a microporous structure and is composed of solid nodes connected by thin fibrils of PTFE. This internodal separation has an average internodal space of 22 μm, allowing for tissue incorporation. The ePTFE is a soft, comfortable microporous material that is available in two configurations: nonreinforced and reinforced with fluorinated ethylene propylene (FEP, which makes a more rigid yet still soft product).

This material is available in 1- to 4-mm nonreinforced sheets, 4.5- to 7-mm reinforced sheets, threads, 1.8 to 6.5-mm tubular strands, and also three-dimensional shapes used for chin, nasal, and malar implants. Threads can be used alone or in multiples, and a patch can be easily shaped, carved to fit the exact dimensions of the effect, and stacked to obtain the required thickness, then tapered at the edges. It is commercially named Gore-Tex or Soft Form. It may be obtained preset for implantation or in the appropriate shape and threaded into position as described under "Technique," below.

Technique

During the consultation and preoperative visit, the goals of the procedure, patient's expectations, risks, possible

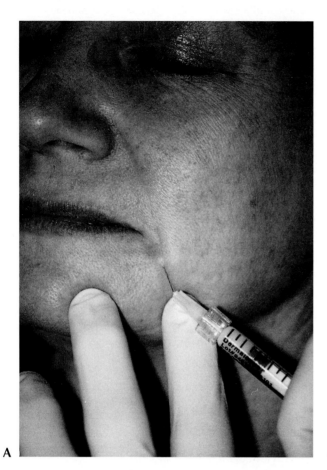

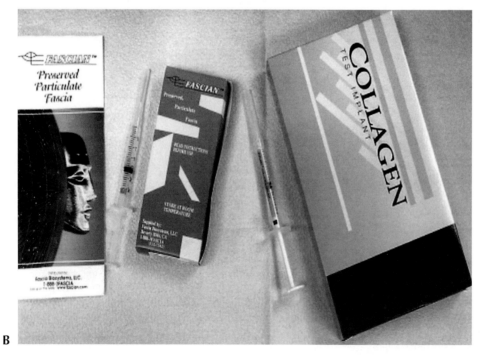

Figure 9-6   (**A**) Dermalogen injection.
(**B**) Bovine collagen, human fascia.

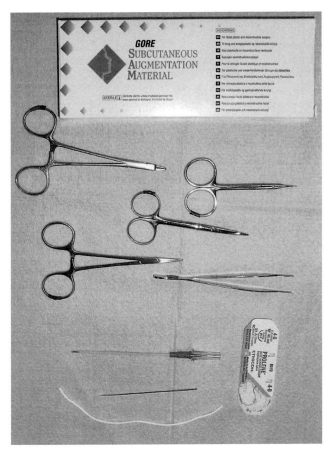

Figure 9-7 The PTFE in tubular form, Keith needle, 14- to 16-gauge angiocath, suture, and appropriate instrumentation to trim and thread.

complications, and alternative treatments are discussed. On the day of the procedure, the patient is marked while seated in an upright position. The patient is then placed supine and the face is prepared for sterility and draped. Local anesthesia is administered. Our most commonly employed technique for oral commissures is linearly running 1 or more ePTFE threads immediately beneath the skin using a straight needle. Once the threads pass through, the skin is slightly gathered or wrinkled like an accordion, and both ends are cut. This allows the cut ends to return to their subdermal position.

The same process is repeated for the upper and/or lower lip. We tend to use the thread or small tubular implants, depending upon the desired effect. For tubular implants, a 14- to 16-gauge angiocath is inserted under the vermilion border and the implant tips are angle-cut for tapering (Fig. 9-7). The trochar is then removed from the catheter and the suture passed through, pulling along the implant. Finally, the catheter is removed and the implant positioned. The ends are trimmed with the skin slightly bunched together, so that there is no implant protrusion upon relaxation.

For glabellar furrows and nasolabial folds, we often favor the tubular implant material as opposed to cutting strips from a sheet. The appropriate-size implant is chosen and the technique described above using a 14- to 16-gauge angiocath is employed. It is again necessary to ensure complete coverage of the ends of the implant material upon completion of the procedure so as to avoid contamination of the material during healing. Antibiotic ointment is applied to the skin puncture sites (Fig. 9-8). The patient is instructed to keep the area dry for 24 h and to avoid exercise and perspiration for 3 days.

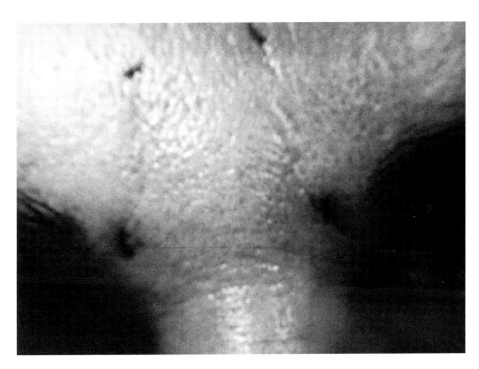

Figure 9-8 The puncture sites from angiocath trocar being dressed with antibiotic ointment.

Results

Typical results are satisfying to both patient and surgeon. As with any cosmetic procedure, patient expectations must be realistic. Esthetic improvement is reliable, usually attaining correction in the 40 to 60 percent range, depending on the severity of the defect, with an estimated 3- to 7-year duration. That is because, although ePTFE is permanent implant material, the ongoing effects of time and gravity will diminish the enhancement. Complications include transient bruising, swelling, and paresthesia. More serious complications, although rare, may include infection of the implant site, fistula formation, induration, implant extrusion, discoloration, and scarring. Malpositioning of the implant is improbable, but removal of the implant is not difficult should it become necessary. (Fig. 9-9; Fig. 9-10; Fig. 9-11; Fig. 9-12; Fig. 9-13)

Discussion

The ideal augmentation material should provide for a predictable, permanent enhancement without visible scars. It should be inert, pliable, malleable, noncarcinogenic, and easily removed if necessary. Expanded polytetrafluoroethylene closely fits this description. It is a highly porous structure that allows penetration of cells and vessels, infiltration of fibroblasts, and leukocytes, and collagen incorporation, resulting in effective anchoring to the tissue. In the event of complications, removal of the implant should be considered, since antibiotic eradication of graft-adherent bacteria may be difficult.

At the subdermal level, implant extrusion is highly unlikely, since fibrous ingrowth into the material occurs. Our preference for tubular material as opposed to strips in certain areas is based on greater implant-tissue interface strength. It has been shown in animal models that tubular implant ePTFE develops a greater attachment to surrounding soft tissues, increasing fixation strength and decreasing extrusion rate but still allowing easy removal.

Summary

Expanded polytetrafluoroethylene is a significant advancement in the treatment of facial rhytids, yielding good to excellent results. The use of this material and that of similar implant materials is likely to increase in the future.

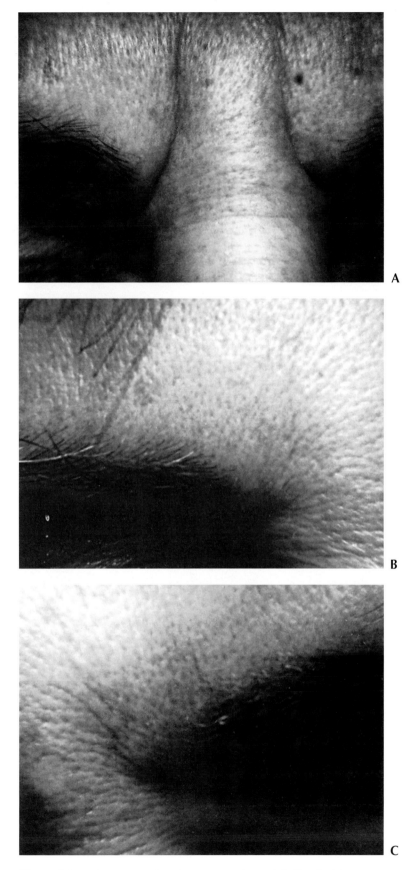

Figure 9-9 (*A*) Preoperative photo—note deep glabellar rhytids. (*B*) Postoperative photo 1 week later—right rhytid. (*C*) Postoperative photo 1 week later—left rhytid.

117

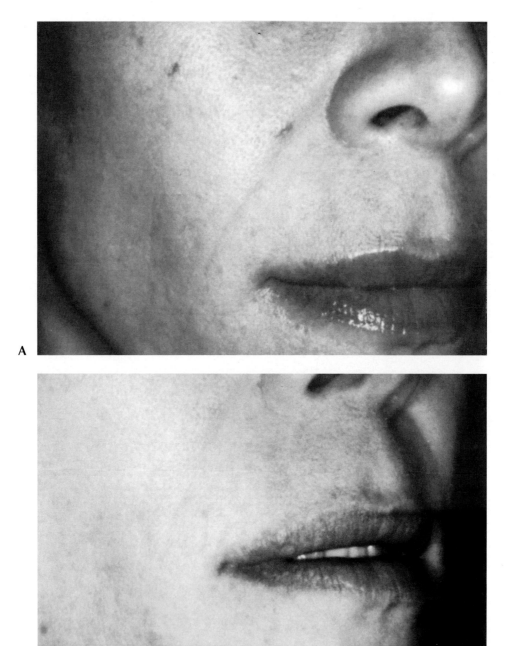

Figure 9-10 (**A**) Right mesolabial rhytid preoperatively. (**B**) Right mesolabial rhytid postoperatively.

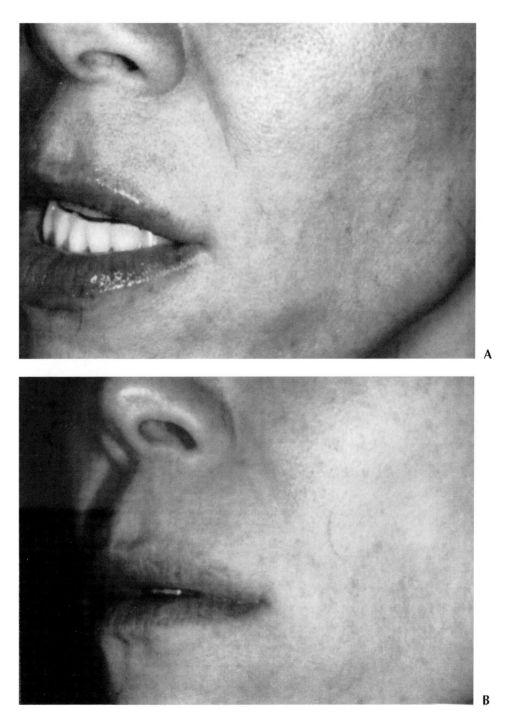

Figure 9-11 (*A*) Left mesolabial rhytid preoperatively. (*B*) Left mesolabial rhytid postoperatively.

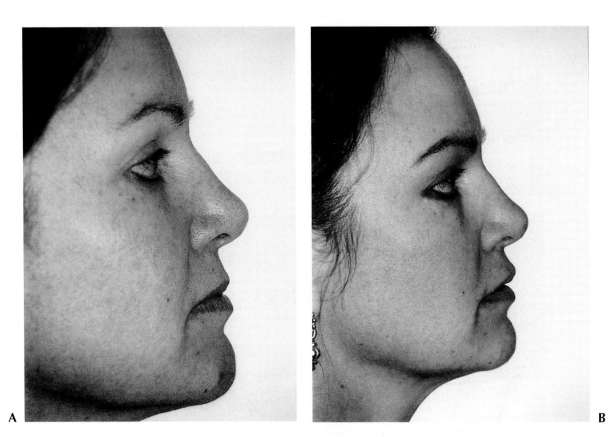

Figure 9-12   (*A*) Right lip, lateral view, preoperatively. (*B*) Right lip, lateral view, postoperatively.

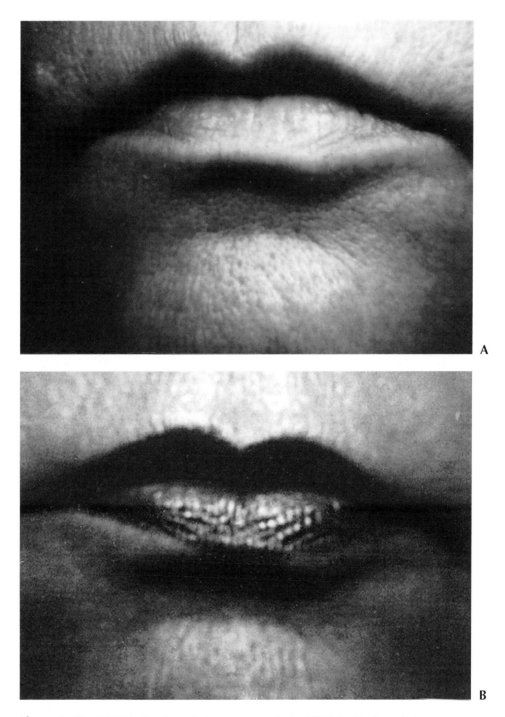

Figure 9-13   (**A**) Right lip, frontal view, preoperatively. (**B**) Right lip, frontal view, postoperatively.

References

1. Austin HW, Weston GW. Rejuvenation of the aging mouth. *Aesthetic Surg Face* 1992; 4:511–523.

2. Maloney BP. Cosmetic surgery of the lips. *Facial Plast Surg* 1996; 12:265–278.

3. Scarborough DA, Bisaccia E. CO$_2$ laser resurfacing with fat grafting for rhytids and acne scars. *Cosmet Dermatol* 1997; 10:7–12.

4. Isenberg JS. Permanent lip augmentation using autologous breast implant capsule. *Ann Plast Surg* 1996; 37:121–124.

5. de Benito J, Fernandez-Sanza I. Galea and subgalea graft for lip augmentation revision. *Aesthet Plast Surg* 1996; 20:243–248.

6. Bisaccia E, Scarborough DA. The esthetic correction of the aging mouth. *Cosmet Dermatol* 1992; 11:8–11.

7. Neuber F. Fat grafting, *Chirurgie* 1893; 22:66 1893 (German).

8. Brunings P, In: Broeckaert TJ: Contribution à l'etude des greffes adipeueses. *Bull Acad Med Belg* 1919; 28:440.

9. Peer LA. Loss of weight and volume in human fat grafts. *Plast Reconstr* 1950; 5:217.

10. Illouz YG. Communications at the Societe Francaise de Chirurgie. *Esthetique* June 1978, 1979.

11. Newman J, Ftaihaz, Special issue on fat transplant surgery. *Am J Cosmet Surg* 1987; 4(2):85–87.

12. Devore DP, Kelman CD, Fagien S. Autologen: Autologous, injectable dermal collagen. In: Bosniak S, ed. *Principles and Practices of Ophthalmic Plastic and Reconstructive Surgery* Philadelphia: Saunders; 1994.

13. Elson ML. The role of skin testing in the use of collagen injectable materials. *J Dermatol Surg Oncol* 1989; 15(3): 301–303.

14. Drake LA, Dinehart SM, Farmer ER. Guidelines of care for soft tissue augmentation: Gelatin matrix implant. *J Am Acad Dermatol* 1996; 34:695–697.

15. Drake LA, Dinehart SM, Farmer ER. Guidelines for care for soft tissue augmentation: Collagen implants. *J Am Acad Dermatol* 1996; 34:698–702.

16. Millikan L. Long-term safety and efficacy with Fibrel in the treatment of cutaneous scars—Results of a multicenter study. Multicenter study group. *J Dermatol Surg Oncol* 1989; 15(8):837–842.

17. Artz JS, Dinner ML. The use of expanded polytetrafluoroethylene as a permanent filler and enhancer: An early report of experience. *Ann Plast Surg* 1994; 32:457–462.

18. Cisneros JL, Singla R. Intradermal augmentation with expanded polytetrafluoroethylene (Gore-Tex) for facial lines and wrinkles. *J Dermatol Surg* 1993; 19:539–542.

19. Conrad K, Reifen E. Gore-tex implant as tissue filler in cheek-lip groove rejuvenation. *J Otolaryngol* 1992; 21:218–222.

20. Conrad K, MacDonald MR. Wide polytef (Gore-Tex) implants in lip augmentation and nasolabial groove correction. *Arch Otolaryngol Head Neck Surg* 1996; 122(6):554–570.

21. Gore WL and Associates. Gore subcutaneous Augmentation Materials product information. Flagstaff, AZ.

22. Scalafani AP, Thomas JR, Cox AJ: Clinical and histologic response of subcutaneous expanded polytetrafluoroethylene (Gore-Tex) and porous high-density polyethylene (Medpore) implants to acute and early infection. *Arch Otolaryngol Head Neck Surg* 1997; 123(3):328–336.

23. Bergamini TM, McCurry TN, Bernard JD, et al. Antibiotic efficacy against *Staphylococcus epidermis* adherent to vascular grafts. *J Surg Res* 1996; 60(1):33–36.

24. Greene D, Pruitt L, Maas CS: Biomechanical effects of ePTFE implant structure on soft tissue implantation stability: A study in the porcine model. *Laryngoscope* 1997; 107(7):977–962.

25. Dabrowski JM, Adour KK, Hilsinger RL Jr: Expanded PTFE patch for suspension in facial paralysis. In: Stucker FJ, ed. *Plastic and Reconstructive Surgery of the Head and Neck. Proceedings of the Fifth International Symposium.* Philadelphia: Decker; 1991:561–564.

Patient Information

Collagen

Collagen is a natural protein that forms the support structure of your skin. When natural collagen thins, wrinkles begin to appear. This loss is attributed mainly to aging, but exposure to the sun, pollution, health, heredity, and lifestyle also play roles. Without enough collagen, wrinkles and lines start to form. Your own collagen can be replaced by collagen implantation, whereby collagen is injected into wrinkles with a needle and syringe to restore the fullness and tension of the skin. Collagen works best for wrinkles around the eyes and mouth; however, it may also be used to give the lips greater fullness. The results are immediate.

Collagen implants, taken from cattle, are natural products derived from highly purified bovine collagen that is injected just under the surface of the skin. Like your own collagen, your body eventually breaks down and absorbs this collagen, so ongoing treatments are necessary to maintain results. If collagen treatments are discontinued, your face will gradually return to its natural contours.

Many people return to work the same day of treatment. People absorb collagen at varying rates, but repeat treatments are usually required every 3 to 6 months.

Preoperative Instructions

Please do not wear make-up to the office; if worn, please plan to remove it upon arrival.

To minimize the chance of bruising, please plan on doing the following:

Avoid aspirin or aspirin-containing products once you are scheduled for the procedure.

Preferably stay off aspirin or aspirin-containing products for 10 days prior to your treatment.

Avoid alcohol for 24 hours prior to the procedure.

Be sure to discuss with the doctor any bleeding tendencies and current medications being used.

Ice will be applied immediately following treatment. If you normally bruise easily, plan to go home and apply ice to the area(s) for an extra few hours.

Get a good night's sleep before the procedure.

Eat a *light* meal (breakfast or lunch) the day of treatment prior to the appointment.

Although the treatments are well tolerated by most patients, to minimize any discomfort you may apply a topical over-the-counter anesthetic agent (Ela-max 4%) to the area(s) to be treated for 1 hour prior to your visit. This may be purchased at your local pharmacy; follow the instructions that come with this product.

Collagen Setup Tray

Patient
1. Makeup remover
2. Gauze

Doctor and Staff
1. Clean gloves

Materials
1. Small tray
2. 5–6 gauze
3. Alcohol prep
4. Two 30-gauge needles
5. Collagen syringes
6. Ice in a bag
7. Paper towel for ice bag

Postoperative Instructions

The treatments are well tolerated by most patients. You may use Tylenol or Extra-Strength Tylenol for any discomfort. It is best not to take aspirin or alcohol for 24 hours after the procedure.

Ice will be applied immediately following treatment. If you normally bruise easily, plan to go home and apply ice to the area(s) for a few hours.

Avoid strenuous exercise (perspiring) for 24 hours following treatment. You may otherwise resume normal activities.

You may apply makeup upon leaving the office. Showering and facial cleansing are not restricted, but facial massage is to be avoided for 24 hours.

Dermalogen

What Is Dermalogen?

Dermalogen is an injectable human tissue matrix (HTM) implant, procured from donor tissue, that has undergone a patented process. It is injected into facial contour defects.

WHAT TYPES OF CONDITIONS CAN BE TREATED WITH DERMALOGEN?

Dermalogen can be used to treat facial contour defects. The most common treatments involve:

Nasolabial folds (sides of the nose)

Perioral lines (above the lips)

The vermillion ridge (top of the lip)

Glabellar frown lines (between the eyebrows)

Oral commissures ("smile lines")

Depressed scars (e.g., acne)

Consult your physician to determine if you are a potential candidate for Dermalogen treatment.

HOW LONG DOES A DERMALOGEN TREATMENT LAST?

The company's results to date with its similar autologous human tissue matrix show significant correction for several months after final treatment for most patients. Ongoing clinical studies are being conducted with Dermalogen.

IS DERMALOGEN TREATMENT A REPLACEMENT FOR LASER SKIN RESURFACING, CHEMICAL PEELS, OR DERMABRASION?

No, but it can be efficacious when used alone or in concert with these procedures for the treatment of facial contour defects.

HOW MANY TREATMENTS ARE REQUIRED?

Typically two to three treatments are required over a 3-month period to correct most dermal depressions. Improvements with Dermalogen are progressive. After the first treatment, you may not see much change, but each additional treatment yields more improvements.

ARE THE TREATMENTS PAINFUL?

Your doctor will inject Dermalogen with a fine-gauge needle. Most patients have found these injections uncomfortable and prefer to be given some anesthetic. If this is the case in your situation, ask your physician about local anesthetics such as those used in facial or dental surgery.

WHAT WILL I LOOK LIKE RIGHT AFTER TREATMENT?

Some patients find that their skin at the injection sites is red or blanched for about 48 hours after treatment. If you have a history of bruising, a bruise may result that could take a few weeks to heal. Your physician will discuss other potential side effects with you during your consultation.

WHERE DOES THE DONOR TISSUE COME FROM?

Tissue comes from donors in much the same way donated organs do. Recovered donor tissue is processed by methods that follow the federally mandated tissue recovery guidelines and those of the American Association of Tissue Banks (AATB). Other applications for processed donor tissue include burn surgery, periodontal (gum) surgery, and bone implants. These number in the hundreds of thousands of implants per year.

IS DONATED TISSUE SAFE?

Tissue donors are very carefully screened and tested to reduce the risk of disease transmission. The tissue banks follow federally mandated guidelines and those of the AATB. The only tissue processed into Dermalogen is tissue from donors who have passed all tests.

In addition, during the processing of Dermalogen, safeguards against viral transmission are used by treating the tissue with powerful antiviral agents.

WHAT IS THE DIFFERENCE BETWEEN DERMALOGEN AND BOVINE (COW) COLLAGEN?

Dermalogen contains intact collagen fibrils, elastic network, and proteoglycans similar to native dermis. Bovine collagen contains digested cow collagen in small segments.

Preoperative Instructions

Please do not wear makeup to the office; if worn, please plan to remove it upon arrival.

To minimize the chance of bruising, please plan on doing the following:

Avoid aspirin or aspirin-containing products once you are scheduled for the procedure.

Preferably stay off aspirin or aspirin-containing products for 10 days prior to your treatment.

Avoid alcohol for 24 hours prior to the procedure.

Be sure to discuss with the doctor any bleeding tendencies and current medications being used.

Ice will be applied immediately following treatment. If you normally bruise easily, plan to go home and apply ice to the area(s) for an extra few hours.

Get a good night's sleep before the procedure.

Eat a *light* meal (breakfast or lunch) the day of treatment prior to the appointment.

Although the treatments are well tolerated by most patients, to minimize any discomfort you may apply a topical over-the-counter anesthetic agent (Ela-max 4%) to the area(s) to be treated for 1 hour prior to your visit. This may be purchased at your local pharmacy; follow the instructions that come with this product.

Dermalogen Setup Tray

Patient
1. Makeup remover
2. Gauze

Doctor and Staff
1. Clean gloves

Materials

1. Small tray
2. 5–6 gauze
3. Alcohol prep
4. Two 30-gauge needles
5. One dermalogen syringe
6. Ice in a bag
7. Paper towel for ice bag

Postoperative Instructions

The treatments are well tolerated by most patients. You may use Tylenol or Extra-Strength Tylenol for any discomfort. It is best not to take aspirin or alcohol for 24 hours after procedure.

Ice will be applied immediately following treatment. If you normally bruise easily, plan to go home and apply ice to the area(s) for a few hours.

Avoid strenuous exercise (perspiring) for 24 hours following treatment. You may otherwise resume normal activities.

You may apply makeup upon leaving the office. Showering and facial cleansing are not restricted, but facial massage is to be avoided for 24 hours.

Fascian

WHAT IS FASCIA?

Fascia is the medical name for the sheets of thick, white connective tissue that are located throughout the human body. All doctors, especially surgeons, are familiar with these important fascia layers because they wrap around many muscles and internal structures, packaging them and giving them support. Surgeons often sew layers of fascia together because they are strong and hold sutures well.

Fascia is living tissue that is largely composed of the protein collagen and the fibroblast cells that make collagen, although other materials, such as the protein elastin, are also present. The protein collagen is found in many tissues besides fascia, such as skin, cartilage, and tendons.

WHAT IS FASCIAN?

Fascian is a special preparation of human fascia. To make Fascian, preserved fascia grafts are procured in the traditional manner and then processed under sterile conditions to different particle sizes. The material is then supplied to doctors in a form which easily can be stored and then rehydrated and injected when it is needed.

IS FASCIAN NEW?

Yes and no. The use of preserved fascia as a graft material is an accepted procedure that began in the 1920s. Fascian, an injectable form of preserved fascia, has only recently become available to physicians.

WHAT HAPPENS WHEN FASCIAN IS INJECTED?

Fascian is a very thick suspension of solid bits of fibrous material. Once it is injected into an area, the liquid in the suspension is absorbed and the residual particles may aggregate locally. This thick material fills the defect into which it is placed.

WHERE CAN FASCIAN BE INJECTED?

Your physician must be the one to decide if Fascian is an appropriate material for injection in each instance. Fascian is intended for the repair of small tissue defects resulting from aging or from medical or surgical conditions—those in which preserved fascia would otherwise be considered an appropriate treatment option.

WHAT TYPE OF PREEVALUATION IS REQUIRED?

Check with your doctor about his or her own requirements for preevaluation before Fascian injection.

WHAT ARE THE RISKS OF INJECTING FASCIAN?

Routinely, the local reaction to the site of injection is mild and pain-free; however, many factors may influence the extent of bruising and swelling—the amount of material injected, the depth at which it is injected, the area of needle dissection performed by the doctor to create a pocket for implantation, the particle size selected, etc. Fascian may feel thick or lumpy in the area, especially for the first few weeks after injection, but typically the graft site will eventually soften.

Some reabsorption of the material is to be expected. This will depend on many factors, including the size of areas being treated and the amount of material placed in the area. Your doctor may choose to overcorrect the area in anticipation of some reabsorption.

Infection is possible with any injection or implant, although it is very uncommon. Often, the contaminant is a bacterium from the patient's own skin surface. Injection into an area that is already infected or inflamed is not advised. A local infection may result in tissue damage and scarring.

In patients with systemic diseases, e.g., AIDS, there may be specific reservations about Fascian use.

Scar tissue may develop at the injection site; to some extent, this may be an acceptable part of the correction of the defect. An overt scar reaction, (e.g., hypertrophic scar or keloid) is unlikely but should be considered.

An adverse reaction of any other kind to this graft material—e.g., a local or systemic allergic response—would be unusual, but the possibility must be considered.

Preoperative Instructions

Please do not wear make-up to the office; if worn, please plan to remove it upon arrival.

To minimize the chance of bruising, please plan on doing the following:

Avoid aspirin or aspirin-containing products once you are scheduled for the procedure.

Preferably stay off aspirin or aspirin-containing products for 10 days prior to your treatment.

Avoid alcohol for 24 hours prior to the procedure.

Be sure to discuss with the doctor any bleeding tendencies and current medications being used.

Ice will be applied immediately following treatment. If you normally bruise easily, plan to go home and apply ice to the area(s) for an extra few hours.

Get a good night's sleep before the procedure.

Eat a *light* meal (breakfast or lunch) the day of treatment prior to the appointment.

Although the treatments are well tolerated by most patients, to minimize any discomfort you may apply a topical over-the-counter anesthetic agent (Ela-max 4%) to the area(s) to be treated for 1 hour prior to your visit. This may be purchased at your local pharmacy; follow the instructions that come packaged with this product.

Fascian Setup Tray

Patient

1. Makeup remover
2. Gauze

Doctor and Staff

1. Clean gloves

Materials

1. Small tray
2. 5–6 gauze
3. Alcohol prep
4. Two 22-gauge needles
5. One Fascian syringe
6. Ice in a bag
7. Paper towel for ice bag

Postoperative Instructions

The treatments are well tolerated by most patients. You may use Tylenol or Extra-Strength Tylenol for any discomfort. It is best not to take aspirin or alcohol for 24 hours after the procedure.

Ice will be applied immediately following treatment. If you normally bruise easily, plan to go home and apply ice to the area(s) for a few hours.

Avoid strenuous exercise (perspiring) for 24 hours following treatment. You may otherwise resume normal activities.

You may apply makeup upon leaving the office. Showering and facial cleansing are not restricted, but avoid facial massage for 24 hours.

Gore-Tex

WHAT IS GORE-TEX MADE OF?

Gore-Tex is made of a material whose scientific name is "expanded polytetrafluoroethylene" (ePTFE); some configurations may also include fluorinated ethylene propylene (FEP). Both are nontoxic polymers that are used in many different kinds of medical products that are implanted throughout the body. Unlike some other materials, ePTFE is not "rejected" by the body, so implants made with it can remain in place permanently, and no "antirejection" treatment is necessary after the implantation surgery. In addition, among the 4 million ePTFE implants to date, there have been no confirmed cases of an allergic reaction to the material.

Unlike a silicone implant, an ePTFE implant is a porous, solid material. Its porosity allows the body's tissue to grown into it. Flexible and soft to the touch, ePTFE is very strong and extremely unlikely to stretch or tear.

Gore-Tex is indicated for facial plastic and reconstructive surgery; it is inserted subcutaneously (deep beneath the skin) to augment the contour of the face.

HOW IS GORE-TEX MATERIAL INSERTED?

Your surgeon will make a small incision at the implantation site. Tissue from the area will be gently lifted and a small tunnel or pocket created for the implant. While ensuring that the implant remains sterile, the surgeon will trim it to fit your facial contours, insert it into the pocket, and, if needed, secure it in place. The time required for this procedure will depend on which area of your face is being treated. The incision may be closed with stitches that your surgeon will remove in a week of so.

HOW WILL MY FACE FEEL AFTER MY OPERATION?

Your surgeon will discuss with you what you can expect as you recover from your specific operation. Generally, some discomfort, aching, stiffness, numbness, and swelling should be expected after any kind of facial implant surgery. These feelings may last for a week or more.

Although the Gore-Tex is compatible with your body's natural tissue, it is an artificial material and not the same as that tissue. As a result, the area of your face where the implant has been inserted may feel somewhat different to the touch after surgery, even after the swelling from the procedure has gone down.

WHAT ARE THE POSSIBLE SIDE EFFECTS OF FACIAL IMPLANT SURGERY?

All operations carry some risks, including those resulting from anesthesia, which your surgeon will discuss with you. Scientific studies have found Gore-Tex to be a very safe product that is supplied sterile to your surgeon. Specific complications associated with its use are unlikely, but they can occur. Possible adverse effects include excessive swelling and bruising on or below the skin, infection, formation of a fistula (an abnormal opening between tissues), extrusion (part of the implant comes through the skin), induration (hardening), formation of seroma (a dense pocket of fluid below the skin), inadequate healing, and inadequate or excessive facial contouring.

Your surgeon will give you detailed instructions and guidelines to follow as you recover from your operation. The best way to prevent complications from surgery is to follow your surgeon's instructions carefully. If a problem begins to develop or your have any concerns at all about the results of your operation or the healing process, call your surgeon immediately. There are many effective treatments for complications that may occur. Early consultation with your doctor is extremely important.

Preoperative Instructions

Please do not wear makeup to the office; if worn, please plan to remove it upon arrival.

To minimize the chance of bruising, please plan on doing the following:

> *Avoid aspirin* or aspirin-containing products once you are scheduled for the procedure.
>
> Preferably stay off aspirin or aspirin-containing products for 10 days prior to your treatment.
>
> *Avoid alcohol* for 24 hours prior to the procedure.
>
> Be sure to discuss with the doctor any bleeding tendencies and current medications being used.
>
> Ice will be applied immediately following treatment. If you normally bruise easily, plan to go home and apply ice to the area(s) for an extra few hours.

Get a good night's sleep before the procedure.

Eat a *light* meal (breakfast or lunch) the day of treatment prior to the appointment.

Take all medications as prescribed *prior* to treatment. These normally will include an antibiotic, an antiviral (if the lip is being treated), and a diazepam (Valium) (you must arrange for a driver if this is taken).

The fee is to be paid in full at the preoperative visit, which must be 7 to14 days prior to surgery.

Gore-Tex Setup Tray

Patient

1. Cape
2. Sterile hat
3. White drape sheet

Doctor

1. Yellow isolation gown
2. Sterile gloves
3. Mask

Materials

1. Betadine solution
2. Mayo stand
3. Two 18-in. sterile drapes (for headrest and chest)
4. Sterile gauze pack
5. Sterile light handle cover
6. Keith needle
7. 14-gauge angiocath (have 2, open 1)
8. 4-0 prolene P-3 (have 2, open 1)
9. Needle holder with scissors
10. Bishop-Harmon forceps
11. Gradle scissors
12. ⅛-in. Steri-Strips
13. 5-mL syringe
14. 1% Lidocaine with epinephrine, buffered
15. 21-gauge needle to draw
16. 30-gauge needle to numb
17. Gore-Tex implant
18. 48-in. white drape across chest
19. Alligator forceps

Postoperative Instructions

You may use Tylenol or Extra-Strength Tylenol for any discomfort. It is best not to take aspirin or alcohol for 24 hours after the procedure.

Steri-Strips may be applied to the site(s) treated. If so, keep them dry for 72 hours, then remove.

Occasionally, fine sutures are used at the site(s) treated. If so, use a cotton swab to gently cleanse the wound with tap water or saline solution once a day. Do not use hydrogen peroxide, alcohol, or soap.

Pat the wound dry and apply an antibiotic ointment liberally twice daily, in the morning and at bedtime. You may leave the wound uncovered. You will be given further instructions when you return for suture removal.

Avoid strenuous exercise (perspiring) for a minimum of 1 week following surgery.

Avoid the application of makeup or washing your face for 24 hours following the procedure.

Avoid facial massage and excessive facial motion for 2 weeks.

Should minor bleeding occur, apply firm constant pressure for 15 to 20 minutes. It is not unusual for mild, red-tinged drainage to occur up to 48 hours after surgery.

Should you have any questions or problems with infection, pain or discharge, please call (____) _____.

Fat Transfer

Over the years, time and gravity help shape our faces in ways we may not appreciate. When we were younger, our faces were not affected by gravity in the same way because they were cushioned by fat, which provides a good foundation for smooth and creaseless skin. As we age and our muscles and skin lose some of their elasticity, this fat cushion dissipates. We may develop deep creases, receding lips, or sunken cheeks, which detract from our appearance.

Facial creases and depressions as well as depression in other areas of the body can be corrected with an extraordinary procedure called fat transplantation. This procedure enables your surgeon to enhance your facial or body contour by extracting fat from one portion of your body and injecting it into another. It is effective in minimizing creases and grooves and also used to augment the lips, cheeks, or chin. An increasingly common use of fat transfer is for lip enhancement. Thinned lips with little lines are supported and redefined, producing a much more youthful appearance. Fat transfer is also used for earlobe augmentation. This helps minimize the earlobe's susceptibility to tearing when large earrings are being worn.

During the fat transfer procedure, the fat is taken from your own body—unlike the case with other procedures used to correct depressions. This eliminates any allergic reactions and the possibility of rejection.

The cosmetic surgeons of this center help people develop and maintain a healthy, more attractive, younger appearance. Our skilled surgeons specialize in fat transfers and have used their knowledge, skill, and experience for over a decade to help numerous patients combat the effects of aging and look more attractive.

The Procedure   Fat transplantation is performed in your doctor's office. The areas on your face or body to and from which the fat is moved are treated with a local anesthetic.

The donor site is often chosen based upon patient preference. The hip, buttocks, thighs, or lower abdomen are all areas in women from which fat can easily be withdrawn. In males, the donor region is often the flank area, right above the hips. During the procedure, your surgeon injects a local anesthetic agent into the site with the thick fat layer. Fat cells are drawn into a syringe and carefully reinjected into the recipient site. Your doctor repeats this process until the desired amount of fat is transferred and the crease or depression is corrected.

There is little discomfort associated with the procedure; the patient can bathe the next day. Makeup can be worn on treated facial areas after 24 hours. A small amount of bruising is not uncommon. Patients usually resume normal activities within a day but should avoid strenuous exercise such as jogging, swimming, and tennis for a week.

The Results   Fat transfer is a safe, effective way to counteract the effects of time and gravity. Most patients who use the procedure to correct deep creases, grooves, or depressions or to augment an area are delighted with the results. Ask for a consultation to find out how fat transfer can help you improve your appearance.

Preoperative Instructions

Please do not wear makeup to the office; if worn, please plan to remove it upon arrival.

To minimize the chance of bruising, please plan on doing the following:

Avoid aspirin or aspirin-containing products once you are scheduled for the procedure.

Preferably stay off aspirin or aspirin-containing products for 10 days prior to your treatment.

Avoid alcohol for 24 hours prior to the procedure.

Be sure to discuss with the doctor any bleeding tendencies and current medications being used.

Ice will be applied immediately following treatment. If you normally bruise easily, plan to go home and apply ice to the area(s) for an extra few hours.

Get a good night's sleep the night before surgery.

Take a normal shower the morning of procedure.

If you are not using the services of our anesthetist, a light breakfast is suggested.

Begin vitamin E 400 IU (this can be easily obtained at any drug store) twice daily for at least 1 week prior to the procedure.

Take all medications as prescribed prior to treatment. These normally will include an antibiotic, an antiviral (if the lip is being treated), and a diazepam (Valium) (you must arrange for a driver if this is taken).

Bring a panty girdle, support hose, or tight elastic shorts with you on surgery day; they will help to provide compression over the donor site and should be worn 7 days following your procedure.

The fee is to be paid in full at the preoperative visit, which must be 7 to 14 days prior to surgery.

Fat Transfer Setup Tray

Patient
1. Cape
2. Sterile surgical hat
3. Photo pants

Doctor and Staff
1. Sterile gloves
2. Mask
3. Yellow gown

Materials
1. Black and purple skin marker
2. Two packets of sterile 3×3 gauze
3. Betadine solution
4. One #11 blade
5. Small undermining scissors
6. Sterile bowl
7. Sterile regular scissors
8. Syringes
   A. One 3-mL LL
   B. Four to six 10-mL LL
   C. One 60-mL LL
9. Cannulae
   A. Small infusion
   B. Small accelerator or neck harvester
10. Four to six 18-gauge needles
11. One 30-gauge 1-in. metal hub needle
12. One 21-gauge 1-in. needle
13. Two 30-mL bottles lidocaine 1% with epinephrine, buffered
14. Six 30-mL bottles of saline
15. One fat box
16. Small ice pack
17. Two medium drapes (sterile)

18. One sterile small bath towel
19, Steri-Strips, ½-in.
20. Wide micro foam tape
21. Sterile light handle cover

Postoperative Instructions

Go home and relax.

Avoid aspirin and alcohol for 48 hours (may use Tylenol).

Avoid vigorous washing and/or massaging of the face for 48 hours. You may cleanse gently, and makeup can be worn after 24 hours.

After 24 hours you may remove the gauze dressing at the donor site, leaving the Steri-Strip in place for 10 days. The panty girdle should be worn to compress the area for 24 hours a day for the first 3 days, then during the daytime only for 7 days.

If any discomfort or bruising occurs, apply an ice pack to the area(s) for 15 to 20 minutes four times daily.

Restrict strenuous activities (no perspiring) for 7 days following the procedure (e.g., no jogging, aerobics, tennis, swimming, hard physical work, etc.).

Some swelling and bruising are expected. If signs of infection occur (excessive redness, swelling, pain, pus), call the office immediately.

Remember, bruising may appear at the donor and/or injection sites, and may take 7 to 10 days to fade, sometimes longer.

Occasionally, multiple treatments are necessary before satisfactory correction is completed. Touch-ups are required to maintain long-term correction. There is a fee for each treatment and touch-up.

Sun exposure should be limited for 2 weeks following the procedure, especially if bruising is present.

CONSENT FOR COLLAGEN IMPLANT

Patient's name_____

Date_____

		YES	NO
A.	Have you had or have your brother, sister, mother, or father had an autoimmune disease such as rheumatoid arthritis, lupus erythematosis, thyroiditis, or ulcerative colitis?	____	____
B.	Are you allergic to Xylocaine (lidocaine)?	____	____
C.	Have you had asthma or atopic dermatitis?	____	____
D.	Are you allergic to anything else?	____	____
E.	Do you have hives or an active skin rash now?	____	____
F.	Have you ever had silicone injections?	____	____
G.	Are you pregnant?	____	____

PRIOR TO BEGINNING TREATMENT, YOU MUST BE AWARE OF THE FOLLOWING:

You must agree that your skin problem is serious enough that the potential benefit of Zyderm implantation outweighs known and unknown risks from this material.

1. There is a remote possibility that problems, including impairment of vision, could develop as a result of the injection process.

    Initial_____

2. If you have had facial herpes simplex at the site where you are to receive Zyderm, the injection could cause another herpes simplex eruption.

    Initial_____

3. Unforeseen results—such as infection of the Zyderm implantation sites, skin ulcerations, permanent scarring and disfigurement and/or unusual allergic reactions—may occur that may jeopardize or impair your health and well-being.

    Initial_____

4. Transient bruising, swelling, induration, and discomfort may occur.

    Initial_____

5. Even after a normal test dose, you may develop an allergic reaction at the injection site in the face, which may take many months to resolve. (Studies show that this may occur in up to 3 percent of patients.)

    Initial_____

6. The correction that is achieved will diminish over time and require additional treatment to be maintained.

    Initial_____

7. For the purpose of advancing medical education, I consent to the admittance of authorized observers to the operating room.

    Initial_____

8. I understand that elective surgical procedures are most often delayed until after the termination of a pregnancy. My signature attests that, to the best of my knowledge, I am not pregnant at this time.

    Initial_____

9. The nature and effects of the operation, the risks and complications involved, as well as alternative methods of treatment have been fully explained to me. I understand these explanations, have been given the opportunity to ask questions, and all questions have been answered to my satisfaction.

    Initial_____

10. I understand that the practice of medicine and surgery is not an exact science and that reputable practitioners cannot guarantee results. No guarantee or assurance has been given to me by the doctor or anyone else as to the results that may be obtained.

    Initial_____

11. I understand that the two sides of the human body are not exactly the same and can never be made the same.

    Initial_____

12. I give permission to _____ to take still or motion clinical photographs with the understanding such photographs remain the property of the center. If in the judgment of the center medical research, education, or science will be benefited by their use, such photographs and related information may be published and republished in professional journals or medical books or used for any other purpose which the center may deem proper. It is specifically understood that in any such publication or use I shall not be identified by name.

    Initial_____

My signature indicates that I have read this "Consent for Collagen Implant" and I understand and accept the risks involved with this operation. I hereby authorize _____ _____ and/or the surgical team to perform this surgical procedure on me.

Date	Signature—Patient/ Responsible Party	Signature— Parent/Guardian

CONSENT FOR DERMALOGEN IMPLANT

Patient's name_____
Date_____

You are being treated with injectable Dermalogen, which is material derived from human skin. The same type of human tissue material from tissue banks has been used for many years to treat burns and other trauma. The donors of the skin from the tissue bank were screened for their social history. They have been tested for viral infections including HIV (the AIDS virus) and hepatitis.

PRIOR TO BEGINNING TREATMENT YOU MUST BE AWARE OF THE FOLLOWING:

1. If you have had facial herpes simplex at the site where you are to receive Dermalogen, the injection could cause another herpes simplex eruption.

   Initial_____

2. Unforeseen results—such as infection of the Dermalogen implantation sites, skin ulcerations, permanent scarring and disfigurement, and/or unusual allergic reactions—may occur that may jeopardize or impair your health and well-being.

   Initial_____

3. I understand that three treatments at 2 to 4 week intervals over a 3-month period *are usually required* to achieve initial correction of most depressions or defects.

   Initial_____

4. The correction that is achieved will diminish over time and require additional treatment to be maintained.

   Initial_____

5. Soft tissue augmentation is an art as well as a science, and although the doctors at _____ are considered experts in this field, no guarantees are made regarding outcome of the procedure or longevity of correction.

   Initial_____

6. I understand that elective surgical procedures are most often delayed until after the termination of a pregnancy. My signature attests that, to the best of my knowledge, I am not pregnant at this time.

   Initial_____

7. I understand that the two sides of the human body are not exactly the same and can never be made the same.

   Initial_____

8. For the purpose of advancing medical education, I consent to the admittance of authorized observers to the operating room.

   Initial_____

9. I have read the brochure titled *Dermalogen* and this consent form and have discussed the risks and benefits of injectable Dermalogen tissue matrix with the doctors at _____. I fully understand such explanations, have been given the opportunity to ask questions, and all questions have been answered to my satisfaction.

   Initial_____

10. I give permission to _____ to take still or motion clinical photographs with the understanding such photographs remain the property of the center. If in the judgment of the center medical research, education, or science will be benefited by their use, such photographs and related information may be published and republished in professional journals or medical books or used for any other purpose that the center may deem proper. It is specifically understood that in any such publication or use, I shall not be identified by name.

    Initial_____

My signature indicates that I have read this "Consent for Dermalogen Implant" and I understand and accept the risks involved with this operation. I hereby authorize _____ and/or the surgical team to administer Dermalogen as described.

Date	Signature—Patient/ Responsible Party	Signature— Parent/Guardian

CONSENT FOR FASCIAN

Patient's name_____

Date_____

I hereby authorize _____ and/or the surgical team to perform a Fascian operation upon me (or my _____) to: (description of procedure) _____

_____

_____

	YES	NO
A. Have you had collagen injections?	____	____
B. Are you allergic to Xylocaine (lidocaine)?	____	____
C. Are you allergic to anything else?	____	____
D. Do you have hives or an active skin rash now?	____	____
E. Are you pregnant?	____	____

PRIOR TO BEGINNING THERAPY, YOU MUST BE AWARE OF THE FOLLOWING:

1. You agree that your skin problem is serious enough that the potential benefit of Fascian implantation outweighs known and unknown risks from this material.

   Initial_____

2. There is a remote possibility that problems, including impairment of vision, could develop as a result of the injection process.

   Initial_____

3. If you have had facial herpes simplex at the site where you are to receive Fascian, the injection could cause another herpes simplex eruption.

   Initial_____

4. Unforeseen results, such as infection of the Fascian implantation sites, skin ulcerations, permanent scarring and disfigurement, and/or unusual allergic reactions may occur that may jeopardize or impair your health and well-being.

   Initial_____

5. Transient bruising, swelling, hardness, and discomfort may occur.

   Initial_____

6. The correction that is achieved will diminish over time and require additional treatment to be maintained.

   Initial_____

7. I understand that elective surgical procedures are most often delayed until after the termination of a pregnancy. My signature attests that, to the best of my knowledge, I am not pregnant at this time.

   Initial_____

8. The nature and effects of the operation, the risks and complications involved, as well as alternative methods of treatment have been fully explained to me and I understand them.

   Initial_____

9. I understand that the practice of medicine and surgery is not an exact science and that reputable practitioners cannot guarantee results. No guarantee or assurance has been given to me by the doctor or anyone else as to the results that may be obtained.

   Initial_____

10. I understand the two sides of the human body are not exactly the same and can never be made the same.

    Initial_____

11. I give permission to _____ to take still or motion clinical photographs with the understanding such photographs remain the property of the center. If in the judgment of the center medical research, education, or science will be benefited by their use, such photographs and related information may be published and republished in professional journals or medical books or used for any other purpose that the center may deem proper. It is specifically understood that in any such publication or use, I shall not be identified by name.

    Initial_____

My signature indicates I have read and understood the above information, that the explanations referred to therein were made to my satisfaction, that I fully understand these explanations and the above authorization, that I have discussed this with my physician, and that I have decided to have this procedure based on the information provided.

Date	Signature—Patient/ Responsible Party	Signature— Parent/Guardian

CONSENT FOR GORE-TEX FACIAL IMPLANT

Patient's name_____

Date_____

I hereby authorize _____ and/or the surgical team to perform a Gore-Tex operation upon me (or my _____) to: (description of procedure) _____

_____

_____

	YES	NO
A. Are you allergic to Xylocaine (lidocaine)?	____	____
B. Have you ever had silicone injections?	____	____
C. Are you pregnant?	____	____
D. Have you had collagen injections?	____	____
E. If so, any adverse reactions	____	____

PRIOR TO BEGINNING TREATMENT, YOU MUST BE AWARE OF THE FOLLOWING:

1. You must agree that your skin problem is serious enough that the potential benefit of the Gore-Tex facial implantation outweighs known and unknown risks from this material.

    Initial_____

2. There is a remote possibility that problems—including infection, scarring, and discoloration—could develop as a result of the injection process and that the Gore-Tex implant may need to be removed.

    Initial_____

3. If you have had facial herpes simplex at the site where you are to receive the Gore-Tex implants, the injection could cause another herpes simplex eruption.

    Initial_____

4. Unforeseen results—such as infection of the Gore-Tex facial implantation sites, skin ulcerations, permanent scarring, and disfigurement and/or unusual allergic reactions—may occur that may jeopardize or impair your appearance and well-being.

    Initial_____

5. Transient bruising, swelling, induration, and discomfort may occur.

    Initial_____

6. The correction that is achieved will diminish over time and may require additional treatment to be maintained.

    Initial_____

7. I understand that elective surgical procedures are most often delayed until after the termination of a pregnancy. My signature attests that, to the best of my knowledge, I am not pregnant at this time.

    Initial_____

8. The nature and effects of the operation, the risks and complications involved, as well as alternative methods of treatment have been fully explained to me and I understand them.

    Initial_____

9. For the purpose of advancing medical education, I consent to the admittance of authorized observers to the operating room.

    Initial_____

10. I understand that the practice of medicine and surgery is not an exact science and that reputable practitioners cannot guarantee results. No guarantee or assurance has been given to me by the doctor or anyone else as to the results that may be obtained.

    Initial_____

11. I have been given the opportunity to ask questions and all my questions have been answered to my satisfaction.

    Initial_____

12. I understand the two sides of the human body are not exactly the same and can never be made the same.

    Initial_____

13. I give permission to _____ to take still or motion clinical photographs with the understanding such photographs remain the property of the center. If in the judgment of the center medical research, education, or science will be benefited by their use, such photographs and related information may be published and republished in professional journals or medical books or used for any other purpose which the center may deem proper. It is specifically understood that in any such publication or use, I shall not be identified by name.

    Initial_____

My signature indicates that I have read this "Consent for Gore-Tex Facial Implant" and I understand and accept the risks involved in this operation. I hereby authorize _____ and/or the surgical team to perform this surgical procedure on me.

_____   _____
Signature (Patient/Responsible Party)   Date

_____   _____
Signature (Witness)   Date

If patient is a minor, complete the following:
Patient is a minor _____ years of age, and we, the undersigned, are the parents or guardian of the patient and do hereby consent for the patient.

_____   _____
Signature (Parent/Guardian)   Date

CONSENT FOR FAT TRANSFER

Patient's name_____
Date_____

I hereby authorize _____ and/or the surgical team to perform a fat transfer operation upon me (or my _____) to: (description of procedure) _____
_____
_____

1. The nature and effects of this operation, the risks and complications involved, as well as alternative methods of treatment have been fully explained to me and I understand them. I have been given the opportunity to ask questions and all questions have been answered to my satisfaction.

    Initial_____

2. I authorize the doctor(s) to remove fat from the "donor" area. I understand that although it is unlikely, there may be dimpling or unevenness of skin in this area.

    Initial_____

3. I consent to the administration of anesthetics by the doctor or under the direction of the anesthetist responsible for this service.

Initial_____

4. Unforeseen severe bruising, swelling, infection, pain, discoloration, disfigurement, muscle and/or nerve damage and scarring, although rare, are possible. I understand the practice of medicine and surgery is not an exact science and that reputable practitioners cannot guarantee results. No guarantee or assurance has been given to me by the doctor or anyone else as to the results that may be obtained.

Initial_____

5. I understand the two sides of the human body are not exactly the same and can never be made the same.

Initial_____

6. For the purpose of advancing education, I consent to the admittance of authorized observers to the operating room.

Initial_____

7. I give permission to _____ to take still or motion clinical photographs with the understanding such photographs remain the property of the center. If in the judgment of the center medical research, education, or science will be benefited by their use, such photographs and related information may be published and republished in professional journals or medical books or used for any other purpose which the center may deem proper. It is specifically understood that in any such publication or use, I shall not be identified by name.

Initial_____

8. I understand it is mandatory for me to have made prior arrangements to be driven to and from the doctor's office by a responsible adult.

Initial_____

9. I understand that elective surgical procedures are most often delayed until after the termination of a pregnancy. My signature attests that, to the best of my knowledge, I am not pregnant at this time.

Initial_____

10. I understand that fat transfer will not bring about permanent correction. Touch-ups may be needed at 3- to 6-month intervals to maintain the result. There will be additional cost for each touch-up procedure.

Initial_____

11. Improvement, not perfection, is the goal; average correction may vary from 20 to 80 percent.

Initial_____

12. Lumpiness or irregular contour may occur at the site of fat implantation; this may very rarely be permanent.

Initial_____

13. I agree to discontinue smoking entirely for a period of 2 weeks prior to surgery and 2 weeks immediately following surgery.

Initial_____

My signature indicates that I have read this "Consent for Fat Transfer" and I understand and accept the risks involved in this operation. I hereby authorize _____ and/or the surgical team to perform this surgical procedure on me.

First Treatment: _____ _____ _____
Signature (Patient/   Signature (Witness)   Date
Responsible Party)

Second Treatment: _____ _____ _____
Signature (Patient/   Signature (Witness)   Date
Responsible Party)

Third Treatment: _____ _____ _____
Signature (Patient/   Signature (Witness)   Date
Responsible Party)

Fourth Treatment: _____ _____ _____
Signature (Patient/   Signature (Witness)   Date
Responsible Party)

Fifth Treatment: _____ _____ _____
Signature (Patient/   Signature (Witness)   Date
Responsible Party)

Sixth Treatment: _____ _____ _____
Signature (Patient/   Signature (Witness)   Date
Responsible Party)

CHAPTER 10

Utilization of Botulinum Toxin in Cosmetic Dermatology

In the field of cosmetic dermatology, the physician can call upon botulinum A exotoxin[1] to temporarily block the impact of muscle hypersensitivity on facial expression and thereby improve the patient's esthetic appearance. Botox is now used routinely in cosmetic surgery for the temporary reduction of lines and wrinkles on the upper face (Fig. 10-1) by affecting the underlying muscle function.

Most wrinkles and esthetically undesirable facial lines are worsened by repeated muscle use and the hypertonic condition of the underlying muscular structure of the face. Botox can diminish the muscular contractions that create these undesirable lines in the upper face by temporarily paralyzing some groups of facial muscles. However, not all parts of a muscle group should be treated.[2]

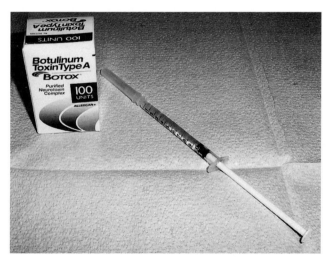

Figure 10-1   Botulinum toxin reconstituted in a PPD syringe with a 30-gauge needle.

Botox (Botulinum Toxin Type A) Purified Neurotoxin Complex is a sterile, vacuum-dried form of purified botulinum toxin type A, produced by the bacterium *Clostridium botulinum.* Eight subtypes are described; of these, types A, B, and E are associated with botulism in humans. Type A is presently the most effective subtype available for human use, and recently type B has become available. The effects of botulinum toxin have been known since the early 1900s, but it was not until 1980 that the toxin was found to be valuable for the treatment of a number of medical disorders.

Treatment of the aging face has long been an interest of the cosmetic surgeon using surgical and nonsurgical rejuvenation methods to treat aging skin and its supporting structures. Aging of the upper face is characterized by varying degrees of forehead laxity, with brow ptosis, horizontal creases in the middle forehead, and deepening glabellar furrows. It is often these furrows, or frown lines, that prompt the patient to visit the cosmetic surgeon. This chapter examines the treatment options for frown lines within the context of upper facial aging.

The Vertical Frown Line System

The formation of frown lines results from a complex set of variables. The inevitable aging process, hastened by excessive sun exposure and smoking, undermines dermal integrity, and the lax skin becomes redundant and tends to bunch up. The obvious loss of elasticity, the decreased supportive body of subcutaneous tissue, and the increased bony reabsorption cause the glabellar furrows to deepen. The procerus muscle pulls the interbrow skin inferiorly, creating horizontal creases at the root of the nose and between the brows. With age, the eyebrows often drop below the level of the supraorbital margins, and the angle of the brow to the root of the nose takes on a horizontal configuration rather than the more delicate youthful angle. The activity of the frontalis muscle helps elevate the plunging brows and thus causes both transient and, later, permanent horizontal creases. The corrugator supercilii muscle, which can be hyperactive, draws the ends of the brow together medially. This produces the characteristic vertical frown lines. Also, the skin type, texture, and previous acne scarring with atrophy and/or fibrosis influence the depth and character of frown lines.

Botox is not currently approved by the U.S. Food and Drug Administration for cosmetic purposes; therefore all such uses are considered off-label usage. It is important to note that Botox's greatest cosmetic success comes from injection into the upper portion of the face. In 1987, researchers first began using botulinum toxin in the glabellar area because there was no other satisfactory treatment for "frown lines."[3] The temporary paralysis caused by Botox is acceptable in this area because the treated muscles of the upper face are not needed for any essential function. The use of Botox is generally restricted to particular muscle groups, including "frown lines," or vertical glabella forehead furrows, and "crow's feet," or lateral canthal rhytids. It has also been shown that in the case of certain muscles, the use of Botox appears to be consistently more suitable than skin resurfacing, soft-tissue fillers, and/or surgical resection.[4] One major factor in the growing use of Botox is that it is a minimally invasive procedure that produces very refined esthetic results, although these results are only temporary. But this very impermanence can be seen as an advantage in that it minimizes the associated risk and gives both the physician and patient an opportunity to reconsider the results.[5]

Botulinum toxin is a nerve impulse "blocker." Specifically, Botox blocks neuromuscular conduction by binding to the receptor sites on motor nerve terminals, entering the nerve terminals, and inhibiting the release of acetylcholine. When Botox is injected intramuscularly, it produces a denervation muscle paralysis. Cosmetic benefits can be obtained by utilizing this effect, and with minimal complications. Therefore one can achieve a reduction of vertical glabellar furrows and lateral rhytids, horizontal brows, deep frown lines, expressive lines, and crow's feet. Photographic examples are given below. The most significant complication of Botox injection into the frontalis muscle is brow ptosis. However, it is important for the physician who is still mastering this procedure to remember that these complications can be minimized when one preselects patients for "preinjection" of the brow depressors as necessary.[6] Botox works especially well for deep wrinkles that are resistant to filler substances because it denervates the muscles that cause these depressions. Also, Botox can render resurfacing more effective because it can further diminish the rhytids that still remain after resurfacing.

Dilution and Storage

Each vial of Botox contains 100 U of (mouse) toxin, 0.5 mg of (human) albumin, and 0.9 mg of sodium chloride in a sterile, vacuum-dried form without preservative.

However, different physicians use various different dilutions. The preferred ones are usually based on the size of the defect and the number of affected areas to be treated. The manufacturer of Botox provides a dilution table up to 8 mL.

Klein[7] points out that many clinicians utilize 1 mL to dilute the vial, resulting in an ultimate concentration of 1 U/0.01 mL, but this yields only a small amount of solution (1 mL). However, he reports a range of dilutions from 1.0 to 10 mL per vial, with a mean dilution of 3 mL per vial.

When storing the vials, it is important to leave them freeze-dried. However, the length of viability of the reconstituted product is contested. The package insert recommends using the product within 4 h; but, as reported by Klein,[7] the actual longevity seems to be significantly greater. It is recommended that the reconstituted product be used within a 24-h period even though several physicians use it from 1 week to a month after reconstitution. Once reconstituted, the product should be stored at 28°C (under refrigeration).

The manufacturer recommends normal saline without preservatives for the dilution of Botox. However, some physicians report using preserved saline (0.9% benzoyl alcohol) with equal effectiveness.[8] It is important to note that preserving the solution in saline can "deactivate" the toxin. Botulinum toxin is fragile; therefore, the dilutent must be added slowly, as forceful squirting can damage the toxin, and the vial should not be shaken.

Botulinum toxin usually takes full effect within 1 to 2 weeks. However, the nerve endings usually grow new connections to the muscles at sites that have not been exposed to the toxin. To maintain the desired effects, therefore, Botox treatment is often repeated two to four times a year. During the consultation process, one must stress that there is a gradual and inevitable recurrence of laugh lines and crow's feet. Reduction of these defects is a continuous process that the patient must be willing to undergo. If not, the possibility of resurfacing or "filling" should be discussed and considered.

Botox purified neurotoxin complex has been recognized by the American Academy of Dermatology, American Academy of Ophthalmology, and National Institutes of Health as a safe and effective treatment. Its widest use has been for blepharospasm associated with dystonia (eyelid muscle spasms). The clinical data indicate that, in over 10 years of use involving thousands of patients, there have been few adverse side effects that might outweigh the potential esthetic benefits of the treatment. It should be noted that the degree of correction will vary from person to person.

When Botox is used for blepharospasm, the most widely reported side effects are drooping of the eyelid (ptosis), 11 percent; irritation of the injected area or tearing, including dry eye, opening of the eyelid (lagophthalmos), and sensitivity to light (photophobia), 10 percent; or an outward or inward turning of the eyelid (ectropion or entropion), inflammation of the cornea (keratitis), or "double vision" (diplopia), less than 1 percent.[4] It is important to note that these side effects are uncommon in cosmetic treatment. However, ptosis of the upper lid is a significant complication that some patients may encounter. This is due to the involvement of the levator palpebrae superioris muscle. If this unlikely complication should occur,it is generally transient in nature. The ptosis may last for 2 to 6 weeks and can be treated with apraclonidine 5% (Iopidine, from Alcon).[9] Botox is well tolerated by the vast majority of patients.

Other adverse effects of Botox injections may include some loss of facial expression, pain upon injection, edema, erythema, ecchymosis, and muscle soreness and weakness, including weakness of adjacent muscles caused by spreading of the toxin.[9] Some of these side effects may be avoided in the following ways:

1. The patient should avoid pressure or massage to the treated area. This may help preventing spread of the toxin.
2. The patient should avoid aspirin or aspirin-like products for 2 weeks prior to treatment.
3. The physician should keep the injection volume to the minimal effective dose.
4. The physician should be careful to stay within the anatomic boundaries.

Botox therapy is generally not appropriate for the lower face. It is used most effectively to treat deepening frown lines, forehead creases, and deepening crow's feet. It does not accomplish the same esthetic effect as cosmetic surgery. That is, both in regard to permanence and overall appearance, cosmetic surgery, usually a more costly and invasive procedure, can provide a longer-lasting result.

Generally, those patients who have hyperfunctioning muscles in the central brow and corrugator supercilia/procerus complex can expect a softening of their stern appearance.[6] In treatment of the brow, the beneficial effects of Botox are twofold: first, it relaxes the muscle that underlies the facial defect. These defects are brought about partly by the experience of physical and emotional tension over many years. The Botox treatment not only relieves the physical tension of the muscle but may also release the emotional and psychological tensions brought on by the defect, thus reenforcing the defect's development.

Pretreatment Consultation with the Patient

A thorough pretreatment consultation between patient and physician is extremely important.

In general, some experts suggest that, initially, the number of injections and amount of Botox utilized should be minimal, since the response to treatment varies on a case-by-case basis. Others suggest one to three treatments a few weeks apart. This span will allow for maximal correction.

It is important to review prospective patients' medical history in the context of their presumed results and expectations as a way of gauging and setting realistic expectations. Any patient with a history of a neuromuscular disorder or who is pregnant or lactating or anyone with a sensitivity to albumin should not be treated with Botox. In terms of drug interaction, aminoglycoside antibiotics and drugs that interfere with neuromuscular transmission may potentiate the effects of Botox and therefore should be used with caution in those patients.

Patients must also realize that both personal and environmental factors can affect the reappearance of their defects

and that they will not be able to predict exactly when repeated injections will be needed. After multiple treatments, over a period of time, many patients report that the effects of Botox become prolonged and that it is possible to allow more time is between treatments.

Technique

A typical treatment visit takes only about 10 min. Initially, the areas to be treated are prepped and the sites injected. The treated areas are then iced for 5–10 minutes. Slight redness and mild bruising are not uncommon; however, the avoidance of aspirin and antiplatelet medication for 2 weeks prior to treatment tends to decrease bruising. The patient is told that she may reapply cosmetics shortly after being treated but is also advised to avoid strenuous exercise for approximately 24 h. In most cases, results may be seen within the first few days, but in rare cases a week or two may go by before the full effect becomes apparent.

THE GLABELLA

Glabellar folds are not due to a single muscle contraction but rather to the combined effects of the corrugator supercilia, procerus, and orbicularis oculi.[10] This muscle group may be identified by asking the patient to frown. Individuals with these hyperfunctional lines may appear hostile, angry, or depressed.

For the glabellar region, a total of approximately 20 U is used. This solution is divided between the procerus (5 to 6 U), medial corrugators (4 U × 2), and orbicularis oculi (3 U × 2) above the corrugators. For repeat treatments, a slightly smaller dose—approximately 15 U per treatment—is generally used.

CROW'S FEET

Treatment of the lateral orbital area (crow's feet) modifies wrinkles in this area. These lines are diminished by weakening the lateral periorbital orbicularis oculi muscle through subcutaneous (not necessarily intramuscular) injections of Botox (Fig. 10-2A through D). The patient is asked to squint to better localize the muscle. Currently most authorities use approximately 12 U to this area. Specifically, 6 U are placed 1.5 cm lateral to the orbital rim at the level of the canthus. An additional 6 U is injected slightly inferior and medial to the previous injection. Slight adjustments may be made to these dosing recommendations based on the amount of wrinkling in this area.

FOREHEAD LINES

The forehead is another very popular area for Botox injections. Current treatment recommendations are a total of 16 to 20 U. This is usually divided equally between the hairline area and 1 cm above the eyebrows. The patient is asked to raise the brow in order to identify the muscle creases (Fig. 10-3A and B). The toxin is then injected intramuscularly. Multiple small injections, equally spaced, should adequately cover the forehead region. Carruthers[6] suggests avoiding injections lateral to the midpupillary line so as not to compromise expressivity. Slight variations in technique are necessary for individuals with brow ptosis.

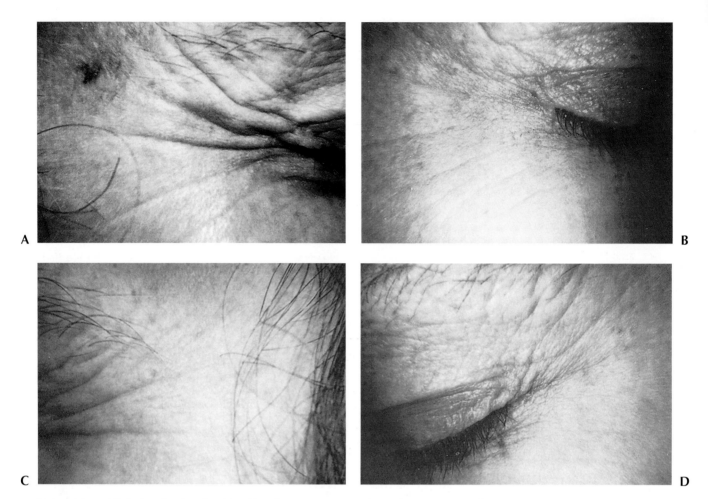

Figure 10-2 (*A*) Periocular rhytids, right side. The patient is actively smiling. (*B*) Periocular rhytids, left side. Patient is actively smiling. (*C*) Four weeks postinjection, right side. The patient is actively smiling. Note the reduction of wrinkling. (*D*) Four weeks postinjection, left side. The patient is actively smiling. Note the reduction of wrinkling.

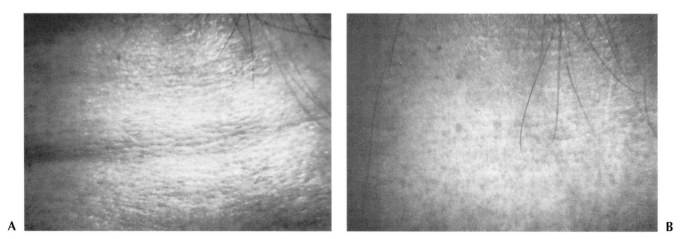

Figure 10-3 (*A*) Forehead rhytids. (*B*) Postinjection reduction.

OTHER FACIAL AREAS THAT MAY BE TREATED WITH BOTOX

Various additional anatomic locations on the face have been treated with Botox, but none of these are commonplace widely accepted, or treated as often as the areas to the forehead, crow's feet, and glabella. When Botox is used in these additional locations, the physician should proceed cautiously and with an "ideal patient." Some physicians inject into the platysmal bands of the aging neck; into the nasalis and base of the procerus to obliterate the "bunny lines" of the nose; into the levator labii superioris alaeque nasi (LLSAN) to soften the superior aspect of the nasolabial folds; and into the depressor anguli oris (DAO) to relieve wrinkling of the upper lip; and into the DAO, mentalis, and orbicularis oris to correct perioral lip wrinkling.

COMBINING BOTOX WITH OTHER TREATMENTS

Botox is often used in combination with CO_2 laser resurfacing. While the laser resurfaces the rhytids, the Botox treats the active muscles that exacerbate the facial lines. Botox has also been used before, during, and after an endoscopic eyebrow and forehead lifts to decrease the effect of the corrugator and procerus muscles, and it may be combined with almost all other cosmetic procedures used in combination with collagen.

OTHER USES

Hyperhidrosis of the axillar and palmar surfaces has been treated with Botox. Multiple and often painful injections are often necessary to treat this difficult condition.[10,11]

Conclusion

Use of Botox for the temporary treatment of hyperkinetic facial lines and furrows is a viable and effective primary and secondary therapy for patients with cosmetic problems. The unwanted side effects are minimal and can be reduced with proper understanding of the facial soft tissue anatomy, proper patient selection, and administration of the lowest effective doses with a minimal volume of delivery. Botox injections are not a replacement for surgery, skin resurfacing, or soft tissue augmentation. However, they have been shown to be of value when used as outlined above or in conjunction with a variety of other treatment options[5] (Fig. 10-4A through D and Fig. 10-5A and B).

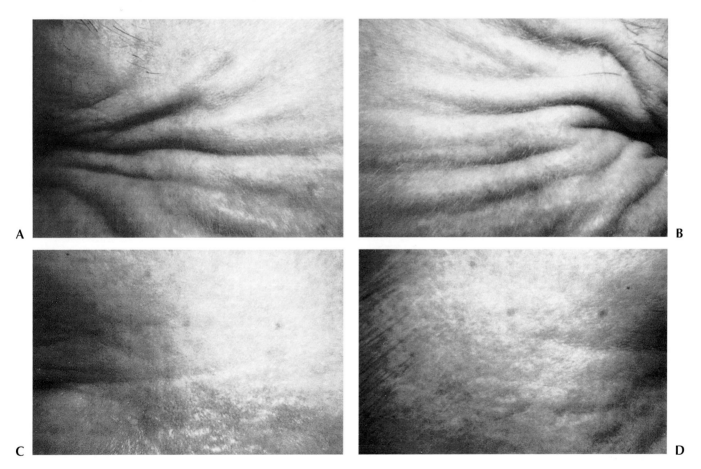

A   B

C   D

Figure 10-4 (*A*) Left side of patient post–laser resurfacing. The patient is actively smiling. (*B*) Right side of patient post–laser resurfacing. The patient is actively smiling. (*C*) Left side of patient postinjection. The patient is actively smiling. Note reduction of muscles bunching. (*D*) Right side of patient postinjection. The patient is actively smiling. Note reduction of muscles bunching.

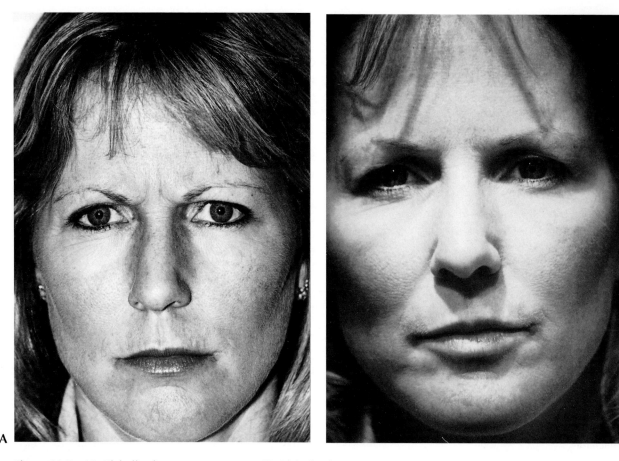

Figure 10-5 (*A*) Glabellar furrows pretreatment. (*B*) Glabellar furrows posttreatment.

References

1. Carruthers A, Kiene K, Carruthers J. Botulinum A exotoxin use in clinical dermatology. *J Am Acad Dermatol* 1996; 34:788–797.

2. Matarasso SL. Complications of botulinum A exotoxin for hyperfunctional lines. *Dermatol Surg* 1998; 24:1249–1254.

3. Carruthers J, Carruthers A. Botulinum A exotoxin use in clinical ophthalmology. *Can J Ophthalmol* 1996; 30:389–400.

4. Edelstein C, Shorr N, Jacobs J, et al. Oculoplastic experience with the cosmetic use of botulinum A exotoxin. *Dermatol Surg* 1998; 24:1208–1212.

5. Faigan S. Botox for the treatment of dynamic hyperkinetic facial lines and furrows: Adjunctive use in facial aesthetic surgery. *Plast Reconstr Surg* 1999; 103:107.

6. Carruthers A, Carruthers J. Clinical indications and injection technique for the cosmetic use of botulinum A exotoxin. *Dermatol Surg* 1998; 24:1189–1194.

7. Klein AW. Dilution and storage of botulinum toxin. *Dermatol Surg* 1998; 24:1179–1180.

8. Hankins CL, Strimling R, Robers GS. Botulinum A toxin for glabellar wrinkles. *Dermatol Surg* 1998;24:1181.

9. *Med Lett* 1999; 41:105.

10. Naumann M, Hofmann U, Bergmann I, et al. Focal hyperdrosis: Effective treatment with intracutaneous botulinum toxin. *Arch Dermatol* 1998 (3):301–304

11. Odderson IR. Hyperhidrosis treated by botulinum A exotoxin. *Dermatol Surg* l998; 24(11):1237–1241.

Patient Information

Botox

Botox (Botulinum Toxin Type A) Purified Neurotoxin Complex is a protein produced by the bacterium *Clostridium botulinum*. The effects of botulinum toxin have been known since the turn of the century, but not until 1980 was the toxin found to be therapeutically valuable for a number of medical disorders. Botox is used in cosmetic surgery for the temporary reduction of lines and wrinkles on the upper face.

How Does It Work?

Botulinum toxin is a nerve impulse "blocker." It binds to nerve endings and prevents the release of chemical transmitters that activate muscles. These chemicals carry the "message" from the brain that causes a muscle to contract; if the message is blocked, the muscle does not contract.

Botulinum toxin usually takes full effect within 1 to 2 weeks. However, the nerve endings usually grow new connections to the muscles at sites that have not been exposed to the toxin. Therefore, to maintain the effects of Botox therapy, treatment is often repeated about two to four times a year, as directed by your physician.

Is It Safe?

Botox Purified Neurotoxin Complex has been recognized by the American Academy of Neurology, American Academy of Ophthalmology, and National Institutes of Health as a safe and effective treatment. Its widest use has been for blepharospasm associated with dystonia (eyelid muscle spasms). More than 10 years of clinical experience involving thousands of patients testify to the potential benefits of this treatment.

It is important to understand that Botox is an effective, ongoing treatment for the improvement of wrinkles; it is not a cure. And, because every patient is different, the degree of correction will vary from person to person.

As with any therapy, some patients may experience side effects from the administration of Botox. The most frequent of such effects are drooping of the eyelid (ptosis), 11 percent; irritation of the injected area or tearing, including dry eye, opening of the eyelid (lagophthalmos), and sensitivity to light (photophobia), 10 percent; or an outward or inward turning of the eyelid (ectropion or entropion, respectively), inflammation of the cornea (keratitis), or "double vision" (diplopia), less than 1 percent. These side effects are uncommon in cosmetic treatments. Should they occur, they are usually transient in nature, and Botox is generally well tolerated by patients.

In addition, the effects of Botox may be increased with the use of certain antibiotics or other drugs that interfere with neuromuscular transmission.

Is Botox Therapy For Me?

If you want to know what Botox therapy can do for you, you should check with your doctor. Precisely how or if it can help depends on your doctor's judgment, your medical history, and the areas you would like to have treated.

For example, Botox therapy is not generally appropriate for smile lines or for the lower face. It is used most successfully for deep frown lines, forehead creases, and deep crow's feet. And it does not do what cosmetic surgery does. Your doctor can describe how the various procedures differ and which is best for your needs.

How Do I Get Started?

The first step is to have a pretreatment consultation with a physician who is trained in the use of Botox therapy. Your doctor will evaluate whether Botox treatment is appropriate for you, discuss the risks and benefits, and answer any questions you may have. No skin testing is needed, so treatment can begin immediately.

For your first treatment, the number of small injections you will need to get good initial results will depend on which areas are treated. Since the response to Botox may vary, you may need one to three treatments a few weeks apart in order to get maximal correction.

Which Areas Can Be Treated?

Botox therapy can make a remarkable difference in the treatment of depressions between the brows, on the forehead, and around the eyes.

Botox provides excellent results in softening certain deep frown lines and crow's feet, which are the furrows produced by frowning and smiling. Your doctor will review the appropriate use of Botox to achieve the result that is best for you.

What Is Involved?

You will find Botox therapy to be quick, easy, and generally painless. And you have to do it only two to four times a year. A typical treatment visit takes about 10 minutes. After your makeup is removed and your face is thoroughly cleaned, it takes just a few minutes to administer the drug.

Aside from the initial needle prick, you should feel little discomfort. The areas are then iced for a few minutes. Slight redness and mild bruising are unlikely but possible. Usually makeup can be reapplied before leaving the office, and normal activities can be resumed. Strenuous exercise should be avoided for 24 hours. The results can sometimes be seen within the first few hours, but it may take 1 to 2 weeks for the full effect to become apparent.

CONSENT FOR TREATMENT WITH BOTOX

Patient's Name _____

Date_____

You have the right to be informed and educated about your treatment(s). This will allow you to make an informed decision as to whether or not you wish to undergo the actual treatment. You have the right to read this consent form, ask any questions you may have, and have them answered to your satisfaction prior to receiving any treatment.

Botox therapy for wrinkles is an injection treatment designed to reduce facial expression lines. Botox is the trade name for Botulinum Purified Neurotoxin Complex. Botox is approved by the U.S. Food and Drug Administration (FDA) for the treatment of strabismus and blepharospasm, which are disorders of the muscles of the eyes. The use of Botox for other conditions, including Botox therapy for wrinkles, is considered "off-label." This means the FDA has not specifically approved Botox for this use. Botox therapy for wrinkles is a commonly performed cosmetic procedure throughout the world.

When Botox therapy for wrinkles is performed, tiny amounts of the toxin are injected into the facial muscles responsible for movement-associated lines and wrinkles. This injection weakens the muscle, thus reducing the associated lines and wrinkles.

Initial _____

Botox therapy for wrinkles works best for "dynamic" lines and wrinkles, that means those lines that are directly associated with the muscle movement. Botox therapy is less effective for fine textural changes on the skin surface, and for those lines present at rest.

Botox therapy is temporary; meaning that it will have to be repeated on a regular basis to remain effective. How long each treatment lasts will depend on many individual factors, including the degree of sun damage present on the skin, the depth of the lines, the size of the muscles, the amount and strength of Botox used, the frequency of retreatment, and the speed of neuromuscular repair. An average response is 3–6 months of diminished muscle contraction. Individual responses may be longer or shorter, depending on the above factors.

After Botox is placed into the targeted muscles, the weakening effect begins gradually over 3 to 5 days and is not complete for 2 weeks. Therefore optimal results are not seen for at least 2 weeks and sometimes longer. During this period, you may notice asymmetry or unevenness within the treated areas. This asymmetry will usually correct itself as the Botox takes effect.

There is no known permanent side effect of Botox therapy for wrinkles. There are, however, several well-known side effects that are temporary. These include the following:

Bruising—Usually at or near the injection site, may be increased with the use of aspirin or aspirin-like products, including vitamin E. This effect generally clears within 7 to 10 days. No treatment is necessary.

Headache—Related to the actual injections. This is uncommon, mild, and transient, lasting less than 24 hours. It may be relieved with Tylenol.

Pain at the injection site—Similar to headach, this is usually mild, transient, and relieved with Tylenol.

Asymmetry—As described above, if present, asymmetry is noticed within the first 2 weeks of therapy. It may possibly be corrected with "touch-up" injections, if necessary.

Muscle twitching—This is unusual, transient, and, if persistent, may possibly be corrected with "touch-up" injections.

Numbness—Actually a change in sensation noticed by some Botox patients in the treated areas, this is better described as a "dullness." It is usually noticed for only a few days after treatment. Further treatment is not necessary.

Eyebrow or eyelid ptosis (drooping) and double vision (diplopia)—Seen in 1 to 2 percent of patients receiving Botox therapy. This is temporary, lasting 2 to 4 weeks, and is usually mild. It may be treated with special eyedrops or, if necessary, patching of the affected eye.

Initial _____

Also, for reasons not fully understood, some patients may be less sensitive or more "resistant" to the effects of Botox. In these patients, Botox will not work as well or for as long as would ordinarily be expected. As the patient, I understand that the practice of medicine and surgery is not an exact science and that no results are guaranteed, including those of Botox therapy for wrinkles and lines.

Botox treatments are not recommended if you are pregnant or breast-feeding.

If you have a history of neurologic (nervous system) disease, especially if it is currently active, you may not be a good candidate for Botox therapy. This should be discussed with your treating neurologist or the physician caring for your neurologic disease prior to receiving Botox therapy.

If you are currently taking aminoglycoside antibiotics or penicillamine, you may need to discuss further your ability to receive Botox therapy with the doctor. Be sure to list all medications, including nonprescription and alternative that you are currently taking.

There are alternatives to Botox therapy for wrinkles, including no treatment, topical cream treatments, chemical peels, laser peeling, surgical face lifting, and surgical destruction of the muscles involved in the formation of dynamic lines.

I give permission to _____ to take still or motion clinical photographs with the understanding such photographs remain the property of the center. If, in the judgment of the center, medical research, education, or science will be benefited by their use, such photographs and related information may be published and republished in professional journals or medical books or used for any other purpose that the center may deem proper. It is specifically understood that in any such publication or use, I shall not be identified by name.

Because Botox therapy for wrinkles is considered a cosmetic procedure, insurance does not pay for treatment. Payment at the time of service is requested for all patients. You may ask for a price quote before your treatment. We request a 48 hour notice of cancellation for all scheduled Botox appointments.

I have been given the opportunity to ask questions and all my questions have been answered to my satisfaction.

Initial _____

My signature indicates that I have read this "Consent for Botox" and I understand and accept the risks involved with this procedure. I hereby authorize _____ and/or his delegated associates to treat my wrinkles and lines with Botox therapy.

First Treatment: _____ _____ _____
Signature (Patient/   Signature (Witness)   Date
Responsible Party)

Second Treatment: _____ _____ _____
Signature (Patient/   Signature (Witness)   Date
Responsible Party)

Third Treatment: _____ _____ _____
Signature (Patient/   Signature (Witness)   Date
Responsible Party)

Fourth Treatment: _____ _____ _____
Signature (Patient/   Signature (Witness)   Date
Responsible Party)

Fifth Treatment: _____ _____ _____
Signature (Patient/   Signature (Witness)   Date
Responsible Party)

Sixth Treatment: _____ _____ _____
Signature (Patient/   Signature (Witness)   Date
Responsible Party)

Preoperative Instructions

Please do not wear makeup to the office; if worn, please plan to remove it upon arrival.

To minimize the chance of bruising, please plan on doing the following:

Avoid aspirin or aspirin-containing products once you are scheduled for the procedure.

Preferably stay off aspirin or aspirin-containing products for 10 days prior to your treatment.

Avoid alcohol for 24 hours prior to the procedure.

Be sure to discuss with the doctor any bleeding tendencies and current medications being used.

Ice will be applied immediately following treatment. If you normally bruise easily, plan to go home and apply ice to the area(s) for an extra few hours.

Get a good night's sleep before the procedure.

Eat a *light* meal (breakfast or lunch) the day of treatment prior to the appointment.

Although the treatments are well tolerated by most patients, you may, to minimize any discomfort, apply a topical over-the-counter anesthetic agent (Ela-max 4%) to the area(s) to be treated for 1 hour prior to your visit. This can be purchased at your local pharmacy; follow the application instructions provided with this agent.

Botox Setup Tray

Patient

1. Makeup remover

Doctor

1. Clean gloves

Materials

1. 30 ml vial saline
2. One vial Botox from freezer (mix as directed)
3. One TB/insulin syringe
4. One 30-gauge needle
5. Gauze
6. Alcohol prep
7. Ice pack

Postoperative Instructions

The treatments are easily tolerated by most patients. You may use Tylenol or Extra-Strength Tylenol for any discomfort. It is best not to take aspirin or alcohol for 24 hours after procedure.

Ice will be applied immediately following treatment. If you normally bruise easily, plan to go home and apply ice to the area(s) for a few hours.

Avoid strenuous exercise (perspiring) for 24 hours following treatment. You may otherwise resume normal activities.

You may apply makeup upon leaving the office. Showering and facial cleansing are not restricted, but avoid facial massage for 24 hours.

CHAPTER 11

Chemical Peels

Chemical peeling refers to the application of a chemical agent to cause selective injury to the epidermis and upper dermis with the aim of rejuvenating the skin. Depending on the depth of penetration, this rejuvenation results in removal of superficial skin lesions, decrease of solar elastosis, and an increase in new collagen. Thus, the skin takes on a more uniform appearance as it becomes smoother in texture, with fewer rhytids and less dyschromia. While the advances in laser technology—with its unmatched predictability and precision—over the past decade has made it our resurfacing method of choice, alternative, more cost-effective resurfacing procedures, including chemical peels, remain important parts of a cosmetic surgeon's armamentarium.

History of Chemical Peel

The beginning of modern-day chemical peeling begins in 1882, with the first description by the German dermatologist Unna.[1] In the American medical literature, the first documentation is ascribed to Eller and Wolff[2,3] in 1941, with their publication on "skin peeling and scarification." It is of interest that MacKee and Karp[2,4] claimed to have used a comparable method in 1903. But it was not until the early 1960s that physicians' renewed interest led to the further evolution of this technique. Ayres[2,5] reported his work with trichloroacetic acid (TCA), and Baker[2,6] and Litton[2,7] introduced the use of phenol formulas to allow for medium-depth and deep chemical peeling, respectively. In 1984, Van Scott and Yu[8] presented the idea of superficial chemical peels with alpha-hydroxy acids. Next, the concept of combination medium-depth peels arose. Brody and Hailey[9,10] described the use of solid carbon dioxide in combination with 35% TCA in 1986, while others[9,11] established the use of Jessner's solution and 35% TCA in 1989. The history of chemical peels continues with the recent addition of the glycolic acid-TCA peel by Coleman and Futrell[9,12] as a new medium-depth peel.

Classification of Peeling Agents

The agents used for chemical peeling are categorized as superficial (epidermal), medium (epidermal/dermal), and deep (deep papillary, papillary/reticular), depending on the depth of the wound created by their application to the skin as measured in histologic studies. These anatomic depths merely present averages that may be greatly influenced by many variables, such as the agent in use, the epidermal barrier, skin thickness, and occlusion. Superficial chemical peeling agents include TCA (10 to 25%), Combe's (Jessner's) solution, alpha- and beta-hydroxy acids, Unna's paste, and carbon dioxide "snow." Phenol 88% and TCA (35 to 50% ± CO_2), Jessner's solution, and glycolic acid make up the medium-depth peeling agents. Finally, the Baker-Gordon phenol formula (occluded/nonoccluded) represents the only agent for deep chemical peels and is now mostly of historical value.[2]

Indications

Among the superficial chemical peeling agents, the best known is glycolic acid, an alpha-hydroxy acid. The most common indication for a glycolic acid peels is facial rejuvenation. In particular, it may succesfully treat manifestations of dyschromia such as melasma, lentigines, and postinflammatory hyperpigmentation secondary to acne. Also, early rhytids respond somewhat to these peels, as does mild acne scarring, especially when the treatment is carried out in a serial fashion. Furthermore, these peels may be succesfully used to treat a small to moderate number of actinic keratoses, early seborrheic keratoses, and flat warts. Finally, serial glycolic acid peels may serve as adjuncts to the treatment of various inflammatory diseases, including acne vulgaris, psoriasis, and even dermatophyte infections of the palms and soles. Besides these clinical indications, one should also consider—in terms of the patient's needs—other more practical factors like the low cost and relatively minor amount of postprocedural recovery time.[13,14]

The various strengths of TCA range from 25 to 100% (Fig. 11-1). TCA at a strength of 35% is the predominant agent for medium-depth chemical peels. Owing to its depth of penetration, TCA may be successfully used for facial rejuvenation in patients beyond the early manifestations of aging and photo damage. Thus, this peel may help with mild to mod-

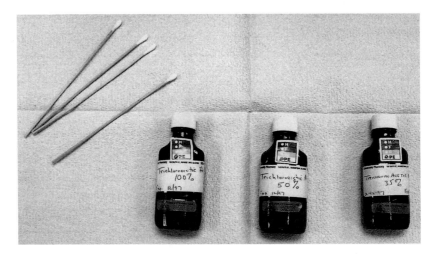

Figure 11-1   The various strengths of trichloroacetic acid (TCA) with applicator tips.

erate mobile rhytids noted around the eyes and on the cheeks. Deeper fixed rhytids of the perioral skin and nasolabial folds simply do not respond. Signs of photo damage such as moderate or even extensive involvement with actinic keratoses and lentigo simplex respond well to this peel. Other forms of dyschromia like melasma and postinflammatory hyperpigmentation may be improved, but the response is variable, such that a test site may be recommended. The 35% TCA peel helps with mild to moderate superficial acne scarring and has even been reported to improve the inflammatory diseases rosacea and seborrheic dermatitis. While some physicians claim that this type of chemical peel decreases the pore size, in our clinical experience there is no such effect. Finally, patients must be aware of the longer recovery time associated with this peel; that alone may militate against its use despite appropriate clinical indications.[15,16]

Deep chemical face peeling with phenol is rarely used today owing to its higher risk of serious complications and increased recovery time. In the past it has been primarily used to treat heavy wrinkling, marked photo damage in the form of actinic keratoses and solar lentigines, and even severe acne scarring. Although phenol peels can effect a dramatic smoothing of advanced rhytids, outcomes with prolonged or permanent erythema, hypopigmentation, and porcelain scarring occur all too commonly. Secondary to the systemic risks of phenol peeling, preexisting cardiac, hepatic, or renal disease is a definite contraindication.[2]

Preoperative Considerations

Appropriate patient selection is the most important aspect of achieving a good outcome with chemical peeling. This selection process is based on both physical and psychological findings. A patient may have all the proper physical requirements but lack the psychological makeup needed to ensure a result satisfactory to the patient and the physician—or just the opposite may be the case. The physical findings important to the outcome of chemical peeling are determined by a detailed history and physical examination, while psychological findings become apparent in the consultation interview when the appropriate questions are asked.

Historical aspects that need to be reviewed include the following.[13] Does the patient have a sensitivity to topical medications or perfume? If this is the case, the patient has a higher risk of complications such as contact dermatitis, irregular pigmentation, prolonged healing, and even scarring. What medications does the patient take? Both steroids and antimetabolites decrease the ability to heal. Estrogens and birth control pills enhance the risk for hyperpigmentation, especially if the patient has a history of melasma. Does the patient smoke? Chronic smokers are poor healers and carry a greater risk for scarring. Is there a history of poor wound healing or keloidal scarring? The presence of one or the other may increase the risk for scarring. Baseline laboratory tests are important in ruling out diabetes, thyroid dysfunction, and anemia, all of which may retard healing. Does the patient have a history of recurrent herpes simplex? Even without such a history, prophylactic treatment with an antiviral is indicated. Does the patient have a high level of anxiety? An anxious patient is less likely to hold still or follow instructions, such that a preoperative oral benzodiazepine taken 1 h prior to the procedure may be useful. Does the patient have a history of prior peels? If the answer is yes, how long ago did this occur and how did the patient react to it? This knowledge aids in choosing the best peel for the patient. Does the patient have a history of prior isotretinoin (Accutane) use or irradiation to the face as used in the past for the treatment of acne? Both isotretinoin and irradiation lead to a decreased number of sebaceous glands, which may result in poor healing and a higher likelihood of scarring, as it is the pilosebaceous unit that acts as the source of reepitheliazation.

Physical findings of importance are the patient's skin type in terms of tanning ability and photo aging, as outlined below.[2] Fitzpatrick's scale of tanning ability ranges from I to VI and denotes the ability to react to sun exposure with erythema, or tanning, or both. The white-skinned, light-haired, and light-eyed type I patient who never tans is ideal, as he or she is basically at no risk for developing pigmentary dyschromia. The white-skinned type II patient who rarely tans is also a good candidate, with a very low risk of pigmentary alterations. On the other hand, there is a notable risk of post-inflammatory hyperpigmentation or hypopigmentation in the type III patient, who sometimes burns mildly and usually tans. This risk turns into almost certain predictability with type IV skin, as seen in the dark-skinned Hispanic or Asian patient with dark hair and dark eyes. And patients with type V or VI skin, who are even darker, are not good candidates for chemical peeling.

Beyond Fitzpatrick's scale of tanning ability, one must also consider Glogau's classification of photo aging, which ranges from types I to IV.[17] Type I denotes the patient with basically no wrinkles who shows early signs of photo aging (pigmentary changes, no keratoses, mild wrinkling), is usually in his or her twenties or thirties, and wears minimal or no makeup. This patient will achieve notable improvement with just a superficial chemical peel. Type II refers to the patient with wrinkles in motion who has early to moderate photo aging (lentigines, palpable keratoses, parallel smile lines), is in their thirties or forties, and usually feels the need to wear foundation. While superficial peels may be of help in this patient, medium-depth peels will usually lead to the desired marked facial rejuvenation. Type III is identified as the patient with wrinkles at rest who presents with obvious photo aging (dyschromia, telangiectasias, visible keratoses, wrinkles even when not moving). Such a patient is usually in her fifties and uses heavy foundation makeup. While most of these patients would achieve a marked improvement from deep chemical peeling, they may get a satisfactory result from medium-depth peels alone or in combination with other resurfacing methods. Type IV is classified as the patient with only wrinkles and no normal skin who has severe photo aging (yellow-gray skin color, prior skin cancers, wrinkles throughout), is age 70 or older, and is unable to wear makeup, as it cakes and cracks. Even deep peels will not fully correct a patient with photo aging of this severity.

The following questions must be addressed in evaluating the patient's psychological makeup. Does the patient have realistic expectations? If not, even an objectively good outcome from the chemical peel may be unsatisfactory to the patient and consequently to the physician. What is the patient's level of tolerance in terms of expected sequelae such as erythema, flaking, and crusting? Patients with a low level of tolerance will require a lot of hand-holding by the physician and office staff and likely cause undue grief. Is the patient able and willing to follow instructions? Patients who are not compliant with postoperative care instructions have a higher risk of complications even if they are otherwise good candidates for chemical peeling. Does the patient have a history of depression? If this is the case, the patient may be more likely to have unrealistic expectations, a low level of tolerance, and be unable or unwilling to follow instructions (see Chap. 5).

To ensure a good outcome from chemical peeling, the preoperative consultation must address all of the above aspects of medical history as well as physical and psychological findings. If this is not done, both patient and clinician will risk disappointment.

Chemical Peeling Technique

The art of chemical peeling requires close adherence to several preparatory steps and detailed knowledge of peeling depth and application technique.

The first step in chemical peeling is the prepeel treatment of the skin. This step is not without controversy.[2] The use of retinoic acid once or twice a day for 1 to 2 weeks prior to the actual chemical peeling procedure does appear to debride the stratum corneum, allowing for increased and more even penetration of the peeling agents as well as possibly a more rapid reepitheliazation. However, the effectiveness of retinoic acid alone or in combination with hydroquinone and a mild topical steroid in a prepeel program intended to diminish the incidence of postpeel hyperpigmentation has not been proven to date.

The next step consists of preparing the skin on the day of treatment. To permit an effective and even chemical peeling independent of the type of agent used for the peel, the sebaceous oils of the skin must be thoroughly removed. Repeated facial cleansing by the patient with soap and water may be adequate. The most aggressive defatting regimen involves using cotton balls soaked with acetone to clean the skin for several minutes. As the endpoint of this preparation is reached, the skin surface feels slightly rough, like fine sandpaper, and individual small scales take on a white color owing to the lack of oils. With this type of thorough defatting of the skin, an otherwise mild peeling agent may be transformed into a deeper resurfacing tool.

After the skin has been prepared, the issue of anesthesia must be addressed. With a superficial or medium-depth peel, the use of an oral or intramuscular sedative 1 h before the procedure may be helpful, especially if the patient is anxious. Topical anesthesia is also recommended. A deep chemical peel with phenol, on the other hand, is best performed under conscious sedation and/or local nerve blocks with 1% plain lidocaine; postoperatively, oral analgesics may be advised for pain control. Without adequate anesthesia, the patient can expect a moderate amount of a stinging or burning during the procedure, which gradually increases and then culminates at the halfway point during the procedure. This discomfort can be kept to a minimum with the help of dry cold compresses and fanned cool air.

Once the skin has been prepped and anesthesia administered, the patient's safety must be assured. With any chemical peel, the patient's eyes must be protected. An antibiotic ointment applied to the eyes under a protective gauze pad or goggles is usually sufficient as a mechanical barrier. By keeping the patient's head erected at a 30-degree angle, the pull of gravity will keep the chemical agent from leaking into the eyes. It is also mandatory to have a container with sterile water at the bedside and an emergency eye shower close by so that the eyes can be flushed properly if the unexpected should happen. In the case of a deep phenol peel, the required safety measures include intravenous access, cardiac monitoring, and the presence of certified advanced cardiac life support (ACLS) medical health professionals at all times (see Chap. 8).

Now, after following all of the above steps, the actual chemical peel may take place. The art in chemical peeling lies in the evaluation of peel depth and use of the proper application technique.[18] The depth of peel is determined on the basis of color, time, and palpation, as follows. The skin in a superficial peel to the level of the epidermis takes on a diffusely pink-white frosted appearance that reblanches in 10 to 15 min; palpation reveals boggy edema. In a medium-depth chemical peel to the level of the papillary dermis, the skin turns a uniform light cloudy-white color that clears in 15 to 20 min; palpation demonstrates "parchment paper-like feeling" with any peel creating injury to the dermis. Deep peels to the level of the deep papillary-reticular dermis cause the skin to assume a dense, cloudy-white frosting that resolves in 40 to 45 min. If the skin turns a gray-yellow frosted color that does not blanch after 40 min, there has been injury to the deep reticular dermis and a prolonged healing time is to be expected. Equipped with this knowledge in evaluating the peel depth, the physician may proceed with the chemical peel after making sure that the tray has been correctly set up. For any chemical peel, the tray must have bottles containing peeling agent, with a small quantity placed into an easily accessible container, plenty of cotton-tipped applicators, and a stacked supply of 3 × 3 square cotton gauze pads next to a container of ice water. A cotton-tipped applicator is first dipped into the container with the peeling agent and then rolled against the rim to drain excessive amounts, which might otherwise roll down the patient's face in an uncontrolled fashion. The peeling agent is put on a small defined area, about 2.5 × 2.5 cm, by rolling the damp applicator up and down with steady pressure and without covering the same area twice. A gauze pad is used to blot away any excess of the peeling agent. Each treated site requires the use of a new cotton-tipped applicator and gauze pad. The treated skin should take on a frosted appearance. The actual color of the frost and the time it takes to appear varies according to the type of peeling agent used, as outlined above. This application technique is used to peel the anatomic units of the face in order, beginning with the forehead and then proceeding to the cheeks, chin, nose, lips, and eyelids. Dry, cold gauze compresses are used throughout the procedure to minimize discomfort in the treated sites.

Postoperative Care

The postoperative care after a peel may be considered under the headings of immediate, intermediate, and late.[18] Immediate care occurs right after the peeling agent has been removed. By definition, intermediate care takes place within 1 to 10 days of a peel. And late care is the management after completion of reepithelialization.

Immediate postoperative care involves an occlusive dressing with a bland emollient, antibiotic ointment, or mild topical steroid; it varies with the individual physician's preference. Immediate postpeel stinging may be controlled with ice-water compresses or topical analgesic ointment.

Intermediate postoperative care includes twice-daily application of a bland ointment, gentle cleansing under the shower head on day 3, complete avoidance of rubbing, and follow-up on days 1, 3, and 7. Pain may be caused by a secondary bacterial, viral, or fungal infection. Accordingly, a skin culture must be obtained and the patient started on appropriate medications. Intense irritation without obvious signs of an infectious process may be helped with antihistamines and a short course of a topical or oral steroid. Milia are frequent and can be quite easily removed with the help of a no. 11 blade and a comedone extractor.

Late postoperative care consists of avoidance of sun exposure and the strict use of sun protection for the first 3 to 6 months, as the new skin is still relatively fragile during this time. The presence of hyperpigmentation may require treatment with retinoin (Retin-A), hydroquinone, and a mild topical steroid, often in combination, and/or cosmetic coverage. Hypopigmentation may also benefit from cosmetic coverage. Prolonged erythema after a chemical peel (<3 months) is best treated with bland topical ointments and steroids. Follow-up at 6 weeks and 3 months completes the postoperative care.

Complications

Not all skin changes following a chemical peel are considered complications. Postoperative changes are classified as category I and category II.[19] Category I refers to expected sequelae of the postoperative period that will resolve completely and represent procedural side effects. Category II entails sequelae that are characteristic of the individual peeling agent, are independent of the patient setting, and can be due to incorrect use of a treatment or a lapse in postoperative care. The last of these are true complications.

Procedural side effects and their proper treatment have been addressed above, in the section on postoperative care. They encompass postpeel stinging, secondary infections (bacterial, viral, and fungal), milia, pigmentary alterations, and prolonged erythema (<3 months).[2,15,19]

The list of true complications includes permanent pigmentary changes, prolonged erythema (>3 months), hypertrophic scarring, atrophy, and systemic effects such as the hepatic, renal, and cardiac abnormalities sometimes seen with phenol.[19–21]

Permanent pigmentary changes are seen most frequently with phenol, followed by 50% TCA peels. While persistent hyperpigmentation or hypopigmentation is rare in 35% TCA peels or combination peels, they may even occur in higher-strength alpha-hydroxy acid peels.

Prolonged postpeel erythema (>3 months) is a rare complication that may occur after any type of chemical peeling. It presents as early as the second week postpeel as erythema, pruritus, and textural changes. These symptoms are the result of an inflammatory reaction that can be due to both intrinsic and extrinsic causes. Sensitivity to the peeling agent, contact dermatitis (allergic or irritant), and a preexistant inflammatory skin disorder (rosacea, systemic lupus erythematosus, or atopic eczema) make up the intrinsic causes. Extrinsic causes are prepeel treatment with glycolic acid and/or retinoin, peeling technique (aggressive preparation and/or application technique), and, again, contact dermatitis (allergic or irritant). Proper treatment includes avoidance therapy, meticulous wound care, bland topical ointments, steroids, and frequent reassurance of the patient. If left untreated, this prolonged postpeel erythema may result in postinflammatory hyperpigmentation, textural changes, or scarring.[1]

Hypertrophic scarring has been most commonly reported with phenol and 50% TCA peels, but it may also occur with medium-depth and even superficial chemical peels when a high-strength glycolic acid is used. Sites of predilection are the mandible and the periorbital region. The incidence of this dreadful complication can be held to a minimum by avoiding chemical peels in patients who have a history of hypertrophic scarring or use of isotretinoin less than 18 months earlier and those who have had a major facial plastic surgery procedure less than 6 months earlier. If hypertrophic scarring does occur, early intervention is the key to success. High-potency topical steroids, steroids injected intralesionally, and application of steroid-impregnated tape or silicone sheeting may, alone or in combination, serve to treat this complication. Q-switched pulsed-dye laser treatment may also be of some benefit when used early.

Atrophy is a rather uncommon complication. It is more likely to occur after repeated phenol peels than with either a single phenol or a TCA peel. Cosmetic coverage is the only treatment option.

The systemic effects of phenol are well known. This chemical is directly toxic to the heart, inactivated in the liver, and excreted by the kidneys. Consequently, the use of phenol is contraindicated in patients with a known history of cardiac, hepatic, or renal problems. To minimize the occurrence of systemic complications, every patient undergoing a phenol peel must have cardiac monitoring, proper IV fluid administration, adequate diuresis, and well-controlled application of the chemical.[2,22]

Conclusion

While the unsurpassed precision of laser technology makes it today's "gold standard" among skin resurfacing methods, chemical peeling should not be cast aside as an outmoded resurfacing procedure. In fact, in the hands of the knowledgeable physician, chemical peeling is a valuable alternative to laser resurfacing and a useful adjunct to other cosmetic procedures. Its relative advantages over laser resurfacing are as follows. First, it enables the physician to be more in control of the resurfacing process, as its success is based actual know-how more than dependence on a computer chip. Second, it is a relatively simple procedure, involving less technical complexity and lower cost. Then, aside from the more antiquated use of phenol, light and medium chemical peeling rarely requires intravenous or general anesthesia. Last, it has a wide scope of application with both medical and cosmetic appeal, as its indications range from the treatment of precancerous lesions, flat warts, and mild acne to reversal of the signs of aging and facial scarring. The results of deep peels with TCA (Figs.11-2A and B, 11-3A and B, and 11-4A and B) and phenol (Fig. 11-5A and B) can be quite remarkable when the treatment is appropriately performed on the proper type of patient.

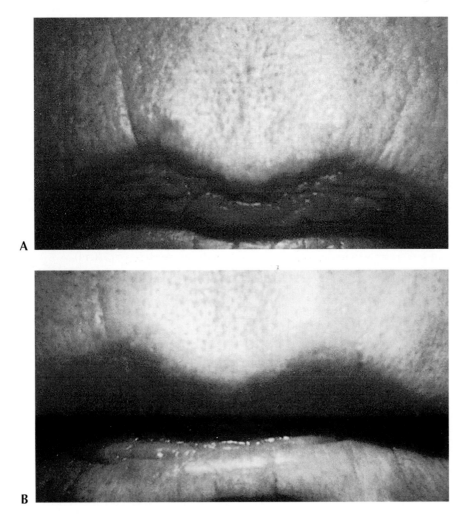

Figure 11-2 (*A*) Preoperative photo of patient undergoing 35% TCA peel. (*B*) Postoperative photo of the same patient.

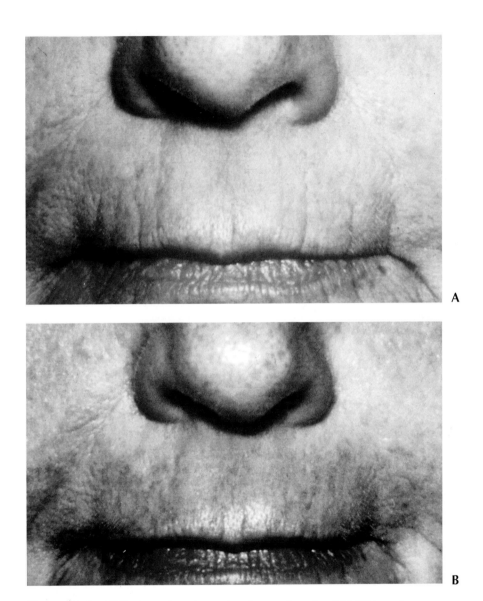

Figure 11-3 (*A*) Preoperative photo of patient undergoing 50% TCA peel.
(*B*) Postoperative photo of the same patient.

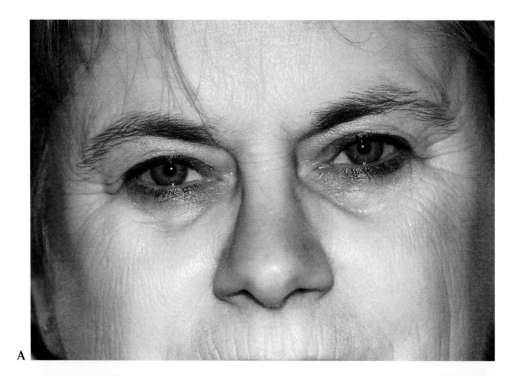

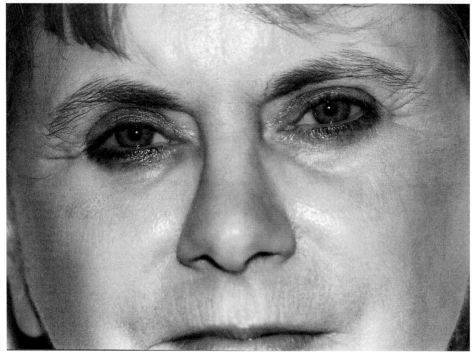

Figure 11-4   (*A*) Preoperative full-face photo of patient undergoing TCA peel and upper blepharoplasty. (*B*) Postoperative photo of the same patient.

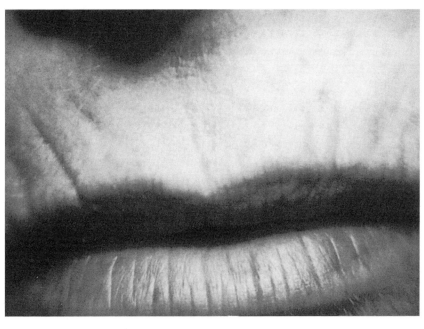

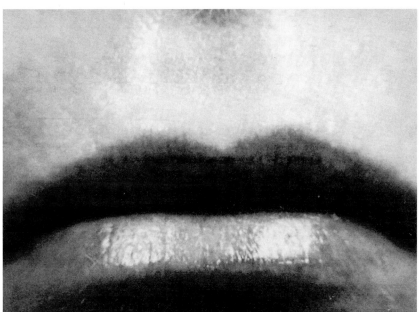

Figure 11-5 (*A*) Preoperative photo of patient undergoing phenol peel. (*B*) Postoperative photo of the same patient.

References

1. Maloney BP, Millman B, Monheit G, et al. The etiology of prolonged erythema after chemical peel. *Dermatol Surg* 1998; 24:337–341.

2. Glogau RG, Matarasso SL. Chemical peels: Trichloroacetic acid and phenol. *Dermatol Clin* 1995; 13:263–275.

3. Eller JJ, Wolff S. Skin peeling and scarification. *JAMA* 1941; 116:934.

4. MacKee G, Karp F. The treatment of post-acne scars with phenol. *Br J Dermatol* 1952; 64:465.

5. Ayres S. Superficial chemosurgery in treating aging skin. *Arch Dermatol* 1962; 85:385.

6. Baker T. The ablation of rhytides by chemical means. *J Fla Med Assoc* 1961; 47:451–454.

7. Litton C. Chemical face lifting. *Plast Reconstr Surg* 1962; 29:371.

8. Van Scott EJ, Yu RJ. Alpha-hydroxy acids: Procedures for use in clinical practice. *Cutis* 1989; 43:222–228.

9. Yarde T, Ostad A, Hyun-Soo L, et al. A clinical and histologic evaluation of medium-depth peels. *Dermatol Surg* 1996; 22:781–786.

10. Brody HJ, Hailey CW. Medium-depth chemical peeling of the skin: A variation of superficial chemosurgery. *J Dermatol Surg Oncol* 1986; 12:1268–1275.

11. Monheit GD. The Jessner's + TCA peel: A medium-depth chemical peel. *J Dermatol Surg Oncol* 1989; 15:945–950.

12. Coleman WP III, Futrell JM. The glycolic acid trichloroacetic acid peel. *J Dermatol Surg Oncol* 1994; 20:76–80.

13. Slavin JW. Considerations in alpha hydroxy acid peels. *Clin Plast Surg* 1998; 25(1):45–52.

14. Murad H, Shamban AT, Premo PS. The use of glycolic acid as a peeling agent. *Dermatol Clin* 1995; 13:285–307.

15. Roenigk RK, Brodland DG. A primer of facial chemical peel. *Dermatol Clin* 1993; 11:349–359.

16. Lober CW. Chemoexfoliation—Indications and cautions. *J Am Acad Dermatol* 1987; 17:109.

17. Glogau RG. Chemical peeling and aging skin. *J Geriatr Dermatol* 1994; 2:30–35.

18. Dinner MI, Arzt JS. The art of the trichloroacetic acid chemical peel. *Clin Plast Surg* 1998; 25:53–62.

19. Resnik SS, Resnik BI. Complications of chemical peeling. *Dermatol Clin* 1995; 13:309–312.

20. Brody HJ. Complications of chemical peeling. *J Dermatol Surg Oncol* 1989; 15:1010–1019.

21. Goldman PM, Freed MI. Aesthetic problems in chemical peeling. *J Dermatol Surg Oncol* 1989; 15:1020–1024.

22. Botta SA, Straith RE, Goodwin HH. Cardiac arrhythmias in phenol face peeling: A suggested protocol for prevention. *Aesthet Plast Surg* 1988; 12:115–117.

Patient Information

Chemical Peel

In order to look their best, people throughout the ages have tried to improve their skin's appearance by various methods.

Records show that, for centuries, ancient Egyptians used alabaster and pumice to minimize facial imperfections. Today, there are safer and more effective procedures that can improve wrinkled, scarred, or damaged skin and help you achieve a more attractive appearance.

The chemical peel is one of these procedures. Chemical peels are most effective on skin with mild acne scarring, freckles, age spots, melasma, or other irregular pigmentation and skin wrinkled by age or the sun. Thick, rough, red, precancerous growths called keratoses can also be removed with the chemical peel.

During this procedure, chemical agents that remove the damaged skin's outer layer are applied. Thin scabs form over the treated areas and fall off a few days later, revealing smoother, younger-looking skin. Most scars, lines, or irregular pigmentation will be minimized, and the "new" skin will be smooth and fresh looking. Three types of chemical peels are available: a light peel, which is used to lighten superficial age spots and fine wrinkles; a medium peel, for more advanced sun-damaged skin and age lines; and a deep peel, which uses the chemical phenol to help correct more severe conditions. Your doctor will determine which technique will be most effective for you.

The cosmetic surgeons of this center help people develop and maintain a healthy and attractive appearance. Our skilled surgeons specialize in the chemical peel procedure and have used their knowledge, skill, and experience for more than a decade to help numerous patients achieve smoother skin.

The Procedure

The medium and deep peel procedures take about 30 to 45 minutes. Generally, you are given a light sedative orally to relax you prior to surgery or, if you prefer, intravenous anesthesia can be administered. After your skin is cleaned with an antibacterial cleanser and your eyes and hair are protected, the chemical is applied to a small area of your face with a cotton-tipped applicator. This process is repeated on the other areas of your face.

Few side effects are associated with the lighter chemical peels. You may experience a slight burning sensation, which may last a short time, when the doctor applies the solution. Immediately after the procedure, your skin may feel as if it had been slightly sunburned.

After the peel, your skin becomes red and moist and thin scabs begin to form. You may experience some tingling and slight itching as these crusts form and your skin heals. You can help speed the healing process by using the special cleansers and ointments your doctor will recommend. Your "new" skin will have a pink cast, which will fade within 4 to 6 weeks. For several months following your procedure, you should wear a sunscreen whenever you are outdoors and avoid exposing yourself to direct sunlight. Most patients resume normal activities within a day to a few weeks, depending upon the depth of the peel.

The Results

The chemical peel is very effective in minimizing wrinkles, scars, age spots, and other skin irregularities. The new skin exposed by the peel is tight and smooth, which gives you a younger and fresher appearance.

Most patients who undergo this procedure are pleased with the results, and many patients experience a significant improvement in their skin's appearance. Depending upon the extent of their skin imperfections, some patients may require more than one treatment to achieve maximum results.

Ask for a consultation to discuss how the chemical peel procedure can help you achieve smoother, younger-looking skin.

Preoperative Instructions

Wash your face thoroughly on the morning of your surgery and do not apply any moisturizers or other cosmetics.

Wear no makeup to the office. Be sure eyelashes are free of mascara.

Wash your hair the night before surgery or on the morning of surgery.

Get a good night's sleep.

Eat a *light* breakfast or lunch on the day of surgery.

Contact lenses must be removed before surgery. If you wish to remove them in the office, please bring your case.

Wear loose clothes that either zip or button and do not have to be pulled over your head.

Do not wear any jewelry to the office on the day of surgery.

Arrange for a ride to and from the office. (You will not be allowed to drive, since your face may be swollen.)

You may apply a topical over-the-counter anesthetic agent (Ela-max 4%) to the area(s) to be treated for 1 hour prior to your visit. This product may be purchased at your local pharmacy, and you may follow the application instructions packaged with it.

Obtain Aquaphor ointment from your local pharmacy prior to surgery (this is a nonprescription item) for postoperative use. If the area around the mouth or lips will be treated, it may be useful for you to obtain the following items before surgery: a baby toothbrush, "Ensure" shakes—nutritional drinks in cans, and straws.

Be sure to discuss with the doctor any history of herpes infection (cold sores) or allergies to medications and review all medicines currently being taken or used.

Take all medications as prescribed *prior* to treatment. These normally will include an antibiotic, an antiviral (if the lip is being treated), and a Valium.

The fee is to be paid in full at the preoperative visit, which must be 7 to 14 days prior to surgery.

Chemical Peel Setup Tray

Patient

1. Cape
2. Nonsterile surgery hat

Doctor

1. Clean gloves

Materials

1. Clean cotton balls
   A. 2 to 4 if small areas
   B. 8 to 10 for large areas
2. Sterile bowl for tap water
3. Acetone
4. 4 cotton-tipped applicators
5. Small stack of clean 3 × 3 gauze
6. Tap water
7. Trichloroacetic acid 25% or 35%
8. Aquaphor ointment
9. Physician's hand towel
10. Nonsterile white drape
11. Small squirt bottle with tap water

Postoperative Instructions

Go home and relax. The sedative used for the chemical peel may last several hours postoperatively.

Do not be alarmed if swelling appears around your eyes and mouth. It can be severe but will gradually subside. Sit up as much as possible and sleep in a head-elevated position for 3 to 5 days, either on three pillows or in a reclining chair. This will help reduce the natural swelling that occurs after this type of procedure.

Pain medication may be taken every 3 to 4 hours as needed, but no aspirin. The burning sensation may last for several hours or days but will gradually ease. Continue any other medications as prescribed.

Pronounced swelling is common. This is normal, and will gradually subside over the first 6 to 10 days. Apply Aquaphor ointment liberally and keep the skin moist throughout the day by reapplying ointment as necessary. The skin should not be allowed to dry out. At bedtime, reapply Aquaphor ointment liberally.

You may shower daily, but avoid the treated areas for 3 days. After 3 days, the face may be rinsed lightly with water. Use *no soap* or any other product (this includes makeup) on treated areas for 2 weeks.

Any excessive bleeding, redness, tenderness, swelling, or pus should be reported immediately to our office at (___) _____.

Your first postoperative visit should be between 7 and 14 days following your procedure.

Your new skin will appear red. This is normal and should be expected.

At this time, a determination will be made as to whether use of makeup can be resumed. If stinging occurs when you resume using makeup, remove it and try again in 5 to 7 days.

After 2 weeks, you should begin wearing sunscreen daily. Discontinue if stinging occurs.

Avoid Retin-A and glycolic acid products for 6 weeks following the procedure.

You should be seen in the office 6 weeks after your peel for another checkup.

Direct sun exposure *must* be avoided completely for at least 3 months postoperatively because of the increased photosensitivity and pigmentation of the chemically peeled areas. Remember, sunscreen with an SPF of 15 or higher must be applied prior to sun exposure. Avoid sun exposure especially between the hours of 10 AM and 5 PM.

Avoid physical exertion for 2 weeks so as not to perspire. Also avoid exposure to strong wind and extreme cold for 2 weeks.

You may shampoo your hair after the third postoperative day. For men, no shaving for 7 to 10 days.

Occasionally, additional peel treatments are necessary to achieve the desired result.

Glycolic Acid Peels

WHAT IS A GLYCOLIC ACID PEEL?

Skin peeling is a process in which a chemical is applied to the skin in order to produce an improvement in appearance. The procedure is primarily used for the removal of fine wrinkles in facial skin, mild acne scarring, some pigmentation problems, and other minor skin blemishes. The procedure is done on an outpatient basis in the office.

HOW MUCH IMPROVEMENT CAN I EXPECT?

The amount of improvement depends on each person's skin. Those who expect perfect skin will be disappointed. The ideal skin type is best described as a fair nordic skin that has had very little exposure to the sun. At the opposite extreme would be a tawny skin that has been further darkened by constant exposure to the sun and the elements. Maximal improvement generally occurs after four to six glycolic acid peels usually given at 1- to 2-week intervals.

How Long Will I Be Incapacitated or How Much Time Will I Lose from Work?

You will probably want to avoid public contact for a period of 24 hours following the procedure. Although bandages are not worn, you would have to avoid exposure to excessive wind, heat, or cold during this time. After the peeling occurs, a faint pinkness will be apparent; this usually fades within 4 to 6 weeks. If you have a strong history of recurrent facial herpes simplex, a glycolic acid peel may not be for you.

How Long Will the Procedure Take?

It depends on the area to be treated. Treatment for the entire face takes 30 minutes.

Will It Hurt?

As the chemical is applied with a cotton applicator, a burning/stinging sensation will develop. This may become very intense and will last for 3 to 5 minutes, until the chemical is neutralized. Immediately after the procedure, you may feel as if you had a warm sunburn. The skin may feel somewhat tight as the peeling occurs during the next 2 to 5 days.

How Soon Can I Have Another Glycolic Acid Peel?

It depends on a number of factors, including type of skin, your individual reaction to the first glycolic acid peel, and the severity of the problem. Follow-up glycolic acid peels are usually done at 1- to 2-week intervals after the first peel. It is normal to wait 3 to 6 months to see the final result.

Chemical Exfoliation Preoperative Instructions

Wash your face thoroughly on the morning of your surgery and do not apply any moisturizers or other cosmetics.

Wear no makeup to the office. Be sure your eyelashes are free of mascara.

Wash your hair the night before surgery or on the morning of surgery.

Get a good night's sleep.

Eat a *light* breakfast or lunch on the day of surgery.

Contact lenses must be removed before surgery. If you wish to remove them in the office, please bring your case.

Wear loose clothes that either zip or button and do not have to be pulled over your head.

Do not wear any jewelry to the office on the day of surgery.

Arrange for a ride to and from the office. (You will not be allowed to drive, since your face may be swollen.)

You may apply a topical over-the-counter anesthetic agent (Ela-max 4%) to the area(s) to be treated for 1 hour prior to your visit. This product may be purchased at your local pharmacy, and you may follow the application instructions packaged with it.

Obtain Aquaphor ointment from your local pharmacy prior to surgery (this is a nonprescription item) for postoperative use. If the area around the mouth or lips will be treated, it may be useful for you to obtain the following items before surgery: a baby toothbrush, "Ensure" shakes—nutritional drinks in cans, and straws.

Be sure to discuss with the doctor any history of herpes infection (cold sores) or allergies to medications and review all medicines currently being taken or used.

Take all medications as prescribed *prior* to treatment. These normally will include an antibiotic, an antiviral (if the lip is being treated), and a Valium.

The fee is to be paid in full at the preoperative visit, which must be 7 to 14 days prior to surgery.

Chemical Exfoliation— Glycolic Acid Peel Setup Tray

Patient
1. Clean washed face
2. Clean hat

Nurse
1. Clean gloves

Materials
1. 50% or 70% glycolic acid
2. Two cotton balls
3. Small plastic container with lid
4. Two clean wet washcloths
5. Aquaphor ointment (optional)
6. Kitchen timer

Postoperative Instructions

Go home and relax. The sedative used for the chemical peel may last several hours postoperatively.

Do not be alarmed if swelling appears around your eyes and mouth. It can be severe but will gradually subside. Sit up as much as possible and sleep in a head-elevated position for 3 to 5 days, either on three pillows or in a reclining chair. This will help reduce the natural swelling that occurs after this type of procedure.

Pain medication may be taken every 3 to 4 hours as needed, but no aspirin. The burning sensation may last for several hours or days but will gradually ease. Continue any other medications as prescribed.

Pronounced swelling is common. This is normal, and will gradually subside over the first 6 to 10 days. Apply Aquaphor ointment liberally and keep the skin moist throughout the day by reapplying ointment as necessary. The skin should not be allowed to dry out. At bedtime, reapply Aquaphor ointment liberally.

You may shower daily, but avoid the treated areas for 3 days. After 3 days, the face may be rinsed lightly with water. Use *no soap* or any other product (this includes makeup) on treated areas for 2 weeks.

Any excessive bleeding, redness, tenderness, swelling, or pus should be reported immediately to our office at (___) _____.

Your first postoperative visit should be between 7 and 14 days following your procedure.

Your new skin will appear red. This is normal and should be expected.

At this time, a determination will be made as to whether use of makeup can be resumed. If stinging occurs when you resume using makeup, remove it and try again in 5 to 7 days.

After 2 weeks you should begin wearing sunscreen daily. Discontinue if stinging occurs.

Avoid Retin-A and glycolic acid products for 6 weeks following the procedure.

You should be seen in the office 6 weeks after your peel for another checkup.

Direct sun exposure *must* be avoided completely for at least 3 months postoperatively because of the increased photosensitivity and pigmentation of the chemically peeled areas. Remember, sunscreen with an SPF of 15 or higher must be applied prior to sun exposure. Avoid sun exposure especially between the hours of 10 AM and 5 PM.

Avoid physical exertion for 2 weeks so as not to perspire. Also avoid exposure to strong wind and extreme cold for 2 weeks.

You may shampoo your hair after the third postoperative day. For men, no shaving for 7 to 10 days.

Occasionally, additional peel treatments are necessary to achieve the desired result.

CONSENT FOR CHEMICAL PEEL

Patient's Name _____
Date_____

I hereby authorize _____ and/or the surgical team to perform a surgical procedure commonly known as "face peeling" on _____.
(Patient Name) or (Myself)

1. The procedure listed in paragraph 1 has been explained to me by the above doctor(s), and I completely understand the nature and consequences of the procedure. The following points have been specifically made clear:

   a. That the process involves the application of chemicals to the face, which may require the use of a face mask following said chemical application.

   b. That during the "face peeling" process, I will experience discomfort and swelling and my face will be covered with a crust, which will usually separate within 5 to 10 days.

   c. That the skin will have a reddish appearance, which may persist for several weeks; that at the juncture of the treated and untreated areas there may be a difference in color, pigmentation, and texture of skin.

   d. Scarring can occur, causing permanent disfigurement.

   e. Blotching of pigmentation can occur, which may be permanent.

   f. Infection can occur.

   g. I may not see any improvement.

   h. Avoidance of sun exposure is necessary for several weeks or months.

   Initial_____

2. I am aware that the practice of medicine and surgery is not an exact science, and I acknowledge that no guarantees have been made to me as to the results of the operation or procedure.

   Initial_____

3. I give permission to _____ to take still or motion clinical photographs with the understanding such photographs remain the property of the center. If in the judgment of the center medical research, education, or science will be benefited by their use, such photographs and related information may be published and republished in professional journals or medical books or used for any other purpose which the center may deem proper. It is specifically understood that in any such publication or use, I shall not be identified by name.

   Initial_____

4. For the purpose of advancing medical education, I consent to the admittance of authorized observers to the operating room.

   Initial_____

5. I understand it is mandatory for me to have made prior arrangements to be driven to and from the doctor's office by a responsible adult.

   Initial_____

6. I am not known to be allergic to anything except: (list):_____
   _____

7. I understand that elective surgical procedures are most often delayed until after the termination of a pregnancy. My signature attests that to the best of my knowledge I am not pregnant at this time.

   Initial_____

8. I agree to discontinue smoking entirely for a period of 2 weeks prior to surgery and 2 weeks immediately following surgery.

   Initial_____

9. I have been given the opportunity to ask questions and all questions have been answered to my satisfaction.

   Initial_____

My signature indicates that I have read this "Consent for Chemical Peel" and I understand and accept the risks involved with this operation. I hereby authorize _____ and/or the surgical team to perform this surgical procedure on me.

_____   _____
Signature (Patient/Responsible Party)   Date

_____   _____
Signature (Witness)   Date

If patient is a minor, complete the following:

Patient is a minor _____ years of age, and we, the undersigned, are the parents or guardian of the patient and do hereby consent for the patient.

_____   _____
Signature (Parent/Guardian)   Date

CONSENT FOR CHEMICAL EXFOLIATION

Patient's Name _____

Date_____

1. I hereby authorize _____ and/or his delegated associates to perform a procedure or series of procedures commonly known as "chemical exfoliation" or glycolic acid peel.

   _____
   (Patient Name) or (Myself)

2. The procedure listed in Paragraph 1 has been explained to me by the above doctor(s), and I completely understand the nature and consequences of the procedure. The following points have been specifically made clear:

   a. That the process involves the application of chemicals to the face. Infrequently, crusting can occur.

   b. That the skin will have a reddish appearance that may persist for several weeks; that at the juncture of the treated and untreated areas there may be a difference in color, pigmentation, and texture of skin.

   c. During the exfoliation process, I may experience discomfort.

   d. Scarring can occur, causing permanent disfiguration.

   e. Blotching of pigmentation can occur that may be permanent.

   f. Avoidance of sun exposure and other sources of ultraviolet rays is recommended.

   g. Infection can occur.

   h. I may not see any improvement.

   Initial_____

3. I am aware that the practice of medicine and surgery is not an exact science, and I acknowledge that no guarantees have been made to me as to the results of the operation or procedure.

   Initial_____

4. I give permission to _____ to take still or motion clinical photographs with the understanding such photographs remain the property of the center. If in the judgment of the center medical research, education, or science will be benefited by their use, such photographs and related information may be published and republished in professional journals or medical books or used for any other purpose which the center may deem proper. It is specifically understood that in any such publication or use, I shall not be identified by name.

   Initial_____

5. I agree to keep the above doctors informed of any change of address so that he or she can notify me to any late findings, and I agree to cooperate with the above doctors in my care after surgery until completely discharged.

   Initial_____

6. I am not known to be allergic to anything except (list):_____

   _____

7. I do not have a history of cold sores/fever blisters on my face. If I am prone to cold sores/fever blisters, I have made arrangements with the doctor to have a prescription for medicine in the event an outbreak should arise following treatment.

   Initial_____

8. I have been given the opportunity to ask questions and all my questions have been answered to my satisfaction.

   Initial_____

My signature indicates that I have read this "Consent for Chemical Exfoliation" and I understand and accept the risks involved with this procedure. I hereby authorize _____ and/or the delegated associates to perform a procedure or series of procedures commonly known as "chemical exfoliation" or glycolic acid peel.

First Treatment: _____ _____ _____
Signature (Patient/   Signature (Witness)   Date
Responsible Party)

Second Treatment: _____ _____ _____
Signature (Patient/   Signature (Witness)   Date
Responsible Party)

Third Treatment: _____ _____ _____
Signature (Patient/   Signature (Witness)   Date
Responsible Party)

Fourth Treatment: _____ _____ _____
Signature (Patient/   Signature (Witness)   Date
Responsible Party)

Fifth Treatment: _____ _____ _____
Signature (Patient/   Signature (Witness)   Date
Responsible Party)

Sixth Treatment: _____ _____ _____
Signature (Patient/   Signature (Witness)   Date
Responsible Party)

CHAPTER 12

Microdermabrasion

Microdermabrasion is a rejuvenation technique that was introduced in the United States fairly recently. In Europe, there has already been more than 10 years of experience with this technique. Several studies establish microdermabrasion as a well-accepted rejuvenation technique, which is usually bloodless, noninvasive, and—in contrast to chemical peels—chemical-free. Microdermabrasion fulfills the expectations of many cosmetic surgery patients. It is associated with a minimum of downtime; therefore, patients can have lunchtime treatment and return to work without problems.[1]

Microdermabrasion was developed in an era when open dermabrasion was found to possibly release infectious viral particles—especially HIV and hepatitis B—within the abraded tissue fragments, which were too small to be eliminated by any available filter (see Chap. 13). To reduce the exposure of the staff and operators, a closed-circuit dermabrading system was developed.[2]

A compressor and an aspirator are the essential components of this system. Aluminum oxide crystals (Fig. 12-1) and/or sodium chloride salt (Fig. 12-2) are projected from a reservoir via a tubing system and handpiece onto the patient's skin. These crystals and loosened skin debris are evacuated from the treatment surface into a second tubing system and finally deposited in another closed container, thereby preventing contamination.

Indications

The depth of the peel depends on the projectile pressure and intensity of the aspirator. With low-pressure settings, the

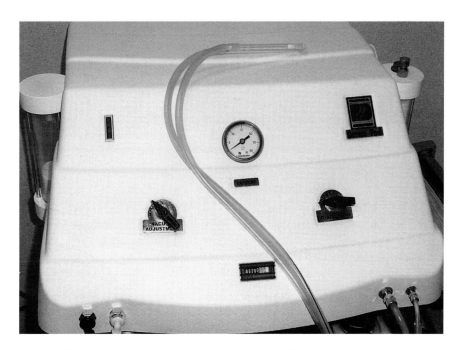

Figure 12-1 Microdermabrador utilizing sodium chloride.

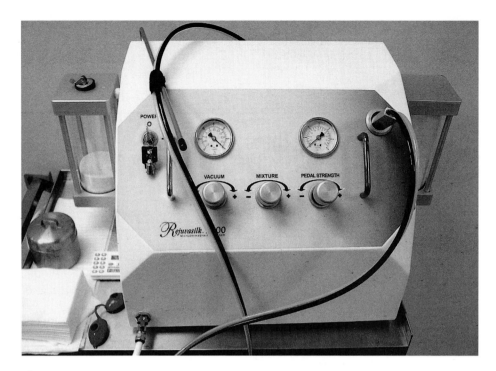

Figure 12-2 Microdermabrador utilizing aluminum oxide crystals.

skin is gently exfoliated; higher-pressure settings can induce deep dermal layer abrasions. The reported indications include treatment of fine rhytids, photo aging, active acne and mild acne scarring, closed and open comedones, dyschromia, as well as a sallow complexion. Microdermabrasion is effective in the treatment of patients ranging from Fitzpatrick skin type I to IV.[1,3] (See Chap. 11 for discussion of skin types.)

Furthermore, notoriously difficult-to-treat areas like the neckline and backs of the hands are treated successfully with a lower-pressure setting. Microdermabrasion of the photo-aged neck in patients who have previously undergone facial laser resurfacing helps diminish the often pronounced contrast between the rejuvenated facial skin and the untreated neck without adverse sequelae. In contrast, deep rhytids, melasma, deep scars, telangiectases, or actinic keratosis will not disappear with microdermabrasion.

The physician-trained skin care specialist conducts an initial evaluation of the patient. The patient completes a dermapeel analysis sheet and past medical history and skin condition are reviewed. A consent form is signed and all questions are answered. It is important to ask the patient specifically about his or her use of antioxidants like vitamin E and ginkgo biloba as well as anticoagulants or any other antiplatelet agent (including aspirin). These medications can increase posttreatment edema and erythema and even lead to petechiae.

The patient is instructed to discontinue all alpha-hydroxy acid-containing products as well as tretinoin (Retin-A) cream, and benzoyl peroxide preparations 2 days prior to the microdermabrasion appointment. Patients are allowed to resume their usual cosmetic routine 2 days posttreatment.

If a patient has had a recurrent herpes simplex infection within the past year, he or she must start on an antiviral agent 1 day prior to treatment and continue this for 7 to 10 days. Treatment isotretinoin (Accutane) may be a relative issue with respect to time, since the drug must be discontinued before starting microdermabrasion. The procedure is either performed by a physician or a specially trained nurse or esthetician.

Technique

The treatment area must be thoroughly cleansed with water before the procedure begins. The skin surface is then prepped with alcohol to remove makeup residue and oil. A headband is worn by the patient in order to avoid hair pulling during treatment. The patient's eyes are covered with goggles or tape to prevent irritation from the aluminum oxide/sodium chloride crystals. If a patient uses contact lenses, he or she is instructed to remove them prior to the treatment. The patient's clothes are protected with a large towel, exposing only the treatment areas. It is advised that the operator wear a mask and goggles or glasses.

Treatment areas are microdermabraded in smooth, stroking movements with a minimum of two passes. After each pass, there is a change in direction, with emphasized treatment of certain problem areas. Depending on the indication, the treatment intensity can be modified by shortening or lengthening the treatment time or by varying the amount of projectile and aspiration pressure and also by changing the handpiece. Although it is possible to dermabrade the skin deeply by pressing a foot paddle, which increases all variables including projectile and aspiration pressure, it is difficult to achieve an evenly abraded surface in this way. Because of this lack of control, the foot paddle–aided deeper abrasion mode is rarely used.

Results

For the best esthetic results, six consecutive treatments 2 weeks apart are recommended. As the treatment is usually painless and well tolerated, there is no need for topical anesthetics. Patients regularly report some discomfort on initial treatment. However, this "discomfort" is generally transient. Yet, all patients experience some erythema. This is, in fact, the treatment endpoint and only lasts an hour or two. Some patients develop streaking, which usually fades within a day or two. Sometimes transient edema, especially in the periorbital areas, has been observed. Cool compresses help resolve it within a few days. To date, there has been no scarring, blistering, or pigmentary change in any of our patients. Two patients with an undisclosed past medical history of herpes simplex developed a new breakout after the procedure. They were treated successfully with an antiviral agent without residual scarring or the development of dyschromia. For further treatments, antiviral prophylaxis was required for patients.[4] Posttreatment care includes a bland moisturizer and the generous use of chemical-free sunscreen.

However, before any of these results can be achieved, patients considering skin resurfacing need to decide how dramatic an effect they want and how much time they have for a given procedure. There are some microdermabrasion peels that give minimal results and cause the least disruptions to patients' lives. Other patients, with severe scarring or damaged skin, may conclude that they need a greater, more pronounced effect and are therefore willing to deal more readily with severe disruptions in their personal lives.

Microdermabrasion is an effective and nonsurgical solution for younger, smoother looking skin. There is still controversy over microdermabrasion versus dermabrasion, acid peels, and laser resurfacing. However, microdermabrasion has the advantages of little or no discomfort, no anesthesia, minimal to no recuperation time and an immediate return to normal activities. Finally, this technique is suitable for all skin types. The associated use of Renova, Kinerase, and glycolic acid products can enhance the appearance of patients with mild rhytids (Fig. 12-3). The fact that this is a nonsurgical procedure carried out in a nonmedical setting helps patients to feel relaxed (Fig 12-4).

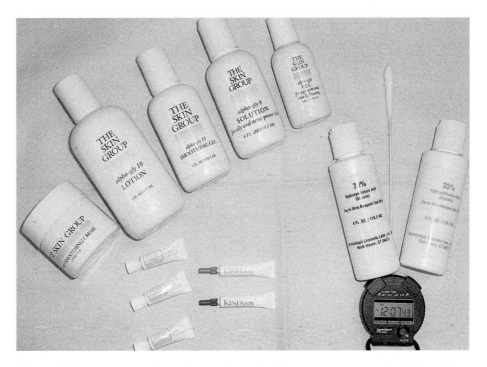

Figure 12-3 Various products that can be utilized between treatments, including alpha-hydroxy acid, Renova, Kinerase, vitamin C serum.

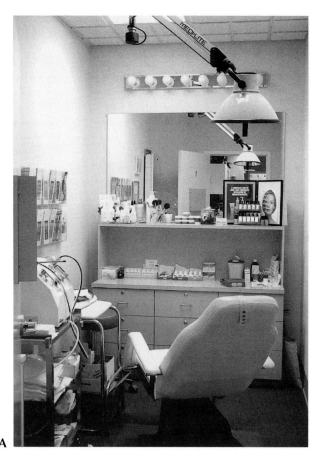

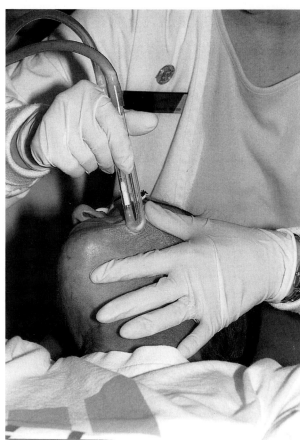

A   B

Figure 12-4 (*A*) A treatment suite without a "medical look." However, cosmetic surgical brochures and other booklets are appropriately displayed. (*B*) Patient receiving treatment.

References

1. Hopping S. The power peel: Its emergency and future in cosmetic surgery. *Int J Cosmet Surg* 1998-1999; 6(2): 98–100.

2. Newman J, Hopping S, Patterson R, et al. Power peeling (micro skin abrasion). *Int J Cosmet Surg* 1998-1999; 6(2): 101–105.

3. Tsai RY, Wang CN, Chan HL. Aluminum oxide crystal microdermabrasion. A new technique for treating facial scarring. *Dermatol Surg* 1995; 21(6):539–542.

4. Warmuth IP, Bader R, Scarborough DA, et al. Herpes simplex infection after microdermabrasion. *Cosmet Dermatol* 1999; 127(7):13.

Patient Information

Microdermabrasion

We were all born with smooth, baby-soft skin. As we go through life, our skin becomes a road map, showing the effects of where we have been and what we have done. Even if we have taken care of our skin, many of us are affected by childhood and adolescent diseases, while heredity and gravity always take their toll.

Exposure to the sun, use of alcohol, smoking, and nutrition all accelerate the signs of aging. Moles, warts, keratoses, scars from disease, or facial trauma may further affect our skin and may even affect the way we perceive ourselves. Chemical peels and dermabrasion have been the primary means of reducing these undesirable effects.

Dermapeel is a revolutionary new skin restoration process, commonly referred to as "the lunchtime peel" because the procedure takes only minutes to perform and most people can return to work immediately. Used at exclusive European spas for over 5 years, this unique skin rejuvenation technique has recently received clearance from the U.S. Food and Drug Administration (FDA).

The Procedure

A highly controlled vacuum and pressure are used to move microscopically abrasive crystals over the surface of the skin. This action causes little or no discomfort while it gently removes the outer layer of the skin. By repeating this process over the course of several weeks or months, the younger, softer skin moves to the surface, revealing significant textural and color changes.

Dermapeel—as opposed to dermabrasion, acid peels, and laser resurfacing—offers the following advantages:

Little or no discomfort

No anesthesia

No recuperation period

Patients return to activities immediately

Reasonable prices

Treats all skin types

Treatment time and frequency may vary, depending on the severity of the skin problem(s) and the area being treated. Most patients require 3 to 10 treatments, after which a maintenance program can be established.

Because the procedure is noninvasive and nonsurgical, you may return to your normal activities immediately. You may notice an immediate improvement in the treated area and your skin may feel softer, and appear smoother and younger-looking. These desirable effects should increase over the course of the treatment series. Treatable conditions are sun damaged skin, enlarged pores, oily and acne-prone skin, acne scars, blackheads and whiteheads, age spots and superficial pigmentation, fine wrinkles, post-laser enhancement, neck and décolleté.

Preoperative Instructions

Please do not wear makeup to the office; if it is worn, please plan to remove it upon arrival.

Sign the consent form.

Be sure to wash face after signing in for your appointment.

Once a staff member has taken you to a room, you will be given a clean hat to wear.

Your face will be gently wiped with face toner.

You will then be asked to wear the supplied protective eye goggles during the procedure.

Once back in the room, you will be asked to lie flat on the table (or as close that as is comfortable). Your shoulders will then be covered with a drape. The sterilized glass wand will then be moved back and forth over the facial surfaces, then repeated in a perpendicular pattern, avoiding the eyelids and soft tissue beneath the eye.

Once the peel is complete, the crystals will be lightly brushed from your face with a dry gauze. Your face will then be wiped gently with a cold cloth. You will then be asked to apply moisturizer to the skin surfaces. This completes the procedure. You may apply your makeup if you wish.

Microdermabrasion Setup Tray

Patient

1. Clean hat
2. Goggles
3. Drape sheet
4. Clean washed face

Nurse

1. Clean gloves
2. Mask
3. Glasses (optional)

Materials

1. Aloe toner
2. Sterile wand
3. Clean wet washcloth
4. Moisturizer with SPF 24 sunscreen

Postoperative Instructions

Do not do strenuous exercise for 12 hours after the initial dermapeel, since this may cause excessive redness.

Be sure to continue use of your moisturizer to the peeled skin surfaces. You may resume your normal skin care products on the morning following your treatment. You may be slightly more sensitive to vitamin A–acid creams (Retin-A) and alpha-hydroxy acids (glycolic acid) for a few days following treatment.

You may resume normal bathing and facial cleansing immediately following treatment. Avoid harsh cleansing products for 5 to 7 days.

You may be slightly more sun-sensitive for 5 to 7 days following treatment. Please take the normal precautions of wearing sun block and a hat.

Consent for Microdermabrasion

Patient's name_____
Date_____

I hereby authorize _____ and/or delegated associates to perform a microdermabrasion procedure on me, which works on the epidermis and removes a portion of same using a combination of controlled suction concomitantly with air abrasion and aluminum oxide particles. I understand that it may take multiple treatments to achieve the desired effect. It is important to note that for the treatment of acne scars, stretch marks (stria) and/or other scars, 12 or more treatments may be required. However, most patients experience some improvement after 1 treatment.

The following points have been discussed with me:

1. The potential benefits of the proposed procedure
2. The possible alternative medical procedure(s)
3. The probability of success
4. The reasonably anticipated consequences if the procedure is not performed
5. The most likely possible combinations/risks involved with the proposed procedure and subsequent healing period, including but not limited to temporary redness and temporary tightness, which generally resolves within 4 to 24 hours after the procedure. If aggressive treatment of acne scars and stretch marks were performed, then additional aftercare management similar to the dermabrasion/laser resurfacing protocol would be utilized.

6. The possibility of ancillary services/fees including but not limited to anesthesia, laboratory and/or surgical facility use.
7. I may not see any improvement.

Initial_____

I am aware of the following possible experiences/risks with particle-beam resurfacing:

Discomfort. If discomfort is experienced, I shall simply inform the operator. I give my permission for the administration of anesthesia when deemed appropriate by the physician. (This is necessary only when aggressively treating scars and/or stretch marks and generally requires only topical or local anesthesia.)

Wound healing. This is generally not an issue, as no open wound exists. In the advent of an aggressive treatment, crusting and inflammation may occur. This is only associated with scar and stria treatments.

Bruising/swelling/infection. Bruising and swelling generally are nonexistent. Finally, skin infection is a possibility any time a skin procedure is performed. However, in this case, the epidermis has only been partially removed so unless otherwise noted this is highly unlikely to occur.

Pigment changes (skin color). As the outer portion of skin is being removed, there is a possibility of the treated area becoming somewhat different in color than the surrounding skin.

Scarring. Scarring is a rare occurrence, but it is a possibility where the skin's surface is disrupted. To minimize the chances of scarring, it is important that you follow all postoperative instructions carefully.

Eye exposure. Protective eyewear (shields) will be provided. It is important to keep those shields on and keep the eyes closed during the treatment in order to protect your eyes from particle exposure. It would feel as if grit or sand had gotten into your eye.

Lines/Streaking. Although uncommon, you may have temporary lines or streaking of the skin, which could last for several days.

I am aware that the practice of medicine and surgery is not an exact science, and I acknowledge that no guarantees have been made to me as to the results of the operation or procedure.

I have been given the opportunity to ask questions and all questions have been answered to my satisfaction.

I give permission to _____ to take still or motion clinical photographs with the understanding such photographs remain the property of the center. If in the judgment of the center, medical research, education, or science will be benefited by their use, such photographs and related information may be published and republished in professional journals or medical books or used for any other purpose which the center may deem proper. It is specifically understood that in any such publication or use, I shall not be identified by name.

Initial_____

My signature indicates that I have read this "Consent for Microdermabrasion" and I understand and accept the risks involved with this procedure. I hereby authorize _____ and/or the delegated associates to perform this procedure on me.

First Treatment: _____ _____ _____
Signature (Patient/   Signature (Witness)   Date
Responsible Party)

Second Treatment: _____ _____ _____
Signature (Patient/   Signature (Witness)   Date
Responsible Party)

Third Treatment: _____ _____ _____
Signature (Patient/   Signature (Witness)   Date
Responsible Party)

Fourth Treatment: _____ _____ _____
Signature (Patient/   Signature (Witness)   Date
Responsible Party)

Fifth Treatment: _____ _____ _____
Signature (Patient/   Signature (Witness)   Date
Responsible Party)

Sixth Treatment: _____ _____ _____
Signature (Patient/   Signature (Witness)   Date
Responsible Party)

DERMAPEEL ANALYSIS SHEET

Patient's name: _____
Date_____

In order to have us tailor the dermapeel to your needs, please answer the following questions:

	YES	NO
• Have you had dermapeels or power peels in the past?	____	____
• If so, how many?	____	____
• Have you had a laser peel or dermabrasion? When? _____	____	____
• Have you had a herpes or cold sore infection? With what frequency? _____	____	____
• Have you taken Accutane for acne treatment? When did that treatment end? _____	____	____
• Do you smoke?	____	____
• Are you currently using any of the following prescription or over-the-counter products?		
Retin A	____	____
Renova	____	____
Avita	____	____
Differin	____	____
Alpha Gly Products	____	____
Beta-Hydroxy Acid	____	____
Glycolic/Alpha-Hydroxy Acid	____	____
• Have you ever had a glycolic acid peel? Salon _____ Doctor's office _____	____	____
• Are you wearing contact lenses?	____	____
• Are you using aspirin, Advil, or vitamin E? Purpose:_____	____	____

CHAPTER 13

Dermabrasion

Dermabrasion has been the "gold standard" with which all other resurfacing techniques are compared. Forms of dermabrasion have existed since Egyptian times, when skin was sanded with pumice, papyrus, or various types of sandpaper in order to improve its appearance and texture. Dermabrasion as we know it today was initially introduced in 1905 by a German dermatologist who experimented with planing the skin to various levels using a burr attached to dental equipment. At this time dermabrasion was shown to be particularly effective for the improvement of acne scarring when wounding was carried out to the reticular dermis.[1–3] In 1953, Kurtin developed modern dermabrasion utilizing a wire brush, motor-driven abraders, and topical refrigerants.[4] Also in 1953, Robbins developed and introduced the diamond fraise.[5] Since then several modifications, refinements, and diverse techniques utilizing dermabrasion have been introduced.

Mechanism of Action

Dermabrasion results in the removal of tissue down to the level of papillary dermis, with reepithelialization occurring via the underlying adnexal structures. Therefore, dermabrasion tends to be more useful than other techniques for superficial scars, which can often be greatly improved. Deeper scars or lesions with dermal elements tend to improve with dermabrasion but are less responsive. Cutaneous areas such as the face, which have more adnexal structures and richer blood supplies, tend to recover quickly. In treating areas other than the face, there will usually be a certain amount of scarring. Since reepithelialization occurs via the adnexal structures, patients who lack these or have altered adnexal structures or sebaceous glands may not be good candidates for dermabrasion. It is thought that dermabrasion alters primary scar formation by creating a repair zone of new, more organized collagen within the papillary dermis. New collagen tends to show an increase in collagen bundle density and size, with a unidirectional orientation of collagen fibers that tends to be more parallel to the epidermal surface. In addition, there appears to be an upregulation of tenascin expression throughout the papillary dermis and the expres-

sion of alpha-6/beta-4 integrin subunit on the keratinocytes throughout the stratum spinosum.[6] Additional evidence in dermabraded photo-aged skin demonstrates an increase in the production of procollagen I mRNA that appears to correlate with the clinical improvement of wrinkled skin.[7]

Indications for Dermabrasion

Although initially developed for the treatment of postacne scarring, the indications for dermabrasion have expanded over time, with at least 50 reported entities having been treated with dermabrasion with relative success. Some of the more important indications are listed in Table 13-1. Many of these entities can currently be treated more readily with new technology. However, dermabrasion remains a valuable approach. The alternative treatments for photo aging, skin appendageal growths, as well as some forms of scarring include CO_2 lasers, while pigmented lesions and tattoos can be removed utilizing either the alexandrite, Q-switched neodymium aluminum–garnet (Nd:YAG) (see Chap. 14), or ruby lasers in a relatively bloodless manner with minimal risk of scarring. Today multiple actinic keratoses may be less traumatically treated with 5-FU (fluorouracil) photodynamic therapy; however, dermabrasion remains a viable treatment option. With the advent of isotretinoin (Accutane), the incidence of resistant acne, acne rosacea, and even acne scarring has decreased dramatically. Certainly the treatment of acne scarring via dermabrasion immediately before or after isotretinoin therapy is contraindicated. Despite these alternatives, acne scarring, rhytids, and postsurgical scars (such as those seen after Mohs' surgery) remain the most enduring indications for the use of dermabrasion. Even today a newer technology, microdermabrasion, is challenging the use of traditional dermabrasion for the treatment of acne scarring and mild rhytids. Microdermabrasion utilizes aluminum oxide crystals to gently and progressively abrade the skin.[8] As compared with dermabrasion, microdermabrasion is a relatively bloodless procedure with fewer complications, less morbidity, and better patient compliance; it also requires

Table 13-1
Indications for Dermabrasion[a]

Scarring	Growths with dermal component
Acne scarring	Angiofibromas (tuberous sclerosis)
Surgical scars/posttraumatic scars/skin grafts	Neurofibromas
Deep thermal burn scars	Syringomas
Pigmentary lesions	Trichoepitheliomas
Congenital pigmented nevi/nevi	Xanthelasma
Lentigines	Other
Tattoos—decorative and posttraumatic	Photoaging—solar elastosis-rhytids
Epithelial-derived growths	Resistant acne/acne rosacea
Actinic keratoses	Rhinophyma
Seborrheic keratoses	

[a]See References 15 to 37.

less surgical skill. Treatments are typically performed without anesthesia, although topical anesthetics may be used with more aggressive treatments (see Chap. 12). Multiple treatments, necessitating minimal healing and downtime, are required. In addition, nonablative laser technology has recently been demonstrated to have a role in these conditions (see Chap. 14).

Technique

ANESTHESIA

The following techniques have been utilized independently or in combination to provide anesthesia for patients undergoing dermabrasion: general anesthesia, intravenous conscious sedation, nerve blocks, and cryoanesthesia. Typically a firm skin surface is desired, so an even planing of the skin is the goal. In the past this has been accomplished by the use of refrigerant sprays such as Fluro Ethyl (dichlorotetrafluoroethane, Freon 75%, and ethylchloride 25%) and Frigiderm (Freon 114) (Fig. 13-1). As the sale of fluorocarbons has now been restricted, some have advocated the use of tumescent anesthesia. This not only provides anesthesia but also eliminates the need to freeze the skin by creating a firm surface for skin planing. In addition, tumescent anesthesia may limit the need for sedatives, narcotics, and more invasive forms of anesthesia while also providing hemostasis.[5] Some argue that infiltration may distort the contours of the skin to be dermabraded and result in less than optimal outcomes. Ultimately, each physician must determine the techniques and types of anesthesia with which he or she feels most comfortable.

EQUIPMENT

Several motor-driven dermabraders exist. Today the most commonly used ones are electrically driven and can achieve up to 60,000 rpm (Fig. 13-1). The two main types of abrasive surfaces utilized are the wire brush and the diamond fraise. The wire brush consists of multiple wires fixed to a stainless steel wheel. The wire caliber may be fine, medium, or coarse. Wire brushes are available in a standard diameter of 17 mm and a width of either 3 or 6 mm. The wire brush tends to cut faster, with less friction than the diamond fraise. Unwanted gouging or catching of the skin can occur more readily with the wire brush, thus calling for greater skill on the part of the surgeon.

Patient Selection

In any surgical procedure, proper patient selection is imperative. As with laser resurfacing, patients with Fitzpatrick skin types I or II tend to be ideal candidates for either a full-face or localized dermabrasion, as they pose a lower risk of postinflammatory hyperpigmentation. Patients with Fitzpatrick skin types III and higher are at increased risk for either hyperpigmentation or depigmentation. As in the case of laser resurfacing, postinflammatory hyper- and hypopigmentation may be temporary or permanent. Alt and coworkers report experience with treating Native Americans and dark-skinned African Americans without incurring pigmentary disturbances.[9] Patients should be fully informed of these risks and, along with their physician, determine whether the benefits of dermabrasion outweigh the potential risks.

As previously mentioned, patients who lack dermal appendageal structures, including an absolute decrease in the number of adnexal structures as seen in radiodermatitis, may not heal adequately and therefore may not be good candidates for dermabrasion. In addition, a decrease in the function of the sebaceous glands, as seen after isotretinoin use, is also a relative contraindication for dermabrasion, specifically owing to the increased risk of scarring postprocedure. Experience has revealed atypical epidermal healing after isotretinoin use.[10] Initially it was recommended to wait at least 6 months after a course of isotretinoin before performing dermabrasion. However, even after that time, the effects on healing may be prolonged and idiosyncratic. Atypical healing has occurred in some patients undergoing dermabrasion even after 38 months. Therefore, it is recommended to delay dermabrasion for as long as practically possible. Before dermabrasion, some advocate performing a biopsy to assess the presence and size of sebaceous glands. A test site or spot dermabrasion prior to full-face dermabrasion may be useful to determine who may be at risk for inadequate healing.[9] As new retinoids appear on the market, such as etretinate and acitretin, the same precautions are expected to apply to patients undergoing dermabrasion who have been treated with these medications.

After undergoing a successful course of isotretinoin, many patients are eager to correct the facial scars that remain. Typically, it may be prudent to wait for a period of time prior to pursuing less aggressive cosmetic procedures, including alpha/beta hydroxy peels or microdermabrasion.

Certainly patients with a known blood-borne infectious disease or a weakened immune system may not be good candidates for dermabrasion. It has been demonstrated that dermabrasion and CO_2 laser resurfacing result in aerosolization of the patient's blood and tissue particles, so that the operating physician and staff may have intimate contact with patients' body fluids.[11,12]

All patients, whether or not they have a known history of herpes simplex, should be treated prophylactically with an antiviral medication. This will minimize the incidence and severity of postoperative herpetic infection. Even patients with no reported history of previous outbreaks of oral herpes may develop postoperative herpetic infections.[13,14]

Other potential contraindications include a history of keloidal or hypertrophic scar formation, a koebnerizing disease such as psoriasis, a collagen vascular or systemic disease that may affect healing.

Sun avoidance for several weeks prior to and after surgery is required. It is known that the sun can influence postinflammatory hyper- and hypopigmentary changes; therefore regular use of high sun protection factor (SPF) sunscreens is mandatory.

If a physician has a concern regarding a particular patient's healing/pigmentary response to dermabrasion, it may prove judicious to perform a spot dermabrasion prior to full-face treatment. Greater predictability may be achieved with this preliminary test.

Preoperative Treatment

Patients who are interested in dermabrasion must first have realistic expectations and also be adequately prepared in terms of healing course and results. Education must be provided regarding the outcomes to be expected; intra- and postoperative healing photographs, although graphic, can be especially useful in this regard. Certainly a patient can expect improvement, but the degree of improvement may vary from individual to individual in both subjective and objective terms. A full description of the procedure, any preoperative requirements, and the expected postoperative course should be discussed. Any potential risks as well as benefits should be reviewed.

A complete medical history—including acute and chronic medical problems, current and past medications (oral retinoid use), and allergies—should be obtained. Questions regarding previous history of healing problems or scarring should be pursued. It is important to discuss previous cosmetic or surgical treatments. Has the patient ever had the lesions of concern previously treated? Previous treatment

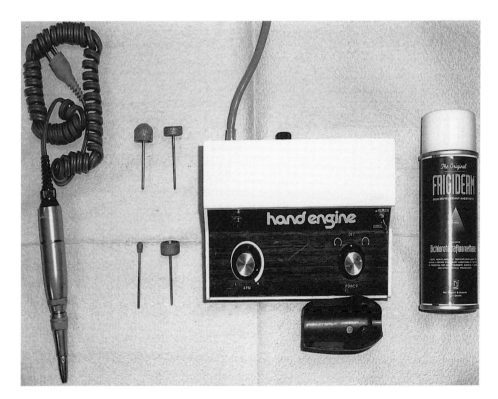

Figure 13-1   The typical hand engine for dermabrading in the treatment of fraises, along with cryorefrigerant.

with either dermabrasion, phenol peels, or CO_2 laser may result in the unmasking of hypopigmentation after subsequent treatment with dermabrasion. Certainly if a patient has undergone previous blepharoplasty, careful evaluation of the periocular area should be performed to decrease the risk of ectropion formation. If a less than optimal "snap" test is revealed, it may be prudent to avoid treatment of this area.

Appropriate preoperative medications are prescribed. As previously mentioned, prophylactic antiviral medication is prescribed to all patients. Acyclovir (Zovirax), famcyclovir (Famvir), and valacyclovir (Valtrex) are all acceptable options. Prophylactic oral antibiotic treatment may also be utilized, especially if larger surfaces are to be treated. Postoperative pain medication and sleeping aids are prescribed. Patients are instructed to obtain all items necessary for treatment prior to surgery and to bring their pain medication with them on the day of the procedure.

Any preoperative screening tests and medical clearance necessary for anticipated anesthesia should be obtained. Physicians are recommended to obtain a serology test for HIV, hepatitis B, and hepatitis C and, if positive, to counsel patients of the attendant risks and contraindications to the procedure. Preoperative and postoperative instructions should be thoroughly reviewed with the patient prior to treatment. All agents that may decrease hemostasis such as aspirin, ibuprofen, naproxen, and vitamin E should be stopped 2 weeks prior to the procedure.

Clinical photographs should be taken preoperatively. It is common for patients to forget their preoperative appearance. Having photo documentation of preexisting lesions and asymmetrical features may prove useful for both the patient and the practitioner. Additional photographs may be taken during the course of healing so that patients can monitor their progress.

Consent forms are reviewed and signed. It is preferable to do this on one of the preoperative visits before the administration of any medications that can influence the patient's ability to reason or fully understand the surgical release form.

Each surgical procedure should be carefully assessed and planned for. Postsurgical scars are usually reviewed 6 to 8 weeks postoperatively in order to blend and contour scar edges. Treatment of acne scars may require a combination approach using punch grafting or surgical scar revision. These steps are usually taken prior to dermabrasion. The proper sequencing of procedures and adequate allotment for healing between procedures should be determined and planned for prior to dermabrasion.

The Procedure

The face is cleansed with an antibacterial cleanser. Scars are marked with a marking pen or 1% gentian violet while the patient is in an upright position, so as not to distort the facial contours. The mandible or the perimeter of the area to be treated may be marked so that the surgeon does not lose these important landmarks when the patient becomes supine. When limited areas are to be treated, it is possible to sedate the patient with an anxiolytic such as diazepam (Valium) and refrigerant spray alone. Marking should be done before sedation or anesthesia is given. The choice of particular fraise wheels is really one of personal preference. However, the diamond fraise, particularly the pear-shaped one, is preferred to sculpt scar edges and blend in the surrounding skin, while the larger cylindrical fraises are useful to quickly abrade larger areas.

The skin to be treated is sprayed with the refrigerant spray to form a firm surface. Tumescent anesthesia can accomplish a similar effect. The rigid surface will not become distorted when external pressure is applied by the dermabrador. Dermabrasion is much more accurate and effective when performed on a firm surface. Because cryorefrigerant may be difficult to obtain, tense stretching of the skin by an assistant can accomplish the same firmness for dermabrasion of small areas. If a refrigerant is used, the assistant holds the spray 1 to 2 in. above the skin surface and sprays for approximately 4 to 8 s, or the assistant may apply opposing traction while the physician dermabrades the area. Small facial segments are treated at a time, so that dermabrasion can be performed before the area thaws.

Dermabrasion is performed until pinpoint bleeding is achieved, which indicates wounding of the papillary dermis. Pinpoint bleeding comes from the capillary loops in the papillary dermis and serves as a useful marker of skin depth. The appearance of yellow globular structures indicates that the sebaceous glands have been exposed and that wounding has extended to the upper reticular dermis. Beyond this point, fat may appear, indicating treatment into and beyond the deep reticular dermis, at which point a greater risk of atypical healing and scarring may exist. When dermabrasion is limited to the papillary dermis, there is less risk of scarring. In addition, spot treatments performed to this level may blend imperceptibly with untreated areas. When not treating full cosmetic units, treatment limited to the papillary dermis may be useful in preventing a noticeable mismatch in skin color between the treated and untreated segments. Where a deep dermabrasion is expected, it may be better to treat the entire cosmetic unit to avoid an obvious mismatch. Feathering at the edges of the dermabraded skin may help to prevent an obvious transition zone between the treated and the untreated skin.

Immediately postoperatively the patient's face is cleansed with sterile saline. The wounds should be kept moist. This can be accomplished either with a healing ointment such as Aquaphor or petroleum jelly or by using a biological occlusive dressing such as Vigilon or Flexan. If an occlusive ointment is utilized, it should be applied generously to the treated areas and covered with a nonstick bandage such as Telfa. A pressure bandage is applied on top of this to aid in hemostasis. Depending on the extent of treatment, the area may be wrapped with a Kling bandage to help stabilize the dressing and also provide pressure for hemostasis. Patients are discharged to a responsible adult with a copy of their postoperative instructions, which have been previously reviewed on several preoperative visits.

POSTOPERATIVE WOUND CARE

Liberal application of ice packs to the treated areas and the use of an oral anti-inflammatory medication such as acetaminophen may help reduce the erythema and edema that may ensue over the first few postoperative days. Again, aspirin and like products are to be avoided. Patients are encouraged to sit upright as much as possible and to sleep with their heads elevated on several pillows or in a reclining chair to help further reduce the swelling. Excessive drainage is expected. Patients are forewarned about this and are instructed not to remove the bandages under any circumstances. Bandages may be reinforced with extra gauze. Excessive bleeding should be reported to the office immediately.

Bandages are removed at the office on the day after surgery. At this visit, the physician will inspect the treated tissue, especially if large surface areas have been treated. If spot treatment has been performed, explicit directions may be given to the patient for home care. In the office, the bandages are gently removed after soaking them in sterile saline, and the face is gently cleansed with sterile saline. Any crusts that have formed may be gently debrided. If an occlusive ointment is being used, it is reapplied in a thin layer, and then the outer bandages are reapplied for one more day. After that, the ointment can be applied without an overlying dressing. The biological dressing may typically be discontinued after 2 to 5 days. Usually an occlusive or antibiotic ointment is then started. Ointments are continued until reepithelialization occurs. Typically, this may take 7 to 10 days. Patients may then use bland emollients. They may shampoo their hair after the second or third postoperative day. They are warned that their skin will be extremely friable and minor trauma may abrade it. The dermabraded areas may be splashed with tap water and patted dry with a clean soft cloth starting on postoperative day 3 or 4. A mild cleansing lotion such as Cetaphil may be started on day 7. Shaving should be avoided for at least 7–10 days.

Patients should be closely monitored during the first postoperative week to assess the skin for evidence of infection or poor wound healing and provide appropriate intervention. Medications that are to be continued should be reviewed with the patient on all office visits.

After reepithelialization occurs, makeup can be utilized to disguise erythema. Camouflage may be achieved with yellow or green concealer placed under foundation. Makeup should be water-based and noncomedogenic.

Physical exertion should be avoided for at least 2 weeks to avoid perspiration. Sun avoidance is encouraged for at least 2 to 3 months postoperatively to protect against photosensitivity and pigmentary alterations.

Patients should be seen by the physician at 2- to 3-week intervals. If any sites appear to be more erythematous

and/or elevating, early intervention with either topical or intralesional steroids or even the pulsed-dye laser may be useful. Bleaching creams may be started if hyperpigmentation is noted.

Side Effects and Complications

Some side effects following dermabrasion are expected. As already discussed, postoperative erythema and edema are the norm. The formation of ointment crusts should not occur, as they may result in scarring. Milia formation and acne flare may be seen. Incision and drainage may be performed as necessary and topical or oral antibiotics may be used. The patients are advised to not pick at any lesions.

Transient hypo- or hyperpigmentation may be seen. Sun avoidance cannot be overemphasized. If persistent hyperpigmentation occurs, agents that may hasten the lightening of the skin may be used. These include bleaching agents with hydroquinone or kojic acid or glycolic, azelaic, retinoid, and ascorbic acid products. Care must be taken, for the skin may be very sensitive and irritant reactions can easily occur. Light glycolic or salicylic acid peels may also be performed. As with laser resurfacing, permanent hypopigmentation may occur, but it may not be detected until 6 to 12 months after the procedure. Permanent hyperpigmentation is rare.

Infection is a negative sequela that can be avoided if the patient is compliant in taking prophylactic medications and frequent evaluation for the presence of infection is performed during the first two postoperative weeks. If evidence of infection is found, aggressive treatment should commence to prevent scarring. Hypertrophic scarring can be treated with a combination of topical steroids, intralesional steroid injections, silicone gel sheeting, and pulse-dye laser treatments.

Summary

In general, dermabrasion remains a viable option for the treatment of many dermatologic lesions as well as facial scarring and rhytids. With proper patient evaluation, preparation, and postoperative care, the risk of complications is decreased. Physicians without experience in this procedure should seek appropriate training or understudy with experts. Adequate physician training, skill, and experience will result in the most optimal outcome (Figs. 13-2*A* and *B* and 13-3*A* and *B*).

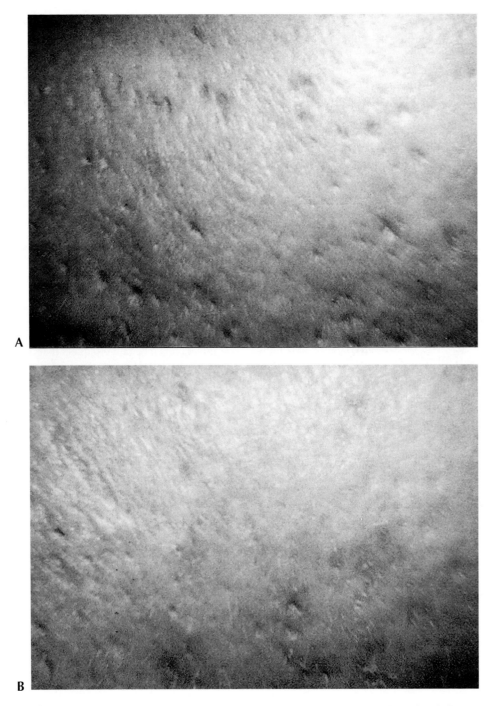

Figure 13-2 (*A*) Closeup of area to be dermabraded. (*B*) Closeup of dermabraded area after treatment.

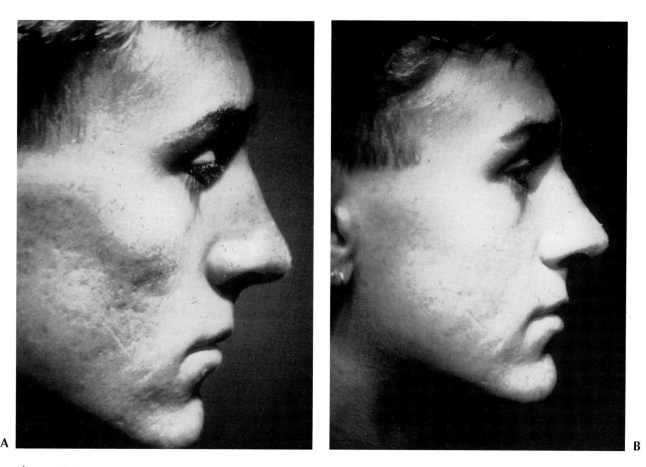

A

B

Figure 13-3   (**A**) Preoperative photo of acne scarring. (**B**) Photo of same area 6 months after dermabrasion.

References

1. Kromayer E. Die Heiung der Akne durch in Neves narbenlases Operations verfahren. Daz Stanzen. *Illustr Monatsschr Aertz Polytech* 1905; 27:101.

2. Kromayer E. Rotioninstrumente: Ein neues Technisches in der dermatologischen Kleinchirurgie. *Dermatol Z* 1905; 12:26.

3. Kromayer E. *Cosmetic Treatment of Skin Complaints.* New York: Oxford University Press, 1930.

4. Kurtin A. Corrective surgical planing of the skin. *Arch Dermatol Syphil* 1953; 68:389.

5. Lawrence N, Mandy S, Yarborough J. History of dermabrasion. *Dermatol Surg* 2000; 26:2.

6. Harmon CB, Zelickson BD, Roenigk RK, et al. Dermabrasive scar revision. Immunohistochemical and ultrastructural evaluation. *Dermatol Surg* 1995; 21:503–508.

7. Nelson BR, Majmudar G, Griffiths CE, et al. Clinical improvement following dermabrasion of photoaged skin correlates with synthesis of collagen I. *Arch Dermatol* 1994; 130:1136–1142.

8. Tsai RY, Wang CN, Chan HL. Aluminum oxide crystal microdermabrasion. A new technique for treating facial scarring. *Dermatol Surg* 1995; 21:539–542.

9. Alt TH, Coleman WP, Hanke CW, et al. Dermabrasion. In: Coleman WP, Hanke CW, and Alt TH, Asken S (eds): *Cosmetic Surgery of the Skin: Principles and Techniques,* 2d ed. St. Louis: Mosby–Year Book, 1997: 114, 121.

10. Rubenstein R, Roenigk HH Jr, Stegman SJ, et al. Atypical keloids after dermabrasion of patients taking isotretinoin. *J Am Acad Dermatol* 1986; 15:280–285.

11. Wentzell JM, Robinson JK, Wentzell JM Jr, et al. Physical properties of aerosols produced by dermabrasion. *Arch Dermatol* 1989; 125:1637–1643.

12. Weber PJ, Wulc AE. The use of a contained breathing apparatus to isolate the operator and assistant from aerosolizing procedures including dermabrasion and laser surgery. *Ann Plast Surg* 1992; 29:182–184.

13. Silverman AK, Laing KF, Swanson NA, et al. Activation of herpes simplex following dermabrasion. Report of a patient successfully treated with intravenous acyclovir and brief review of the literature. *J Am Acad Dermatol* 1985; 13:103–108.

14. Perkins SW, Sklarew EC.: Prevention of facial herpetic infections after chemical peel and dermabrasion: New treatment strategies in the prophylaxis of patients undergoing procedures of the perioral area. *Plast Reconstr Surg* 1996; 98:427–433.

15. Burks JW. Abrasive removal of scars. *South Med J* 1955; 48:452–459.

16. Yarborough JM Jr. Ablation of facial scars by programmed dermabrasion. *J Dermatol Surg Oncol* 1988; 14:292–294.

17. Katz BE, Oca AG. A controlled study of the effectiveness of spot dermabrasion ("scarabrasion") on the appearance of surgical scars. *J Am Acad Dermatol* 1991; 24:462–466.

18. Collins PS, Farber GA. Postsurgical dermabrasion of the nose. *J Dermatol Surg Oncol* 1984; 10:476–477.

19. Robinson JK. Improvement of the appearance of full-thickness skin grafts with dermabrasion. *Arch Dermatol* 1987; 123:1340–1345.

20. Harashina T, Iso R. The treatment of leukoderma after burns by a combination of dermabrasion and "chip" skin grafting. *Br J Plast Surg* 1985; 38:301–305.

21. Onur Erol O, Atabay K. The treatment of burn scar hypopigmentation and surface irregularity by dermabrasion and thin skin grafting. *Plast Reconstr Surg* 1990; 85:754–758.

22. Floccard B, Tixier F, Chatot-Henry D, et al. Early dermabrasion of deep dermal burns with sandpaper. Case reports. *Scand J Plast Reconstr Surg Hand Surg* 1998; 32:415–419.

23. Imagawa I, Endo M, Morishima T. Mechanism of recurrence of pigmented nevi following dermabrasion. *Acta Derm Venereol* 1976; 56:353–359.

24. Johnson H. Permanent removal of pigmentation from giant hairy nevi by dermabrasion in early life. *Br J Plast Surg* 1977; 30:321–323.

25. Miller CJ, Becker DW Jr. Removing pigmentation by dermabrading nevi in infancy. *Br J Plast Surg* 1979; 32:124–126.

26. Rompel R, Moser M, Petres J. Dermabrasion of congenital nevocellular nevi: Experience in 215 patients. *Dermatology* 1997; 19:261–267.

27. Wilder LW, Smith B. Benign Lentigo of the face. Treatment with a diamond abrader: A case report. *J Kansas Med Soc* 1970; 71:196.

28. Iverson PC. Surgical removal of traumatic tattoos of the face. *Plast Reconstr Surg* 1947; 2:247.

29. Clabaugh W. Removal of tattoos by superficial dermabrasion. *Arch Dermatol* 1968; 98:515–521.

30. Notaro WA. Dermabrasion for the management of traumatic tattoos. *J Dermatol Surg Oncol* 1983; 9:916–918.

31. Burks JW, Marascalco J, Clark WH. Half-face planing of precancerous skin after five years. *Arch Dermatol* 1963; 88:572–585.

32. Coleman WP, Yarborough JM, Mandy SH. Dermabrasion for the prophylaxis and treatment of actinic keratoses. *Dermatol Surg* 1996; 22:17–21.

33. Brown GR, Burks JW, Farber GA. Dermabrasion for showers of seborrheic keratoses. *J Dermatol Surg Oncol* 1976; 2:258–259.

34. Menon PA. Dermabrasion for the management of angiofibromas in tuberous sclerosis. *J Dermatol Surg Oncol* 1982; 8:984–985.

35. Hanke CW, Conner AC, Reed JC. Treatment of multiple facial neurofibromas with dermabrasion. *J Dermatol Surg Oncol* 1987; 13:631–637.

36. English DT, Martin GC, Reisner JE. Dermabrasion for nodular cutaneous elastosis with cysts and comedones. Favre-Racouchot syndrome. *Arch Dermatol* 1971; 104:92–93.

37. Roenigk HH Jr. Dermabrasion of miscellaneous cutaneous lesions (exclusive of scarring from acne). *J Dermatol Surg Oncol* 1977; 3:322.

Patient Information

Dermabrasion

Throughout the ages, people with facial imperfections have sought effective ways to make their skin smoother. Dermabrasion is a modern surgical procedure that helps men and women achieve the smoother, more even skin contour they desire. This procedure is very effective in minimizing acne scars, wrinkles caused by aging or the sun, pox marks, age spots, and scars caused by accidents or previous skin grafts.

Dermabrasion can also dramatically improve the appearance of fine lines and wrinkles around the mouth and eyes.

Dermabrasion was first introduced in the 1940s and has been highly refined over the last few decades. During this procedure, the surgeon "sands" the damaged areas with a rotary instrument. This planing action removes the outer damaged skin layers that give the skin an uneven appearance. A smoother, more pleasing facial contour and improved skin texture is the result.

Dermabrasion tends to be most effective when performed in the late fall or early winter, because the procedure makes the skin sensitive to sunlight for several months.

The cosmetic surgeons of this center help people develop and maintain a healthy and more attractive appearance. Our skilled surgeons specialize in dermabrasion and have used their knowledge, skill, and experience for more than a decade to help numerous patients achieve smoother, more attractive looking skin.

The Procedure

Your surgeon usually performs dermabrasion in the office on an outpatient basis. After your doctor cleans your face with an antiseptic cleansing agent, the areas to be treated will be numbed with a cold spray. The abrading instrument, which has a rapidly spinning diamond fraize wheel, is then applied to the skin and the appropriate skin layers are carefully sanded off. The amount of time required to perform dermabrasion depends upon the areas to be treated. It usually takes 10 to 20 minutes to treat a few wrinkles or acne scars, 25 to 35 minutes to treat both cheeks, and 45 minutes to treat the entire face.

For the first few days after surgery, you may experience some swelling and feel as if you had a mild sunburn. Most of this discomfort can be alleviated with medication. Two to three days following surgery, a crust will begin to form over the treated area. This will begin to loosen on the fifth or sixth day and fall off within six to eight days. During this healing period, it is important to keep the area moist with cool tap-water compresses and an ointment your doctor will recommend. Your "new" skin will have a slightly pink cast, which will gradually fade. Most patients resume normal activities within 2 weeks.

Sometimes, to produce optimum results, dermabrasion is used in conjunction with other procedures such as punch grafting. This is particularly effective for minimizing "ice pick" scars, which are generally several skin layers deep. During the punch grafting procedure, your doctor excises the ice pick scars with a 1- to 4-mm biopsy punch and replaces them with the same-size grafts of normal skin. The normal skin is usually taken from the back of the ear. After they heal, these areas are smoothed by dermabrasion.

For several weeks following dermabrasion, it is important to avoid becoming sun- or wind-burned. You will also need to use a strong sunscreen daily during the summer following the procedure to protect your younger, smoother skin.

The Results

Most people are delighted with the results of dermabrasion; however, those who expect perfect skin will be disappointed. The amount of improvement patients experience depends on the condition of their skin.

People who undergo dermabrasion to reduce wrinkles can often achieve a significant improvement in their appearance. Those who use the dermabrasion procedure combined with punch grafting or excisional surgery to treat acne scars usually experience a significant improvement. The procedure can be repeated, if necessary, to achieve maximum results.

Preoperative Instructions

Wash your face thoroughly on the morning of your surgery.

Wash your hair the night prior to surgery.

Get a good night's sleep.

Eat a *light* meal (breakfast or lunch) on the day of treatment prior to the appointment. (Do not eat anything if intravenous sedation is being considered.)

Wear clothing that does not have to be pulled over your head.

Please do not wear makeup to the office; if it is worn, please plan to remove it upon arrival.

Do not wear any jewelry to the office on the day of surgery.

Contact lenses must be removed before surgery. If you wish to remove them in the office, please bring your case.

Bring your pain medication with you on surgery day.

Bring someone with you. Your face will be bandaged following the procedure, and under no circumstances should you plan to drive yourself home.

Obtain Aquaphor ointment from your local pharmacy prior to surgery (this is a nonprescription item) for postoperative use. If the area around the mouth or lips will be treated, it may be useful for you to obtain the following items before surgery: a baby toothbrush, "Ensure" shakes—nutritional drinks in cans, and straws.

Be sure to discuss with the doctor any history of fever blisters, facial herpes infection, or allergies to medication, and review all medicines currently being used.

Take all medications as prescribed *prior* to treatment. These normally include an antibiotic, an antiviral (if the lip is being treated), and a Valium.

Write down any last-minute questions or personal or medical history notes and bring this memo with you.

The fee is to be paid in full at the preoperative visit, which must be 7 to 14 days prior to surgery.

Dermabrasion Setup Tray

Patient

1. Sterile surgical hat
2. Cape

Doctor and Staff

1. Mask with facial shield
2. Sterile gloves
3. Surgical hats
4. Yellow isolation gloves

Materials

1. Purple skin marker
2. Alcohol
3. One sterile 18" drape
4. Sterile bowl
5. One 1-g packet of 3 × 3 gauze
6. 0.25% Lidocaine with epinephrine tumescent solution
7. Dermabrader
   A. Foot pedal
   B. Burrs
8. Solution
   A. Saline (spot derm)
   B. Mixture of ½ lidocaine with epinephrine, buffered, and ½ saline, 30 mL each (large areas)
9. Telfa pads 3 × 4" or 3 × 8" (size depends on area to be covered)
10. Two rolls of Kling
11. Tape
12. Aquaphor ointment
13. Sterile light-handle cover
14. Nonsterile white drape (nonanesthesia day)

Postoperative Instructions

Go home and relax. The sedative used for the dermabrasion may last several hours postoperatively.

Do not be alarmed if swelling appears around your eyes and mouth. This will gradually subside. Sit up as much as possible and sleep in a head-elevated position, either on three pillows or in a reclining chair. This will help reduce the natural swelling that occurs after this type of operation.

The dermabraded areas often produce excessive drainage, occasionally enough to saturate the dressing. *Under no circumstances should this dressing be removed.* It can be reinforced with additional gauze bandages, or a Turkish towel may be used to protect your clothing or bedding. If you have had a full-face dermabrasion, the nurse will remove the dressing at the office the following day.

Any excessive bleeding should be reported immediately to our office at (___) _____.

Pain medication may be taken every 3 to 4 hours as needed, but no aspirin.

The day following a full-face dermabrasion, the initial dressing will be removed at the office. The area will be cleansed and a light dressing applied over Aquaphor. This should be removed the next day. Patients having partial dermabrasion or a long distance to travel will remove their dressing the day after surgery at home. No dressing will be worn from this point on.

Avoid letting your face dry out. Always keep it covered with the Aquaphor. Do not wash or clean your face for the first 72 hours. After this initial period, cool tap-water compresses may be applied for 20 to 30 minutes, three to five times a day, and you may stand in the shower to let a gentle flow of lukewarm water flow over the facial areas for 10 minutes. This is followed immediately by a liberal application of Aquaphor. Use no soap on your face for 10 days.

As the dermabraded area heals, crusts will gradually separate themselves. **DO NOT** pull off tightly adherent crusts.

You should be seen for a postoperative checkup 7 to 10 days following the procedure.

Direct sun exposure *must* be avoided for at least 3 months postoperatively because of the increased photosensitivity and hyperpigmentation of the dermabraded area.

Avoid physical exertion for 2 weeks, to avoid perspiration. For men, no shaving for 7 to 10 days.

Avoid exposure to strong wind or extreme cold for 2 weeks.

You may shampoo your hair after the third postoperative day.

Use Basis soap for sensitive skin or Dove soap for washing the face beginning 10 days after procedure.

For several weeks following dermabrasion, a few acne-like lesions may appear. These are not true acne lesions but represent new pores coming to the surface of your skin. Do not pick them. They will disappear on their own.

Occasionally, a second dermabrasion is necessary to achieve the desired result.

CONSENT FOR DERMABRASION

Patient's name_____

Date_____

I hereby authorize _____ and/or the surgical team to perform a surgical procedure commonly known as dermabrasion on _____.

(Patient's name or "myself")

1. The procedure listed in paragraph 1 has been explained to me by the above doctor(s), and I completely understand the nature and consequences of the procedure. The following points have been specifically made clear:

   a. That the process involves the application of a diamond fraise or wire brush wheel to the face, which may require the use of a face mask following said application.

   b. That the dermabrasion process will cause discomfort and swelling, and my face will be covered with a crust, which will usually separate within 5 to 10 days.

   c. As the skin heals it will have a reddish appearance, which may persist several months; and at the juncture of the treated and untreated areas, there may be a difference in color, pigmentation, and texture of skin.

   d. That scarring can occur, causing permanent disfigurement.

   e. That blotching of pigmentation can occur, which may be permanent.

   f. That infection can occur.

   g. That I may not see any improvement.

   h. That avoidance of sun exposure will be necessary for several weeks or months.

   Initial_____

2. I recognize that, during the course of the operation, unforeseen conditions may necessitate additional or different procedures than those set forth above. I therefore further authorize and request that the above-named surgeon, assistants, or designees perform such procedures as are, in his professional judgment, necessary and desirable, including but not limited to procedures involving pathology and radiology. The authority granted under this paragraph shall extend to remedying conditions that are not known to the above doctors at the time the operation is commenced.

   Initial_____

3. I consent to the administration of anesthesia to be applied by or under the direction and supervision of the above doctors or such anesthetists as they shall select and to the use of such anesthetics as they may deem advisable with the exception of

   _____

   (None or a particular one)

   Initial_____

4. I am aware that the practice of medicine and surgery is not an exact science, and I acknowledge that no guarantees have been made to me as to the results of the operation or procedure.

   Initial_____

5. I give permission to _____ to take still or motion clinical photographs with the understanding such photographs remain the property of the center. If, in the judgment of the center, medical research, education, or science will be benefited by their use, such photographs and related information may be published and republished in professional journals or medical books or used for any other purpose which the center may deem proper. It is specifically understood that in any such publication or use, I shall not be identified by name.

   Initial_____

6. I agree to cooperate with the above doctors in my care after surgery until completely discharged.

   Initial_____

7. I understand that no two sides of the face are exactly the same and can never be made to look the same. I understand that bone and muscle structures help create overall shape and are never identical on both sides of the body, and that these will remain unchanged by the surgery.

8. For the purpose of advancing medical education, I consent to the admittance of authorized observers to the operating room.

   Initial_____

9. I understand it is mandatory for me to have made prior arrangements to be driven to and from the doctor's office by a responsible adult.

   Initial_____

10. I am not known to be allergic to anything except: (List) _____

    _____

11. I understand that elective surgical procedures are most often delayed until after the termination of a pregnancy. My signature attests that to the best of my knowledge I am not pregnant at this time.

    Initial_____

12. I agree to discontinue smoking entirely for a period of 2 weeks prior to the surgery and 2 weeks immediately following surgery.

    Initial_____

13. I have been given the opportunity to ask questions and all questions have been answered to my satisfaction.

    Initial_____

My signature indicates that I have read this "Consent for Dermabrasion" and I understand and accept the risks involved with this operation. I hereby authorize _____ and/or the surgical team to perform this surgical procedure on me.

_____   _____
Signature (Patient/Responsible Party)   Date

_____   _____
Signature (Witness)   Date

If patient is a minor, complete the following:
Patient is a minor _____ years of age, and we, the undersigned, are the parents or guardian of the patient and do hereby consent for the patient.

_____   _____
Signature (Parent/Guardian)   Date

CHAPTER 14

Laser Surgery

Over the past decade, the use of laser applications in dermatologic and cosmetic surgery has experienced an ever-increasing growth. The combination of patient demand and expectations for advanced technology, the societal interest in cosmesis, and the practical application of the principle of selective photothermolysis has led to the rapid development of an array of new laser systems. These target the different components of the skin with a precision unsurpassed by any other form of surgery. Because of this uncanny precision, the current lasers make it possible to provide patients with highly reproducible results with a high safety margin in the treatment of a variety of medical conditions. Among the medical conditions targeted by the current laser systems are dermatoheliosis as well as vascular, pigmented, tattooed, and scarred lesions, rhytids, and hair. As with every form of surgery, the results of laser surgery still remain operator-dependent despite the precision and wide safety margin offered by the currently available lasers. Hence, every dermatologic and cosmetic surgeon should have a good understanding of laser physics, laser interaction with tissue, laser profiles, laser safety, and the indications and limitations of laser surgery in the treatment of various medical conditions to obtain the best possible results.

LASER PHYSICS

The term *laser* is actually an acronym formed from the first letters of the following words: *light amplification* by the *stimulated emission of radiation*. The concept of stimulated emission, introduced by Einstein in 1927, led to the development of a ruby laser by Maiman[1] in 1959. Several years later, in 1963, the dermatologist Leon Goldman[2] became the first physician to test the effects of this laser on human skin.

Since that time there has been an unparalleled growth in the development of new lasers, based on the unique properties of laser light. The physical properties of laser light include the following: monochromacity, coherence, collimation, high intensity, and compressibility into pulses of ultrashort duration. *Monochromacity* refers to the capability of laser light to selectively target chromophores with a corresponding single wavelength. In contrast, most light sources other than lasers are composed of a variety of different wavelengths. *Coherence*

means that the light waves of lasers travel in time with respect to both time and space. In other words, lasers show an alignment of the nonstationary peaks and valleys of its light waves. *Collimation* is described as the ability of lasers to transmit parallel rays of light without divergence and loss of intensity despite increasing distance. Light of *high intensity* is required to allow for transmission of maximal energy to the site of irradiation. And *compressibility* into pulses of ultra-short duration make it possible to deliver localized energy with minimal heat diffusion to areas surrounding the intended target, thus increasing the precision and margin of safety of laser treatment. The combination of these unique characteristics of laser light allow for selective target destruction with extraordinary precision and consequently a high margin of safety if the appropriate wavelength, light intensity, and pulse duration are applied.[3,4]

In order to achieve consistency in performing laser surgery, the laser surgeon must have knowledge of two basic laser parameters, *irradiance* and *energy* fluence. Both irradiance and energy fluence are means of measuring laser output.[3,5] The term *irradiance* refers to the rate of energy absorption and is used to describe the output from continuous-wave (CW) lasers.[6] This means of measuring laser output is calculated with the following formula:

$$\text{Irradiance} = \frac{\text{laser output (watts)}}{\pi r^2 \text{ (area of laser beam)}}$$

In examining this formula, it becomes apparent that the irradiance is inversely related to spot size of the CW laser beam and specifically to its radius. Therefore the smaller the radius of the laser beam and thus its spot size, the larger the exerted irradiance. On the other hand, *energy fluence* is defined as the amount of energy put out in a single pulse from pulsed and Q-switched lasers.[6] The formula to calculate energy fluence is as follows:

$$\text{Energy fluence} = \frac{\text{laser output (watts)} \times \text{exposure time (seconds)}}{\pi r^2 \text{ (area of laser beam)}}$$

This formula indicates that energy fluence, as a measure of pulsed and Q-switched laser output, is also inversely related to the area of the laser beam and thus its radius. Consequently, the smaller the radius of the laser beam and thus its spot size, the larger the exerted energy fluence. In addition, energy fluence is directly related to the exposure time or pulse duration of the energy delivered by the laser. Hence, the shorter the pulse duration, the less the wielded energy fluence. In other words, the shorter the pulse duration, the more localized the delivery of energy with a lesser degree of heat diffusion to surrounding tissues. In view of the above, knowledge of the two basic laser parameters of irradiance and energy fluence and the factors influencing them allows the laser surgeon to perform treatment of different conditions with consistency and precision.

LASER INTERACTION WITH TISSUE

The basic level of laser interaction with tissue, and its resultant effects, consists of laser light penetrating the skin in the form of energy-carrying protons that are absorbed by chromophores with a corresponding absorption spectrum. As the energy of these photons is absorbed, an excitation of the targeted chromophores ensues. When this energy is released, three possible modes of laser effects may take place, namely photothermal, photomechanical, and photochemical. Photothermal effects are due to the absorbed energy causing kinetic excitation that is released directly as heat. In fact, almost all of the energy absorbed by any wavelength is released in the form of heat. Photomechanical effects are the result of the absorbed energy, leading to quickly expanding thermal activity, waves of pressure and shock, transfer of momentum, or vaporization. And photochemical effects are due to the absorbed energy leading to electronic excitation capable of activating native or photosensitizer-induced photochemical reactions. The latter are only seen with ultraviolet and visible light, since infrared light carries insufficient quantum energy. While all three of these laser effects can take place simultaneously, usually one or two are predominant. Among these laser effects, all of which play important roles in dermatology, photothermal effects are the most commonly applied in clinical use, followed by photomechanical and photochemical effects.[7]

Photothermal effects are both temperature- and time-dependent. The majority of cells become injured or nonviable when exposed to temperatures of approximately 40 to 45°C as denaturation of enzymes and structural proteins occurs. Temperatures above 50 to 60°C lead to coagulation of serum proteins in blood, with subsequent hemostasis. Type I collagen in the skin is known to respond to temperatures of about 65°C with a melt (helix coil) transition. This transition of collagen generates an irreversible coagulation and shrinkage of connective tissue matrix that is visible as local skin contraction. Once temperatures exceed 100°C (the boiling point of water), tissue water is vaporized. Eventually, if the desiccated tissue continues to be heated, carbonization takes place.[6] And the longer the time of tissue exposure to such temperatures, the more extensive is the thermal damage surrounding the target tissue. CW and pulsed lasers utilize these photothermal effects differently. While CW lasers cause thermal destruction of tissue, this process is nonselective, as prolonged times of exposure to CW laser light give rise to thermal destruction that spreads significantly beyond the site of treatment. Examples of the nonselective photothermal effects of CW lasers are the use of the carbon dioxide (CO_2) laser as an excisional tool because of its outstanding hemostatic capacity and usefulness for the vaporization of warts, seborrheic keratoses, lentigines, actinic cheilitis, and other epidermal lesions.[7-9] However, pulsed lasers are based on the principle of selective photothermolysis. The term *selective photothermolysis* as conceived by Anderson and Parrish[10] in 1983 refers to the concept of targeting a chromophore in a specific manner utilizing light energy to cause temperature-mediated localized injury in a precise fashion so as to avoid or keep to a minimum damage to surrounding regions. This concept of laser-tissue interaction is based on a target's thermal relaxation time, defined as the time required for an object to cool down to 50 percent of the temperature experienced right after laser exposure. To achieve the maximal precision seen with selective photothermolysis, the pulse duration (exposure time) of the beam emitted must be shorter than the intended target's thermal relaxation time. If the pulse duration exceeds the intended target's thermal relaxation time, heat will spread notably beyond the target site to cause nonspecific thermal damage to surrounding tissues. The thermal relaxation time of individual targets varies with the type of chromophore involved and its size, ranging from macroseconds to nanoseconds in duration.[11,12]

Next to the photothermal effects discussed above, photomechanical effects are second in terms of clinical use in dermatology. Photomechanical effects, also known as photoacoustic effects, consist of destruction of organelles, membranes, and cells by expanding thermal activity, waves of pressure and shock, transfer of momentum, or vaporization as induced by the absorption of high-energy pulsed-laser light. Mechanical injury actually represents an undesired side effect in the treatment of vascular lesions and the removal of tissue with pulsed laser systems. However, mechanical effects are among the main mechanism responsible for successful tattoo removal via selective photothermolysis. At the cutaneous level, tattoos are made of small, insoluble ink particles that the body immediately attempts to phagocytose with cells designated to this purpose. Treatment of these tattoos with pulsed lasers increases the ink particle's temperature at such an extraordinarily fast rate that these pigment granules and the cells containing them are literally shattered into millions of tiny pieces. This explosion of ink particles into such tiny pieces aids the body significantly in their phagocytosis, as it allows for more efficient and therefore faster removal of the foreign pigment.[7,13,14]

As previously stated, photochemical effects have been the most underdeveloped in terms of their use in clinical dermatology. Nevertheless, photochemical effects have found their niche with the use of photodynamic therapy of skin cancers, in particular basal and squamous cell carcinomas. Photodynamic therapy requires the use of a photosensitizing drug to be preferentially taken up by the targeted skin cancer. In the past, the photosensitizing drug of choice was systemic dihematoporphyrin ether (DHE), a hematoporphyrin derivative. But in recent years, topical aminolevulinic acid (ALA) has been shown to be very effective, as it is a porphyrin precursor that induces cells to generate an excess of protoporphyrin IX. Once the cancerous cells have been photosensitized with DHE or ALA, they are exposed to a 630-nm red-light laser that produces an excited state of the drug, which then results in the formation of singlet oxygen. These singlet oxygen molecules lead to the demise of cancerous cells via oxidation of their cell membranes.[7,15–18]

Cutaneous optics are defined by absorption of light with its resultant effects on the skin, as discussed above, and scattering of light by the skin with ensuing reflection. *Absorption* relates to the energy of a photon being entirely taken up by a chromophore, the absorbing molecule. *Scattering* refers to light returned from the skin due to a change in the path of photon travel. Both of these processes determine the depth of penetration of light into the skin. In general, as more light is absorbed by chromophores, it becomes less capable of penetrating deeper into the skin. And scattering relates inversely to wavelength, thereby allowing light to penetrate deeper as its wavelength increases.[7,11,19,20]

In the epidermis, most of the entering light is actually absorbed by chromophores, not scattered. For wavelengths less than 320 nm, the main absorbing molecules are proteins, nucleic acids, and melanin. Melanin becomes the most significant epidermal chromophore for light in the 320 to 400 nm (UVA), 400 to 720 nm (visible), and 720 to 1000 nm (near infrared) range. However, this changes with wavelengths greater than 1000-nm (mid and far infrared) for which water becomes the predominant chromophore[7,11,19,20]

The dynamics of skin optics change in the dermis, where scattering dominates over absorption. This is due to the masses of light-scattering collagen fibers in the dermis, which demonstrates limited absorption of light by blood, specifically the chromophores oxyhemoglobin and hemoglobin. The combination of low absorption and low scattering with light in the 630- to 1000-nm (red and near infrared) region generates an "optical window," permitting deeper penetration of light into the dermis.[7,11,19,20]

LASER PROFILES

In general, lasers can be characterized by the type of beam emitted, their specific wavelength, and the chromophore targeted. With respect to the type of beam emitted, they are referred to as continuous-wave (CW) or pulsed lasers. CW lasers emit a constant beam of light that remains unchanged for as long as the operator depresses the foot pedal. Despite modifications such as mechanical shutters and automated scanning devices to minimize the exposure time of the skin at any one point of time, CW lasers are unable to provide pulse durations shorter than the thermal relaxation times of the majority of cutaneous targets. Hence, CW lasers do not operate on the principle of selective photothermolysis. While these lasers target specific chromophores, they are incapable of limiting the thermal damage to the intended target and consequently are associated with a much higher risk of scarring than the pulsed lasers. Examples of CW lasers include the argon, krypton, older Nd:YAG, and original CO_2 lasers. In contrast, pulsed lasers function on the principle of selective photothermolysis as they are indeed capable of bursts of high-energy light that are shorter than the thermal relaxation

times of their intended target. The category of pulsed lasers includes the pulsed-dye laser as well as the Q-switched (QS) ruby, QS-Nd:YAG, and QS-alexandrite laser. The term *Q switching* alludes to a specialized technique involving an optical polarizer and a Pockel cell to allow for a tremendous amount of energy to develop prior to its release in a sudden powerful burst.[3–5]

A laser's specific wavelength is another important factor as diverse cutaneous targets absorb different wavelengths of light with a variable intensity. The degree to which light is absorbed by cutaneous targets or chromophores determines the effectiveness and potential downfalls of the different lasers in treating various skin conditions, as explained below.

Ablative Resurfacing Lasers

CO_2 Laser CO_2 lasers have taken on great importance in the field of dermatologic surgery owing to their versatility in clinical applications, thereby making them one of the most commonly used laser systems on the market today. These lasers can be employed in an excisional, vaporizational, and superpulsed/ultrapulsed mode to achieve different effects. All of these modes of CO_2 laser function are based on the emission of light at a wavelength of 10,600 nm, which is primarily absorbed by intracellular and extracellular water. Absorption of this light results in the rapid conversion of the targeted tissues into steam and smoke, as water makes up more than 80 percent of skin. It also, at the same time, effectively seals the blood vessels of the treated tissues and thus decreases the degree of intraoperative bleeding, postoperative ecchymosis, and edema.[5,8,21]

Conventional (CW) CO_2 laser therapy utilizes a small beam with high power for the excisional mode and a large beam with low power for the vaporizational mode. The excisional mode allows for precise incision of tissue with excellent hemostasis, a function widely employed for upper and lower blepharoplasty,[22–24] creation of recipient sites in hair transplantation surgery,[25] scalp reduction,[26] rhinophyma reduction,[5,27,28] and surgical removal of keloids.[5,29,30] The vaporizational mode has proven itself as a particular valuable tool in the treatment of actinic cheilitis,[8,31,32] epidermal nevi,[8,31–34] rhinophyma,[8,35,36] and resistant warts of the periungal, subungal, and plantar variety.[8,37–39] Further cosmetic applications of the CO_2 laser in its vaporizational mode include the treatment of appendiceal tumors (adenoma sebaceum,[40] syringomas,[41] trichoepitheliomas,[42] apocrine hydrocystomas,[43] vellous hair cysts,[44] neurofibromas[45]), pigmented lesions (lentigines[46]), vascular lesions (lymphangioma circumscriptum,[47,48] port-wine stain,[49] and pyogenic granulomas[50,51]), and other miscellaneous conditions (xanthelasma,[52,53] tattoos,[54] pitted acne scarring,[55] digital mucous cyst,[56] and pearly penile papules[57]). In using the CW CO_2 laser in either of these two modes, the most commonly noted side effect is hypertrophic scarring.

More recently, superpulsed/ultrapulsed CO_2 lasers have been developed that deliver high-intensity pulsed light of short duration. These pulsed CO_2 lasers follow the principle of selective photothermolysis to allow for specific tissue ablation while minimizing thermal destruction of surrounding areas. This highly specific tissue destruction has popularized the use of these pulsed lasers for cutaneous resurfacing of rhytids, especially in the periorbital and perioral areas, and acne scarring. From a clinical perspective, the improvement of even severe rhytids and acne scarring is based upon re-epithelialization and notable collagen contraction of up to 25 percent.[58,59] Although the essentially bloodless CO_2 laser resurfacing with its selective photothermolysis markedly reduces the risk of adverse scarring as compared with the use of CW lasers and is often touted as a safe cosmetic procedure, it is still fraught with potential complications. The spectrum of complications noted with this procedure ranges from mild (prolonged erythema, milia, acne flare) to moderate (transient hyperpigmentation, delayed hypopigmentation, contact dermatitis, local infection) and severe complications (hypertrophic scarring, ectropion, systemic infection).[60] While the complication rate is relatively low and without doubt operator-dependent, even the most experienced laser surgeons are not exempt from having their patients develop complications.

Erbium:YAG Laser The pulsed erbium:YAG laser, introduced to the United States in 1996, represents the newest ablative resurfacing tool available to the dermatologic surgeon. Similar to the CO_2 laser, it primarily targets water, but with infrared light at a wavelength of 2940 nm. As this wavelength approximates the peak absorption spectrum of water far better than that the CO_2 laser wavelength of 10,600 nm, the erbium light is 12 to 18 times more efficiently absorbed by tissue.[60,61] Consequently, the erbium laser demonstrates less depth of penetration (2 to 5 μm rather than 20 to 30 μm) and less residual thermal damage to surrounding areas (20 to 50 μm instead of 25 to 100 μm) than the CO_2 laser in a pass-for-pass comparison.[60–63] Hence, the erbium light allows for more superficial surface ablation than the CO_2 laser. While both types of lasers may be used for cutaneous resurfacing, the erbium laser is generally less effective in bringing about clinical improvement, as it causes only 1 to 2 percent collagen contraction, which is far less than the shrinkage of up to 25 percent seen with the CO_2 laser.[60,64] Therefore the erbium laser may be indicated for the treatment of mild to moderate rhytids and acne scarring, unlike the CO_2 laser, which can be used for even severe wrinkling and atrophic scarring.

In looking at the recovery period and side-effect profile of the two resurfacing lasers, certain differences are noted. The recovery period of both the erbium and the CO_2 laser are characterized by serous discharge, crusting, and a burning sensation. Yet patients treated with the erbium laser generally experience faster reepithelialization and shorter duration of erythema than is seen with the CO_2 laser, depending upon the energy settings used. Accordingly, edema and pruritus are of notably shorter duration with erbium laser resurfacing. One drawback of erbium laser resurfacing is the high incidence of spot bleeding experienced by patients throughout the initial 24 to 48 h of recovery. In comparison, the CO_2 laser allows for essentially bloodless resurfacing, as its wider zone of thermal destruction effectively seals blood vessels. With respect to complications of cutaneous resurfacing, it appears that they are similar and occur at a relatively low rate with either type of laser. Albeit improvement is more limited, it is likely that the complication rate may turn out to

be even lower for the patient treated with the erbium laser, since its lesser depth of penetration and spread of thermal destruction make for a less invasive procedure.[60]

Nonablative Resurfacing Lasers

Cool Touch Laser The Cool Touch laser is a 1320-nm Nd:YAG laser that utilizes high fluences around 28 to 38 J/cm^2 and a short pulse duration of 200 ms in combination with cryogen cooling of the epidermis to improve the appearance of skin with mild to moderate wrinkling and mild atrophic acne scarring. This unique constellation of laser parameters is aimed at causing low-grade nonspecific damage of the upper dermis to induce a response of increased new collagen production while sparing the epidermis. For optimal clinical results, three to six treatments spaced several weeks apart are probably needed. Since there is no ablation of the epidermis, this laser avoids a prolonged recovery period related to reepithelialization. And when carried out appropriately, side effects and complications are to date minimal to nonexistent.[65,66]

NLite Laser The NLite laser is another nonablative laser that may be used to reduce mild to moderate wrinkling in particular and potentially may be useful for mild atrophic acne scarring also. The combination of a 585-nm wavelength at a low fluence in the range of 2 to 4 J/cm^2 and a short pulse duration of 250 to 400 μs produce a light beam that in theory is selectively absorbed by vessels of the upper dermal plexus. Selective targeting of these upper dermal vessels induces a low-grade inflammation and growth response that ultimately results in production of new collagen. As this laser uses low fluences that specifically target a chromophore in the upper dermis and largely bypasses the epidermis, it does not require cryogen cooling for epidermal protection, like the Cool Touch laser. Consequently, this nonablative technique is characterized by an immediate recovery with minimal to no side effects or complications, all of which are features valued by patients and physicians alike.[67]

Continuous-Wave (CW) and Quasi-Continuous-Wave (QCW) Lasers

Argon Laser The argon laser, characterized by a continuous blue-green light beam, has wavelength peaks at 488 and 514 nm. The energy of the argon laser is absorbed by two chromophores of the skin, namely hemoglobin and melanin. Historically, it has been primarily applied in the treatment of vascular lesions. In particular, this laser was commonly used in targeting vascular lesions consisting of larger blood vessels or those with high flow rates,[3] such as telangiectasias of the nasal alae,[68] angiofibromas,[69] venous lakes,[70] spider nevi, pyogenic granulomas,[71] and port-wine stains.[72] in the treatment of vascular lesions, the improvement seen varies with the amount of pigment present in the patient's skin. The light penetrates deeper in light-skinned individuals, allowing it to reach the level of tissue in which blood vessels are present. Thus, if there is a recent history of suntan or prolonged sun exposure, the patient with vascular lesions may have to be rescheduled.

Because of the outstanding absorption of melanin by its green-light wavelengths, the argon laser has also been used to target various pigmented lesions. Among these are benign nevi, nevus of Ota, melasma, Becker's nevus, café-au-lait macules, lentigines, and early seborrheic keratoses.[3,73]

Whether the intended target is hemoglobin or melanin, the argon laser actually works by causing nonspecific tissue thermal injury as the pulse duration exceeds the thermal relaxation times of vessels. Even with the use of an automated scanning device to release 1-mm spots in a hexagonal pattern, the pulses prevail too long to accomplish selective photothermolysis. As with any laser, the outcome is to a certain degree operator-dependent. But the imprecision associated with the failure to adhere to the principle of selective photothermolysis results in an increased risk for complications like hypopigmentation, textural changes, and even hypertrophic scarring, ranging from 5 to 20 percent in the treatment of port-wine stains. Thus, the treatment of young patients and/or those with lesions on the upper lip, mandible, nasolabial folds, eyelids, neck, or extremities (at high risk for scarring) should be avoided altogether. Another disadvantage of the argon laser is that its use is very time-consuming owing to its small spot size. Consequently, the argon laser is generally regarded as a secondary choice, used in select cases only, in the treatment of these patients.[3,5]

Copper Vapor Laser The copper vapor laser can be configured to produce yellow light at 578 nm or green light at 511 nm. It does so by heating elemental copper or copper salts in the optical cavity. The created energy is released in the form of rapid low-energy pulses with a frequency of 10 to 15 kHz. The pulse duration varies from 20 to 40 ns, and the use of an electronic shutter device can generate pulses 0.075 to 0.3 s in duration.[73] Nevertheless, as with any CW laser, the pulse duration remains too long to produce selective photothermolysis at its target site. Rather, it causes nonselective thermal tissue damage.

Clinical applications of this laser include the treatment of both vascular and pigmented lesions. The copper vapor laser with its yellow light at 578 nm can be used much like the argon laser in the treatment of vascular lesions. These include larger-sized telangiectasias, cherry angiomas, spider angiomas, venous lakes, pyogenic granulomas, deeply red to blue and cobblestoned port-wine stains, angiokeratomas, Kaposi's sarcoma, and even blue-rubber-bleb nevi. The pigmented lesions amenable to treatment with the copper vapor laser with its green light at 511 nm include benign lesions like café-au-lait macules, lentigines, and early, still flat seborrheic keratoses. The targeting of epidermal melanin induces epidermal necrosis with resultant dermoepidermal separation.[3–5,73]

Not only the clinical applications but also the results are for the most part the same as those of the argon laser. In order to limit the potential for scarring secondary to adjacent thermal destruction, it is recommended to use energies below 15 J/cm² and to learn from an experienced laser surgeon before starting out on one's own.

Potassium Titanyl Phosphate Laser The potassium titanyl phosphate laser (KTP) uses Nd:YAG and potassium titanium phosphate crystals to generate a light beam of 532 nm. Using fluences of 15 to 20 J/cm² at these longer, 10- to 50-ms pulses, it effectively targets telangiectasias without rupturing them, thus avoiding postoperative purpura. Fol-

lowing treatment, there is only some erythema and swelling that generally disappears within 24 h. Purpura-free treatment of vascular lesions is appealing to adult patients, and they may choose the KTP laser over the pulsed-dye laser even if it is less efficient. One disadvantage of this laser is that its wavelength of 532 nm is well absorbed by melanin, thereby exposing darker-pigmented individuals to a significantly higher risk of epidermal tissue damage. Clinical applications and results are equivalent to those of the other CW lasers mentioned above. The use of newer cooling devices—which lower skin temperature as an adjunct to the laser treatment of vascular lesions—is proving to be useful in that it allows a greater target effect while limiting thermal damage. The combination of lower-energy fluences and operator experience will ensure the best possible outcome, keeping the potential for scarring to a minimum.[3,4,74–76]

Krypton Laser Energy is emitted by this laser in CW fashion, either a yellow light at a wavelength of 568 nm to treat vascular lesions or a green light at wavelengths of 521 and 530 nm to treat pigmented lesions. While an electronic shutter can break the beam up into shorter pulses, the skin still perceives it as a continuous beam of light, which is therefore unable to achieve selective photothermolysis. It can be used to treat the same range of cosmetically important lesions as the argon laser. The major benefits and disadvantages of this laser are the same as with the previously described CW lasers: purpura-free treatment of vascular lesions with only mild swelling and erythema but also increased risk of scarring secondary to nonselective thermal damage.[4,5,73]

CO_2 *Laser* The traditional CW CO_2 laser allows for vaporization that can be utilized in treating a wide range of epidermal and dermal lesions. Among these are actinic cheilitis, epidermal nevi, rhinophyma, resistant warts, appendiceal tumors, pigmented lesions, vascular lesions, and other inflammatory conditions. To ensure an optimal outcome in the treatment of these lesions, the operator must have a thorough understanding of the indications as well as proper technique.

Conventional laser vermilionectomy is effective at eradicating actinic cheilitis, and the risk of scarring is lower when it is appropriately applied. Usually a single pass at a low-power setting of 3 to 7 W, extended over the vermilion border, is sufficient to cause the epidermis to "bubble up"; it is then removed with a wet gauze pad. Prior to treatment, antiviral prophylaxis is indicated. Following treatment, the use of petrolatum or aquaphor will help to reduce the associated discomfort and speed the healing process, which may take 2 to 4 weeks to reach completion.[8,31,32]

In treating epidermal nevi, one must be aware of the relatively narrow margin of safety. If only the epidermis is taken away, the nevus soon return. Should the treatment extend as far as the reticular dermis, it can result in hypertrophic scarring. Thus, the aim is to keep the level of treatment at the papillary dermis to avoid recurrence and prevent scarring. Hypopigmentation may be anticipated after complete healing of a successfully treated epidermal nevus.[8,31,32]

The hypertrophied sebaceous glands of rhinophymas can be effectively debulked with the help of the conventional CO_2 laser. While the use of a scalpel or dermabrasion is also effective at debulking tissue, their use is characterized by substantial bleeding (with the scalpel) and blood aerosolization (in the case of dermabrasion). The CO_2 laser has the distinct advantage of simultaneously coagulating and vaporizing the tissue, thus avoiding any problems with bleeding. With a setting of 10 to 20 W in the defocused mode, the aim is to vaporize the excessive sebaceous tissue until a prerhinophyma shape, as verified with an old picture, has been attained. It is important to remain conservative with regard to the amount of tissue removed, as there is significant amount of posttreatment slough of thermally damaged dermis beyond the site that has actually been treated. In particular, the area of the nasal ala is susceptible to scarring. The healing process is usually completed within a month, while postoperative erythema may persist for several months.[8,35,36,77,78]

Owing to the cost, pain, and prolonged healing process associated with the CO_2 laser, less aggressive methods of destruction are preferred in the treatment of warts. However, the vaporization mode of the CO_2 laser is very useful in targeting resistant warts, such as those in a periungual, subungual, or plantar location, as the presence of a nail or thick stratum corneum does not present a hindrance, as with other destructive modalities. The response rate of these recalcitrant warts varies from 56 to 81 percent.[8,37–39,79]

Appendiceal tumors, such as syringomas, trichoepitheliomas, apocrine hydrocystomas, and others are easily vaporized with the CO_2 laser. A low-power setting is recommended, around 3 to 5 W, with a spot size matching that of the lesion to be treated. Vaporization of these lesions should extend into the dermis without removing them entirely, as one has to keep in mind the extension of residual thermal damage. In treating a large number of lesions, deepithelialization of the entire cosmetic unit should precede vaporization of the individual lesions. Reepithelialization normally occurs within 2 weeks. Although scarring is rarely seen, mild hypopigmentation may sometimes develop.[8,40–45]

There is no question that pigmented lesions do respond to treatment with the CO_2 laser. The question is whether it is wise to treat them in this way. Following CO_2 laser vaporization of melanocytic nevi, no tissue remains to confirm the diagnosis histologically. Thus, the CO_2 laser should not be used at all in a pigmented lesion if there is clinical doubt about its benign nature. Furthermore, it is not a good idea to treat medium to larger-sized congenital nevi, though benign in designation, as they have the potential to develop malignant melanomas within them. Laser vaporization fails to eradicate congenital nevi in their entirety, and they then become more difficult to follow clinically. Also, melanocytic nevi can recur and mimic a melanoma, a condition referred to as pseudomelanoma. Finally, there remains the question of whether exposure of nevomelanocytes to sublethal laser irradiation may increase their risk for malignant transformation.[8,19,80,81]

Vascular lesions that have been treated with vaporization using the CO_2 laser include port-wine stains, pyogenic granulomas, and lymphangioma circumscriptum. The last of these may be limited to the upper dermis but is often associated with a deep component. The significant lymphatic drainage resulting from the superficial component of the lesion, experienced by many patients, can be effectively treated with the CO_2 laser. During the healing process, a superficial layer of fibrosis develops that prevents further drainage. Thus, treatment of lymphangioma circumscriptum

with the CO_2 laser can be curative when the lesion is limited to the superficial dermis and palliative when it has a deeper dermal component.[8,47–51]

A number of inflammatory conditions have been treated with success using the CO_2 laser, as evidenced by occasional case reports. This list of inflammatory conditions includes Hailey-Hailey disease, granuloma faciale, chondrodermatitis nodularis helicis, keratoderma, porokeratosis, balanitis xerotica obliterans, Zoon's balanitis, and lichen sclerosus et atrophicus. Laser vaporization of these conditions should be done only if other, more conventional therapies have failed. To avoid scarring, it is a good idea to limit treatment to a test site before proceeding to treat the entire lesion. And when treating the lesion, it is vital to limit tissue injury to the level of the superficial dermis.[8]

Pulsed Lasers

Flashlamp-Pumped Pulsed-Dye Laser (585 nm) The vascular laser produces a light beam with a wavelength of 585 nm that is delivered as pulses of a short, 450-µs duration. This short pulse duration is less than the known relaxation time for microvessels. Therefore it follows the principle of selective photothermolysis to allow for highly specific targeting of blood vessels while avoiding thermal damage to the adjacent tissue. The consequent rupture of the targeted blood vessels results immediately in purpura, which usually resolves over a 1- to 2- week period. Scaling and crusting may also be observed. However, complications such as blistering and scarring are quite rare, estimated to be less than 1 percent.[3–5,82]

The pulsed-dye laser (PDL) was initially developed for the treatment of port-wine stains.[83] Since then, it has proven itself effective in the treatment of a wide range of vascular lesions, including telangiectasias,[84] spider angiomas,[85] cherry angiomas,[86] venous lakes,[86] pyogenic granulomas,[87] poikiloderma of Civatte,[88] angiofibromas,[89] Kaposi's sarcoma,[90] lymphangioma circumscriptum,[91] blue-rubber-bleb nevi,[92] verrucae,[93] inflammatory linear verrucous epidermal nevi,[94] and scars.[95] Variables in the treatment of these lesions are the spot size (5 to 10 mm) and the fluence (4 to 9 J/cm^2). Deeper tissue penetration can be achieved with a larger spot size. To achieve a similar tissue depth of penetration with a smaller spot size, it is necessary to increase the fluence. Even when using the proper parameters, treatment of these vascular lesions may have to be repeated several times at 4- to 8-week intervals to remove them entirely, as the vessels are often not uniform, varying in diameter and flow rate.[4]

Flashlamp-Pumped Pulsed-Dye Laser (510 nm) This pigment-specific laser emits green light at a wavelength of 510 nm partnered with a 300-ns pulse duration and a fluence between 2 and 3.5 J/cm^2 that is very well absorbed by melanin in the epidermis. Thus, it is very effective in treating epidermal pigmented lesions. However, as the penetration of this wavelength is limited to the superficial dermis, it is of no help in the treatment of dermal pigmented lesions. Side effects are limited to transient postoperative erythema, edema, and rarely purpura. The last of these side effects is related to absorption by oxyhemoglobin. Potential complications consist of transient pigmentary alterations, including hypo- and hyperpigmentation.[3–5,96]

Q-Switched Lasers The group of Q-switched lasers belongs to the category of pulsed lasers that work on the principle of selective photothermolysis. Among them are the Q-switched ruby, the Q-switched alexandrite, and the Q-switched Nd:YAG laser. As previously explained, the term *Q-switching* refers to a specialized technique not found in other lasers, involving an optical polarizer and a Pockel cell. This configuration allows for a large amount of energy to build up prior to its release in a sudden powerful burst.[5]

The Q-switched ruby laser emits a visible red light at 694 nm with a short pulse duration of 28 to 50 ns. It is preferentially absorbed by melanin and blue to black tattoo pigments. Hence, it has been successfully used in the treatment of various epidermal and dermal pigmented lesions. Also, it has been used in the past in the treatment of excessive terminal hair.[3–5,97]

The alexandrite laser is also of the Q-switched type, but emits a red light with a wavelength of 755 nm and a longer pulse duration at 100 ns. It is similar to the Q-switched ruby laser in that it also targets melanin and tattoo pigment, allowing for the treatment of the same type of pigmented lesions. With regard to tattoo pigment, it is especially effective at removing green pigment. Also, the red light of the alexandrite laser is utilized in the newer generation of hair removal lasers. The longer wavelength of the alexandrite laser as compared with the Q-switched ruby laser penetrates the skin more deeply with less epidermal absorption, which may be an advantage in treating dermal pigmented lesions, professional tattoos, and terminal hair in more heavily pigmented individuals.[3–5,98]

The Nd:YAG laser differs from the other Q-switched lasers in that it emits an invisible, near infrared light beam with a wavelength of 1064 nm as well as a green light with a wavelength of 532 nm when a frequency-doubling crystal is used. This unique capability allows for selective targeting of chromophores. Melanin is well absorbed by both wavelengths of the Nd:YAG laser, though somewhat better at 532 nm. The longer wavelength of 1064 nm allows for deeper dermal penetration and, thus, may be more effective in treating dermal melanocytoses, such as nevi of Ota and Ito. With regard to treatment of tattoos, the Nd:YAG at 1064 nm predominantly targets black pigment, while its wavelength of 532 nm is primarily absorbed by red pigment. Despite lacking the specificity of the other two Q-switched lasers in targeting melanin, the Nd:YAG has been used in the removal of unwanted hair, often with assistance of a topical carbon suspension acting as an exogenous target chromophore when introduced to the hair follicle. The multiple applications possible with this laser make it an effective tool for the laser surgeon.[3–5,99]

Diode Laser

High-Power Diode Laser Array The Lightsheer Diode laser is a high-power diode laser array that was recently approved by the U.S. Food and Drug Administration (FDA) for hair removal. Like all diode lasers, it utilizes semiconductor technology to emit light in the near infrared range, allowing for miniaturization and high efficiency. In particular, this high-power diode array emits light at a wavelength of 800 nm with a pulse width of 5 to 30 ms, a 9×9 mm spot size, a 1-Hz repetition rate, and fluences between 10 to 40 J/cm.[2] The resultant light beam targets melanin within hair follicles, while contact cooling with a patented sapphire handpiece provides epidermal protection. This constellation of features offers long-lasting and possibly permanent hair reduction that may even be used to treat darker-skinned individuals with relative safety.[100–102]

LASER SAFETY

Working with lasers exposes the patient and the laser surgeon to potential health hazards. These include the following: (1) accidental eye injury, (2) ignition of fire, and (3) aerosolization of hazardous particles. Keeping these hazards in mind, there are several steps the responsible laser surgeon can take to minimize such unfortunate accidents. The possibility of eye injury due to exposure to the laser light is a real health risk to both the patient and the surgeon, but it can be essentially avoided by applying some common-sense measures. To begin with, the patient, the surgeon, and anyone else in the treatment room must wear the appropriate laser safety glasses with side shields before the laser is used. Next, care must be taken to remove any reflective jewelry and surgical instruments from the laser field to prevent reflection of the laser light. Along the same line, the surgical instruments ideally should be nonreflective. Before starting laser treatment, it is necessary to make sure that the door to the treatment room is closed, marked with a clearly posted laser warning sign on its exterior side. Furthermore, the windows should be dressed with a nontranslucent cover to keep innocent bystanders from being injured by a reflected laser beam. Also, skin preparation with chlorhexidine is contraindicated, as it may cause irreversible damage to the cornea when vaporized. Last, once active treatment starts, the laser surgeon should be highly aware of the direction in which the laser beam is pointing and keep it at standby or off and away from the patient and bystanders when resting.[8,103]

Ignition of fire is another potential health hazard, particularly in working with the CO_2 laser. To prevent fire injury, it is important to be aware of potentially inflammable subjects and keep them away from the surgical field and surroundings. Thus, skin preparation with alcohol is contraindicated, as it is flammable. Dry gauze should never enter the surgical field during treatment with the CO_2 laser, and drapes in the surgical field must be wet. Also, as oxygen is a highly flammable substance, particular care should be applied to removing the oxygen mask in CO_2 lasering of the perinasal region and using a nonflammable endotracheal tube or one that is covered with nonflammable and nonreflective material in resurfacing the skin of a patient under general anesthesia. And once again, the laser should be at standby or off when the patient is not being actively treated.[104]

Aerosolization of hazardous particles can affect exposed individuals in two ways. Laser treatment of warts and CO_2 laser resurfacing of the intact skin of an HIV-positive individual leads to a laser plume containing human papillomavirus (HPV) and human immunodeficiency virus (HIV), respectively; this poses a risk for transmission. However, to date there has been no documented case of HIV infection due to exposure to a CO_2 laser plume containing the virus. The other exposure risk is that to a plume of carbonized particles, which carries a higher carcinogenicity than cigarette smoke. Safety measures to ensure against exposure to such infectious and carcinogenic particles start with checking the patient's HIV status prior to treatment with the CO_2 laser. Next, the laser surgeon and anyone present during the procedure must wear a laser mask that filters particles of at least 0.1 μm diameter. And the individual operating the high efficiency smoke evacuator has to keep the smoke evacuator tube as close as possible to the laser treatment site. To gain the best possible smoke evacuation, the tube should not be more than 1 cm away from the site being treated, as an increase in the distance to 2 cm has been shown to diminish the smoke evacuation efficiency by 50 percent.[7,8,105,106]

LASER SURGERY

Ablative Cutaneous Resurfacing: CO_2 Laser and Erbium:YAG Laser

Patient Selection The basis of successful laser resurfacing lies in proper patient selection. This requires a systematic approach during the consultation visit, involving a thorough history, physical examination, and laboratory workup as well as patient education focused on the controlled cutaneous wounding achieved with the laser resurfacing.

A thorough history must examine the medical, surgical, psychological, and social aspects of each potential candidate. As laser resurfacing causes controlled cutaneous wounding, it is important to make sure that the patient does not have a medical history of collagen vascular disease, thyroid dysfunction, diabetes, other immune disorders, or isotretinoin use in the recent past. Also, a medical history of viral, bacterial, and yeast infections may necessitate an adjustment in the antiviral, antibiotic, and antiyeast regimen. A prior history of various cosmetic procedures, including various forms of resurfacing (chemical, mechanical, and laser) and blepharoplasty may predispose the patient to a higher risk for fibrosis and ectropion, respectively. Next, a positive psychological profile should be of concern, especially if the condition is not well medicated, as this may predispose the patient to unrealistic expectations and may be a setup for patient dissatisfaction irrespective of how good the actual outcome of the procedure may be. In reviewing the patient's social history, it is important to focus on smoking and the presence of a social support system. Tobacco use is detrimental to wound healing; therefore the patient should be encouraged either to stop smoking or at least markedly reduce the daily nicotine abuse before undergoing laser resurfacing. The presence of a good social support system is vital to proper postoperative care and ultimately to a good outcome from both the patient's and physician's perspective. Moral support by the surrounding family makes the prolonged healing phase of laser resurfacing a less arduous ordeal to the patient and will require less "hand-holding" by the physician.[107–110]

The physical examination consists of two parts. One is the cutaneous examination, which concentrates on indications and contraindications of laser resurfacing. The indications are slightly different for the two resurfacing lasers. The ideal skin type for either type of resurfacing laser is fair (Fitzpatrick type I or II), as patients with darker skin tones (Fitzpatrick type III or IV) need to be treated far more cautiously to avoid pigmentary alterations. Although both resurfacing lasers aim at skin rejuvenation, the CO_2 laser, with

its far more extensive collagen-tightening effects, works better for patients with moderate to extensive photo damage in the form of rhytids and dyspigmentation in the perioral and periorbital regions and the cheeks. The erbium:YAG laser is more limited to treatment of patients with mild to moderate photo damage in the same distribution. Neither type of laser works particularly well for movement-associated rhytids of the forehead, glabellar region, and nasolabial folds, making them a secondary indication. In fact, movement-associated rhytids will be significantly improved only when they are treated with laser resurfacing in combination with another cosmetic procedure, such as facial rhytidectomy. Facial scarring, often the result of severe acne, will also be more responsive to the CO_2 laser than the erbium:YAG. In particular, atrophic acne scarring responds well to the collagen-tightening effects of the CO_2 laser, while deeply pitted scars may necessitate an approach in combination with punch excision and grafting to achieve any considerable improvement. Contraindications evident on the cutaneous examination include evidence of ongoing UV exposure, hyperelastic or keloidal skin, koebnerizing diseases, fibrosis from prior cosmetic procedures of the face, skin changes secondary to collagen vascular diseases or prior radiation exposure, concurrent cutaneous bacterial or viral infection, and ectropion. The presence of an ongoing cutaneous infection and an ectropion both are absolute contraindications, while the other contraindications are all relative. And medical clearance by an internist or family physician to undergo conscious sedation for laser resurfacing makes up the other part of the physical examination. It must be obtained well in advance of the surgical appointment.[60,107,111–113]

The laboratory workup in preparation for laser resurfacing is primarily directed toward detecting underlying medical disorders that may prove inhibitory to wound healing, as mentioned above, or a risk to the physician. Thus, for every one of our patients scheduled for laser resurfacing, we request a complete blood count, chemistry panel, thyroid function tests, liver function tests, HB_sAg, and HIV test. In addition, every female patient should have a pregnancy test just prior to the scheduled surgery time, as the patient may attribute any negative outcome regarding the pregnancy to the laser resurfacing procedure even if there is no evidence-based connection.

Finally, patient education is of paramount importance to the outcome of this surgical procedure. This is twofold. First, there must be a review what the laser resurfacing procedure entails, including anesthesia and its potential risks, controlled cutaneous ablation, length of procedure from start to finish, postoperative recovery time from reepithelialization to resolution of erythema, postoperative care, potential complications, clinical follow-up regimen, and the cost involved. Second, patient education must be directed toward setting realistic patient expectations. Hence, the physician should talk to patients about the expected range of improvement, how long after the resurfacing they are likely to achieve their maximal improvement, and how long the laser resurfacing effects last. Reviewing results with "before and "after" photographs of several previously treated patients can be very helpful in this respect. These aspects of patient education should be reiterated during the consultation session and documented in the form of a consent form signed by the patient. If the patient appears to have unrealistic expectations for this procedure despite proper patient education, the physician should decline service to them. Such patients are not going to be satisfied with the outcome of the laser resurfacing no matter how good the actual results are, and an unhappy patient makes for a very unhappy physician.

Preoperative Regimen The result of newly resurfaced skin is an open wound with exposed dermis, as the epidermis has been obliterated. The goal with any open wound is to achieve rapid healing with a good cosmetic appearance while also preventing infection. Consequently, there is an abundant literature on the subjects of skin care preparation and anti-infectious prophylaxis in laser resurfacing.

The skin care preparation used by many of the physicians attempting to achieve the best possible outcome of laser resurfacing is mistakenly based on the lightweight literature of preconditioning of the skin for chemical peeling and dermabrasion. The idea behind preconditioning the skin is that it establishes a more homogenous wound during resurfacing, allowing for more rapid reepithelialization while minimizing postinflammatory hyperpigmentation. The topical agents used for such skin care preparation include the vitamin A derivative tretinoin, alpha-hydroxy acids, and hydroquinone. Tretinoin became the primary preconditioning agent when studies pointed to its ability to accelerate wound healing in chemical peeling and dermabrasion. The mechanism behind tretinoin's effect on wound healing may relate to retinoids' ability to enhance the production of mucopolysaccharides, collagen, and fibronectin, curtail collagenase production, and incite both epidermal mitotic activity and migration. Alpha-hydroxy acids have also been used in preconditioning skin based on their ability to decrease corneocyte adhesion and stratum corneum thickness and to expand production of glycosaminoglycans and collagen. But there are no studies to demonstrate that alpha-hydroxy acids result in improved wound healing when used in priming skin for chemical peeling or dermabrasion. And hydroquinone is frequently used in preconditioning of the skin in chemical peeling, as it is thought to diminish the appearance of postinflammatory hyperpigmentation by lessening melanosome formation, changing melanosome structure, and enhancing melanosome degeneration via tyrosine inhibition.[114–118]

However, these priming principles do not necessarily apply to laser resurfacing. In fact, there are no data to uphold the usefulness of tretinoin, alpha-hydroxy acids, or hydroquinone as preconditioning agents in laser resurfacing. Experts have noted that patients with skin types I to III pretreated with topical glycolic acid or combination tretinoin/hydroquinone failed to show a statistically significant difference in postoperative hyperpigmentation as compared with those patients who did not get any pretreatment. Accordingly, we do not recommend the use of any skin care preparation for our patients undergoing laser resurfacing. Patients may be on a skin care program prior to resurfacing that contains the aforementioned agents, and they may use such agents until the morning of their procedure. They may rightfully expect a follow-up skin care regimen based upon their previous inquiries and a desire for a certain degree of control over their care. This will be instituted postoperatively at the physician's discretion. The physician may use the patient's ability to follow a skin care program as a gauge of his or her likely compliance with postoperative care instructions, which are so vital to good cosmesis following laser resurfacing. Tretinoin and alpha-hydroxy acids may help to reduce the appearance of milia or acne lesions postoperatively, but they must be introduced gradually, generally no sooner than 3 to 6 weeks postoperatively.[107,119]

As with any other type of wound, there is always a concern about the potential development of infection following resurfacing that may mar its results despite otherwise flawless technique. Thus, the great majority of laser surgeons do prescribe drugs for antiviral and antibacterial prophylaxis.

Latent herpes reactivation, particularly in the perioral region, is a clearly identified risk that occurs in approximately 2 to 7 percent of all laser resurfacing patients.[120] Even patients with no prior history of herpes simplex infection may develop an extensive viral infection of the resurfaced area. Since a high percentage of the population has been exposed to the herpes simplex virus independent of any prior history of herpetic infection, the prescription of antiherpetic agents for any patient undergoing laser resurfacing is recommended. We prescribe famcyclovir at a dose of 500 mg orally two times daily, starting 24 h before the procedure and continuing for a total of 10 days. Other commonly used antiherpetic regimens used include acyclovir 400 mg orally three times daily and valacyclovir (Valtrex) 500 mg orally twice a day.

On the other hand, the use of prophylactic antibiotics is not as well established. There are no controlled studies supporting the common practice of prescribing antibiotic agents to patients undergoing laser resurfacing.[112] This practice is upheld for two reasons. Newly resurfaced skin is likened to a superficial burn, generating abundant drainage and mild to moderate crusting, which offer optimal conditions for colonization with bacteria. Also, thermal injury results in local immunosuppression, which may further increase the risk of a bacterial infection. But recent studies[121,122] on burn patients have demonstrated that the use of oral prophylactic antibiotics did not reduce the incidence of infection as compared with that of untreated controls, and it may lead to a higher incidence of infection with resistant bacterial organisms and colonization with *Candida*. In fact, despite the use of oral prophylactic antibiotics in laser resurfacing, infections have been noted to occur in 1 to 4.3 percent of patients—the identified responsible organisms usually are *Staphylococcus aureus* and *Pseudomonas aeruginosa*,[117,120,123,124] the latter occurring most frequently in patients undergoing "closed" wound healing. Nevertheless, given the cosmetic nature of the laser resurfacing procedure and the potential threat of scarring secondary to bacterial infection, most laser surgeons do make use of prophylactic antibiotics. It has been our practice to give our patients a 2-g intravenous dose of cephalexin because of its excellent coverage against gram-positive organisms. Other commonly used antibiotics that offer a similar effective coverage against gram-positive organisms are dicloxacillin, azithromycin, and ciprofloxacin.

Resurfacing Procedure and Technique To allow for effective laser resurfacing, patients must be well anesthetized.

Involuntary movements due to pain may result in injury or scarring. For laser resurfacing, the types of anesthesia vary from topical to local anesthesia to regional anesthesia with nerve blocks to intravenous sedation or general anesthesia. In our opinion, topical anesthesia with a eutectic mixture of lidocaine 2.5% and prilocaine 2.5% (EMLA cream) is not effective for resurfacing beyond the epidermal level. Local anesthesia may be carried out with success for small cosmetic units, such as the periorbital region or upper lip. And nerve blocks, if done correctly and after allowing for enough time for diffusion of the anesthetic, can be used to achieve anesthesia for larger cosmetic units, like the forehead, medial cheeks, and chin. Many experts have found the use of intravenous sedation ideal for laser resurfacing. The combination of short-acting intravenous sedative agents such as propofol, fentanyl, and midazolam provides rapid and adequate anesthesia. And while general anesthesia may work well, it suffers from decreased patient acceptance and does not permit as rapid a recovery as intravenous sedation.[107,125,126]

With the patient anesthetized, care is taken to ensure that appropriate safety measures are in place before turning to the actual resurfacing and the technique involved. In particular, eye protection is accomplished by employment of nonreflective laser eye shields lubricated with ophthalmic ointment. These are placed in the eyes like contact lenses after the application of tetracaine drops and removed only upon completion of the resurfacing procedure. Then, as an initial step, cosmetic units to be treated are clearly marked; additional markings may be used to outline the extent of wrinkles and scars. Thereafter, the skin may be cleansed with an antiseptic like Septisol, followed by rinsing with normal saline. Unlike the case with other surgical procedures, lengthy skin preparation and cleansing are not necessary, as laser resurfacing sterilizes the skin and agents like chlorhexidine and alcohol actually pose a fire hazard.[8] Now the focus is on the resurfacing technique.

Although there are differences in resurfacing technique between the CO_2 laser and the erbium:YAG laser, certain rules apply to both. The setting of the laser parameters differs from case to case, depending on the area to be treated, the patient's skin type, prior cosmetic procedures, the depth of the lesion, and the surgeon's comfort level. A mindful approach employing conservative energy values and/or fewer passes should be taken when facing anatomic areas prone to scarring (malar and periorbital regions, upper lip, mandible, and neck). This also applies to patients with skin types III and above or patients with a history of radiation, dermabrasion, or chemical peeling, as they are at a higher risk for complications. Next, in laser resurfacing, the energy density for either type of laser must match or exceed the critical threshold of irradiance (5 J/cm²), since lower irradiances increase the risk for undue thermal damage and charring. Also, it is essential to treat various anatomic regions as the different cosmetic units they represent, avoiding a sharp transition from one unit to the other or to untreated skin by feathering along the borders of these cosmetic units. This feathering can be achieved by using lower energy per pulse or a lower pulse density or by keeping the laser beam at an oblique angle to soften its impact on the skin. In resurfacing rhytids, the goal is to achieve effacement by carrying ablation

throughout the entire length and depth of these wrinkles. Another important point is that the shoulders of scars may need additional laser passes to achieve satisfactory results. And meticulous laser technique requires that pulse overlap or scan stacking be minimized, as such excess thermal injury is associated with a higher risk for scarring. Throughout the resurfacing process, ablation to prevent scarring, attention must be paid to the depth of ablation. The endpoint of treatment is defined by varying degrees of effacement of wrinkles or scars while limiting depth of ablation to the papillary or upper reticular dermis. Resurfacing beyond this point increases the risk of scarring.[60,104,107,113,127,128]

Before proceeding with CO_2 laser resurfacing, the laser surgeon must have a thorough understanding of its capabilities, know how to vary its parameters and application with the nuances of different anatomic sites, and possess the ability to use clinical findings to aid in recognizing the clinical endpoint. The CO_2 systems, of which there are several, ordinarily vaporize 20 to 60 μm of tissue on the first pass, completely obliterating the epidermis. The depth of residual thermal damage reaches 20 to 100 μm after a few passes. Following the first pass, each subsequent pass vaporizes lesser amounts of tissue owing to the effects of progressive desiccation. But on average, most CO_2 systems ablate down to the papillary dermis after only two passes and reach the upper reticular dermis with three passes. And it has been shown that more than three passes do not by guarantee a better clinical and histologic outcome. Keeping in mind this power of ablation, the operator must vary the energy parameters and the number of passes according to the thickness of the skin and its susceptibility to scarring. Commonly, using an Ultrapulse CO_2 laser with the 8-mm computer pattern generator (CPG) scan at settings of 250 to 300 mJ, 60 W power, and a density 5, resurfacing would proceed. Thin areas of the skin that are also generally prone to scarring—including the eyelids, malar region, upper lip, mandible, and neck—may receive one or rarely two passes, while thicker areas of the skin, like the cheeks and forehead, may be treated with as many as three or four passes. This applies especially if the forehead and cheeks show signs of heavy photo damage or significant atrophic acne scarring but are otherwise healthy. In making multiple passes during resurfacing, it is our preference to use a pattern similar to dermabrasion, where the first pass may be vertical while the second pass is oblique, followed by a pass that is horizontal, and so on. For the purpose of feathering of transition zones, in particular along the mandible and the preauricular region (especially when treated in combination with facial rhytidectomy), the laser beam is held at an oblique angle. And between laser passes it is usually desirable to carefully remove coagulated debris with a wet gauze, as it may serve as a heat sink that diminishes tissue vaporization while at the same time leading to increased thermal injury. Also, removal of this keratinous debris makes for better visualization of clinical findings. Clinical findings in the form of changes in the skin color help in the recognition of the depth of the achieved ablation. Removal of the debris after one pass reveals the pink color of the dehydrated papillary dermis. Subsequent passes result in a transition to a chamois color at the level of the deeper papillary dermis and a yellowish hue at the level of the reticular dermis. Consideration of all these factors allows for successful CO_2 laser resurfacing without untoward risk for the patient.[60,104,107,113,127–129]

In comparison, erbium:YAG lasers vaporize on average only 2 to 5 μm of tissue with one pass. With the erbium:YAG laser, unlike the CO_2 lasers, there is no decrease in the depth of ablation with subsequent passes, as there is a relatively small zone of thermal damage, ranging from 20 to 50 μm. The depth of ablation relates directly to the energy density used. The latter can be varied from 5 J/cm² in treating the thin skin of the periorbital area to 15 J/cm² for areas of thicker, more actinically damaged skin. Therefore erbium: YAG lasers allow for a greater range of adaptability than CO_2 lasers in targeting mild to moderate actinic damage or acne scarring. However, due to their shallower depth of ablation, erbium:YAG lasers are less able than CO_2 lasers to deal with more severe photodamage or acne scarring. It actually takes three to four passes with an erbium:YAG laser to ablate the same amount of tissue as with one pass of a CO_2 laser. In clinical terms, this translates to two to three passes with an erbium:YAG laser at the irradiance threshold (5 J/cm) to completely obliterate the epidermis as compared with one pass with a CO_2 laser. And to gain the same depth of ablation

as with three passes with a CO_2 laser—namely the level of the upper reticular dermis—it takes a total of nine to ten passes with an erbium:YAG laser. Furthermore, the photomechanical injury produced by an erbium laser effectively removes the desiccated tissue on each pass, leaving behind whitened areas of skin that fade fast and make it difficult to judge the depth of ablation by the skin color, as with a CO_2 laser. Instead, the amount of bleeding encountered during the resurfacing helps to determine the depth of ablation. The pinpoint bleeding achieved after several passes indicates that the level of the papillary dermis has been reached. Thereafter, keeping track of the number of passes is the only guide to the depth of ablation beyond the development of brisk bleeding. Brisk bleeding also indicates the endpoint of treatment, independent of whether rhytids or scars are fully ablated. In summary, while an erbium:YAG laser allows for more fine tuning in the treatment of mild to moderate rhytids and acne scars, it is more time-consuming and less effective in terms of deep ablation than a CO_2 laser.[60,107]

The results of ablative laser resurfacing are second to none in reversing the effects of cutaneous aging and sun damage. Both physician and patient are often elated with the outcome (see Figs. 14-1 through 14-11).

(text continues on page 197)

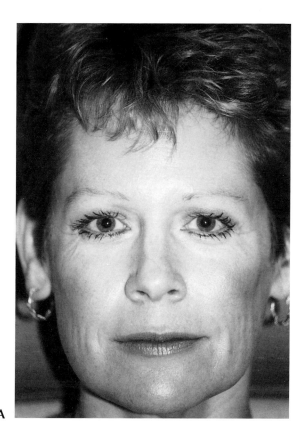 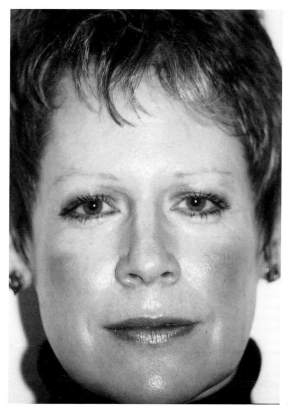

A   B

Figure 14-1 (*A*) This 42-year-old patient had mild dermatoheliosis with early rhytid formation due mainly to inherited tendency. (*B*) A CO_2 laser resurfacing was performed. The patient is seen 6 weeks postoperatively.

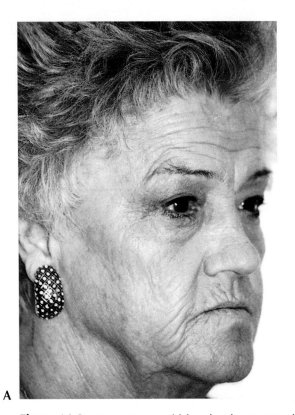
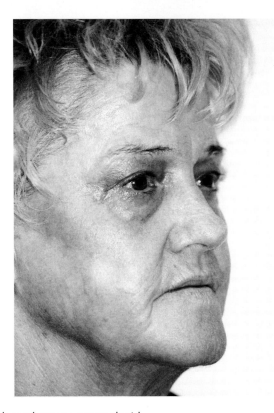

A   B

Figure 14-2 (*A*) A 68-year old-female who presented with moderate to severe rhytid formation. (*B*) The postoperative view, obtained 4 months following CO_2 laser resurfacing.

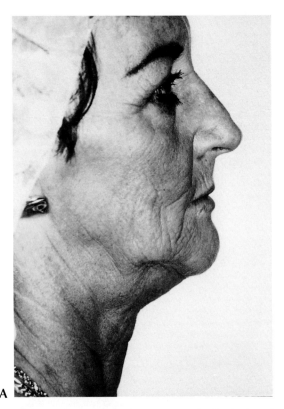
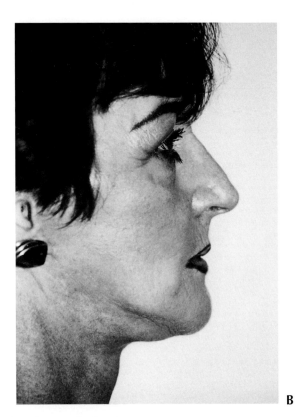

A   B

Figure 14-3 (*A*) Another patient who had a long history of smoking and solar damage. (*B*) The 6-month postoperative view shows good improvement following CO_2 laser resurfacing, with a slight line of demarcation at the jaw line easily coverable with makeup. The patient also had neck and jowl liposuction.

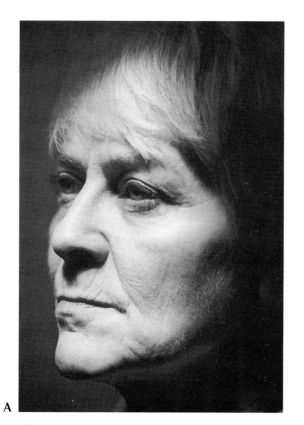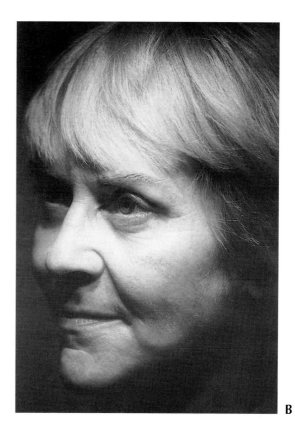

Figure 14-4 (**A**) This 61-year-old patient's greatest concern were rhytids in the perioral zone. (**B**) Excellent correction is noted following a CO_2 laser peel; however, patients are clearly told to expect only 40 to 80% improvement on average.

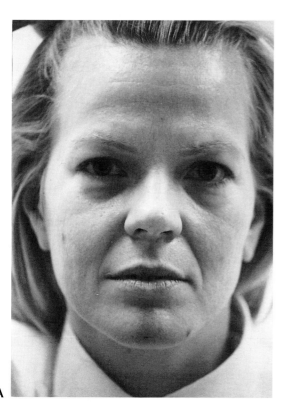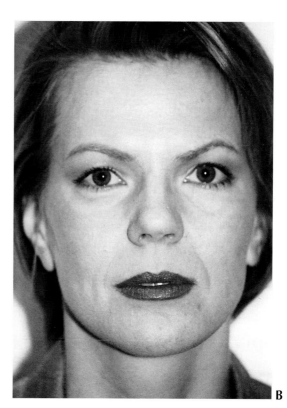

Figure 14-5 (**A**) A 41-year-old patient with early rhytid formation and mild acne scarring who requested maximal improvement. (**B**) The CO_2 laser can be used at various settings to allow for blending and customizing the resurfacing process. The patient was very pleased with the result 3 months postoperatively.

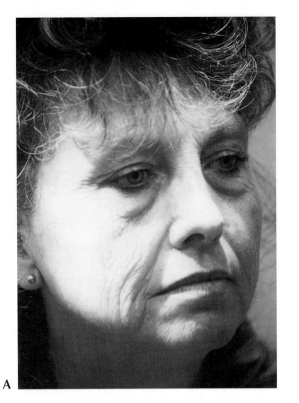
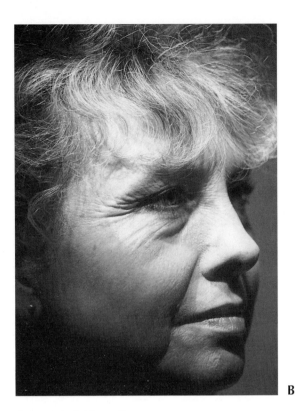

A   B

Figure 14-6 (*A*) This 51-year-old professional was concerned about rhytid formation on her cheeks. She had limited time off. (*B*) Significant improvement can be noted 3 months following an erbium:YAG resurfacing procedure. The periorbital zone and chin did not respond as well to this "kinder and gentler" procedure.

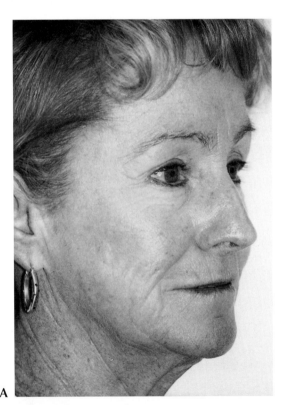
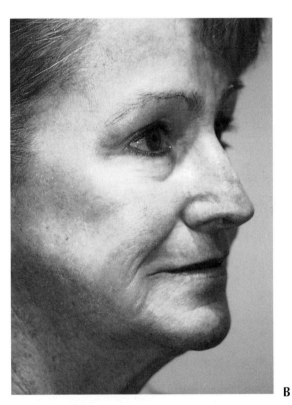

A   B

Figure 14-7 (*A*) Another 57-year-old woman wanted improvement of her wrinkles but often traveled and did not have much time for recovery. (*B*) An erbium:YAG laser treatment was performed. At 3 months, very good improvement can be seen in the glabellar, periocular, and periorbital zones.

194

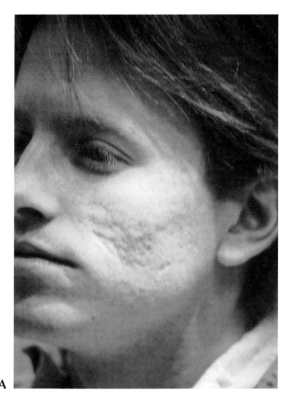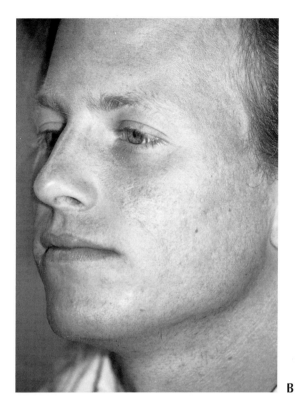

A   B

Figure 14-8 (*A*) This 28-year-old man presented with widespread facial scarring. (*B*) Excellent improvement is seen 6 months following CO$_2$ laser resurfacing. For acne scarring, average improvement is usually in the 20 to 80 percent range.

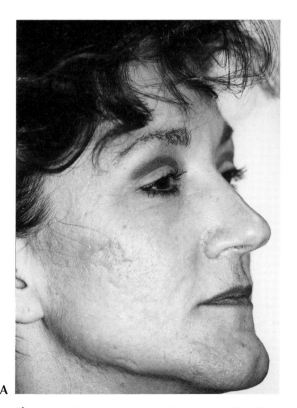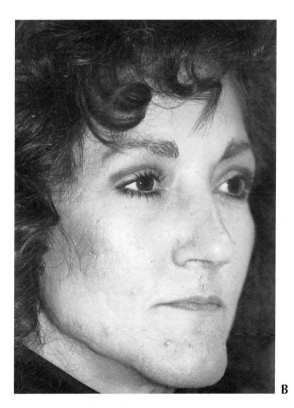

A   B

Figure 14-9 (*A*) A 38-year-old woman with a history of acne is concerned about the irregular skin contour of her cheeks. (*B*) At 3 months, significant improvement is noted. For acne scarring, average improvement is usually in the 20 to 80 percent range.

195

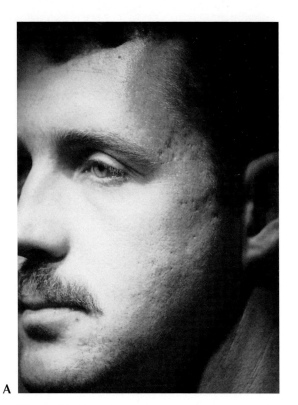
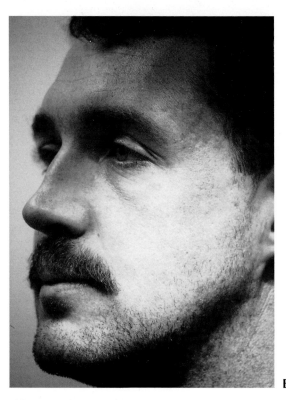

A   B

Figure 14-10 (*A*) Acne scarring was present in this 34-year-old man with an outdoor profession. Resurfacing with an erbium:YAG laser was planned to minimize recuperative time. (*B*) Good improvement was seen at 4 months postoperatively.

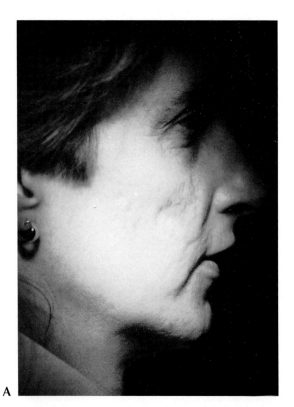
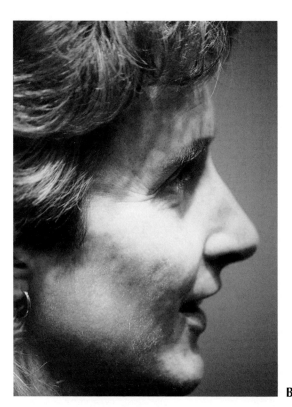

A   B

Figure 14-11 (*A*) Facial scarring in a 39-year-old professional speaker. After discussing options, she underwent erbium:YAG laser resurfacing. (*B*) At 3 months postoperatively, she was pleased with results. Injectable filler substances were later used to enhance the results.

196

Postoperative Regimen Postoperative care can be divided into two parts. The first takes place in the initial 7 to 14 days, the time it takes to achieve reepithelialization, and should address the choice of wound dressing, pain management, and whether to use systemic steroids. The second part of postoperative care takes place after completion of reepithelialization and consists of preventive skin care measures.

The subject of what constitutes the best postoperative wound care until reepithelialization has occurred is beset with controversy yet remains adaptable to physician preference. It certainly has been established that the partial-thickness wound of laser resurfacing benefits from a moist environment, as this promotes reepithelialization. Yet dry crusts and eschar formation hinder keratinocyte migration and thus the healing process.[130] However, the question remains whether this moist environment is best achieved with an open or closed technique of wound dressing.

The open technique of wound dressing involves frequent soaking with distilled water or normal saline (with or without the addition of some white vinegar) and subsequent application of a topical antibiotic or a bland emollient. This technique offers the advantage of being cheap, providing patients with a sense of control over their own care, and allowing for early recognition of an infectious process. Disadvantages evolve from the dependence on patient compliance. The patient's failure to apply sufficient amounts of antibiotic ointment or emollient may result in dryness, crusting, bleeding, and pain. On the other hand, excessive application of ointment or emollient may lead to acne, milia, and even a higher risk for bacterial and yeast infections. Thus, patients must often be instructed thoroughly in order to ensure compliance.[107] If one is utilizing an open technique of wound dressing, bland emollients are preferable over antibiotic ointments. Topical antibiotics may diminish the amount of bacteria colonizing the wound surface, but they are often the cause of contact dermatitis and should be avoided.[131] And studies[117] have failed to show a significant difference in the incidence of infection and in the healing time between wounds treated with an occlusive emollient (petrolatum) and those treated with a topical antibiotic. Care should be taken in choosing among the different types of plain emollient for wound care, as they may affect wound healing. Commonly used emollients that are recommended include white petrolatum, Crisco, and Aquaphor (our personal choice). An inert lotion containing propylene glycol and white petrolatum cream has actually been shown to increase wound healing by 15 and 24 percent, respectively. In contrast, a preparation containing USP petrolatum diminished wound healing by 17 percent.[132]

The closed technique of wound dressing consists of a totally occlusive or a semiocclusive dressing to promote a moist healing environment. Semiocclusive dressings, such as hydrogels and silicone polymer films, are preferable over a totally occlusive dressing, as they not only absorb exudate but also allow for a certain degree of wound inspection. Wound healing has been demonstrated to be equivalent or possibly improved with these dressings in comparison with topical antibiotics or some bland emollients alone. Furthermore, closed dressings can be well liked by patients owing to the sense of comfort they may provide. However, some patients dislike them, as they may make them feel claustrophobic or cause difficulty in sleeping. Additional drawbacks are significant: they may include 24-h dressing changes that are often time-consuming and high in cost because of the materials alone and the consumption of nursing time; they may also pose a risk of denuding fragile reepithelium owing to their tendency to stick. Finally, leakage of exudate and a loss of such a dressing's integrity may occur after prolonged use, causing a change in the wound's metabolic environment and possibly posing a higher risk of infection—and the start of an infection may be missed because of the the occlusive or semiocclusive nature of the dressing.[107,117]

There is no consensus as to which type of dressing best maintains the moist environment required for optimal wound healing. Yet many laser surgeons favor the open technique for the reasons outlined above, especially because it lacks the higher risk for infection and diminished visibility for wound inspection associated with the closed technique. The utilization of a semiocclusive dressing for the first 24 to 48 h after surgery and, thereafter, making use of a bland emollient seems to be the ideal approach.

Besides the choice of wound dressing, the first part of postoperative care must consider pain management and the question of whether to use systemic steroids. In our experience, the discomfort a patient experiences is similar in nature to varying degrees of sunburn but does not last beyond 1 to 3 postoperative days. Any significant pain generally responds to nonsteroidal anti-inflammatory agents, with the occasional use of an oral narcotic analgesic. Complaints of burning beyond this time period or the prolonged use of analgesics may indicate a more serious underlying problem, such as a herpetic or bacterial infection or a contact dermatitis. If a patient has trouble sleeping, the addition of a mild sedative may be helpful. With regard to the use of systemic steroids following laser resurfacing, there are no studies in the literature that document their effectiveness. And steroids may actually be responsible for side effects such as sleeping problems and mood swings.[107,133] Still, many laser surgeons will routinely give their patients systemic steroids after laser resurfacing for the purpose of decreasing swelling.

The second part of postoperative care consists of preventive skin care measures to protect the newly formed epithelium. Rules that patients should abide by are as follows: (1) Strictly avoid sun for the first 3 months or until complete resolution of postoperative erythema. (2) Make use of UVA and UVB blocking agents to prevent burning and postinflammatory hyperpigmentation (titanium dioxide and zinc oxide are recommended if sunscreen is applied before 6 weeks postoperatively). (3) Wash the face only with mild synthetic detergents. (4) Moisturize the skin with products that are free of oils, perfumes, or preservatives and are not too occlusive. (5) Avoid the use of tretinoin and alpha-hydroxy acids until 6 to 12 weeks after laser resurfacing, as prior application may result in irritation. (6) Do not start the use of foundation makeup until completion of reepithelialization (usually 7 to 14 days postoperatively), as its adherence to the oozing skin hinders the healing process. Thereafter, foundation makeup helps with the coverage of postoperative erythema (particularly when it has a yellow or green base) and offers the benefit of additional sun protection.[107]

Side Effects, Complications, and Their Management Despite the best efforts at proper patient selection, flawless laser technique, and optimal postoperative care, side effects and complications may develop. These occur at a relatively low rate with either method of laser resurfacing. They may be less likely with the use of the erbium:YAG laser for reasons previously discussed; however, additional treatments may be required owing to the erbium:YAG's less effective nature. Side effects must be distinguished from true complications.

Side effects are expected sequelae of the postoperative period that resolve over time. To begin with, every patient undergoing the laser resurfacing procedure will initially experience a certain degree of serous discharge and crusting as well as associated mild pain and a burning sensation; these resolve upon completion of reepithelialization. Frequent application of ice packs and pain control medications will help the patient through this period. In addition, spot bleeding is a sequela frequently noted with the erbium:YAG laser, as this technique cannot cauterize blood vessels during the ablation process, as the CO_2 laser can. If spot bleeding remains persistent, pressure, pinpoint application of aluminium chloride 20% in anhydrous ethyl alcohol 93%, or, if necessary, low-level cautery can be used to resolve the problem. And as a normal part of the inflammatory process, patients experience a variable amount of postoperative erythema and edema, followed by pruritus. The postoperative erythema is always noticeable with the onset of the newly formed skin and generally lasts from several weeks to 6 months with the CO_2 laser and 1 to 6 weeks with lower settings of the erbium:YAG laser. It is thought to be due to a combination of factors including lack of epidermal maturity, diminished melanin absorption of light, lessened dermal optical scattering, and enhanced postsurgical blood flow. Accordingly, the intensity and duration of this postoperative erythema correlate with the level of depth achieved during the ablation process. Other potential contributing factors are frictional trauma from excessive rubbing between laser passes, wound infection, and improper postoperative care, including lack of emollient use, contact dermatitis from topical preparations, and early use of alpha-hydroxy acids or tretinoin. Sparing use of mild topical corticosteroid cream or ointment may aid in the resolution of this erythema. Postoperative edema goes hand in hand with the erythema and resolves along with it. If the laser peel is performed in combination with other procedures (e.g., face-lift or blepharoplasty), swelling may be enhanced. And pruritus, frequently noted in the first several postoperative weeks, may persist for up to 3 months. It normally responds well to treatment with emollients and mild topical steroids as well as cool compresses. Oral antihistamines and occasionally systemic steroids may be needed to address more significant pruritus.[107,112,134,135]

True complications differ from side effects in that they represent an aberrant process or event resulting from the surgical procedure without being a development essential to it. Complications of laser resurfacing are categorized as minor, moderate, and severe.

Minor complications include acne and milia, contact dermatitis, and prolonged erythema. The formation of acneiform pustules and milia is fairly common after laser resurfacing, afflicting up to 83.5 percent of patients in one study,[123]

though in our experience the incidence is much lower. This development is attributed to the fact that the laser peeled skin becomes hypersebaceous and to the follicular plugging that occurs as a result of the occlusive postoperative care with dressings or emollient ointments. Acne flares, appearing early on in those with a history of acne and between 6 weeks to 6 months in those without such a history, respond well to oral antibiotics and avoidance of the use of ointments that are too occlusive. And milia, which manifest between weeks to months after resurfacing, may be limited in number by not using ointments that are too occlusive in nature; they should be treated with careful manual expression, alpha-hydroxy acids, and the cautious application of tretinoin. The development of contact dermatitis is a minor complication that affects up to 65 percent of patients who use topical antibiotics in their postoperative regimen after laser resurfacing. Soaps, moisturizers, cosmetics, sunscreens, exfoliants, and steroid creams are other potential culprits. This dermatitis is usually irritant in nature, related to the diminished barrier of ablated skin, such that patch testing for allergens is often negative. Avoidance of topical antibiotics markedly reduces the incidence of this complication. As a rule, bland emollients should be used after resurfacing, as they are associated with a far lower incidence of contact dermatitis. If contact dermatitis develops nonetheless, the patient may benefit from switching to another type of bland emollient and the use of a mild topical steroid or even low-dose systemic steroids to resolve the problem, depending on the severity of the case. One other minor complication is prolonged or excessive erythema, which is almost always due to contact dermatitis or a superficial skin infection. If these causes are appropriately addressed, the erythema will resolve without consequences. At times there is no such obvious explanation, and its association with tissue induration may precede the onset of scarring. The latter, although rarely attributed to laser technique (such as using inappropriate energy parameters or inadvertent pulse stacking) can be an enigma. At the first sign of scarring, topical, intralesional, and even systemic steroids may have to be used to salvage the situation.[60,107,109,112,117,120,123,133,136]

The category of moderate complications seen with laser resurfacing consists of infections, severe postinflammatory melasma-like hyperpigmentation, and hypopigmentation. Infections[124] may lead to scarring and thus require the laser surgeon's immediate attention. Even with the common use of prophylactic antibiotic and antiviral medications, bacterial and to a lesser extent herpetic infections may still occur. Bacterial infections, usually due to *Staphylococcus aureus* or *Pseudomonas aeruginosa*, may be kept to a minimum by limiting the duration of the use of occlusive dressings and avoiding postoperative antibacterial prophylaxis. Once a bacterial infection is suspected, a culture specimen should be taken to identify the organism and rule out a resistant species, so as to allow for an adjustment in antibiotic therapy. And while breakthrough herpetic infections are rather rare, they have been reported and are probably due to inadequate absorption or low dosage of the antiviral drug. Viral resistance to the chosen antiviral drug is another possible explanation. In case of a breakthrough herpetic infection, patients should be treated with a higher dose of the medication or changed to an alternative antiviral medication. Even more unusual are candidal infections in the postoperative period. These present as pustules in the perioral and adjacent regions and are ascribed to the use of topical antibiotics or markedly occlusive ointments. Candidal infections are effectively treated with topical ketoconazole or oral fluconazole. Postinflammatory hyperpigmentation is another complication to contend with. Reported in up to 37 percent of patients,[120] this complication commonly presents between 2 weeks and 2 months following resolution of postoperative erythema and lasts for several months. Patients with darker skin tones, Fitzpatrick skin types III and above, are at the highest risk for developing postinflammatory hyperpigmentation, though even fair-skinned patients may be afflicted by it, especially those with dark-colored hair and eyes. The occurrence of postinflammatory hyperpigmentation can be limited by selecting predominantly fair-skinned individuals for treatment, doing more superficial resurfacing in darker-skinned individuals, and ensuring proper postoperative care with strict sun avoidance, use of sunscreens, and keeping away from topical steroids. When hyperpigmentation does present after laser resurfacing, the use of hydroquinone, alpha-hydroxy acids, and tretinoin aid in reducing its severity and duration. Even more severe than postinflammatory hyperpigmentation is the phenomenon of true hypopigmentation. Although the incidence of this after resurfacing is relatively low, it can be quite distressing to patients when it develops, as it is permanent. It can affect both patients with fair skin and those with darker skin tones but is less noticeable in skin types I and II. The risk for postlaser hypopigmentation appears to be higher in patients with a prior history of dermabrasion or phenol peel. This untoward event is caused by an epidermal loss of melanin. It characteristically presents with a delayed onset (6 to 12 months postoperatively) following resolution of postoperative erythema as a porcelain-white discoloration.[137] Once it manifests itself, treatment options are limited to the use of makeup for camouflage or depigmentation of the surrounding pigmented areas to lessen the contrast.[60,107,109,112,117,120,123,133,136]

The most feared complications of laser resurfacing are hypertrophic scarring and ectropion formation. The rare but confounding problem of hypertrophic scarring most commonly involves only certain facial areas, such as the malar and periorbital regions, upper lip, mandible, and neck. Prolonged postoperative erythema in association with tissue induration may precede the onset of hypertrophic scarring in these regions. It can be due to inadequacies in patient selection, laser technique, and postoperative care. Since prevention is the best form of treatment, the laser surgeon should pursue the following steps to actively minimize the problem: (1) In selecting patients, clearly identify individuals with risk factors for scarring, like a history of isotretinoin use, hyperelastic or keloidal skin, prior radiation, or prior cosmetic procedures. (2) Before beginning with laser resurfacing, the physician should take the time to carefully select energy parameters and number of laser passes appropriate for the individual patient. During the actual laser procedure, pulse or scan stacking is to be avoided and the debris between laser passes carefully removed. (3) In the postoperative period it is important to follow-up on patients frequently so as to be able to diagnose an infection early on, thus making it possible to treat such a complication in a timely manner. In the event that scarring does occur despite efforts at prevention, this situation may often be salvaged with potent topical steroids, intralesional triamcinolone, silicone gel sheeting, pulsed-dye laser, or a combination thereof. The other severe complication of laser resurfacing, namely ectropion of the lower eyelid, is fortunately also a rare event. In one series of a 1000 patients, ectropion developed only in 0.3 percent.[138] Acknowledged risk factors for ectropion formation include a prior history of blepharoplasty or rhytidectomy or a delayed "snap" test, denoting excessive lower-lid laxity on preoperative examination. Awareness of these risk factors and laser resurfacing with care around the eyelids goes a long way toward preventing this complication. If ectropion of the lower eyelid does develop, it rarely resolves spontaneously and therefore may have to be corrected surgically.[60,107,109,112,117,120,123,133,136]

Nonablative Cutaneous Resurfacing: Cool Touch Laser and NLite Laser

Patient Selection The nonablative cutaneous resurfacing lasers offer several advantages over the ablative resurfacing methods. Both the Cool Touch and the NLite lasers are virtually painless and thus generally do not require any type of anesthesia. During nonablative resurfacing, these lasers attempt to selectively stimulate collagen production in the dermis while leaving the epidermis entirely intact. Consequently, there is no prolonged recovery period involving 1 to 2 weeks of reepithelialization or several weeks to months of postoperative erythema. Rather, patients may return to work immediately after the procedure, usually without any significant clinical signs of skin damage. Side effects are limited to mild discomfort and mild postoperative erythema with either type of nonablative laser and rarely mild purpura with the NLite laser. Complications are unusual when using appropriate laser parameters and technique.

The postulated mechanism of increased collagen production differs between these two nonablative resurfacing methods. The 1320-nm Nd:YAG irradiation characteristic of the Cool Touch laser is nonspecifically absorbed in the human dermis. The use of high fluences at this wavelength is aimed at raising the dermal temperature just enough, to around 60 to 68°C, inducing mild collagen contraction with subsequent new collagen production. In order to avoid significant epidermal blistering at such high fluences, the Cool Touch laser employs cryogen cooling of the epidermis. On the other hand, the NLite laser utilizes a 585-nm light beam with low fluences at a short enough pulse duration to selectively target a specific chromophore in the dermis—namely, the vessels of the upper dermal plexus—without causing their rupture and coagulation. Instead, the low-energy light interaction within these vessels is supposed to incite a low-grade inflammation and growth response. This response results in the release of inflammatory mediators from endothelial cells that stimulate fibroblast activity, in turn enhancing the production of new collagen.[65,67]

Indications for treatment are the presence of mild to moderate rhytid formation and possibly mild atrophic acne scarring, particularly when present in isolated cosmetic units. Nonablative laser systems may also serve as a supplement to augment and/or maintain the rejuvenating effect of ablative laser systems. Both of these nonablative lasers may be used even in dark-skinned individuals without significant risks for the following reasons. The 1320-nm wavelength of the Cool Touch laser with its high fluences is located outside the absorption spectrum of melanin and coupled with protective cryogen cooling of the epidermis. And the 585-nm wavelength of the NLite laser, although it fits the absorption spectrum of melanin, utilizes very low fluences. Contraindications to the use of these nonablative lasers include retinoid use within the past year, intake of drugs that increase light sensitivity, and pregnancy. During the consultation, the laser surgeon must relate this relevant information to the patient and make sure that the patient has realistic expectations with regard to the degree of improvement that can be achieved. The site of wrinkling or atrophic acne scarring is documented with 35-mm photographs. Thereafter, consent is obtained.[139,140]

Preoperative Regimen There are no pretreatment requirements. The patient just needs to remove all cosmetics before the treatment.

Resurfacing Procedure and Technique As there is only minimal discomfort, described as a slight stinging sensation if any at all, no anesthesia is necessary. After making sure that appropriate safety eyewear is in place, the actual treatment is performed, targeting the reduction of mild to moderate rhytid formation and even mild atrophic acne scarring.

The Cool Touch laser provides the best possible results within specific laser parameters. This 1320-nm-wavelength laser is generally used with a 5-mm spot size; it is set at a fluence of 28 to 38 J/cm^2 and a pulse duration of 200 ms. Cryogen cooling is applied for 20 to 30 ms with a 30- to 40-ms delay before each pulse. A built-in temperature probe provides readings of the cutaneous surface, for which temperatures of 40 to 48°C are sought, as the dermis will be about 20°C warmer, just enough to cause collagen tightening. The laser pulses are delivered with up to 30 percent overlap. The treatment area is covered with one or two passes, depending on when the endpoint of mild reactive erythema is reached. A total of three to six treatments may be given 2 to 4 weeks apart for optimal outcome.[65]

When using the NLite laser, the key laser parameters besides its 585-nm wavelength and the commonly employed 5-mm spot size are an energy density of 2 to 4 J/cm^2 and a pulse duration of 250 to 400 μs. Once these laser parameters are set, the laser surgeon may proceed with the nonablative resurfacing. The entire treatment area, whether it is the full face or selected cosmetic units, is covered evenly with laser pulses, with less than 10 percent overlap of the individual pulses. While the NLite laser's effectiveness in reducing rhytids after a single treatment is modest, the possibility of achieving even better cosmetic results with follow-up treatments is currently being investigated.[67]

Postoperative Regimen There is basically no postoperative regimen to speak of for nonablative laser resurfacing. Some physicians advocate the use of a topical antibiotic ointment or plain emollient following treatment.

Side Effects, Complications, and Their Management
Side effects, defined as expected sequelae, are limited to a mild stinging sensation during treatment and rarely mild purpura with the NLite laser, as well as mild postoperative erythema, more commonly with the Cool Touch laser. Purpura resolves over 1 to 2 weeks. Any postoperative erythema responds to twice-daily applications of mild topical corticosteroids for 1 to several days.

Complications, representing untoward events, are uncommon with nonablative laser systems. In fact, the just published original research on the Nlite laser failed to reveal any complications at all, likely due to its use of very low fluences. However, transient hyperpigmentation and pitted scarring has been noted in some patients undergoing treatment with the Cool Touch laser, as it utilizes characteristically high fluences that necessitate the use of cryogen cooling to protect the epidermis. As with any laser procedure, the complication rate is operator-dependent. If one is using improper laser parameters such as inappropriately high fluences and pulse durations with either type of nonablative laser, there is the potential for blistering, pigmentary changes, and scarring.[66,67]

Treatment of Vascular Lesions

Patient Selection Proper patient selection in the treatment of vascular lesions depends on the laser surgeon's knowledge of the mechanism behind the laser's effect and which lesions are amenable to treatment of the different vascular lasers; it also depends on patient education.

The pulsed-dye laser (PDL), based on the principle of thermokinetic selectivity with a pulse duration shorter than that of most small vessels, is ideally suited to specifically target vessels 0.2 mm or less in diameter and is noted for a low risk of complications; transient purpura is its only drawback. Therefore it is remarkably effective at treating a wide range of vascular lesions, including port-wine stains, facial telangiectasia, rosacea-associated telangiectasia and erythema, spider angiomas, superficial hemangiomas, cherry angiomas, venous lakes, poikiloderma of Civatte, and small pyogenic granulomas,[83–88] most of them requiring only a few treatments. The most troublesome lesions to treat are port-wine stains (PWS), and poikiloderma of Civatte. PWS characteristically take multiple treatments for maximal lightening, and those darker in color and with nodular features may not completely respond. Several factors are thought to favor a positive response of PWS to PDL.[83,141] Among these factors are young age of patient,[142–144] small size,[141,145] light color,[146–148] limited depth of vessels,[149,150] and location on the lateral face, eyelids, or neck (rather than on the central face and distal extremities).[144,145,148,151,152] And despite excellent results in many cases, there is a tendency for some degree of recurrence of PWS. In one study,[151] recurrence was noted at a rate of 50 percent 3 to 4 years after discontinuation of treatment. Besides the need for multiple treatments in extensive poikiloderma of Civatte, there are two other concerns. Owing to its location on the neck, it carries a higher risk of scarring. Also, incompletely treated areas—as a consequence of their having been overlooked or failure of sufficient overlap—result in an obvious demarcation line or unsightly grid pattern, respectively. Thus, we usually avoid treating poikiloderma of Civatte unless the lesion is quite small and localized.

In contrast, the continuous/quasicontinuous lasers are associated with a significantly higher risk of scarring and pigmentary alteration, as they do not comply with the principle of thermokinetic selectivity. Rather, they cause nonspecific tissue damage, making them inferior to the PDL, with its vascular specificity, except for two aspects that may support its occasional use given sufficient operator experience. These lasers are more effective than the PDL when it comes to the treatment of larger-caliber vessels (2 to 4 mm in diameter) and offer the cosmetic advantage of no postoperative purpura. Nevertheless, the PDL is considered the "gold standard" in the treatment of vascular lesions.

After explaining these pro and cons of laser treatment to the patient in detail and setting realistic goals in terms of outcome, consent is obtained and the lesions to be treated are documented with 35-mm photographs.

Preoperative Regimen With the PDL, unlike the case with laser resurfacing, there is no need for skin preparation. However, antiviral prophylaxis is of benefit for patients with or without a history of herpes labialis if treatment targets the skin at or close to the vermilion border. And it is important to advise patients to avoid significant sun exposure in the month prior to laser treatment, as an increase in the background pigmentation does lead to a higher risk for pigmentary alteration, some of which may be permanent.

Laser Procedure and Technique Anesthesia is rarely needed except in children or very sensitive adult patients, as the mild discomfort is likened to the snap of a rubber band. For the purpose of anesthesia, a eutectic mixture of topical lidocaine 2.5% and prilocaine 2.5% (EMLA cream) or topical lidocaine 4% (ELA-max cream) applied 1 h prior to the procedure and/or a topical clear cooling gel throughout the procedure is to be advised.

The PDL is relatively simple to operate. The spot size of the emitted beam ranges from 2 to 10 mm and the fluence varies from 3 to 10 J/cm^2. It is well to remember that when the spot size is decreased, a higher fluence is needed to gain the same result, and that larger spot sizes may provide better penetration for vessels located somewhat more deeply.[153]

In performing the actual procedure, the risk for complications can be minimized by good technique. In anatomic regions prone to scarring—such as the periorbital region, neck, anterior chest, and shoulders[153,154]—this involves application of pulses to the targeted lesion with no more than 10 percent overlap and a 10 to 20 percent reduction in fluence. To the same effect, we like to follow the "just enough" purpura approach, especially in dealing with sites susceptible to scarring. Rather than going with a set combination of fluence and spot size, we generally do several test pulses beginning with a low fluence and progressively increasing the fluence until just the right amount of blue-gray purpura is evident. This approach helps to define the lowest amount of fluence necessary to treat a vascular lesion at these sites successfully with a minimal risk of complications. For all other sites, the combination of 5 to 7.5 J/cm^2 and a spot size of 5 to 7 mm present a safe and effective approach. Treatments are repeated at 6- to 8-week intervals.

On the rare occasion of resorting to the use of a continuous/quasicontinuous laser to treat larger-caliber vessels, it is important to follow a minimal blanching approach. By using just enough energy to get a minimal blanching response, the occurrence of scarring and pigmentary alterations is kept to a minimum.[155]

Improvement ranging from fair to excellent can be expected after proper treatment (see Figs. 14-12 through 14-16). Variables include skin type, lesion size and depth, number of treatments, type of laser used, and setting of parameters.

Postoperative Regimen Postoperative care is relatively simple. Patients apply an antibiotic ointment twice daily to the treatment site followed by a clean dressing for 7 to 14 days until resolution of purpura and/or mild edema and crusting or eschar. Also, they must avoid trauma and sun exposure to the treated site postoperatively, as both are associated with a higher risk of pigmentary alteration. To that end, the use of a sunscreen for several months after completion of wound care is very helpful.

Side Effects, Complications, and Their Management Side effects, or expected sequelae of the postoperative period that resolve over time, differ from complications, or morbid events resulting from the surgical procedure that may be permanent.

There are few side effects with lasers used to treat vascular lesions. The purpura caused by the PDL—its main drawback from the patient's perspective—generally resolves within 1 to 2 weeks. CW lasers—such as the argon, KTP, krypton, and copper vapor/bromide laser—do not cause purpura but rather mild edema and crusting or eschar that disappears on wound healing within 1 to 2 weeks.

In terms of complications, the PDL has without question a better safety profile than continuous/quasicontinuous lasers in the treatment of vascular lesions.[3–5] The risk for scarring with the use of the PDL laser is less than 1 percent. Scarring,[82,86,146,153,156] if it occurs, is commonly atrophic and at times hypertrophic and primarily involves the periorbital region, neck, anterior chest, and shoulder areas. Atrophic-type scarring tends to resolve over time. The most common complication seen with the PDL is hyperpigmentation, reportedly presenting in 10 to 15 percent of cases and usually transient[86,153] It particularly afflicts individuals with naturally darker skin types or tanned skin when they are treated at higher fluences or may occur after posttreatment sun exposure. Hypopigmentation, transient in most cases, is far less common, occurring in 2.5 to 5 percent of patients.[86,153,156] Rarely, persistent hypopigmentation—likened in appearance to nevus anemicus—develops customarily on the neck, chest, and legs. In comparison, the argon CW laser, which was used as the primary laser in the treatment of vascular lesions prior to the development of the PDL, poses a much higher risk for hypopigmentation and scarring. In the treatment of PWS, hypopigmentation has been noted in as many as 28 percent of the cases, and the risk for hypertrophic scarring ranges from 5 to 15 percent.[155,157] Similarly, the other continuous/quasicontinuous lasers (KTP, krypton, and copper vapor/bromide laser) also pose a notably higher risk for these complications than the PDL, as they lack thermokinetic selectivity and thus vascular specificity.

As prevention of these complications is the best form of management, the combination of minimal overlap (10 percent or less) and just enough purpura production with the PDL or minimal blanching with continuous/quasicontinuous lasers is to be recommended. If scarring does occur, the use of 10 to 25 mg/mL of intralesional triamcinolone in small amounts helps to flatten the hypertrophic variant, while the atrophic variant may require the use of filler substances. Silicone gel or sheets may also prove to be helpful. Hyperpigmentation can often be successfully resolved with the application of hydroquinone or other bleaching creams and the avoidance of sun exposure. But it is hypopigmentation that may prove to be the most difficult problem to rectify, particularly in darker-skinned individuals, in whom it is the most apparent. Makeup to camouflage this unsightly complication is often the only remaining solution.

Treatment of Pigmented Lesions

Patient Selection Traditional therapy of pigmented lesions involved various destructive methods—including excision, cryosurgery, or chemical peels—all of which carried a high risk of scar formation or permanent pigmentary alterations. The use of continuous-wave CO_2 and argon lasers was also accompanied by a high risk of scarring and pigmentary changes, as these lasers cause nonspecific thermal injury to normal skin. Later, the principle of selective photothermolysis realized in the form of pulsed and Q-switched lasers made it possible to specifically target melanin without excessively damaging the surrounding collagen.

The mechanism behind the success in laser removal of pigmented lesions can be explained as follows. In accordance with selective photothermolysis, the high-energy light of pulsed and Q-switched lasers is characterized by ultrashort pulse duration, well below the thermal relaxation time of melanosomes (0.5 to 1 µs), thus limiting absorption to melanosomes and with only minimal extension to surrounding tissue. The absorption of this high-energy light results in rapid thermal tissue expansion and consequent rupture of melanosome-carrying cells (melanocytes and keratinocytes), also referred to as photoacoustic mechanical disruption. The fragmented pigment particles are then taken up by phagocytic inflammatory cells and carried away by the lymph system.[158]

Proper patient selection forms the foundation of successful laser treatment of pigmented lesions. Not all pigmented lesions respond in a satisfactory fashion. And even if laser treatment is likely to bring about an excellent outcome, not every patient is a good candidate.

In general, pigmented lesions are classified as epidermal or dermal, which influences the type of laser that can be used to treat them. All the melanin of epidermal pigmented lesions is located within the epidermis. Examples of epidermal pigmented lesions are solar lentigines, labial lentigos, ephelides, café-au-lait macules, Becker's nevi, and epidermal melasma. In contrast, dermal pigmented lesions also demonstrate melanin pigment in the underlying dermis. The list of dermal pigmented lesions includes, among others, nevus of Ota, nevus spilus, dermal melasma, and compound nevi.

(text continues on page 205)

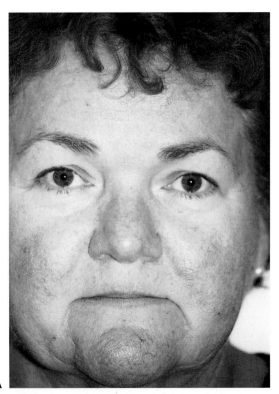

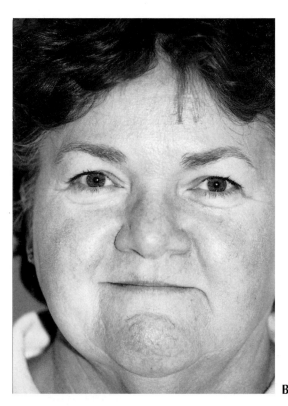

A

B

Figure 14-12   (*A*) A woman with rosacea underwent Q-switched pulsed-dye laser treatment. She had been on various oral and topical therapies for years and wanted further improvement. (*B*) Six weeks postoperatively, good clearing is noted.

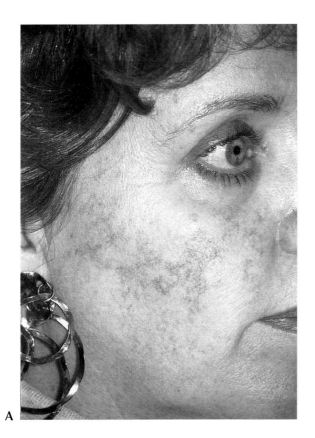

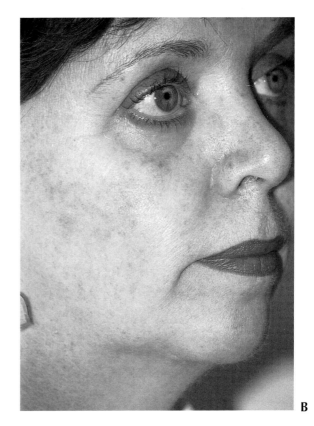

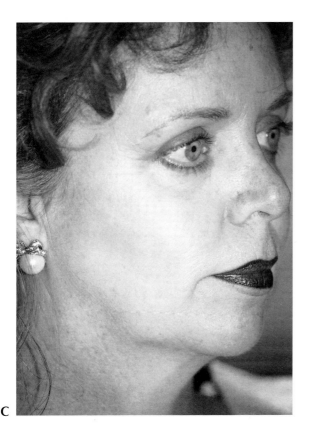

Figure 14-13   (*A*) Prominent telangiectatic matting is present on the cheeks. (*B*) Three months after a single Q-switched pulsed-dye laser treatment, partial resolution is noted. (*C*) Three months after a second Q-switched pulsed-dye laser treatment, complete clearing is noted.

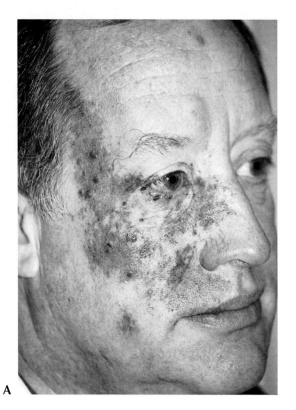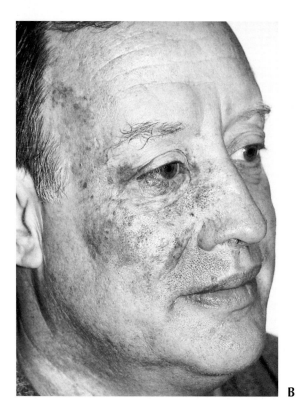

A B

Figure 14-14 (*A*) This patient with a port-wine stain had received argon laser treatment several years earlier, resulting in whitish scarring centrally. (*B*) After four Q-switched pulsed-dye laser treatments, significant improvement can be seen, with the vascular bleb essentially resolved.

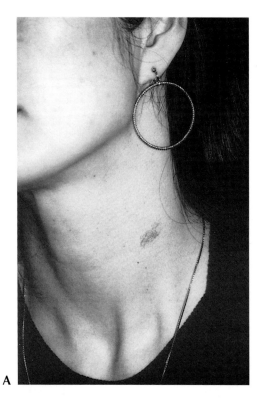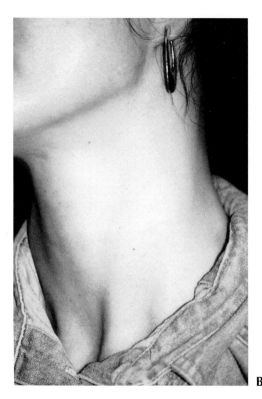

A B

Figure 14-15 (*A*) Small port-wine stains may show remarkable improvement after a single Q-switched pulsed-dye laser treatment. (*B*) Three months later.

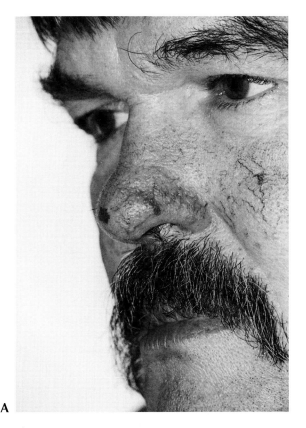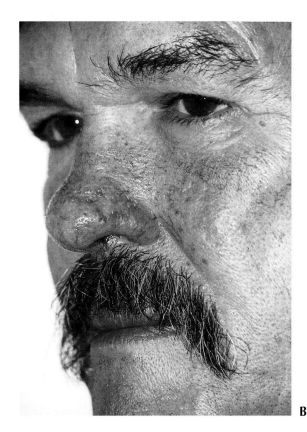

A   **B**

Figure 14-16   (**A**) Unsightly telangiectasias on the central face. (**B**) The KTP laser was used to treat the most prominent lesions; the patient is seen 6 weeks postoperatively.

The choice of laser for these lesions hinges on the location of the melanin pigment. The 510-nm PDL and the 534-nm frequency-doubled Q-switched Nd:YAG laser (both green light-pulsed lasers) are useful in the treatment of epidermal pigmented lesions only, despite a high specificity for melanin absorption, as their short wavelengths limit penetration to the superficial dermis. On the other hand, the 694-nm Q-switched ruby laser and the 755-nm alexandrite laser (red light-pulsed lasers), and the 1064-nm Q-switched Nd: YAG laser (near infrared light-pulsed laser) can be used for both epidermal and dermal pigmented lesions owing to their greater depth of dermal penetration. The 1064-nm Q-switched Nd:YAG laser offers a lesser degree of melanin absorption than the aforementioned red light lasers, allowing for more safety in treating epidermal pigmented lesions in darker-skinned individuals. At the same time, the decreased melanin absorption of the 1064-nm Q-switched Nd: YAG laser is overcome by its longer wavelength, generating a deeper level of dermal penetration, which is particularly effective for treating pigmented lesions with a predominantly dermal location of melanin.[80,159]

Despite the proper choice of laser in the treatment of pigmented lesions, they do not all respond in the same fashion.[19,80,158–160] Among the epidermal pigmented lesions, solar and labial lentigines are effectively cleared with just a few treatments (see Fig. 14-17 through 14-19).[161,162] However,

even after achieving complete clearing with multiple treatments, ephelides, café-au-lait macules, and Becker's nevi are all characterized by a high rate of recurrence, within 6 to 12 months.[162–164] And it is rather rare to clear epidermal melasma, as this condition arises from multiple causes, including sun exposure, hormones, and genetics. With regard to the dermal pigmented lesions listed above, nevus of Ota is most often effectively cleared after multiple treatments and usually does not recur. In contrast, the spilus nevus is difficult to remove, as the junctional nevus portion tends to clear while the café-au-lait macule portion commonly persists.[163] The laser treatment of compound nevi remains controversial. As the dermal portion of compound nevi generally persists, superficial clearing may mask the development of an underlying melanoma. Furthermore, the exact effects of laser irradiation of melanocytes are still unknown.[19,80,81] And dermal melasma shows a variable response, ranging from some clearing to repigmentation or a worsening of pigmentation.

During the consultation process, the laser surgeon can educate the patient on all these aspects of laser treatment, with an emphasis upon potential complications and possible number of multiple treatments required for optimal improvement. It is also important, at this time, to set realistic goals for the patient. "Before" and "after" examples of previously treated pigmented lesions, including the immediate postoperative appearance, help to ensure realistic expectations. If

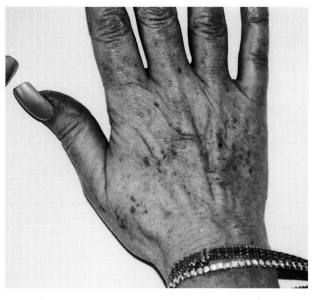

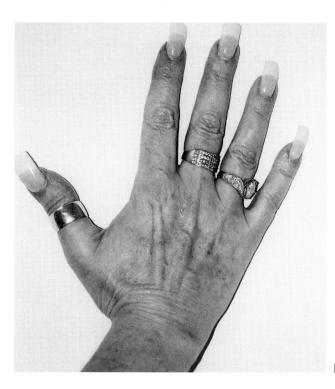

Figure 14-17 (*A*) Solar lentigines on the hands can be very disturbing to some patients. (*B*) A single treatment with the Q-switched Nd:YAG laser (1064 nm) often provides satisfactory results. This patient is seen 6 months postoperatively.

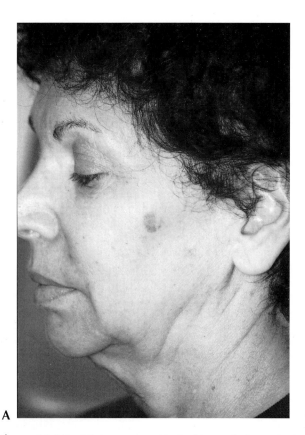

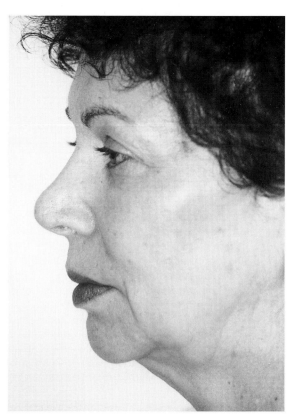

Figure 14-18 (*A*) A woman with the histopathology of seborrheic keratosis–lentigo overlap desired removal of this lesion. (*B*) Three months after treatment with the Q-switched Nd:YAG laser (1064 nm).

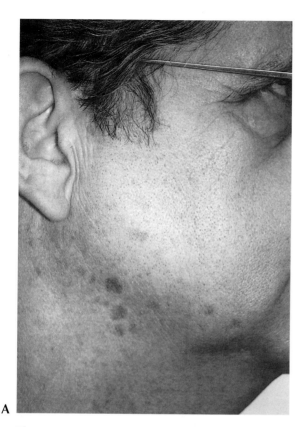
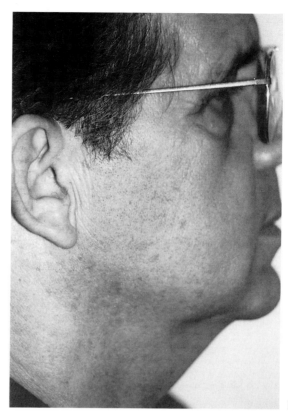

A   B

Figure 14-19 (*A*) Facial "age spots" are often very responsive to laser treatment. (*B*) Satisfactory resolution 3 months after Q-switched Nd:YAG laser (1064 nm) treatment.

patients are unclear on any of these points, treatment is best delayed until thorough understanding is demonstrated. All of this is documented and the consent obtained. The pigmented lesion in question should be recorded with 35-mm photographs prior to attempting any laser treatment, as it will help to demonstrate clinical improvement and thus increase patient satisfaction, especially when multiple sessions are needed.

Preoperative Regimen Ideally, patients are instructed to strictly avoid sun exposure and tanning between the scheduled PLD treatment sessions and also to use sun protection at the site of treatment for several weeks beforehand. A hydroquinone-containing bleaching cream may be used twice daily for 1 to 4 weeks preoperatively by darker-skinned individuals and those with significant tans. If a patient has a history of herpes simplex reactivation at or near the site of treatment, antiviral prophylaxis, starting the day before the scheduled laser session, should be considered.

Laser Procedure and Technique The discomfort experienced with this procedure is mild, commonly described as a rubber band-like snapping sensation. Thus, there is usually no need for anesthesia. However, the treatment of more sensitive areas of skin, especially in children, may require the use of a eutectic mixture of topical lidocaine 2.5% and prilo-

caine 2.5% (EMLA cream) or topical lidocaine 4% (ELA-max cream) applied 1 to 2 h before the procedure under occlusion. Rarely is there any need to use lidocaine 1% with or without epinephrine for local infiltration or a regional nerve block for faster and more complete anesthesia.

As a first step, the laser surgeon must choose the appropriate laser for the pigmented lesion in question. For this purpose, the pigmented lesion to be treated must be categorized as epidermal or dermal. Epidermal lesions will respond to treatment with green light-pulsed lasers (510-nm pulsed dye and 534-nm frequency-doubled Nd:YAG) as well as red light-pulsed lasers (694 nm Q-switched ruby and 755-nm Q-switched alexandrite) and a near infrared-pulsed laser (1064-nm Nd:YAG). But effective treatment of dermal pigmented lesions can be achieved only with the Q-switched ruby, Q-switched alexandrite, or the Q-switched Nd:YAG laser. And for dermal pigmented lesions in patients with skin type III and above, the Q-switched Nd:YAG laser may be the best treatment option owing to its relative sparing of epidermal melanin.[80,159]

Treatment parameters differ between these different lasers and with various pigmented lesions. The 510-nm PDL with a pulse duration of 300 ns can be used to treat ephelides, solar lentigines, and labial lentigos effectively with one to two treatments, generally utilizing a 5-mm spot size at a fluence of 2 to 2.5 J/cm². Café-au-lait macules may require six to eight treatments at a slightly higher fluence of 2.5 to 3.5 J/cm². Similarly, the 534-nm frequency-doubled Nd:YAG with a pulse duration of 5 to 10 ns, another green light-pulsed laser, can be used to resolve ephelides, solar lentigines, and labial lentigines often with one to two treatments, employing a 1- to 3-mm spot size at 10 Hz and a fluence of 2 to 2.5 J/cm². This laser also helps to remove café-au-lait macules after six to eight treatments at an increased fluence of 2.5 to 3.5 J/cm². In comparison, the Q-switched ruby laser and Q-switched alexandrite laser use higher fluences. Fluences in the range of 5 to 6 J/cm² and 6 to 7 J/cm², respectively, are used to effectively eliminate ephelides and solar or labial lentigines after one or two sessions and café-au-lait macules and nevi of Ota usually after four to six treatments. And the Q-switched Nd:YAG laser can be used with a 3-mm handpiece at an even higher fluence, averaging 8 J/cm², to effectively lighten these lesions in about the same number of sessions.[159,165]

After the laser and proper laser parameters are selected, pulses are delivered to the targeted lesions without any to at most 10 percent overlap. The beam should be directed to the site of treatment in a perpendicular fashion to allow for maximal effect. But even with flawless technique, a high recurrence is noted following treatment of ephelides, café-au-lait macules, Becker's nevi, spilus nevi, and dermal melasma.

Postoperative Regimen Wound care must address any areas of bleeding and support wound healing. Pinpoint applications of aluminum chloride 20% in ethyl alcohol 93% right after the laser surgery help to control any bleeding points. Wound healing is promoted by creating a moist environment with twice-daily applications of an antibiotic ointment and a nonstick dressing for 1 to 2 weeks. The use of a plain emollient ointment may suffice for cases of minimal epidermal damage. As makeup may hinder the process of reepithelialization, it should be avoided until healing is complete. If the patient was started on an antiviral medication for prophylaxis, its course should be completed. Following laser treatment, the patient should strictly avoid sun exposure and tanning beds and start sun protection after complete healing to decrease the risk for postinflammatory hyperpigmentation. And a hydroquinone-containing bleaching cream applied twice a day will help to resolve any noticeable hyperpigmentation if it occurs despite these preventive measures.

Side Effects, Complications, and Their Management Side effects, defined as expected sequelae, of pulsed and Q-switched laser treatment of pigmented lesions include immediate tissue whitening, a minimal amount of tissue splatter and bleeding, and subsequent mild erythema and edema. Tissue splatter and bleeding may be prevented or kept at a minimum by lowering the fluence accordingly. Epidermal perforation in the form of tissue splatter heals rapidly in response to proper wound care with antibiotic ointment and a nonstick dressing. Pinpoint application of aluminum chloride 20% in ethyl alcohol 93% (Drysol) controls any noticeable bleeding points. Erythema and edema respond to the application of ice several times a day. Another side effect that may be seen is purpura, limited to the use of

the 510-nm PLD and the frequency-doubled 532-nm Nd:YAG laser, as these wavelengths are also well absorbed by oxyhemoglobin. If purpura develops, the patient can be assured that it will fade within 1 to 2 weeks postoperatively.

The treatment of pigmented lesions with pulsed and Q-switched lasers generally has few complications and those that occur are usually not permanent. Untoward events that may be noted include pigmentary and textural changes.

The most common complication is transient pigmentary alteration. Both transient hypopigmentation and hyperpigmentation may occur, though the former tends to be more common. Hypopigmentation is most noticeable with wavelengths well absorbed by melanin. Owing to limited tissue penetration, the hypopigmentation associated with the 510- and 532-nm wavelengths appears to resolve quickly. On the other hand, the hypopigmentation noted with the 694- and 755-nm wavelengths often lasts for several months and may rarely be permanent. The risk for hypopigmentation has been noted to be somewhat lower for the 755-nm wavelength, as it is not quite as well absorbed by melanin as the 694-nm wavelength and actually penetrates deeper into the dermis. Among the pulsed and Q-switched lasers used in the treatment of pigmented lesions, the Nd:YAG laser at 1064 nm carries the lowest risk for hypopigmentation, owing to its notably lesser degree of absorption by melanin and greater depth of penetration. Hyperpigmentation, if it occurs, may last for months. One source reports it to be around 15 percent for the Q-switched ruby laser[3]; data on its incidence with the other lasers used to treat pigmented lesions are scarce. It appears to be related mainly to skin type, as individuals with darker skin tones are at the greatest risk for developing hyperpigmentation. The preoperative use of hydroquinone as a preventive measure may be of benefit in this group of patients. Treatment-related hyperpigmentation responds well to twice-daily applications of a hydroquinone-containing bleaching cream.

Textural changes may become manifest after the use of high fluences; mild but prolonged erythema or mild atrophy is typically transient. Permanent textural changes in the form of scarring or epidermal atrophy are rather uncommon.[3] If hypertrophic scarring presents postoperatively, the use of intralesional triamcinolone, PDL, silicon gel, and silicon sheeting may lead to its resolution. Atrophic scarring with loss of dermal substance responds to subcutaneous injection of filler substances.

Treatment of Tattoos

Patient Selection Prior to the recent evolution in laser surgery, treatment of tattoos consisted of a variety of destructive modalities, including dermabrasion, excision, cryosurgery, and chemical peels, all of which resulted in scar formation or permanent pigmentary alterations. Initial attempts at laser surgery of tattoos entailed the use of the CW CO_2 and argon lasers but caused the same problems, with scarring and pigmentary changes due to nonspecific thermal injury of normal skin. It was not until the development of Q-switched lasers, based on the principle of selective photothermolysis, that it became possible to specifically target tattoo ink particles without excessively damaging the surrounding collagen.

The success in the laser removal of tattoos is explained for the most part by the following mechanism. Q-switched lasers release high-energy light of ultrashort pulse duration that cause shattering of tattoo ink particles into even tinier fragments while avoiding destruction of adjacent tissue. Some of these fragments are extruded transepidermally. But the great majority of these fragments are removed by phagocytosis and lymphatic drainage. Optical alteration of laser-irradiated tissue further contributes to the fading of tattoos observed clinically.[3,5,166,167]

Despite these advances in laser technology, proper patient selection is essential to any successful laser treatment. Not all tattoos respond in the same manner. The type of tattoo present, its age, and the colors used within it determine in large part what kind of response can be expected with laser therapy.

In general, tattoos can be delineated as professional versus amateur, traumatic, and cosmetic. Professional tattoos are far more difficult to eradicate than the amateur type.[168,169] They are composed of more densely packed and deeply placed multicolored metallic pigments. These pigments are variably found in the papillary dermis, reticular dermis, and at times even the subcutaneous fat; thus they often require 8 to 12 treatment sessions. In contrast, amateur tattoos consist of less densely packed carbon-based particles (India ink, cigarette ash, and pencil graphite) in a more superficial location, usually uniformly deposited in the papillary dermis, and they can often be removed with only four to six laser treatments. Similarly, traumatic tattoos, usually composed of carbon-based pigments implanted into the skin, often clear with only one to four treatments, based upon the amount of pigment deposited.[170,171] On the other hand, cosmetic tattoos can be a challenge. The red, white, and flesh-colored inks used cosmetically to enhance eyebrows, eyelids, cheeks, and lips often result in immediate pigment darkening after pulsed laser treatment. This is likely due to a laser-induced oxidation-reduction reaction of iron or titanium oxide contained within these pigments. Such darkened tattoo pigment does not always respond to subsequent laser treatments.[172]

The age of a tattoo also influences how easily it can be removed. Older tattoos are more likely to respond to fewer treatment sessions with pulsed lasers. This may be ascribed to the passage of time, allowing for more complete phagocytosis of the pigment by the body's scavenger cells, and the increased fragility of pigment particles, which are then more easily shattered by the laser's impact.[80,158]

Besides determining the type of tattoo and its age, it is important to note the colors involved in evaluating a patient for potential pulsed laser therapy of such a lesion. Most black, blue, green, and red tattoo pigment may be removed by one of the Q-switched lasers and/or the 510-nm PDL. Unfortunately, the many newer and brighter colors used in tattoo parlors these days do not always respond to pulsed laser treatment. And, as noted above, pulsed laser therapy of the colored inks used for cosmetic tattoos may actually result in immediate pigment darkening.

Another consideration to be noted is the patient's skin type. Darker-skinned individuals are at a somewhat higher risk for scarring and pigmentary alterations, transient and permanent, with pulsed laser treatment. In these patients, higher wavelengths, lower fluences with larger spot sizes, and cooling of the epidermis are advantageous.

The most serious concern with pulsed laser treatment of tattoos is the occurrence of a systemic allergic reaction, triggered by fragmented tattoo ink particles acting as an allergen. Patients with a localized allergic reaction at the tattoo site appear to be more predisposed to develop a systemic allergic reaction. Consequently, a cutaneous reaction noted within the tattoo of a patient represents a relative contraindication to treatment.[173,174]

Equipped with this knowledge, the laser surgeon is able to educate the patient on all aspects of laser treatment—emphasizing potential complications and costs involved—as well set realistic expectations for the patient. "Before" and "after" pictures of previously treated tattoos, including the immediate postoperative appearance, help to ensure realistic expectations. If patients are unclear on any of these points, treatment must be delayed until they demonstrate a thorough understanding. Thereafter, consent is obtained and the tattoo in question is documented with 35-mm photographs. This photographic documentation, performed before the initial treatment and each subsequent treatment session, serves two important purposes. Since patients tend to forget what their tattoos looked like originally, these photographs are helpful in showing the amount of fading that has taken place following laser treatment. And it provides evidence for any textural changes/scarring related to the tattoo ink placement that the patient might not become aware of until after the ink is removed. Without such documentation, the laser surgeon is at increased risk of having to confront a dissatisfied patient.

Preoperative Regimen Patients should strictly avoid sun exposure and tanning between the scheduled pulsed laser treatment sessions. Individuals with skin types III and above and those who tend to develop hyperpigmentation may be started on a hydroquinone-containing bleaching cream twice daily for 1 to 4 weeks preoperatively. In addition, antiviral prophylaxis is indicated if a patient has a history of herpes simplex reactivation at or near the site of treatment.

Laser Procedure and Technique Frequently there is no need for anesthesia, as the rubber band-like snapping sensation is usually well tolerated. In treating more sensitive areas of skin and especially in treating children, topical anesthesia is achieved with a eutectic mixture of lidocaine 2.5% and prilocaine 2.5% (EMLA cream) or lidocaine 4% (ELA-max cream) applied 1 to 2 h before the procedure under occlusion; this will notably reduce any discomfort secondary to the procedure. If necessary, faster and more complete anesthesia can be achieved with lidocaine 1% with or without epinephrine for local infiltration or a regional nerve block.

Next, the attention turns toward the actual laser procedure. To begin with, the laser surgeon must decide on the type of laser to be used in the treatment of a particular tattoo. This choice is mainly based upon the color of the tattoo pigment and the patient's skin type.

The Q-switched ruby laser effectively eliminates black and blue-black pigment and, to a lesser degree, also green. The Q-switched alexandrite laser is equally effective for black, blue-black, and green tattoos. But neither is capable of removing red, orange, or yellow. However, the Q-switched Nd:YAG laser at 1064 nm is not only effective for the treatment of black tattoos but, in the frequency-doubled mode at 532 nm, can be used to remove red and pink tattoos. The other commonly employed laser in the treatment of tattoo pigment, namely the 510-nm PDL, is effective at removing red pigment and even yellow and orange.

The patient's skin type is another important consideration. Darker-skinned individuals are at a somewhat higher risk for scarring and pigment alterations with pulsed laser treatment. This is particularly the case with the Q-switched ruby laser owing to its strong melanin absorption. The Q-switched alexandrite and especially the Q-switched Nd:YAG laser are better choices for treating individuals with skin types III and above due to the lesser degree of absorption and deeper penetration with their higher wavelengths. These patients will also benefit from epidermal cooling as well as the selection of lower fluences in combination with larger spot size to minimize damage to melanin in the epidermis.

After choosing the appropriate laser, the correct parameters must be established. Depending on the spot size selected, starting fluences for the Q-switched lasers in the treatment of tattoos vary from 4 to 8 J/cm²—even lower if the tattoo to be treated is in a site prone to scarring. The laser parameters are adjusted according to the clinical response. The clinical goal is to achieve immediate whitening of the tattooed skin with minimal to no tissue splatter or bleeding. If the latter does occur, the fluence should be lowered to a level that does not

cause epidermal perforation. After several laser treatments, the fluence may be increased for resistant areas of tattoo pigment on an individual basis if deemed appropriate by the laser surgeon. Keep in mind that the use of larger spot sizes in combination with lower fluences allows for deeper penetration while minimizing the risk for epidermal and textural changes, a particularly important concept in treating darker-skinned individuals. Treatment sessions are scheduled at 8- to 12-week intervals.[165]

Careful considerations of all these aspects of laser treatment of tattoos allows for successful elimination of tattoo pigment while keeping the risk for complications to a minimum (see Figs. 14-20 through 14-24).

Postoperative Regimen Wound care should proceed as follows. Immediately after the procedure, pinpoint applications of aluminum chloride 20% in ethyl alcohol 93% (Drysol) may be used to stop any bleeding. Thereafter, twice-daily applications of an antibiotic ointment and a nonstick dressing for 1 to 2 weeks help to promote wound healing. If there is only mild epidermal damage, a plain emollient ointment is sufficient. The addition of a urea 40% cream (Carmol 40) may aid in transepidermal elimination of pigment. Make-up should not be applied until after reepithelialization. If the patient was started on an antiviral medication for prophylaxis, its course should be completed. Of course, the patient must be instructed to avoid sun exposure and tanning beds strictly so as to diminish the risk of postinflammatory hyper-

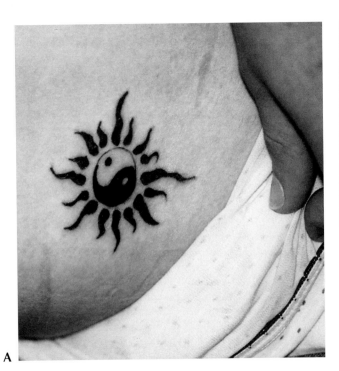
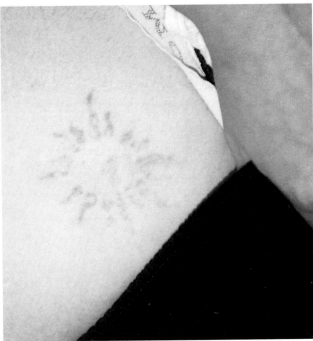

A   B

Figure 14-20 (*A*) A 14-year-old girl presented with her mother for removal of a red-and-black tattoo. (*B*) After three treatments with the Q-switched Nd:YAG laser (1064 nm for black ink, 532 nm for red ink), significant clearing of the black portion is noted and less clearing of the red.

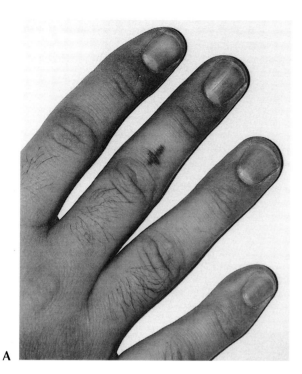

A

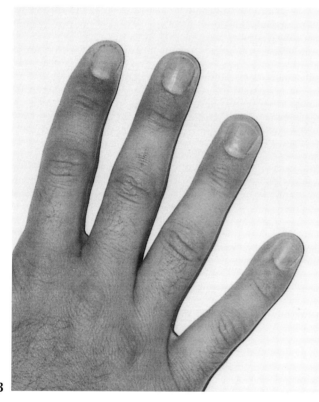

B

Figure 14-21 (**A**) An amateur tattoo is seen on the patient's third finger. (**B**) Although results can be variable for amateur tattoos, excellent clearing was achieved with the Q-switched Nd:YAG laser (1064 nm).

pigmentation. In case hyperpigmentation is noted within the treated site, therapy with hydroquinone-containing bleaching creams applied twice a day is initiated and continued until the hyperpigmentation has resolved.

Side Effects, Complications, and Their Management
Side effects, defined as expected sequelae, of pulsed and Q-switched laser treatment of tattoos include immediate tissue whitening as well as a certain amount of tissue splatter and bleeding and subsequent mild erythema and edema. Lowering the fluence accordingly minimizes the occurrence of tissue splatter and bleeding. Epidermal perforation in the form of tissue splatter heals rapidly in response to proper wound care with antibiotic ointment and nonstick dressings. Pinpoint application of aluminum chloride 20% in ethyl alcohol 93% (Drysol) controls any noticeable bleeding points. And application of ice several times a day helps to resolve erythema and edema. Another side effect that may be seen is purpura, limited to the use of the 510-nm PDL and the frequency-doubled 532-nm Nd:YAG laser, as these wavelengths are also well absorbed by oxyhemoglobin. If purpura develops, the patient can be assured that it will fade within 1 to 2 weeks postoperatively.

Complications are untoward events; in the treatment of tattoos with Q-switched lasers, these entail pigmentary changes, textural changes, immediate pigmentary darkening, and systemic allergic reactions.

Transient pigmentary change represents the most common complication, occurring in up to 50 percent of treated patients, and usually hypopigmentation rather than hyperpigmentation.[175] Hypopigmentation is most noticeable with wavelengths well absorbed by melanin. The hypopigmentation seen with the 510- and 532-nm wavelengths tends to resolve quickly, while the hypopigmentation experienced with the 694- and 755-nm wavelengths is more likely to last for several months and may rarely be permanent. The 1064-nm wavelength is the least likely to cause hypopigmentation owing to a notably lesser degree of absorption by melanin and the greater depth of penetration. Hyperpigmentation lasts for months and appears to be related mainly to skin type. Individuals with darker skin tones are at greatest risk for developing hyperpigmentation; they may profit from the use of hydroquinone in a preoperative regimen as a preventive measure. If hyperpigmentation develops nonetheless, the use of a hydroquinone-containing bleaching cream twice daily will expedite its resolution.[19,158,173]

Textural changes—commonly manifesting as cigarette paper–like wrinkling, mild but prolonged erythema, or a waxy surface—after the use of high fluences are for the most part transient. Permanent textural changes have been noted less than 5 percent of the time. Even rarer is the development of hypertrophic scarring, noted in one large study of Q-switched ruby laser therapy of tattoos[176] to occur in 0.5 percent of cases. The incidence for hypertrophic scarring is even less likely for the other Q-switched laser types. Should hypertrophic scarring develop, it often resolves with the use of intralesional triamcinolone or silicone gel or sheeting.[19]

Immediate pigmentary darkening may occur with tattoo pigments that contain iron oxide or titanium dioxide. It is

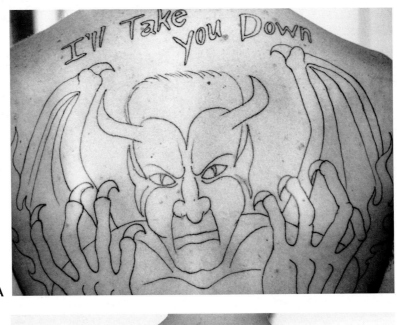

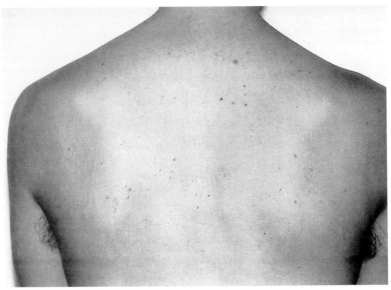

Figure 14-22   (**A**) A young man who was changing careers wanted to remove this grotesque, single-color tattoo. (**B**) Three treatments with the Q-switched Nd:YAG laser (1064 nm), produced excellent results.

believed to result from an oxidation-reduction reaction of these compounds induced by the pulsed laser treatment. This is especially a concern with the red, white, and flesh-colored inks used cosmetically to enhance eyebrows, eyelids, cheeks, and lips. Once this pigmentary darkening develops, it may be permanent, as it does not always resolve with further laser treatments. Consequently, it is recommended to begin by placing a test spot when dealing with tattoo pigment at risk for potential darkening.[172]

Rarely, systemic allergic reactions may develop, attributed to the setting loose of extracellular particles with a high antigenicity (chromium-containing red or yellow inks). Thus, patients with a history or obvious clinical finding of a cutane-

ous reaction within a tattoo, in particular when red and yellow inks are involved, should not be treated. However, if a patient is treated and develops signs of a systemic allergic reaction, the use of epinephrine and/or steroids as well as immediate transfer to a hospital setting may be indicated.[173,174]

Treatment of Scars

Patient Selection Early attempts at the treatment of keloids and hypertrophic scars with lasers consisted of the use of the CO_2 laser, Nd:YAG laser, and argon laser. While the CO_2 laser allows for precise removal of keloids with minimal tissue trauma, studies did show recurrence rates of 37.5 to 92 percent. Similarly, the Nd:YAG laser and the argon

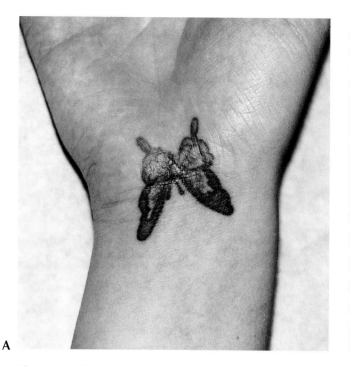

A

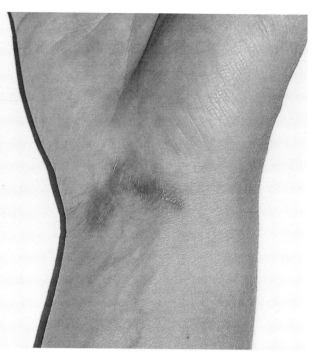

B

Figure 14-23 (*A*) A multicolored (green, yellow, black, blue, and red) butterfly tattoo was placed on the patient's wrist to camouflage a scar. (*B*) The alexandrite and Q-switched Nd:YAG (532 and 1064 nm) lasers brought partial improvement after two treatment sessions.

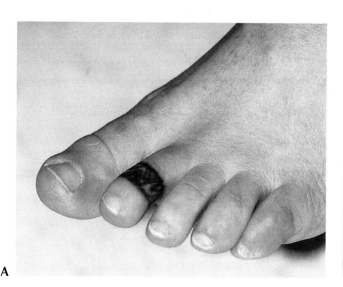

A

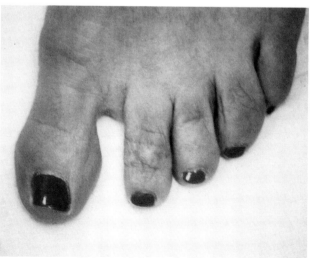

B

Figure 14-24 (*A*) A "toe-band" yellow, green, and black tattoo became obtrusive to this patient, who frequently wore open-toed shoes. (*B*) Slight residual was present after six treatments with the alexandrite and Q-switched Nd:YAG (532 and 1064 nm) lasers.

laser demonstrated promising results initially but were also characterized by high recurrence rates in the range of 53 to 100 percent and 45 to 93 percent respectively.[177–181]

Since that time the PDL has emerged as the gold standard in the laser treatment of keloids, hypertrophic scars, and even striae distensae. PDL treatment of keloids, in particular those of the anterior mediastinum, led to significant improvement in all clinical parameters, including symptomatic responses of pruritus and dysesthesia. In the same fashion, several studies reported improvement of erythematous and hypertrophic scars by 57 to 83 percent following one to two treatments with the PDL. Even long-standing striae have been noted to improve by as much as 60 percent after a single treatment with the PDL. The exact mechanism behind the success of the PDL in ameliorating the appearance of these types of scars is not known. Based on the histologic finding of an increased number of mast cells in tissue after irradiation, it has been proposed that the effect of the PDL on scars is related to the influence of histamine release on collagen turnover.[95,182–186]

Next to the actual laser procedure and technique, the most important factors in optimizing this outcome in the treatment of scars with the PDL are patient selection and patient education. Neglecting the process of patient selection increases the potential for complications and patient dissatisfaction.

Proper patient selection depends on identification of the type of scar, length of time it has been present, associated symptoms, location, prior treatments to it other than the PDL, skin type of patient, and patient expectations. The various types of scars differ in the laser parameters and number of treatments required bringing about the expected improvement. Keloids and hypertrophic scars respond most favorably to a higher energy setting and necessitate at least two or three treatments. Striae, on the other hand, do better with a low energy setting and show remarkable results after only one or two treatments. The length of time a scar has been present must also be considered. Whereas erythema is an expected finding early on and by itself does not call for laser intervention, prolonged erythema within a scar qualifies for such intervention. And treatment of hypertrophy at its earliest stage helps to accelerate clinical improvement and counteract further worsening. Next, the symptoms of pruritus and dysesthesia noted with scars do improve rapidly with PDL irradiation. Also, it is worthwhile to note the location of scars, as those on the chest, shoulders, and upper back are more likely to become hypertrophic, even keloidal, and tend to persist, favoring their laser treatment over scars in other locations. Another aspect to consider is what type of prior treatments the scar has been subjected to. The increase in fibrosis of scars due to previous excision, cryosurgery, and electrocautery may necessitate a greater number of treatments and still fail to bring about the expected improvement in appearance. Yet previous treatment with intralesional triamcinolone or silicone gel or sheets does not alter the surmised response of scars to PDL irradiation. Furthermore, the patient's skin type comes into play, as darker-colored skin absorbs a substantially greater amount of the 585-nm laser light than fair skin, preventing the full delivery of laser energy to scar tissue and increasing the risk of pigmentary alteration. Therefore, patients with Fitzpatrick skin types I and II can expect the greatest benefit from this treatment and are least likely to develop complications. Finally, patients must have realistic expectations in terms of degree of improvement and an understanding of expected sequelae as well as the potential for morbid events due to PDL irradiation; these must be acknowledged in a detailed consent form. Patients who fail to complete such a form should not be treated.[95]

Preoperative Regimen The patient should be advised to keep clear of UV radiation from the sun or a tanning bed in the time preceding the laser irradiation, as the risk for pigmentary alteration increases with higher levels of melanin in the skin. If a patient arrives for treatment with a notable tan, the appointment should be rescheduled.

Laser Procedure and Technique Anesthesia is usually not required with the PDL, as most patients tolerate the discomfort—akin to snapping a rubber band against the skin—very well. However, children and particularly sensitive adult individuals may benefit from topical application of eutectic mixture of lidocaine 2.5% and prilocaine 2.5% (EMLA cream) or lidocaine 4% (ELA-max cream) prior to treatment and/or a cooling gel throughout irradiation.

Independent of the type of scar present, this laser procedure is best carried out by placing pulses with no overlap or at most 10 percent overlap. Yet the laser energy parameters used to treat various scars does make a difference. Keloids and hypertrophic scars do best with a 5- or 7-mm spot size at high energy densities in the range of 6.0 to 7.5 J/cm^2 and should demonstrate an immediate purpuric response. If the scar fails to show such a response, as may be the case with keloids, additional actually overlapping pulses may be applied to achieve purpura. In contrast, striae respond the best with a 10-mm spot size at a lower energy density of 3.0 J/cm^2, followed by a 7-mm spot size at 4.0 J/cm^2. Subsequent treatments at the same energy density are scheduled at 6- to 8-week intervals as needed to gain a satisfactory response.[95,165,186]

Observance of all these aspects in the laser treatment of scars allows for the best possible results (see Figs. 14-25 and 14-26).

Postoperative Regimen Care consists of twice daily application of a topical antibiotic or emollient ointment under a nonadherent dressing. Strict avoidance of sun exposure prevents postinflammatory changes in pigmentation and allows for optimal delivery of laser energy during the next treatment session.

Side Effects, Complications, and Their Management Purpura is the expected sequela of PDL irradiation and resolves on its own within 1 to 2 weeks following the procedure. True complications, including further scarring as well as hyperpigmentation and hypopigmentation, can usually be prevented by applying pulses with minimal to no overlap and appropriate energy densities. Worsening of scars is unlikely to occur with observance of appropriate laser parameters and technique. In the event of increased scarring, the use of intralesional triamcinolone and/or silicone gel or sheets is often effective. Transient hyperpigmentation or hypopigmentation occurs in 10 to 20 percent of the cases.[165] Intervention with hydroquinone, other bleaching creams, and

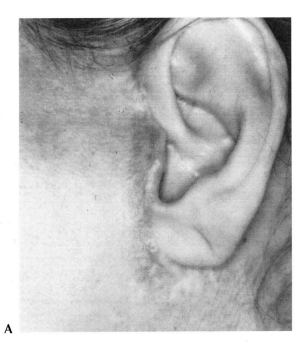

A

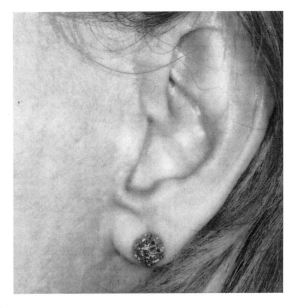

B

Figure 14-25   (*A*) Prominent periauricular scarring is shown immediately following Q-switched pulsed-dye laser treatment. (*B*) Reasonable improvement is seen 3 months later.

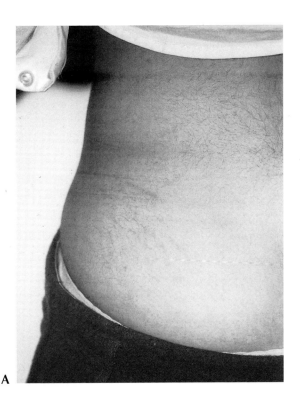

A

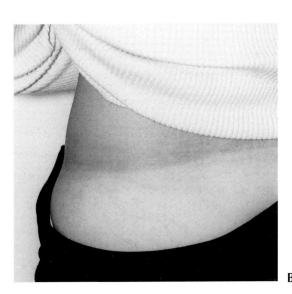

B

Figure 14-26   (*A*) Evolving striae can be significantly improved with Q-switched pulsed-dye laser treatment. (*B*) The patient is pleased with the result seen 3 months after a single treatment.

sun avoidance helps with the occasional case of persistent hyperpigmentation. And makeup masks the presence of obvious hypopigmentation in darker-skinned individuals.

Treatment of Terminal Hair

Patient Selection Laser-assisted hair removal is based on the principle of selective photothermolysis. It utilizes wavelengths in the red and infrared regions to preferentially target follicular melanin, an endogenous chromophore, or an exogenous pigment placed within the follicle to thermally damage the hair shaft and follicle. To limit absorption of these wavelengths by melanin-containing structures outside the follicle (melanocyte, keratinocyte, and nevus) and thus inadvertent epidermal damage and pigmentary changes, hair removal lasers apply a combination of longer wavelengths, longer pulse duration, and cooling devices. This preferential targeting of melanin or an exogenous pigment within the follicle over melanin-containing structures in the surrounding skin is also referred to as thermokinetic selectivity.[98]

Patient selection is the key to successful laser-assisted hair removal. Vital to proper patient selection is a good physical and history, an understanding of the differences in the effectiveness and complications rates of the available hair removal lasers, and, obviously, realistic patient expectations.

The physical examination concentrates on evaluating the skin phototype and the color of the hair to be removed. Ideal candidates combine a fair skin tone (Fitzpatrick skin types I and II) with the presence of dark terminal hair, as they are able to tolerate higher fluences for more effective hair removal while minimizing untoward epidermal damage and pigmentary changes. In contrast, individuals with darker skin tones (natural or due to tanning) and/or hair without much pigment (blond, red, gray, or white) at prospective sites of treatment are far from ideal. These patients fail to provide a well-defined follicular target and therefore increase the risk for blistering or hyper- and hypopigmentation as well as reduce the chance for permanent hair removal. Other than skin and hair color, keloids and hypertrophic scarring noted on examination may point to a higher risk for such scarring in the event of blistering.

History obtained before laser-assisted hair removal should focus on the presence of conditions that may be the cause of hypertrichosis, previous herpes reactivation, prior treatment modalities, and medications. Hypertrichosis, the presence of excess hair, is commonly related to genetic or ethnic factors. However, should history reveal other potential causes of hypertrichosis—such as medications, endocrine disturbances, malnutrition, porphyria, and rarely tumors—it is wise to hold off with laser-assisted removal until these conditions have been adequately addressed. Antiviral prophylaxis, beginning on the day before treatment, is indicated for a strong history of herpes reactivation in the perioral, perianal, and pubic or bikini area before attempting laser hair removal in these regions. Prior treatment modalities must also be considered. Recent plucking, waxing, or epilation gets rid of pigmented hair shafts and thus target melanin within the follicle, resulting in less effective laser hair removal. And the effectiveness, side effects, or complications experienced by the patient with previous laser-assisted hair removal may influence the current choice of laser system and treatment

parameters. One last consideration goes to reviewing the patient's list of medications. Both current intake of photosensitizing medications and use of oral isotretinoin within the past year increase the potential for scarring and pigmentary alterations.[100,101]

The various hair removal lasers differ with regard to effectiveness and risk for complications. The Q-switched Nd:YAG system utilizes a wavelength of 1064 nm in combination with pretreatment of unwanted hair-bearing areas with a topical carbon solution as an exogenous chromophore. The use of the carbon solution offers follicular selectivity irrespective of the presence of endogenous melanin, allowing for treatment of lighter hair colors. Recently, however, Nanni and Alster[187] demonstrated that there is no benefit to laser treatment with carbon suspension application as opposed to laser treatment alone. One additional benefit is that the relatively poor eumelanin absorption at 1064 nm makes the Nd:YAG somewhat safer to use in individuals with skin phototypes III and above than the other hair removal lasers. The downfall of the Q-switched Nd:YAG laser is that it provides only temporary hair reduction, not permanent hair removal. In comparison, the long-pulsed ruby laser system at 694 nm, the long-pulsed alexandrite laser system at 755 nm, and the high-power diode laser array at 800 nm do provide more effective hair removal. While all of these hair removal lasers effectively target melanin (endogenous chromophore) within follicles, certain points of distinction are worth noting. The long-pulsed alexandrite laser system and the high-power diode laser array have a greater depth of penetration and carry a lower risk for epidermal damage and pigmentary alteration than the long-pulsed ruby laser system, secondary to decreased scattering of light and slightly diminished absorption of melanin at their higher wavelengths.[97–99]

As always, the patient has to show an understanding of what results can be realistically expected with laser-assisted hair removal, what side effects and complications are possible, and the ability to comply with preoperative and postoperative regimen. Failure to do so is a contraindication to treatment.

Preoperative Regimen Beginning 4 to 6 weeks before laser treatment, patients should start a skin care regimen as follows. Regular use a broad-spectrum sunscreen—even a topical skin lightener (hydroquinone, tretinoin, azelaic acid, or kojic acid) in darker-skinned individuals—as well as strict avoidance of sun exposure are encouraged. Decreasing the amount of epidermal melanin present in this manner allows for more effective hair removal while minimizing the risk of complications. Plucking, waxing, and electrolysis are discouraged, as they remove pigmented hair shafts, and thus target melanin within follicles. Rather, patients are advised to shave, clip, or depilate hair, in particular on the day before the intended laser treatment. Besides preserving the target melanin in follicles, it helps to minimize epidermal injury by singed surface hairs. Another consideration is to start a prophylactic antiviral (acyclovir, valacyclovir, or famcyclovir) on the day before use of a hair removal laser in the perioral, perianal, pubic or bikini areas if there is a strong history of HSV reactivation in these anatomic regions. And though the risk for bacterial infections is exceedingly low, use of a prophylactic oral antibiotic may be indicated in patients planning to undergo hair removal of the nasal and perianal skin. Finally, patients are instructed to arrive with the area to be treated thoroughly cleansed and without makeup.[100,101]

Laser Procedure and Technique For the most part, laser-assisted hair removal is well tolerated by patients, rarely requiring any anesthesia. Topical anesthesia in the form of a eutectic mixture of lidocaine 2.5% and prilocaine 2.5% (EMLA cream) or lidocaine 4% (ELA-max cream) is recommended for more sensitive areas. Seldom is there a need for local or regional anesthesia.

Before attempting laser hair removal, the area to be treated is thoroughly cleansed with alcohol swabs, getting rid of any remnants of makeup or topical anesthetic creams. And if the patient did not shave the site on the day before, the medical staff must do so in the office preoperatively so as to maximize the effectiveness of laser-assisted hair removal and minimize epidermal injury by singed surface hairs. A red marking pen or ink grid may be used to outline areas of treatment.

After complying with safety measures, the procedure for hair removal with any of the aforementioned lasers progresses as follows. Initially, the spot size and level of fluence to be used for treatment must be determined. The largest available spot size is recommended, as it provides for deeper penetration and is more time-efficient. The largest spot size in combination with the highest tolerable fluence provides for the best results.

Yet the highest tolerable fluence is not easy to establish and varies from patient to patient, depending on the skin type. Individuals with Fitzpatrick skin types IV and above are at a much higher risk for the development of complications, necessitating the use of much lower fluences than in patients with Fitzpatrick skin types I to III. Thus, skin types IV and above are unsuitable for treatment. The approach to establishing the highest tolerable fluence in skin types I to III utilizes single-pulse test fluences, if possible at inconspicuous sites within the area to be treated. Based upon routine predetermined treatment parameters for lasers, these single-pulse test fluences are begun at the lowest fluence within a given range for a skin type and carefully increased (by 0.5 to 1 J/cm^2). Meanwhile, the skin must be monitored for signs of epidermal injury for up to 5 min prior to the next single pulse delivery. If whitening, blistering, ablation, or Nikolsky signs (epidermal separation) are noted at a test site, the fluence must be decreased by about 1 J/cm^2 before treatment of the entire site is begun. Examples of such routine predetermined treatment parameters include the following: (1) Long-pulsed ruby laser: 7-mm spot size and 19 to 40 J/cm^2 for skin types I and II, 10-mm spot size and 10 to 19 J/cm^2 for skin types II and III; (2) long-pulsed alexandrite laser: 12 mm spot size and 20 to 30 J/cm^2 for skin types I and II, 12-mm spot size and 18 to 25 J/cm^2 for skin types II and III. A somewhat safer option is to start treatment of the entire site at the lowest predetermined fluence for a specific skin type. Thereafter, the amount of fluence can be carefully increased with each subsequent treatment session up to the point of notable discomfort and/or noticeable early signs of epidermal injury (whitening or rapid development of perifollicular edema), all of which serve as clinical endpoints of treatment.[97,98,100]

Once the proper spot size and fluence have been chosen, attention turns toward the actual treatment. Laser pulses are placed with up to 10 percent overlap while providing adequate cooling of the epidermis. This cooling of the epidermis aids in limiting the amount of inadvertent epidermal damage and pigmentary change. To achieve adequate cooling of the epidermis, hair removal lasers employ one of three methods: (1) Contact cooling—the sapphire-cooled handpiece is placed firmly in direct contact with the skin; it should be wiped every 5 to 10 pulses to take off debris. (2) Dynamic cooling—automated delivery of short burst of cryogen (5 to 100 ms) provides cooling just prior to laser pulses. (3) Cooling gel—a thick layer of cooled gel (KY jelly or plain aloe vera gel) is put on the skin before placement of laser pulses; the laser tip must be wiped every 5 to 10 pulses to remove buildup of cooling gel containing singed hair. The recommended treatment interval is 6 to 8 weeks, as it coincides with the early anagen phase of the hair cycle during which hairs are small, pigmented, and in a superficial location. Compliance with the technique of laser-assisted hair removal outlined above increases the likelihood of permanent hair removal while minimizing the risk of complications.[101]

Postoperative Regimen Proper care in the postoperative period helps to achieve the best possible outcome. It begins with addressing posttreatment discomfort, for which the use of ice packs and mild topical steroids is usually sufficient. Rarely, analgesics may be needed. In addition to helping with postoperative pain, continued use of ice packs also helps to diminish swelling, while application of mild topical steroids aids in lessening swelling and erythema. Asymptomatic postoperative sites and those with crusts or blistering are treated with twice-daily application of a topical antibiotic to aid healing and prevent postoperative infection. Prophylactic courses of antivirals or antibiotics should be carried to completion. If an infection develops despite these measures, an appropriate culture is taken and the dose or type of antiviral or antibiotic is changed accordingly. Makeup may be applied to the treated site the very next day assuming that there are no crusts or blistering, in which case healing would be impeded by doing so. Moreover, patients are instructed to refrain from picking or scratching of the area, to steer clear of sun exposure, and to practice effective sun protection with an SPF 30 sunscreen. Finally, patients should be reassured that the shedding of treated hair in the first few weeks following laser hair removal does not represent the growth of new hair.[97,100]

Side Effects, Complications, and Their Management The side effects of laser-assisted hair removal, also defined as expected sequelae, are the same for all of the employed laser systems and occur in the great majority of cases. These include treatment pain, perifollicular erythema, and transient erythema. Discomfort related to treatment is usually mild and well tolerated, partially due to concomitant cooling of the epidermis. On occasion it may be necessary to use topical anesthesia for more sensitive areas, like the upper lip and the "bikini" and/or pubic area. Icing of the skin and application of mild topical steroids following the treatment help to resolve any remaining discomfort as well as any perifollicular edema and transient erythema.

Distinct from side effects, the term *complications* refers to morbid events of treatment, and these actually do differ in their incidence among the various hair removal lasers.[188] Complications of laser-assisted hair removal include folliculitis, vesiculation, hyperpigmentation, hypopigmentation, and scarring. The Q-switched Nd:YAG laser tends to produce significantly higher rates of folliculitis (35 percent) and purpura (18 percent) than the long-pulsed ruby and alexandrite lasers. The folliculitis is probably related to pretreatment with wax epilation and carbon solution rather than to the laser itself. On the other hand, more severe complications like blistering and pigmentary changes appear to be rarely observed, and scarring seems to be unusual. In comparison, the long-pulsed ruby and alexandrite lasers are characterized by higher rates of blistering, hyperpigmentation (11 and 19 percent), and hypopigmentation (18 and 17 percent); these are ascribed to the greater degree of melanin light absorption of their wavelengths as compared with the Q-switched Nd:YAG laser. Still, development of scarring is also rather unusual with these long-pulsed lasers, excluding cases of improper (overly aggressive) technique or failure to recognize and treat postoperative infection early on.[189]

Most of the time these complications resolve upon proper management. Irritant folliculitis may benefit from the use of a mild topical steroid cream. In case of blistering, wound care with a topical antibiotic ointment or an emollient ointment twice a day until healing is complete is appropriate. Hyperpigmentation tends to be temporary, lasting 2 to 3 months. The process of clearing it up can be accelerated by twice-daily applications of a bleaching cream containing hydroquinone in combination with a corticosteroid and a mild glycolic acid cream. While hypopigmentation is often transient, lasting for 3 to 4 months, its resolution may be helped by gradual exposure to sunlight (15 to 30 min every other day).

References

1. Maiman TH. Stimulated optical radiation in ruby. *Nature* 1960; 187:439.
2. Goldman L, Blaney DJ, Kindel DJ, et al. Effect of the laser beam on the skin. *J Invest Dermatol* 1963; 40:121–122.
3. Rosenbach A, Alster T. Cutaneous lasers: A review. *Ann Plast Surg* 1996; 37:220–231.
4. Alster TS, Bettencourt M. Review of cutaneous lasers and their applications. *South Med J* 1998; 91:806–814.
5. Wheeland RG. Cosmetic use of lasers. *Dermatol Clin* 1995; 13:447–459.
6. Sliney D. Laser-tissue interactions. *Clin Chest Med* 1985; 6:203–208.
7. Anderson RR, Levins PC, Grevelink JM. Lasers in dermatology. In: Fitzpatrick TB, Eisen AZ, Wolff K, et al, eds. *Dermatology in General Medicine*, 4th ed. New York, McGraw-Hill, 1993:1757–1760.
8. Hruza GJ. Laser treatment of warts and other epidermal and dermal lesions. *Dermatol Clin* 1997; 15:487–506.
9. McKenzie AL. How far does thermal damage extend beneath the surface of CO_2 laser incisions? *Phys Med Biol* 1983; 28:905.
10. Anderson RR, Parrish JA. Selective photothermolysis: Precise microsurgery by selective absorption of pulsed radiation. *Science* 1983; 220:524–527.
11. Anderson RR, Parrish JA. The optics of human skin. *J Invest Dermatol* 1983; 77:13–19.
12. Parrish JA, Anderson RR, Harris T. Selective thermal effects with pulsed irradiation from organ to organelle. *J Invest Dermatol* 1983; 80:75–80.
13. Goldberg DJ. Laser treatment of pigmented lesions. *Dermatol Clin* 1997; 15:397–407.
14. Watanabe S. Putative photoacoustic damage in skin induced by pulsed ArF excimer laser. *J Invest Dermatol* 1988; 90:761.
15. Bissonette R. Current status of photodynamic therapy in dermatology. *Dermatol Clin* 1997; 15:507–519.
16. Henderson BW, Dougherty TJ. How does photodynamic therapy work? *Photochem Photobiol* 1992; 55:145–157.
17. Dougherty TJ, Gomer CJ, Henderson BW, et al. Photodynamic therapy: Review. *J Natl Cancer Inst* 1998; 12:889–905.
18. Oseroff AR, Dozier SE. Lasers and photodynamic therapy. In: Miller SJ, Maloney ME eds. *Cutaneous Oncology.* London: Blackwell Science; 1998:534–541.
19. Levins PC, Anderson RR. Q-switched ruby laser for the treatment of pigmented lesions and tattoos. *Clin Dermatol* 1995; 13:75–78.
20. Anderson RR, Parrish JA. Optical properties of human skin. In: Regan JD, Parrish JA, eds. *The Science of Photomedicine.* New York: Plenum Press; 1982:147.
21. Garden JM, Geronemus RG. Dermatologic laser surgery. *J Dermatol Surg Oncol* 1990; 16:156–168.
22. Seckel BR, Kovanda CJ, Cetrulo CL Jr, et al. Laser blepharoplasty with transconjunctival orbicularis muscle/septum tightening and periocular skin resurfacing: A safe and advantageous technique. *Plast Reconstr Surg* 2000; 106:1127–1141.
23. Lessner AM, Fagien S. Laser blepharoplasty. *Semin Ophthalmol* 1998; 13:90–102.
24. Glassberg E, Babapour R, Lask G. Current trends in laser blepharoplasty. Results of a survey. *Dermatol Surg* 1995; 21:1060–1063.
25. Villnow MM, Feriduni B. Update on laser-assisted hair transplantation. *Dermatol Surg* 1998; 24:749–754.
26. Wheeland RG, Bailin PL. Scalp reduction with the carbon dioxide laser. *J Dermatol Surg Oncol* 1984; 10:565–569.
27. Karim AM, Streitmann MJ. Excision of rhinophyma with the carbon dioxide laser: A ten-year experience. *Ann Otol Rhinol Laryngol* 1997; 106:952–955.
28. Simo R, Sharma VL. Treatment of rhinophyma with carbon dioxide laser. *J Laryngol Otol* 1996; 110:841–846.
29. Lim TC, Tan WT. Carbon dioxide laser for keloids. *Plast Reconstr Surg* 1991; 88:1111.
30. Norris JE. The effect of carbon dioxide laser surgery on the recurrence of keloids. *Plast Reconstr Surg* 1991; 87:44–49.
31. Sexton J. Carbon dioxide laser treatment for actinic cheilitis. *J Oral Maxillofac Surg* 1993; 51:118–121.
32. Zelickson BD, Roenigk RK. Actinic cheilitis. Treatment with the carbon dioxide laser. *Cancer* 1990; 65:1307–1311.
33. Hohenleutner U, Wlotzke U, Konz B, et al. Carbon dioxide laser therapy of a widespread epidermal nevus. *Lasers Surg Med* 1995; 16:288–291.
34. Hohenleutner U, Landthaler M. Laser therapy of verrucous epidermal nevi. *Clin Exp Dermatol* 1993; 18:124–127.
35. Roenigk RK. CO_2 laser vaporization of rhinophyma. *Mayo Clin Proc* 1990; 62:676–680.
36. Wheeland RG, Bailin PL, Ratz JL. Combined carbon dioxide laser excision and vaporization in the treatment of rhinophyma. *J Dermatol Surg Oncol* 1987; 13:172–177.

37. Sloan K, Haberman H, Lynde CW. Carbon dioxide laser treatment of resistant verrucae vulgaris: Retrospective analysis. *J Cutan Med Surg* 1998; 2:142–145.

38. Lim JT, Goh CL. Carbon dioxide laser treatment of periungual and subungual viral warts. *Australas J Dermatol* 1992; 33:87–91.

39. Mancuso JE, Abramow SP, Dimichino BR, et al. Carbon dioxide laser management of plantar verrucae: A 6-year follow-up survey. *J Foot Surg* 1991; 30:238–243.

40. Spenler CW, Achauer BM Vander Kam VM. Treatment of extensive adenoma sebaceum with a carbon dioxide laser. *Ann Plast Surg* 1988; 20:586–589.

41. Wheeland RG, Bailin PL, Reynolds OD, et al. Carbon dioxide laser vaporization of multiple facial syringomas. *J Dermatol Surg Oncol* 1986; 12:225–228.

42. Buecker JW, Estes SA, Zalla JA. Multiple trichoepitheliomas treated with the carbon dioxide laser. *J Ky Med Assoc* 1986; 84:543–544.

43. Bickley LK, Goldberg DJ, Imaeda S, et al. Treatment of multiple apocrine hidrocystomas with the carbon dioxide laser. *J Dermatol Surg Oncol* 19889; 15:599.

44. Huerter CJ, Wheeland RG. Multiple eruptive velus hair cysts treated with carbon dioxide laser vaporization. *J Dermatol Surg Oncol* 1987; 13:260–263.

45. Roenigk RK, Ratz JL. CO_2 laser treatment of cutaneous neurofibromas. *J Dermatol Surg Oncol* 1987; 13:187.

46. Dover JS, Smoller BR, Stern RS, et al. Low-fluence carbon dioxide laser irradiation of lentigines. *Arch Dermatol* 124:1219–1224.

47. Elizieri YD, Sklar JA. Lymphangioma circumscriptum: Review and evaluation of carbon dioxide laser vaporization. *J Dermatol Surg Oncol* 1988; 14:357–364.

48. Bailin PL, Kantor GR, Wheeland RG. Carbon dioxide laser vaporization of lymphangioma circumscriptum. *J Am Acad Dermatol* 1986; 14:257–262.

49. Dover JS, Arndt KA, Geronemus RC, et al. Selecting a laser to treat vascular lesions. In: *Cutaneous and Aesthetic Laser Surgery,* 2d ed. New York: McGraw-Hill; 2000:234.

50. White JM, Chaudhry SI, Kudler JJ, et al. Nd:YAG and CO_2 laser therapy of oral mucosal lesions. *J Clin Laser Med Surg* 1998; 16:299–304.

51. Modica LA. Pyogenic granuloma of the tongue treated by carbon dioxide laser. *J Am Geriatr Soc* 1988; 36:1036–1038.

52. Apfelberg DB, Maser MR, Lash H. Treatment of xanthelasma palpebrarum with the carbon dioxide laser. *J Dermatol Surg Oncol* 1987; 13:149–151.

53. Alster TS, West TB. Ultrapulse CO_2 laser ablation of xanthelasma. *J Am Acad Dermatol* 1996; 34:848–849.

54. Katalinic D. Experience with surgical laser treatment of tattoos and use of the CO_2 laser plastic surgery. *Adv Otorhinolaryngol* 1995; 49:63–66.

55. Garret AB, Dufresne RG Jr, Ratz JL, et al. Carbon dioxide laser treatment of pitted acne scarring. *J Dermatol Surg Oncol* 1990; 16:737–740.

56. Karrer S, Hohenleutner U, Szeimies KM, et al. Treatment of digital mucous cysts with a carbon dioxide laser. *Acta Derm Venereol* 1999; 79:224–225.

57. McKinlay JR, Graham BS, Ross EV. The clinical superiority of continuous exposure versus short-pulsed carbon dioxide laser exposures for the treatment of pearly penile papules. *Dermatol Surg* 1999; 25:124–126.

58. Ross E, Naseef G, Skrobal M, et al. In vivo dermal collagen shrinkage and remodeling following CO_2 laser resurfacing. *Lasers Surg Med* 1996; 18:38.

59. Fulton JE, Barnes T. Collagen shrinkage (selective dermoplasty) with the high-energy pulsed carbon dioxide laser. *Dermatol Surg* 1998; 24:3.

60. Alster TS. Cutaneous resurfacing with CO_2 and erbium:YAG lasers: Preoperative, intraoperative, and postoperative considerations. *Plast Reconstr Surg* 1999; 103:619–631.

61. Walsh JT, Flotte TJ, Deutsch TF. Er:YAG laser ablation of tissue: Effect of pulse duration and tissue type on thermal damage. *Lasers Med Sci* 1991; 6:391.

62. Kaufmann R, Hibst R. Pulsed erbium:YAG laser ablation in cutaneous surgery. *Lasers Surg Med* 1996; 19(3):324–330.

63. Hohenleutner U, Hohenleutner S, Baumler W, et al. Fast and effective skin ablation with an Er:YAG laser: Determination of ablation rates and thermal damage zones. *Lasers Surg Med* 1997; 20:242.

64. Ross EV, Anderson RR. The erbium laser in skin resurfacing. In: Alster TS, Apfelberg DB (eds): *Cosmetic Laser Surgery,* 2nd ed. New York: Wiley; 1999:57–84.

65. Goldberg DJ. Non-ablative subsurface remodeling: Clinical and histologic evaluation of a 1320 nm Nd:YAG laser. *J Cutan Laser Ther* 1999; 1:153–157.

66. Kelly KM, Nelson JS, Lask GP, et al. Cryogen spray cooling in combination with nonablative laser treatment of facial rhytides. *Arch Dermatol* 1999; 135:691–694.

67. Bjerring P, Clement M, Heickendorff L, et al. Selective non-ablative wrinkle reduction by laser. *J Cutan Laser Ther* 2000; 2:9–15.

68. Achauer BM, Vander Kam VM. Argon laser treatment of telangiectasia of the face and neck: 5 years' experience. *Lasers Surg Med* 1987; 7:495–498.

69. Pasyk KA, Argenta LC. Argon laser surgery of skin lesions in tuberous sclerosis. *Ann Plast Surg* 1988; 20:426–433.

70. Neumann RA, Knobler RM. Venous lakes of the lips—Treatment experience with the argon laser and 18 months follow-up. *Clin Exp Dermatol* 1990; 15:115–118.

71. Apfelberg DB, Maser MR, Lash H, et al. Expanded role of the argon laser in plastic surgery. *J Dermatol Surg Oncol* 1983; 9:145–151.

72. Silver L. Argon laser photocoagulation of port-wine stain hemangiomas. *Lasers Surg Med* 1986; 6:24–28.

73. Dover JS, Arndt KA, Dinehart SM, et al. Guidelines of care for laser surgery. *J Am Acad Dermatol* 1999; 41:484–495.

74. Dover JS, Arndt KA. New approaches to the treatment of vascular lesions. *Lasers Surg Med* 2000; 26:158–163.

75. Goldberg DJ, Meine JG. A comparison of four frequency doubled Nd:YAG (532 nm) laser systems for treatment of facial telangiectasias. *Dermatol Surg* 1999; 25:463–467.

76. Bernstein EF, Kornbluth S, Brown DB, et al. Treatment of spider veins using 10 millisecond pulse duration frequency doubled neodymium YAG laser. *Dermatol Surg* 1999; 25:316–320.

77. Haas A, Wheeland RG. Treatment of massive rhinophyma with the carbon dioxide laser. *J Dermatol Surg Oncol* 1990; 16:645–649.

78. Ali KM, Callari RH, Mobley DL. Resection of rhinophyma with CO_2 laser. *Laryngoscope* 1989; 99:453–455.

79. Logan RA, Zachary CB. Outcome of carbon dioxide laser therapy for persistent cutaneous viral warts. *Br J Dermatol* 1989; 121:99.

80. Carpo BG, Grevelink JM, Grevelink SV. Laser treatment of pigmented lesions in children. *Semin Cutan Med Surg* 1999; 18:233–243.

81. Goldman MP, Fitzpatrick RE. Treatment of benign pigmented cutaneous lesions. In: Goldman MP, Fitzpatrick RE, eds. *Cutaneous Laser Surgery: The Art and Science of Selective Photothermolysis.* St Louis: Mosby–Year Book; 1994:109.

82. Swinehart JM. Hypertrophic scarring resulting from flashlamp pulsed dye laser surgery. *J Am Acad Dermatol* 1991; 25:845–855.

83. Katugampola GA, Lanigan SW. Five years' experience of treating port-wine stains with the flashlamp-pumped pulsed dye laser. *Br J Dermatol* 1997; 137:750–754.

84. Scheepers JH, Quaba AA. Clinical experience in the treatment of the "red nose" using the flashlamp-pumped pulsed dye laser (585 nm). *Aesthet Plast Surg* 1994; 18:57–60.

85. Scheepers JH, Quaba AA. Treatment of nevi aranei with the pulsed tunable dye laser at 585 nm. *J Pediatr Surg* 1995; 30:101–104.

86. Lask GP, Glassberg E. 585-nm pulsed dye laser for the treatment of cutaneous lesions. *Clin Dermatol* 1995; 13:63–67.

87. Glass AT, Milgraum S. Flashlamp-pumped pulsed dye laser treatment for pyogenic granuloma. *Cutis* 1992; 49:351–353.

88. Wheeland RG, Applebaum J. Flashlamp-pumped pulsed dye laser therapy for poikiloderma of Civatte. *J Dermatol Surg Oncol* 1990; 16:12–16.

89. Hoffman SJ, Walsh P, Morelli JG. Treatment of angiofibroma with the pulsed tunable dye laser. *J Am Acad Dermatol* 1993; 29:790–791.

90. Alster TS, Kohn SR. Dermatologic lasers: Three decades of progress. *Int J Dermatol* 1992; 31:601–610.

91. Weingold D, White P, Burton CS. Treatment of lymphangioma circumscriptum with tunable dye laser. *Cutis* 1990; 45:365–366.

92. Olson TG, Milroy SK, Goldman L, et al. Laser surgery for blue rubber bleb nevus. *Arch Dermatol* 1979; 115:81–82.

93. Arielle N, Kauvar MD, McDaniel DH, et al. Pulsed dye laser treatment of warts. *Arch Fam Med* 1995; 4:1035–1040.

94. Alster TS. Inflammatory linear verrucous epidermal nevus: Successful treatment with the 585 nm flashlamp-pumped pulsed dye laser. *J Am Acad Dermatol* 1994; 31:513–514.

95. Alster TS. Laser treatment of hypertrophic scars, keloids, and striae. *Dermatol Clin* 1997; 3:419–429.

96. Goldberg DJ. Laser treatment of pigmented lesions. *Dermatol Clin* 1997; 3:397–407.

97. Williams RM, Christian MM, Moy RL. Hair removal using the long-pulsed ruby laser. *Dermatol Clin* 1999; 17:367–372.

98. Ash K, Lord J Newman, McDaniel DH. Hair removal using a long-pulsed alexandrite laser. *Dermatol Clin* 1999; 17:387–399.

99. Rogers CJ, Glaser DA, Siegfried EC, et al. Hair removal using topical suspension assisted Q-switched Nd:YAG and long-pulsed alexandrite lasers: A comparative study. *Dermatol Surg* 1999; 25:844.

100. Ort RJ, Anderson RR. Optical hair removal. *Semin Cutan Med Surg* 1999; 18:149–158.

101. Dierickx C, Alora MB, Dover JS. A clinical overview of hair removal using lasers and light sources. *Dermatol Clin* 1999; 17:357–366.

102. Campos VB, Diedrickx CC, Farinelli WA, et al. Hair removal with an 800-nm pulsed diode laser. *J Am Acad Dermatol* 2000; 43:442–447.

103. Tabor E, Bostwick DC, Evans CC. Corneal damage due to eye contact with chlorhexidine gluconate (letter). *JAMA* 1989; 261:557.

104. Goldbaum AM, Woog JJ. The CO_2 laser in oculoplastic surgery. *Surv Ophthalmol* 1997; 42:255–267.

105. Nezhat C, Winer WK, Nezhat F, et al. Smoke from laser surgery: Is there a health hazard? *Lasers Surg Med* 1987; 7:376.

106. Smith JP, Moss CE, Bryant CJ, et al. Evaluation of a smoke evacuator used for laser surgery. *Lasers Surg Med* 1989; 9:276.

107. Ratner D, Yardy T, Marchell N, et al. Cutaneous laser resurfacing. *J Am Acad Dermatol* 1999; 41:365–389.

108. Katz BE, MacFarlane DF. Atypical facial scarring after isotretinoin therapy in a patient with a previous dermabrasion. *J Am Acad Dermatol* 1994; 30:852–853.

109. Fulton JE. Complications of Laser resurfacing. *Dermatol Surg* 1997; 24:91–99.

110. Smith JB, Fenske NA. Cutaneous manifestations and consequences of smoking. *J Am Acad Dermatol* 1996; 34:717–732.

111. Massey R, Jones D, Diamond J, et al. The importance of patient selection in CO_2 laser resurfacing. *Cosmet Derm* 1997; 10:9–14.

112. Horton S, Alster TS. Preoperative and postoperative considerations for carbon dioxide laser resurfacing. *Cutis* 1999; 64:399–406.

113. Matarasso SL, Hanke CW, Alster TS. Cutaneous resurfacing. *Dermatol Clin* 1997; 15:569–582.

114. Hevia O, Nemeth AJ, Taylor JR. Tretinoin accelerates healing after trichloroacetic acid chemical peel. *Arch Dermatol* 1991; 127:678–682.

115. Mandy SH. Tretinoin in the preoperative and postoperative management of dermabrasion. *J Am Acad Dermatol* 1986; 15:878–879.

116. Van Scott EJ, Yu RJ. Hyperkeratinization, corneocyte cohesion, and alpha hydroxy acids. *J Am Acad Dermatol* 1984; 5:867–879.

117. Duke D, Grevelink JM. Care before and after laser skin resurfacing. *Dermatol Surg* 1998; 24:201–206.

118. Swinyard EA, Pathak MA. Surface acting drugs demelanizing agents: Hydroquinones. In: Gilman AG, Goodman LS, Rall TW, et al, eds. *The Pharmacological Basis of Therapeutics,* 7th ed. New York: Macmillan; 1985:954.

119. West TB, Alster TS. Effect of pretreatment on the incidence of hyperpigmentation following cutaneous CO_2 laser resurfacing. *Dermatol Surg* 1999; 25:15–17.

120. Nanni CA, Alster TS. Complications of carbon dioxide laser resurfacing: An evaluation of 500 patients. *Dermatol Surg* 1998; 24:315.

121. Boss WK, Brand DA, Acampora D, et al. Effectiveness of prophylactic antibiotics in the outpatient treatment of burns. *J Trauma* 1985; 25:224–227.

122. Krizek TJ, Gottlieb LJ, Koss N, et al. The use of prophylactic antibacterials in plastic surgery: A 1980's update. *Plast Reconstr Surg* 1985; 76:953–963.

123. Bernstein L, Kauvar A, Grossman, et al. The short and long-term side-effects of carbon dioxide laser resurfacing. *Dermatol Surg* 1997; 23:519–525.

124. Sriprachya-Anunt S, Fitzpatrick R, Goldman M, et al. Infections complicating pulsed carbon dioxide laser resurfacing for photoaged facial skin. *Dermatol Surg* 1997; 23:527–536.

125. Langdon RC. Anesthesia techniques for facial laser resurfacing. *Cosmet Dermatol* 1998; 11:26–28.

126. Trytko RLK, Werschler P. Total intravenous anesthesia for office-based laser facial resurfacing. *Lasers Med Surg* 1997; 20(suppl 9):34.

127. Alster TS, Nanni CA, Williams CM. Comparison of four carbon dioxide resurfacing lasers. A clinical and histopathological evaluation. *Dermatol Surg* 1999; 25:153–159.

128. Fitzpatrick RE. Laser resurfacing of rhytids. *Dermatol Clin* 1997; 15:431–447.

129. West TB. Laser resurfacing of atrophic scars. *Dermatol Clin* 1997; 15:449–457.

130. Demling RH. Burns. *N Engl J Med* 1985; 313:1389–1398.

131. Fisher AA. Lasers and allergic contact dermatitis to topical antibiotics, with particular reference to bacitracin. *Cutis* 1996; 58:252–254.

132. Eaglestein WH, Mertz PM. "Inert" vehicles do affect wounding. *J Invest Dermatol* 1980; 74:90–91.

133. Weinstein C, Ramirez O, Pozner J. Postoperative care following carbon dioxide laser resurfacing: Avoiding pitfalls. *Dermatol Surg* 1998; 24:51–56.

134. Trelles MA, Mordon S, Svaasand LO. The origin and role of erythema after carbon dioxide laser resurfacing: A clinical and histological study. *Dermatol Surg* 1998; 24:25–29.

135. Ruiz-Espaza J, Gomez JMB, DeLaTorre OLG, et al. Erythema after laser skin resurfacing. *Dermatol Surg* 1998; 24:31–34.

136. Nanni CA, Alster TS. Complications of cutaneous laser surgery: A review. *Dermatol Surg* 1998; 24:209–219.

137. Laws RA, Finley EM, McCollough ML, et al. Alabaster skin after carbon dioxide laser resurfacing with histologic correlation. *Dermatol Surg* 1998; 24:633–636.

138. Roberts TL, Weinstein C, Alexandides JK, et al. Aesthetic CO_2 laser surgery: Evaluation of 907 patients. *Aesthet Surg J* 1997; 17:293–303.

139. Goldberg DJ. Nonablative resurfacing. *Clin Plast Surg* 2000; 27:287–292.

140. Goldberg DJ. Full-face nonablative dermal remodeling with a 1320 nm Nd:YAG laser. *Dermatol Surg* 2000; 26:915–918.

141. Morelli JG. Use of lasers in pediatric dermatology. *Dermatol Clin* 1998; 16:489–495.

142. Ashinoff R, Geronemus RG.: Flashlamp-pumped pulsed dye laser for port-wine stains in infancy: Earlier versus later treatment. *J Am Acad Dermatol* 1991; 24:467.

143. Goldman MP, Fitzpatrick RE. Treatment of port-wine stains (capillary malformations) with flashlamp-pumped pulsed dye laser. *J Pediatr* 1993; 122:71–72.

144. Fitzpatrick RE, Lowe NJ, Goldman MP, et al. Flashlamp-pumped pulsed dye laser treatment of port-wine stains. *J Dermatol Surg Oncol* 1994; 20:743.

145. Morelli JG, Weston WL, Huff JC, et al. Initial lesion size as a predictive factor in determining the response of port-wine stains in children treated with the pulsed dye laser. *Arch Pediatr Adolesc Med* 1995; 149:1142.

146. Achauer BM, Vander Kam VM, Miller Scott R. Clinical experience with the pulsed dye laser in the treatment of capillary malformations (port-wine stains): A preliminary report. *Ann Plast Surg* 1990; 25:344–351.

147. Fitzpatrick R, Lowe N. Flashlamp-pumped pulsed dye laser treatment of port-wine stains. *J Dermatol Surg Oncol* 1994; 20:743–748.

148. Holy A, Geronemus RG. Treatment of periorbital port-wine stains with the flashlamp-pumped pulsed dye laser. *Arch Ophthalmol* 1992; 110:793–797.

149. Fiskerstrand EJ, Daluker M, Norvang T. Laser treatment of port-wine stains: A study comparing therapeutic outcome with morphologic characteristics of the lesion. *Acta Derm Venereol (Stockh)* 1995; 75:92–93.

150. Fiskerstrand EJ, Svaasand L, Kopstad Gg, et al. Laser treatment of port-wine stains: Therapeutic outcome in relation to morphological parameters. *Br J Dermatol* 1996; 134:1039–1043.

151. Orten SS, Waner M, Flock S, et al. Port-wine stains: An assessment of 5 years of treatment. *Arch Otolaryngol Head Neck Surg* 1996; 122:1174.

152. Renfro L, Geronemus RG. Anatomical differences of port-wine stains in response to treatment with the pulsed dye laser. *Arch Dermatol* 1993; 129:182.

153. Ross BS, Levine VJ, Ashinoff R. Laser treatment of acquired vascular lesions. *Dermatol Clin* 1997; 15:385–396.

154. Alster TS. Laser treatment of vascular lesions. In: Alster TS, ed. *Manual of Cutaneous Laser Techniques.* Philadelphia: Lippincott-Raven; 1997:44–77.

155. Sheehan-Dare RA, Cotterill JA. Lasers in dermatology: Review. *Br J Dermatol* 1993; 129:1–8.

156. Levine VJ, Geronemus RG. Adverse effects associated with the 577 and 585 nanometer pulsed dye laser in the treatment of cutaneous vascular lesions: A study of 500 patients. *J Am Acad Dermatol* 1995; 32:613–617.

157. Apfelberg DB, Flores JT, Maser MR, et al. Analysis of complications of argon laser treatment for port-wine hemangiomas with reference to striped technique. *Lasers Surg Med* 1983; 2:357–371.

158. Raulin C, Schoenermark MP, Greve B, et al. Q-switched ruby laser treatment of tattoos and benign pigmented lesions. *Ann Plast Surg* 1998; 41:555–565.

159. Goldberg DJ. Laser treatment of pigmented lesions. *Dermatol Clin* 1997; 15:397–407.

160. Grossman MC. What is new in cutaneous laser research. *Dermatol Clin* 1997; 15:1–8.

161. Nelson JS, Applebaum J. Treatment of superficial cutaneous pigmented lesions by melanin-specific selective photothermolysis using the Q-switched ruby laser. *Ann Plast Surg* 1992; 29:231–237.

162. Shimbashi T, Kamide R, Hashimoto T. Long-term follow-up in treatment of solar lentigo and café-au-lait macules with Q-switched ruby laser. *Aesthet Plast Surg* 1997; 21:445–448.

163. Taylor C, Anderson RR. Treatment of benign pigmented epidermal lesions by Q-switched ruby laser. *Int J Dermatol* 1993; 32:908–912.

164. Kopera D, Hohenleutner U, Landthaler M. Quality-switched ruby laser treatment of solar lentigines and Becker's nevus. *Dermatology* 1997; 194:338–343.

165. Alster TS. Cosmetic laser surgery. *Adv Dermatol* 1996; 11:51–80.

166. Taylor C, Anderson R, Gange R, et al. Light and electron microscopic analysis of tattoos treated by Q-switched ruby laser. *J Invest Dermatol* 1991; 97:131–136.

167. Zelickson BD, Mehregan DA, Zarrin AA, et al. Clinical, histologic, and ultrastructural evaluation of tattoos treated with three laser systems. *Lasers Surg Med* 1994; 15:364–372.

168. Alster TS. Q-switched alexandrite laser treatment (755 nm) of professional and amateur tattoos. *J Am Acad Dermatol* 1995; 33:69.

169. Lowe NJ, Luftman D, Sawcer D. Q-switched ruby laser. Further observations on treatment of professional tattoos. *J Dermatol Surg Oncol* 1994; 20:307–311.

170. Achauer BM, Nelson JS, Vander Kam VM, et al. Treatment of traumatic tattoos by Q-switched ruby laser. *Plast Reconstr Surg* 1994; 93:318.

171. Ashinoff R, Geronemus RG. Rapid response of traumatic and medical tattoos to treatment with the Q-switched ruby laser. *Plast Reconstr Surg* 1993; 91:841.

172. Anderson RR, Geronemus R, Kilmer SL, et al. Cosmetic tattoo ink darkening. A complication of Q-switched and pulsed laser treatment. *Arch Dermatol* 1993; 129:1010–1014.

173. Kilmer SL. Laser treatment of tattoos. *Dermatol Clin* 1997; 15:409–417.

174. Ashinoff R, Levine VJ, Soter NA. Allergic reactions to tattoo pigment after laser treatment. *Dermatol Surg* 1995; 21:291–294.

175. Kilmer SL, Anderson RR. Clinical use of the Q-switched ruby and the Q-switched Nd:YAG (1064 nm and 532 nm) lasers for treatment of tattoos. *J Dermatol Surg Oncol* 1993; 19:330–338.

176. Levins PC. Q-switched ruby laser treatment of tattoos. *Br J Plast Surg* 1991; 11(suppl 3):255.

177. Berman B, Bieley HC. Adjunct therapies to surgical management of keloids. *Dermatol Surg* 1996; 22:126–130.

178. Lawrence WT. In search of the optimal treatment of keloids: Report of a series and a review of the literature. *Ann Plast Surg* 1991; 27:164–178.

179. Norris JCE. The effect of carbon dioxide laser surgery on the recurrence of keloids. *Plast Reconstr Surg* 1991; 87:44–53.

180. Sherman R, Rosenfeld H. Experience with the Nd:YAG laser in the treatment of keloid scars. *Ann Plast Surg* 1988; 24:231–233.

181. Henning JPH, Roskam Y, van Gamert MJC. Treatment of keloids and hypertrophic scars with an argon laser. *Lasers Surg Med* 1986; 6:72–75.

182. Alster TS, Williams CM. Treatment of keloid sternotomy scars with 585 nm flashlamp-pumped pulsed dye laser. *Lancet* 1995; 345:1198.

183. Alster TS. Improvement of erythematous and hypertrophic scars by the 585 nm pulsed dye laser. *Ann Plast Surg* 1994; 32:186.

184. Diedrickx C, Goldman MP, Fitzpatrick RE. Laser treatment of erythematous/hypertrophic and pigmented scars in 26 patients. *Plast Reconstr Surg* 1995; 95:84.

185. Alster TS, McMeekin TO. Improvement of facial acne scars by the 585 nm flashlamp-pumped pulsed dye laser. *J Am Acad Dermatol* 1996; 35:79.

186. McDaniel DH, Ash K, Zukowski M. Treatment of stretch marks with the 585-nm flashlamp-pumped pulsed dye laser. *Dermatol Surg* 1996; 22:332–337.

187. Nanni CA, Alster TS. Optimizing treatment parameters for hair removal using a topical carbon-based solution and 1064 nm Q-switched neodymium:YAG laser energy. *Arch Dermatol* 1997; 133:1546–1549.

188. Nanni CA, Alster TS. A practical review of laser-assisted hair removal using the Q-switched Nd:YAG, long-pulsed ruby, and long-pulsed alexandrite lasers. *Dermatol Surg* 1998; 24:1399–1405.

189. Nanni CA, Alster TS. Laser-assisted hair removal: Side effects of Q-switched Nd:YAG, long-pulsed ruby, and alexandrite lasers. *J Am Acad Dermatol* 1999; 41:165–171.

Patient Information

Laser Peel

Great strides in the understanding of the interactions between laser light and skin tissue have resulted in the development of new-generation laser systems that are improving the treatment of wrinkles, age lines, and acne scars. A new ultrapulsed mode of the carbon dioxide (CO_2) laser offers improved precision and control to perform cosmetic skin resurfacing, sometimes referred to as laser peeling. In contrast to the CO_2 laser systems of the 1960s, this latest generation emits very short bursts of extremely high-energy laser light. This results in char-free and highly targeted vaporization of tissue with a reduced risk of scarring or damage to adjacent tissue areas. Moreover, virtually no blood loss is associated with laser therapy.

Resurfacing with the Ultrapulse CO_2 laser system has proved successful in minimizing wrinkles, improving facial discoloration, smoothing scars, and rejuvenating sun-damaged and aging skin without surgery.

The laser light smooths the high ridges of wrinkles at the surface and peels off the top layer of skin at precisely the correct depth, giving the underlying tissue a fresher, healthier look. Following treatment, which usually lasts about an hour, the patient returns home with a pink, sunburned look, which normally heals in 7 to 10 days. As a promising complement to the chemical peel and dermabrasion, the Ultrapulse CO_2 laser heralds a new era in skin rejuvenation.

Erbium/CO_2 Laser Preoperative Instructions

Please do not wear makeup to the office; if it is worn, please plan to remove it upon arrival.

Wash your face thoroughly on the morning of your surgery.

Wash your hair the night prior to surgery.

Get a good night's sleep.

Take all medications as prescribed prior to treatment. These normally include an antibiotic, an antiviral (if the lip is being treated), and a Valium.

Wear loose clothes that either zip or button and do not have to be pulled over your head.

Obtain Aquaphor ointment from your local pharmacy prior to surgery (this is a nonprescription item) for postoperative use. If the area around the mouth or lips will be treated, it may be useful for you to obtain the following items before surgery: a baby toothbrush, "Ensure" shakes—nutritional drinks in cans, and straws.

Do not wear any jewelry to the office on the day of surgery.

Contact lenses must be removed before surgery. If you wish to remove them in the office, please bring your case.

Bring someone with you. Your face will be bandaged following the procedure and under no circumstances should you plan to drive yourself home.

Be sure to discuss with the doctor any history of fever blisters, facial herpes infection, or allergies to medication, and review all medicines currently being used.

The fee is to be paid in full at the preoperative visit, which must be at least 7 to 14 days prior to surgery.

CO_2 Laser Setup Tray

Patient

1. Cape
2. Nonsterile surgery hat
3. Goggles (provided by laser co.)
4. White drape sheet

Doctor

1. Clean gloves
2. Mask (laser co. brings)
3. Eye wear (laser co. brings)

Materials

1. Alcohol
2. Two 18″ sterile drapes (1 on headrest, 1 on mayo stand)
3. Sterile 3×3 gauze pads
4. Kling rolls
5. Sterile blue bowl
6. Kenalog 40 mg/mL
7. Tongue blade
8. Q-Tip
9. Tetracaine (if doing periorbital)
10. Polysporin ophthalmic ointment (if doing periorbital)
11. Eye shields
12. Telfa pads for face mask dressing
13. Aquaphor ointment

Laser Peel Postoperative Instructions

Go home and relax. The sedative used for the laser peel may last several hours postoperatively.

Do not be alarmed if swelling appears around your eyes and mouth. It can be severe. This will gradually decrease by itself. Sit up as much as possible and sleep in a head-elevated position for 3 to 5 days either on three pillows or in a reclining chair. This will help reduce the natural swelling that occurs after this type of operation.

The treated areas often produce drainage, occasionally enough to saturate the dressing. Under no circumstances should this dressing be removed. It can be reinforced with additional gauze bandages, or a Turkish towel may be used to protect your clothing or bedding.

Pain medication may be taken every 3 to 4 hours as needed, but no aspirin. The burning sensation may last for several hours. This will gradually ease and subside in a few days.

Continue all other medications as prescribed.

Days 1–14

Pronounced swelling is common. This is normal. It will gradually subside over the first 3 to 10 days. The dressing should not be removed for 24 hours. Upon removing the dressing, apply Aquaphor ointment liberally and keep the skin moist throughout the day by reapplying Aquaphor as necessary. The skin should not be allowed to dry out. At bedtime, reapply Aquaphor. Because of the ointment, you may want to use older pillowcases for the first 2 to 3 weeks. Reapply Aquaphor daily for 14 days.

You may shower daily but avoid the laser peel areas for 3 days. After 3 days, the face may be rinsed lightly with water. Use no soap or any other cosmetic product on treated areas for 2 weeks.

You may shampoo your hair after the third postoperative day.

Any excessive bleeding, redness, tenderness, swelling, or pus should be reported immediately to our office at (___) _____.

No physical exertion for 2 weeks, to avoid perspiration. For men, no shaving for 7-10 days.

No exposure to strong wind or extreme cold for 2 weeks.

Your first postoperative visit will be 7 to 14 days following your procedure.

Day 14 to 6 Weeks

Your new skin will appear red. This is normal and should be expected. You may also experience itching, from mild to very intense. This too is normal and medications are available to help.

Makeup should not be applied until after you have been evaluated by the doctor. Discontinue if stinging occurs.

Your daily regimen will consist of rinsing gently with tap water morning and evening. You should begin wearing a chemical-free sunscreen daily. Discontinue if stinging occurs.

Between 14 and 21 days postoperatively, you may begin using Cetaphil or Moisturel moisturizer every morning and Aquaphor at bedtime. Plan to continue this regimen as instructed.

Avoid Retin-A and glycolic acid products for 6 weeks following the procedure.

You should be seen in the office at about 6 weeks postoperatively for a second checkup.

After 6 Weeks

Direct sun exposure *must* be avoided completely for at least 3 months postoperatively because of the increased photosensitivity and pigmentation of the treated area. It is a good idea to always use a sunscreen with an SPF of 15 or higher. This will help prolong the improvement gained by the laser peel. Avoid sun exposure especially between the hours of 10 a.m. and 5 p.m.

Occasionally, follow-up laser peel treatments are necessary to achieve the desired results.

Hair Removal Treatment

Do not come in with a tan. You are encouraged not to tan proposed treatment areas several weeks prior to the procedure, between treatment sessions, and after procedures. Also avoid self-tanning lotions. A broad-spectrum (UVA/UVB) sunscreen of SPF 30 or greater should be applied to the area being treated whenever it is exposed to the sun and throughout your course of treatment.

If you have a history of cold sores in an area to be treated, please let the doctor know.

Epilation, electrolysis, waxing (hot or cold), or bleaching of treatment areas should be avoided 4 to 6 weeks prior to treatment, but you are allowed to shave.

The day before treatment, gently shave areas to be treated and try to avoid skin irritation.

If a topical anesthetic was prescribed, it should be applied **1 hour** prior to treatment.

On the appointment date, the proposed treatment areas are cleaned and makeup is removed.

Baseline photographs may be taken before and after. These photographs will be used for medical purposes only. If this is your first visit, pretreatment photographs will be taken prior to shaving.

A cooling gel will be applied to the treatment area by our staff just prior to laser treatment.

Protective eyewear will be provided to you and every person in the treatment room to be worn at the time of treatment.

After laser treatment, the cooling gel is removed and ice packs may be applied as needed for discomfort. Polysporin ointment is then applied twice a day for several days.

The Skin Group ChemFree SPF 15 or higher should be applied after treatment on a daily basis and every 2 hours if you are outdoors for prolonged periods.

Several treatments may be required, depending on the growth rate and dormancy of hair follicles. These treatments result in a prolonged hair-free interval and/or the reduction of coarseness and/or a lightening of hair color.

Hair Removal Laser Preoperative Instructions

Don't come in with a tan. Pretanning will decrease the effectiveness of your treatment. You must not tan the proposed treatment areas for 6 weeks prior to the procedure, between treatment sessions, and after procedures. Also avoid self-tanning lotions. A broad-spectrum (UVA/UVB) sunscreen of SPF 30 or greater should be applied to the area(s) being treated for 6 weeks prior to and throughout your course of treatment.

If you have a history of cold sores in an area to be treated, please let the doctor know.

Epilation, electrolysis, waxing (hot or cold), or bleaching of treatment areas should be avoided 4 to 6 weeks prior to treatment. You are allowed to shave.

The day before your visit, gently shave all areas to be treated and try to avoid skin irritation. If you do not shave these areas, a separate "skin prep" fee will be charged at the time of your visit.

If a topical anesthetic was prescribed, it should be applied **1 hour** prior to treatment.

On the appointment date the proposed treatment areas are cleaned and makeup is removed.

Baseline photographs may be taken before and after. These photographs will be used for medical purposes only. If this is your first visit, pretreatment photographs will be taken prior to shaving.

A cooling gel will be applied to treatment area by the staff just prior to laser treatment.

Protective eyewear will be provided for you and every person in the treatment room at the time of treatment.

After laser treatment, the cooling gel is removed and ice packs may be applied as needed for discomfort. Polysporin ointment is then applied twice a day for several days.

The Skin Group ChemFree SPF 15 or higher should be applied after treatment on a daily basis and every 2 hours if you are outdoors for prolonged periods.

Several treatments may be required, depending on the growth rate and dormancy of hair follicles. These treatments result in a prolonged hair-free interval and/or the reduction of coarseness and/or a lightening of hair color.

Hair Removal Laser Setup Tray

Patient

1. Shave area 1 to 2 days prior
2. Laser glasses
3. Photo pants, cape, or drape

Nurse/Doctor

1. Laser glasses
2. Clean gloves

Materials

1. Slushy clear aloe vera gel
2. Emesis basin
3. Tongue blade
4. Large towel
5. Ice bags (optional)
6. Polysporin (optional)

Hair Removal Laser Posttreatment Skin Care Instructions

The area being treated cannot be exposed to the sun. You should apply a broad-spectrum (UVA/UVB) sunscreen (SPF 15 to 30) whenever the area is exposed to the sun.

Immediately following treatment, the area(s) will show a slight erythema with some swelling. Blistering may occur.

During the healing phase, the area must be treated delicately. Do not rub, scratch, or pick. If a crust develops, let it fall off on its own.

Apply a thin layer of antibiotic ointment to the treated area several times a day to keep it moist until all blistering and/or crusting has healed.

Do not scrub the area. Wash it gently with water only. Do not use hydrogen peroxide, etc., to cleanse the area. Use soap only after the area is healed. Pat the area dry. Do not shave over the area if swelling, crusting, or scabbing is present.

If swelling occurs, apply ice. Wrap the ice in a soft cloth. Discomfort or stinging may be relieved with Tylenol.

If makeup is used, apply and remove it delicately, avoiding crusted or blistered areas. Excess rubbing can open treated areas and increase the chance of scarring.

Avoid sports and/or strenuous exercise for 2 to 3 days following treatment.

In case of signs of infection (pus, tenderness, fever), contact the office immediately at (___) _____.

The treated hairs will exfoliate or push out in approximately 2 weeks. This is normal.

The above instructions for care of the skin after laser treatment must be followed carefully in order to prevent any complications. Please, contact the office with questions or concerns regarding your treatment.

Pulsed-Dye Laser

Many of us have some type of dark skin pigmentation or small veins that we feel detracts from our appearance. Freckles, age spots, birthmarks, and spider veins are a few of the more common types of naturally occurring pigmented lesions or blemishes. Laser treatment for these spots provides a safe and simple solution.

Tattoos also can be removed. The art of tattooing dates back to 1300 B.C., and through the years people have long sought effective ways to remove tattoos. While tattoos can be removed by excision, dermabrasion, or salabrasion, these conventional methods may leave scars or abnormal pigmentation.

Modern laser surgery can now be performed to effectively remove dark skin pigmentation, vascular blemishes such as birthmarks, and spider veins as well as tattoos. During this remarkable procedure, your doctor uses a specific laser to produce wavelengths of light that easily pass through the skin and are then rapidly absorbed by the dark pigment, vein, blemish, or tattoo, causing them to disintegrate. Laser surgery is much more effective than other methods because it leaves little or no scarring.

For more than a decade, the doctors at this center have helped people develop and maintain a healthy and attractive appearance. Our skilled cosmetic surgeons specialize in laser surgery and use their knowledge and experience to help patients achieve desirable results.

The Procedure

Our doctors perform laser surgery in our offices on an out-patient basis. There is often no need for an anesthetic because little discomfort is associated with the procedure; the laser pulses feel similar to the snap of a thin rubber band against the skin.

The laser emits short flashes of light in high-intensity pulses. These selective wavelengths of light pass through the skin but are absorbed by the dark pigmentation, veins, or tattoos, causing them to disintegrate. The body's natural filtering system then removes the pigment.

The size and darkness of the affected area determine how many treatments are needed. On average, dark pigmentation, like freckles, can usually be removed in one to three office visits. The number of treatments for veins depends on their size and location. For a short period after treatment, the treated veins will appear purplish. This clears in 7 to 10 days and the veins disappear. For best results, amateur tattoos usually require four to seven treatments and professional tattoos require seven to nine treatments. Blue, black, red, orange, and purple tattoo inks respond most favorably to laser surgery. Green and yellow inks are the most difficult to remove and may require additional treatments to produce optimal results.

Laser treatments are usually spaced 4 to 8 weeks apart to allow time for fading. Between visits, treated areas will gradually lighten.

After laser surgery, an antibacterial ointment and dressing are applied to the treated area. A small amount of pinpoint bleeding may occur. Bathing or showering is allowed the day following the procedure. However, scrubbing of the treated areas should be avoided. The areas that received the laser surgery may become slightly red, but the redness will subside and the skin will return to its normal coloring and texture within a few weeks.

Most dark pigmentation, like freckles and age spots, are caused by exposure to the sun. It is therefore important to use a sunscreen after laser surgery to prevent new pigmented lesions from forming.

The Results

Our patients are delighted with the results of laser surgery to remove freckles, age spots, birthmarks, spider veins, and tattoos. In most cases, a substantial improvement can easily be accomplished.

Pulsed-Dye Laser Setup Tray

Patient
1. Photo pants, booties, cape, or drape
2. Eye shields or laser glasses

Doctor and Staff
1. Mask
2. Laser glasses
3. Clean gloves

Materials
1. Handle with sterile No. 15 blade
2. Polysporin
3. Band-Aids, Telfa, tape (either or all)
4. Q-Tips
   Slushy clear aloe vera gel (optional)

Pulsed-Dye Laser Postoperative Instructions

You have been treated with the pulsed-dye laser. The treated area is now bruised, and a crust may form; it can look dark. This is normal and may last 2 to 3 weeks. The area is very delicate and should be treated with care. Please read and follow the instructions below.

PRECAUTIONS TO TAKE
FOLLOWING YOUR LASER TREATMENT

Avoid direct exposure to the sun and tanning booths for 6 to 8 weeks. Sunscreen (15 to 30 SPF) may be applied after healing occurs.

Do not rub, scratch, or pick at the treated area. A protective dressing should be applied if the area is irritated by clothing or jewelry.

Do not apply makeup until the crusting has completely healed.

Avoid swimming and contact sports while bruising is present.

If the treated area shows signs of infection (tenderness, redness, swelling, or pus), please call the office immediately.

CARE OF THE TREATED AREA

Apply antibiotic ointment to the treated area once or twice a day for 5 days or until the surface is totally healed.

The area can be covered during the day if desired but should be left uncovered at night.

Brief showers are permitted, but pat the area dry gently. Do not scrub the area. Do not rub with a towel or washcloth because the area is extremely delicate while any crusting is present. Reapply the antibiotic after area is gently dried.

Any discomfort you may have after the procedure can usually be relieved with Tylenol.

If swelling occurs, an ice pack wrapped in a soft cloth can be applied. If there has been treatment of facial lesions, sleep with your head elevated on a few pillows.

You may return to normal activities within 24 hours and resume vigorous activity in 5 to 7 days.

The treated area is extremely delicate and must be treated with care while any dark discoloration or crusts are present. *It is normal to see dark areas for 2 to 3 weeks following treatment.* Please understand that these will disappear. It takes a few weeks to months for fading of the treated lesion to occur. Further treatment may be necessary to achieve optimal results. If you have any questions or concerns regarding your laser treatment, please contact our office.

YAG Laser Treatment

Q. Who are the best candidates for treatment with the pigmented lesion laser?

A. The YAG pigmented lesion laser can best treat persons having benign pigmented lesions, such as liver or age spots, freckles, café-au-lait (brown) birthmarks, and tattoos. These spots are usually caused by extensive sun exposure or genetic factors. This laser is safe for all ages, from newborns to adults.

Q. How common are benign pigmented lesions in light-skinned persons?

A. 95 percent will develop age spots at some time in their lives. 30 percent between the ages of 20 and 60 have freckles. 10 percent have café-au-lait (or brown) birthmarks.

Q. Why should someone have a pigmented lesion treated?

A. Many people are uncomfortable with the appearance of these abnormal brown lesions, and this may affect their self-confidence. Young children may also suffer psychological problems from teasing by other children regarding their birthmarks. Now that a safe and more effective treatment is available, doctors recommend early treatment for children, before they experience unnecessary embarrassment.

Q. Are benign pigmented lesions cancerous?

A. Benign pigmented lesions are not malignant. The YAG pigmented lesion laser is not designed to treat malignant, cancerous lesions or pre-malignant lesions. In some cases, physicians may require preliminary testing to determine the lesion type.

Q. How does the YAG pigmented lesion laser differ from other lasers?

A. This is the first laser designed to exclusively treat brown and tan spots of the skin. In targeting the brown pigment only, without damaging the surrounding skin, this laser decreases the chance of scarring, unlike other lasers previously used for this problem.

Q. How does the YAG pigmented lesion laser work?

A. The pigmented lesion laser generates a very short flash of high-energy light, which penetrates only the epidermis (top layer of skin) until it reaches the abnormal pigment within the cell. As the undesired lesions are removed, the remaining skin is virtually undisturbed. The chance of scarring and loss of normal skin pigmentation is slight. Pain is mild and healing time is short.

Q. How is the YAG pigmented lesion laser different from other methods of treatment?

A. This laser is more effective than previously available methods such as cryosurgery (liquid nitrogen), acids, retinoin (Retin-A), and other lasers. These other methods have been known to cause scarring, permanent loss of skin color, and skin texture changes, as well as pain and irritation.

Q. What is the treatment procedure?

A. For areas larger than a silver dollar, the physician may test the skin with the laser to determine the most effective power setting. After about 1 month the test spots are evaluated and a treatment setting is selected. For smaller areas, treatment can begin immediately.

Treatment is given without anesthesia. Patients describe this treatment as nearly painless. Some say it feels like a rubber band snapping against the skin.

Temporary changes in the skin may include flakiness, dryness or a white-gray discoloration, a bruise, or a brown crust. But such changes will heal completely within 1 to 2 weeks and are always a temporary stage of the healing process.

Q. Are there precautions that should be taken after treatment?

A. Immediately following treatment, some patients find the application of an ice pack to be soothing. In some instances, the application of a topical antibiotic cream or ointment may be required. Care should be taken, during the first few days following treatment, to avoid scrubbing the area, and abrasive skin cleansers should be avoided. A bandage or patch may help to prevent abrasion of the treated area.

Q. How soon after treatment does fading occur?

A. Fading of the pigmented lesion occurs within 2 to 3 weeks following treatment. Some lesions require more than one treatment to clear completely.

Q. Is it possible to have a lesion treated that was previously treated by another method?

A. Patients with previously treated pigmented lesions can be candidates for the pigmented lesion laser. Pigmented lesions that have not been effectively removed by other treatments may respond well to pigmented lesion laser therapy provided that the prior treatment did not cause excessive scarring or skin damage.

Q. What is the cost of this treatment?

A. The cost of treatment is determined by the number and size of the pigmented lesions. One treatment session costs approximately $150 to $1500. Because this is generally considered a cosmetic procedure, it will, in most cases, not be covered by insurance.

KTP, PDL, and YAG Lasers Preoperative Insructions

Don't come in with a tan. Pretanning will decrease the effectiveness of your treatment. Patients are specifically instructed not to tan the proposed treatment areas for 6 weeks prior to procedure, in between treatment sessions, and after procedures. Also, avoid self-tanning lotions. A broad spectrum (UVA/UVB) sunscreen of SPF 30 or greater should be applied to the area(s) being treated for 6 weeks prior and throughout your course of treatment.

Do not wear make-up over or near any areas to be treated on the day of surgery. Makeup may be worn again 3 to 5 days after surgery or after any crusting/scabbing has resolved.

Do not wear jewelry near areas to be treated on the day of surgery. For example, if spots on the hands will be treated, avoid wearing rings; or if spots on the neck and face will be treated, avoid necklaces and/or earrings.

Get a good night's sleep the night before the surgery.

Eat a light meal (breakfast or lunch) on the day of surgery before your appointment.

Be sure to discuss with the doctor any bleeding tendencies you may have and the medications you are currently taking.

Contact lenses should be removed before surgery if facial areas are to be treated. If you wish to remove them in the office, please bring your case.

Although the treatments are well tolerated by most patients, to minimize any discomfort you may apply a topical over-the-counter anesthetic agent (Ela-max 4%) to the area(s) to be treated for 1 hour prior to your visit. This product may be purchased at your local pharmacy; follow the application instructions packaged with it.

YAG Laser Setup Tray

Patient

1. Photo pants, booties, cape, or drape
2. Eye shields or laser glasses

Doctor and Staff

1. Mask
2. Laser glasses
3. Clean gloves

Materials

1. Handle with sterile No. 15 blade
2. Polysporin

3. Band-Aids, Telfa, tape (either or all)
4. Q-Tips
5. Slushy clear aloe vera gel (optional)

YAG Laser Postoperative Instructions

You have been treated with the YAG laser for the treatment of pigmented lesions. The treated area is now discolored, and a crust may form. This may last 1 to 2 weeks. The area is very delicate and should be treated with care. Please read and follow the instructions below.

PRECAUTIONS TO TAKE FOLLOWING YOUR LASER TREATMENT

Avoid direct exposure to the sun and tanning booths for 6 to 8 weeks. Sunscreen (15 to 30 SPF) may be applied after healing occurs.

Do not rub, scratch, or pick at the treated area. A protective dressing should be applied if the area is irritated by clothing or jewelry.

Do not apply makeup until any crusting has completely healed.

Avoid swimming and contact sports while any crusts are present.

If the treated area shows signs of infection (tenderness, redness, swelling, or pus), please call the office immediately.

CARE OF THE TREATED AREA

Keep dressing in place for 48 hours.

Brief showers are permitted after 48 hours, but pat the area dry gently. Do not rub with a towel or washcloth because the area is extremely delicate while any crusting is present. Reapply antibiotic ointment after area is gently dried.

Keep the site moist with ointment for the first 7 to 14 days. Do not let the area dry out to form thick scabs. This is especially important during the first 48 hours.

Any discomfort you may have after the procedure can usually be relieved with Tylenol.

If swelling occurs, an ice pack wrapped in a soft cloth can be applied.

The skin should heal normally within 10 to 14 days. Contact your doctor should you have any concerns.

You may return to normal activities within 24 hours and resume vigorous activity in 5 to 7 days.

FOR TATTOO TREATMENT

Apply the prescribed urea compound liberally to the treated area twice a day for 7 to 14 days or until the surface is totally healed. Cover with a Telfa or nonstick dressing during the day and leave it open to the air at night. It is not uncommon for initial swelling, weeping, crusting, or flaking to occur.

The tattoo will look foggy and begin its fading process over the next month. Fading is typically 30 to 50 percent with each treatment. The total fading process can take up to

8 weeks. Green inks fade more slowly and can take up to 16 weeks for maximum fading.

The treated area is extremely delicate and must be treated with care while discoloration or crusts are present. *It is normal to see pigment remain initially following treatment.* It takes a few weeks to months for fading of the treated lesion to occur. Further treatment may be necessary to achieve optimal results. If you have any questions or concerns regarding your laser treatment, please contact our office.

KTP Laser Postoperative Instructions

You have been treated with the KTP laser. The treated area may now be slightly scabbed, and a crust may form. This is normal and may last 2 to 3 weeks. The area is very delicate and should be treated with care. Please read and follow the instructions below.

PRECAUTIONS TO TAKE FOLLOWING YOUR LASER TREATMENT

Avoid direct exposure to the sun and tanning booths for 6 to 8 weeks. Sunscreen (15 to 30 SPF) may be applied after healing occurs.

Do not rub, scratch, or pick at the treated area. A protective dressing should be applied if the area is irritated by clothing or jewelry.

Do not apply makeup until crusting has completely healed.

Avoid swimming and contact sports while bruising is present.

If the treated area shows signs of infection (tenderness, redness, swelling or pus), please call the office immediately.

CARE OF THE TREATED AREA

Apply antibiotic ointment to the treated area once or twice a day for 5 days or until the surface is totally healed.

The area can be covered during the day if desired but should be left uncovered at night.

Brief showers are permitted but pat the area dry gently. Do not scrub the area. Do not rub with a towel or washcloth, because the area is extremely delicate while any crusting is present. Reapply antibiotic ointment after area is gently dried.

Any discomfort you may have after the procedure can usually be relieved with Tylenol.

If swelling occurs, an ice pack wrapped in a soft cloth can be applied. If there has been treatment of facial lesions, sleep with your head elevated on a few pillows.

You may return to normal activities within 24 hours, and resume vigorous activity in 5 to 7 days.

The treated area is extremely delicate and must be treated with care while discoloration or crusts are present. *It is normal to see scabbing for 2 to 3 weeks following treatment.* Please understand that this will disappear. It takes a few weeks to months for fading of the treated lesion to occur. Further treatment may be necessary to achieve optimal results. If you have any questions or concerns regarding your laser treatment, please contact our office.

Patient's name_____

Date_____

Laser Resurfacing for Reduction of Rhytids, Wrinkling, or Scarring with the Ultra Pulse CO_2 or Erbium Laser

I hereby authorize _____ and/or the surgical team to perform a surgical procedure commonly known as laser resurfacing on _____.
(Patient's Name) or (Myself)

Laser Peel

a. That the process involves the application of a coherent light beam to the face, which may require the use of a face mask following said application.

b. That during the resurfacing process I shall experience discomfort and swelling and my face will be covered with a crust, which will usually separate within 5 to 10 days.

c. That as the skin heals, it will have a reddish appearance, which may persist several months; at the juncture of the treated and untreated areas, there may be a difference in color, pigmentation, and texture of skin.

d. That scarring can occur, causing permanent disfigurement.

e. That blotching of pigmentation can occur which may be permanent.

f. That infection can occur.

g. That I may not see any improvement.

h. That avoidance of sun exposure is necessary for several weeks or months.

Initial_____

While laser surgery is effective in most cases, no guarantee can be made that a specific patient will benefit from the procedure. Additionally, the nature of laser surgery may require a patient to return for numerous visits in order to achieve the desired results or to determine that laser surgery may not be completely effective at treating the particular condition. I authorize the physician(s) to do any other procedure that in their judgment may be necessary or advisable should unforeseen circumstances arise during the operation.

The following points have been discussed with me:

1. The potential benefits of the proposed procedure

2. The possible alternative medical procedure(s)

3. The probability of success

4. The reasonably anticipated consequences if the procedure is not performed

5. The most likely possible complications/risks involved with the proposed and subsequent healing period; including but not limited to infection, scarring, increased or decreased pigmentation, recurrence of lesion, bleeding and local nerve damage

6. The possibility of ancillary services/fees including but not limited to anesthesia, laboratory and/or surgical facility use

Initial_____

I am aware of the following possible experiences/risks with laser surgery:

Discomfort. Some discomfort may be experienced during laser treatment. I give my permission for the administration of anesthesia when deemed appropriate by the physician.

Wound healing. Laser surgery may result in swelling, weeping, crusting, or flaking of the treated area, which may require 1 to 3 weeks to heal. Once the surface has healed, it may be pink and sensitive to the sun for an additional 3 to 6 months.

Swelling/infection. There may be some swelling, especially when the lips and eyelids have been treated. The swelling may be severe during the first few days but will gradually recede. Finally, skin infection is a possibility whenever a skin procedure is performed. I have been told to take all medications as prescribed to minimize this possible complication.

Pigment change (skin color). During the healing process, there is a possibility of the treatment area becoming either lighter or darker in color than the surrounding skin. This is usually temporary, but may sometimes although rarely be permanent.

Scarring. Scarring is a rare occurrence, but it is a possibility when the skin's surface is disrupted. To minimize the chances of scarring, it is important that you follow all postoperative instructions carefully.

Persistence of lesion. Some growths, birthmarks, and tattoos may respond only partially or not at all to laser surgery. If this situation arises, other treatment alternatives may be available.

Eye exposure. Protective eyewear will be provided. Protective eye shields (contact lens type) will be placed in your eyes by our staff for eye protection. Your vision may be blurry for 24 hours due to the lubricants used for these shields.

Initial_____

ACKNOWLEDGMENT

- Each issue outlined in this consent for laser surgery has been clarified to me.

Initial_____

- I have been satisfactorily informed of the possible experiences, benefits, and risks of the surgery and, if applicable, the administration of anesthesia.

Initial_____

- I have been given the opportunity to ask questions and my questions have been answered to my satisfaction.

Initial_____

- I give permission to _____ to take still or motion clinical photographs with the understanding such photographs remain the property of the center. If in the judgment of the center medical research, education, or science will be benefited by their use, such photographs and related information may be published and republished in professional journals or medical books or used for any other purpose which the center may deem proper. It is specifically understood that in any such publication or use, I shall not be identified by name.

Initial_____

- For the purpose of advancing medical education, I consent to the admittance of authorized observers to the operating room.

Initial_____

My signature indicates that I have read this "Consent for Laser Peel" and I understand and accept the risks involved with this procedure. I hereby authorize _____ and/or the surgical team to perform this surgical procedure on me.

_____ _____
Signature (Patient/Responsible Party) Date

_____ _____
Signature (Witness) Date

_____ _____
Signature (Parent/Guardian) Date

CONSENT FOR HAIR REMOVAL TREATMENT

Patient's name_____
Date_____

1. The purpose of this treatment is to reduce or eliminate unwanted hair. I understand that the results of this treatment vary with each individual.

Initial_____

2. The LPIR/Apogee laser procedure is an intense burst of light that is absorbed by the hair follicle without causing damage to the surrounding tissue. All personnel in the treatment room, including myself, will wear protective eyewear to prevent eye damage from this intense light.

Initial_____

3. I give permission to _____ to take still or motion clinical photographs with the understanding such photographs remain the property of the center. If in the judgment of the center medical research, education, or science will be benefited by their use, such photographs and related information may be published and republished in professional journals or medical books or used for any other purpose which the center may deem proper. It is specifically understood that in any such publication or use, I shall not be identified by name.

Initial_____

4. The sensation of the light is uncomfortable and may feel like a pinprick or burst of heat that lasts a few seconds. The use of anesthesia is at the discretion of the physician; nevertheless, all the options and possible side effects will be discussed with me.

Initial_____

5. Multiple treatments are most often necessary. The hair may not be eliminated entirely even after multiple treatments. Although significant improvement is expected, some types of hair can be difficult to remove. I understand no guarantees have been made as to the success of this treatment.

Initial_____

6. I have been informed that blistering, scarring, hypopigmentation (lightening of the skin), and hyperpigmentation (darkening of the skin) are possible risks and complications of the procedure. I understand that sun exposure and not adhering to postoperative instructions may increase my chance of complications. The area should be treated delicately following treatment.

Initial_____

I have been given the opportunity to ask questions and all my questions have been answered to my satisfaction.

My signature indicates that I have read this "Consent for Hair Removal Laser" and I understand and accept the risks involved with this procedure. I hereby authorize _____ _____ and/or the trained laser staff to perform this procedure on me.

First Treatment: _____ _____ _____
              Signature (Patient/ Signature (Witness)   Date
              Responsible Party)

Second Treatment:_____ _____ _____
              Signature (Patient/ Signature (Witness)   Date
              Responsible Party)

Third Treatment: _____ _____ _____
              Signature (Patient/ Signature (Witness)   Date
              Responsible Party)

Fourth Treatment: _____ _____ _____
              Signature (Patient/ Signature (Witness)   Date
              Responsible Party)

Fifth Treatment: _____ _____ _____
              Signature (Patient/ Signature (Witness)   Date
              Responsible Party)

Sixth Treatment: _____ _____ _____
              Signature (Patient/ Signature (Witness)   Date
              Responsible Party)

CONSENT FOR PULSED-DYE LASER TREATMENT

Patient's name_____
Date_____

The procedure planned is treatment of a lesion (vein, pigmentable spot, scar, wart, etc.) with the pulsed-dye laser using local, topical, or no anesthesia. The purpose of this procedure is to attempt to remove, fade lighten, or improve the presenting lesion.

This form is designed to give you the information you need to make an informed choice as to whether to undergo laser surgery. If you have any questions, please do not hesitate to ask us.

Although laser surgery is effective in most cases, no guarantees can be made that a specific patient will benefit from this type of treatment. Many conditions require a series of treatments to reach the desired level of improvement. These may range from one treatment to as many as six or more, depending on the type of lesion. Some conditions will not completely clear but will become lighter. Some vascular lesions may not respond to this treatment at all.

WHAT IS PULSED-DYE LASER SURGERY?

The pulsed dye laser has been used to treat various skin conditions for over 10 years. It emits an intense beam of light that penetrates the skin to a depth of about 1.5 mm (1/20 in.). This heats the targeted superficial blood vessels almost instantaneously and so precisely that normal surrounding tissue is hardly affected. This laser is used to lighten or remove birthmarks, port-wine stains, facial telangiectasias (prominent blood vessels, often called spider veins), and other vascular growths of the skin, as well as some scars, warts, pigment spots, etc.

WHAT ARE THE SIDE EFFECTS AND POSSIBLE COMPLICATIONS OF LASER SURGERY?

The most common side effects and complications of laser surgery are:

1. **Pain.** Many people feel some pain during treatment. This discomfort may range from moderate to minimal but fortunately is of short duration. A local anesthetic may be used to block pain during the treatment. Most adults and older children can tolerate the discomfort without anesthesia. Younger children may need to undergo intravenous sedation if extensive areas are to be treated.

Initial_____

2. **Healing wound.** Occasionally there is a crust, blister, or superficial wound that requires care. When this occurs, it tends to heal in 5 to 10 days.

Initial_____

3. **Pigmentary changes.** The treated area may heal with increased pigmentation (hyperpigmentation). This occurs most often in darker skin and following exposure of the area to the sun. Some patients have a predisposition to this type of reaction and may have noticed it with minor cuts, abrasions, or acne lesions. It is advised to protect the treated area from exposure to the sun for up to 3 months following treatment in order to minimize the chances of hyperpigmentation. In some patients, hyperpigmentation occurs even though the area has been protected from the sun. Hyperpigmentation spots usually fade away in 3 to 6 months. Prescription bleaching creams usually resolve this problem, should it occur. However, rarely, the pigmentary change can be permanent.

In addition, a few patients may notice a decrease in skin color (hypopigmentation) in the treated area after repeated treatment to the same area. As with hyperpigmentation, hypopigmented spots usually repigment in 3 to 6 months, but the pigmentary change may be permanent.

Initial_____

4. **Bruising.** Laser treatment will cause a blue-purple bruise in the treated area. This bruise will look unsightly and usually lasts 2 to 3 weeks. As the bruising fades, there may be rust-brown discoloration of the skin. This discoloration, which occurs in approximately 30 percent of patients treated with the laser, usually takes 1 to 3 months to fade.

Initial_____

5. **Excessive swelling.** Immediately after laser surgery, there may be swelling of the skin, especially when the cheek or nose has been treated. This is a temporary condition and not harmful in itself, but it may be frightening. It usually subsides in 3 to 7 days and requires frequent applications of ice for treatment.

Initial_____

6. **Fragile skin.** The skin at or near the treatment site may become fragile. The area should not be rubbed, since this may cause tearing of the skin. Makeup should not be applied to or removed from the treated area while the skin is fragile.

Initial_____

7. **Scarring.** There is a very small chance of scarring, including *hypertrophic scars*, which are enlarged scars, and, very rarely, *keloid scars*, which are abnormal, heavy, raised scar formations. Scarring is a very rare occurrence but is a possibility when there is disruption of the skin's surface. Fortunately, this is a rare occurrence, and therefore scarring is very rare. To minimize the chances of scarring, it is important that you follow all postoperative instructions carefully.

Initial_____

8. **Persistence of a lesion.** Some growths or birthmarks may respond only partially or not at all. There can be no guarantee of results obtainable with this therapy.

Initial_____

I understand that the risks of the procedure include possible pain, bleeding, infection, scarring, and damage to nearby structures, drug reactions, and unforeseen complications. In addition, there is risk of accidental eye injury if struck by the laser beam. This is highly unlikely since complete eye protection is provided throughout laser treatment sessions. There is also a possibility that this procedure will be unsuccessful or need to be repeated or may require additional treatment sessions. There may also be change or permanent lightening of skin color, change in skin texture, and easy bruising of the skin after treatment. The risk of scarring (including raised scarring) despite proper treatment exists in all cases, but can be greatly minimized by proper aftercare. Previous treatment by any method may increase any or all of these risks.

I understand that this procedure may fail to remove all of the lesion in some cases, especially with some types of vascular birthmarks. Some vascular discolorations, such as facial spider veins, may be cleared in only a few sessions, while port-wine birthmarks usually require multiple treatments. Loss of skin pigment (usually temporary) is uncommon but may occur. I understand my responsibility for properly following the aftercare instructions as explained by _____ and/or delegated associates or from written or videotaped instructions provided.

Initial_____

WHAT ARE THE POSSIBLE COMPLICATIONS IF I DO NOT HAVE LASER SURGERY PERFORMED?

Most skin conditions amenable to laser treatment are cosmetic in nature and pose no medical threat if they are not treated. Port-wine stains that are not treated may become darker and more nodular with age. Some other blood vessel growths of the skin may tend to enlarge or spread with time if not treated.

Alternative treatment methods include but are not limited to overtattooing in flesh tones, x-ray irradiation, surgery with subsequent skin grafting, cryosurgery, electrocautery, injection of sclerosing agents, chemical peels and other laser modalities, or no treatment.

I give permission to _____ for still or motion clinical photographs to be taken with the understanding such photographs remain the property of the center. If in the judgment of the center medical research, education, or science will be benefited by their use, such photographs and related information may be published and republished in professional journals or medical books or used for any other purpose which the center may deem proper. It is specifically understood that in any such publication or use, I shall not be identified by name.

Although insurance companies may reimburse part or all of the costs for this procedure, some policies/companies may consider the procedure not medically necessary or not covered for various reasons. I understand that I am responsible for all costs of treatment at my preoperative appointment.

I have been given the opportunity to ask questions and all my questions have been answered to my satisfaction. I understand the procedure and accept the risks of not treating my condition, and I hereby consent to have laser surgery performed.

Initial_____

My signature indicates that I have read this "Consent for Pulsed-Dye Laser" treatment and I understand and accept the risks involved with this procedure. I hereby authorize _____ and/or delegated associates to perform this laser procedure on me. The area to be treated is my:

_____.

(area to be treated)

First Treatment: _____ _____ _____
                 Signature (Patient/   Signature (Witness)   Date
                 Responsible Party)

Second Treatment: _____ _____ _____
                  Signature (Patient/   Signature (Witness)   Date
                  Responsible Party)

Third Treatment: _____ _____ _____
                 Signature (Patient/   Signature (Witness)   Date
                 Responsible Party)

Fourth Treatment: _____ _____ _____
Signature (Patient/ Signature (Witness) Date
Responsible Party)

Fifth Treatment: _____ _____ _____
Signature (Patient/ Signature (Witness) Date
Responsible Party)

Sixth Treatment: _____ _____ _____
Signature (Patient/ Signature (Witness) Date
Responsible Party)

CONSENT FOR YAG LASER TREATMENT

Patient's name_____
Date_____

The procedure planned is treatment of brown spots, lesion(s), tattoo, birthmark, etc., with the YAG laser using local topical or no anesthesia. The purpose of this procedure is to attempt to remove, fade, improve, or lighten the presenting skin lesions.

Alternative treatment methods include but are not limited to cryosurgery (freezing), dermabrasion, electrocautery, depigmenting creams, other laser modalities, or no treatment.

This form is designed to provide the information needed to make an informed choice on whether or not to undergo YAG laser surgery. The YAG laser is a type of laser developed to remove certain brown-pigmented growths and birthmarks from the skin and blue, brown, black, and possibly other colors of tattoo pigment. If you have any questions, please do not hesitate to ask.

Although laser surgery is effective in most cases, no guarantees can be made that a specific patient will benefit from the treatment. Treatment of the tattoo or pigmented area will be done in stages. Initially a test does may be done to determine the necessary energy settings of the laser. Once this dose is determined, the entire tattoo or pigmentation will be treated. The tattoo or pigmentation will be reexamined and re-treated if necessary at 6- to 8-week or longer intervals until all the pigment is removed or it is decided that the pigment will not be capable of being removed by this laser. Often a total of 3 to 7 treatments will be necessary, sometimes more.

WHAT ARE THE SIDE EFFECTS AND POSSIBLE COMPLICATIONS OF LASER SURGERY?

The most common side effects and complications of laser surgery are:

1. **Pain.** You will feel some pain during treatment. The pain is mild and it is similar to snapping the skin with a rubber band. Some areas are more sensitive than others. Local or topical anesthesia may be given to minimize discomfort.

   Initial_____

2. **Healing wound.** Laser surgery may cause a superficial burn to the surface of the skin, which may take several days or weeks to heal. This may result in swelling, weeping, crusting, or flaking of the treated area. This area may be unsightly during the healing stages.

   Initial_____

3. **Pigmentary changes.** In most patients the treated area loses pigmentation (hypopigmentation) and becomes a lighter color than the surrounding skin temporarily. This type of reaction tends to gradually fade away and return to normal over a period of 1 to 6 months.

   With repeated treatment, this pigment loss may become more persistent and require longer to heal, as long as 6 to 8 months more. There is some risk of permanent pigment loss in the area of treatment, leaving a white shape similar to the original tattoo or pigment being treated, but this is rare and usually minimized by allowing adequate healing time between treatments.

   There is some risk of increased pigmentation (hyperpigmentation) as a healing reaction. However, this type of change is uncommon with this particular laser. It is important to avoid sun exposure and irritation of the treated area during the healing stages. If hyperpigmentation should occur, the increased pigment usually fades away over a 2- to 6-month period, and may require bleaching creams.

   On occasion, certain pigmented lesions may recur, especially if ongoing significant sun exposure is not avoided (melasma, lentigines, café-au-lait spots).

   Initial_____

4. **Scarring.** There is a very small chance of scarring, including *hypertrophic scars*, which are enlarged scars, and, very rarely, *keloid scars*, which are abnormal, heavy, raised scare formations. Scarring is a very rare occurrence but is a possibility because of the disruption of the skin's surface. To minimize the chances of scarring, *it is important that all postoperative instructions be followed carefully.*

   Initial_____

5. **Eye exposure.** There is also a risk of harmful eye exposure to laser energy. Safeguards have been provided including the use of safety eyewear during laser treatment. It is important that these protective glasses be kept on at all times during treatment to protect the eyes from accidental laser exposure.

   Initial_____

6. **Persistence of tattoo or pigment.** Some tattoo ink or pigment is located too deep in the skin to be removed entirely in spite of repeated treatment and may leave vague spots of color remaining after treatment. There may be some inks that change color prior to removal and others that simply will not respond to this laser. This means that it may not be possible to completely remove all tattoo and skin pigmentations with this laser. However, if this situation arises, there may be other treatment alternatives available.

   Initial_____

I understand that the risks of the procedure include possible pain, bleeding, infection, hyperpigmentation, scarring, and damage to nearby structures, drug reactions, and unforeseen complications. In addition, there is risk of accidental eye injury if struck by the laser beam. This is highly unlikely, since complete eye protection is provided throughout laser treatment sessions. There is also risk of patchy residual pigment, persistence of the skin lesion, change or permanent lightening of skin color, change in skin texture, and easy bruising of the skin after treatment. The risk of complications (including raised scarring) despite proper treatment exists in all cases but can be greatly minimized by proper aftercare. Previous treatment by any method may increase any or all of these risks.

I understand that this procedure may fail to remove all pigment in some cases, especially with some types of brown birthmarks. Pigmented or brown blemishes such as freckles, sunspots, and liver spots may be cleared in only a few sessions, while café-au-lait birthmarks usually require multiple treatments. Loss of skin pigment (usually temporary) is uncommon but may occur. I understand my responsibility for properly fulfilling the aftercare instructions as explained by _____ and/or delegated associates or from written or videotaped instructions provided.

The treatment chosen is the YAG laser. The doctor has explained the theory of this laser and any risks involved, complications, successes, and benefits. Also, alternative treatment methods have been discussed, including no treatment, cryosurgery, excision, dermabrasion, bleaching creams, and treatment with other laser modalities.

The number of treatments with a YAG laser will vary depending on the lesion size, location, color, age of patient, length of time the pigment has been present, and age of the tattoo. The doctor has also explained treatment protocols, laser safety, and any precautions necessary.

I give permission to _____ for still or motion clinical photographs to be taken with the understanding such photographs remain the property of the center. If in the judgment of the center medical research, education, or science will be benefited by their use, such photographs and related information may be published and republished in professional journals or medical books or used for any other purpose which the center may deem proper. It is specifically understood that in any such publication or use, I shall not be identified by name.

This procedure is generally considered not medically necessary and thus may not be covered by insurance. I understand that I am responsible for all costs of the treatment at the preoperative appointment, payable *in full* at that time or earlier.

Initial_____

I have been given the opportunity to ask questions and all my questions have been answered to my satisfaction. I understand the procedure and accept the risks of not treating my condition, and I hereby consent to laser surgery to be performed.

Initial_____

My signature indicates that I have read this "Consent for YAG Laser" treatment and I understand and accept the risks involved with this procedure. I hereby authorize _____ _____ and/or delegated associates to perform and assist in the YAG laser procedure on me. The area to be treated is my: _____.

(area to be treated)

First Treatment: _____ _____ _____
Signature (Patient/ Signature (Witness) Date
Responsible Party)

Second Treatment: _____ _____ _____
Signature (Patient/ Signature (Witness) Date
Responsible Party)

Third Treatment: _____ _____ _____
Signature (Patient/ Signature (Witness) Date
Responsible Party)

Fourth Treatment: _____ _____ _____
Signature (Patient/ Signature (Witness) Date
Responsible Party)

Fifth Treatment: _____ _____ _____
Signature (Patient/ Signature (Witness) Date
Responsible Party)

Sixth Treatment: _____ _____ _____
Signature (Patient/ Signature (Witness) Date
Responsible Party)

CHAPTER 15

Scar Revision

Many modalities are available for the revision of scars. Nonsurgical methods involve less downtime and recovery; however, they also tend to make for a smaller improvement than surgical methods. Very often, a combination of nonsurgical and surgical modalities may be necessary to achieve scar improvement. Each scar must be addressed in terms of depth, location, length, and length of time, and no one approach can be universally applied. An algorithm may help outline the indications of the various modalities. As with every cosmetic intervention, an assessment of the patient's expectations and psychological attitude about the scar and its removal will serve to guide the treatment plan and determine whether any treatment should be attempted (see Chap. 5).

To choose the appropriate scar treatment, a thorough knowledge of scar formation and the techniques available for their removal is helpful. Scars are composed primarily of collagen, synthesized by fibroblasts in response to wounding of reticular dermis. Human fetal wounds show rapid healing—rapid deposition of hyaluronic acid and tenascin.[1] Fetal and adult scar formation is influenced by different rates of proliferation and differentiation of fibroblasts, keratinocytes, endothelial cells, inflammatory cells, and all the various cytokines released at various stages of wound healing. Clinically, the edges of the wound contract maximally between days 5 and 15 after wounding, with movement of the full thickness of the wound edges in a centripetal fashion to accomplish closure of the wound. However, complete healing can range from 6 months to as long as 18 months. One must therefore consider the appropriate time to intervene to best achieve the best result. The final scar can take any of various forms, ranging from a flattened epidermis with subcutaneous atrophy or a raised, hypertrophic scar to a keloidal scar.

Instituting therapy for scar revision appears to be best timed within 6 to 8 weeks after the event. In our experience, intervention before a hypertrophic scar develops into a keloid can result in quite dramatic improvement. Therefore a history of the mechanism of injury resulting in the scar, time elapsed since wounding occurred, and any compli-cations (such as infection, dehiscence, or previous revisions) should be obtained. In addition, the surgical dermatologist should determine the patient's past personal and family history of hypertrophic and keloidal scarring.

Patient Selection

As always, patient selection is the key to a successful outcome. During the initial interview, the patient's level of psychogenic pain, psychologically based problems, and perception of the scar should be assessed. These issues will have a significant impact on the patient's perception of the result. An example is acne scarring, which may cause a patient to carry all the emotional weight of adolescence into adulthood. Such a patient must be thoroughly screened prior to intervention, as his or her hopes must be aligned with realistic expectations. On average, only modest correction of the defect is the rule. It should be clear to the patient that even the best result will not make the scars invisible, and that improvement is the goal, not perfection.

Physical Examination

Initial physical examination of the scar should include location on the body, configuration, measurements, direction or orientation of the scar along body lines, color, texture, elevation or depression, adherence or nonadherence to underlying structures, proximity of the scar to functional landmarks (joints, eyelids, lips, nares), and proximity to other scars.[2] The potential physical disfigurement due to a given scar has a broad range. The minimally significant disfigurement is that cosmetic disturbance which can be seen at a conversational distance of a few feet in either artificial or natural light.[2] Scars that remain within an esthetic skin unit, that are small, oriented along relaxed skin tension lines, flush with the skin surface, and blend in color with the surrounding skin have good features that tend to be minimally noticeable. These are the types of scars most amenable to correction. In

235

contrast, the functionally disruptive, large, long, contracted, raised, hypertrophic, keloidal, depressed atrophic, and discolored scars pose the greatest challenge.

Scar Prevention

All efforts should be made to prevent undue surgical scarring in the first place. Ideal surgical incisions are made parallel to relaxed skin tension lines, where possible, in order to minimize the risk of problems. Tissue ischemia is prevented by placing deep merseline, PDS, or monocryl sutures in the subcutaneous fat, and the muscular and fascial layers to decrease skin tension. The wound edges should be everted with cutaneous sutures to be removed at the earliest time appropriate to the body site. Steri-Strips may be used to support and immobilize the incision.

Tissue Ischemia

Desiccation is prevented by liberal use of petrolatum-based (usually antibiotic) ointment to reepithelialize the incision site optimally. Meticulous intraoperative hemostasis and a light pressure dressing for 24 to 48 h postoperatively may help to prevent hematomas. The rare hematoma is evacuated to prevent disruption of wound closure and infection. If infection during the postoperative course is suspected, the wound is cultured, locally lavaged with sterile saline, and systemically treated with antibiotics.

Table 15-1
Nonsurgical Scar Revision Methods

Pressure
Mechanical (massage)
High-pressure hydrotherapy
Silicone gel sheeting
Topical creams for scar massage
Vitamin E
Corticosteroid creams
Imiquimod
Silicone-containing creams
Intralesional triamcinolone injections
Camouflage makeup
Tattooing for scar camouflage
Chemical peels
Superficial depth (salicylic/glycolic acid for blending scar color)
Medium depth (trichloroacetic acid for scar texture irregularities)
Microdermabrasion to improve scar texture
Botox for smoothing skin in vicinity of scar

Table 15-2
Surgical Scar Revision Methods

Simple excision of scar and closure
Modified excision for depressed scars
Advancement flaps
Transposition flaps
S, Z, running W, geometric broken-line plasty
Expansion of neighboring normal skin
Grafts
Dermabrasion
Subscision
Laser Resurfacing
Carbon dioxide
Erbium:YAG
Pulsed-dye
Cryosurgery
Tissue filler substances
Collagen
Autologous fat transplantation
Gore-Tex

Scars gain strength over the first months of healing, achieving 70 percent maximum tensile strength at 2 months. Scars tend to contract maximally, resulting in decreased thickness of the scar between days 5 and 15. Collagen remodeling continues over the first 2 years. Even when all care of a new wound is optimal, a scar that is noticeable and unacceptable to the patient can occur. Often no identifiable cause may be found. With lack of optimal healing highly possible, accidental and traumatic wounds should ideally be assessed as early as possible so that timely intervention can be instituted. Sometimes an underlying disease state may be adversely affecting wound healing and scar formation (Tables 15-1, 15-2, and 15-3).[3]

Nonsurgical and Surgical Modalities for Scar Revision

ELEVATED SCARS

Scars that are raised reflect light differently than the normal surrounding skin and draw the observer's attention. Raised scars may be among those more commonly encountered by the dermatologic surgeon. All normally healing scars go through an often clinically unapparent, transient phase of elevation in the first month after excision. Hypertrophic, keloid, trap-door, contracted, and webbed scars all represent varieties of elevated scars.

Glucocorticoids are commonly injected intralesionally into elevated and keloidal scars. They can be applied topically as an occlusive tape or an ointment, gel, or cream with or without occlusion to bolster potency. The potency of glucocorticoids is categorized by the relative vasoconstrictive effect of the individual agent. Typically a medium-potency agent like triamcinolone is used for injection into scars at a concentration ranging from 1.5 to 25 mg/mL based on the clinical evaluation of the scar location, characteristic type, and size. The patient must give informed consent to the untoward possibility of hypopigmentation, atrophy, and/or telangiectasis of surrounding normal skin. Risk of these undesirable effects is minimized by careful selection of triamcinolone concentration and care to deliver the injection only within the scar itself.

Many patients ask about the utilization of vitamin E. Unfortunately, vitamin E has been shown to have no beneficial effect on the cosmetic outcome of scars and causes contact dermatitis in 33 percent of patients.[4] Imiquimod has been said to have a therapeutic benefit in several recent reports.[5]

Traditionally, compression and/or occlusive therapy alone, after triamcinolone injection or postsurgical excision of scar has been used to try to soften, flatten, and blanch small raised scars. One example reported to be successful is the Cica-care adhesive gel sheet for keloids and hypertrophic scars.[6] If there is muscular contraction causing skin folds that accentuate the scar, botulinum toxin injections may be effective in smoothing the skin and making the scar appear less prominent (see Chap. 10). In addition, botulinum can immobilize the scar after revision to minimize expressive contour changes. Small, raised postsurgical scars can be derma-

braded to the superficial papillary dermis to blend the profile of the scar with surrounding skin if this is done within several weeks of the initial procedure.

Larger keloid scars usually require surgery plus adjuvant therapies. Intrascar or intramarginal excision to debulk hypertrophic scars where the sutures are placed into a narrow margin of remaining scar has been advocated by many physicians with good results.[7,8] A series of three 500-rad x-ray treatments have been reported to yield a high cure rate when combined with prior surgical excision. Also, cryosurgery of keloids and hypertrophic scars can be attempted alone or in combination with intralesional triamcinolone injections, with reported success.[9]

Raised linear scars can be reexcised and resutured in geometric broken-line fashion to place the cross bars of the closure in favorable directions, with each segment no longer than 6 mm on most areas of the face and 1.5 to 2 mm on the upper lip close to the philtral crest (Fig. 15-1).[10] Facial lesions larger than 20 mm can be closed by rhomboid-to-"W" technique to help hide the scar.[11]

Raised scars that become contracted usually do so because the wound was under tension; often they are oriented perpendicularly to relaxed skin tension lines. Running W-plasty, serial Z-plasty, or S-plasty (Fig. 15-2)[12] and similar advancement flap revisions have been devised to reorient the tension vectors of a scar and to close along favorable relaxed skin tension lines after a widened scar has been removed. The gap created after excision of a widened scar necessitates careful placement of deep sutures to prevent

Table15-3
Disease States Associated with Impaired Wound Healing

Hereditary	Malnutrition
Ehlers-Danlos syndrome	Cushing's syndrome
Prolidase deficiency	Hyperthyroidism
Coagulation disorders	Immunologic deficiency states
Hemophilia	HIV infection
Von Willebrand's disease	Lymphoproliferative
Factor XIII deficiency	disease/cancer
Werner's syndrome	Methotrexate, azathioprine,
Vascular disorders	cyclosporine,
Congestive heart failure	cyclophosphamide
Atherosclerosis	Other
Hypertension	Smoking
Vasculitis	Chronic pulmonary disease
Venous stasis	Chronic liver disease (cirrhosis)
Lymphedema	Malignancy
Metabolic	Myelofibrosis/chronic
Chronic renal failure	thrombocytopenic conditions
Diabetes mellitus	Other chronic illnesses

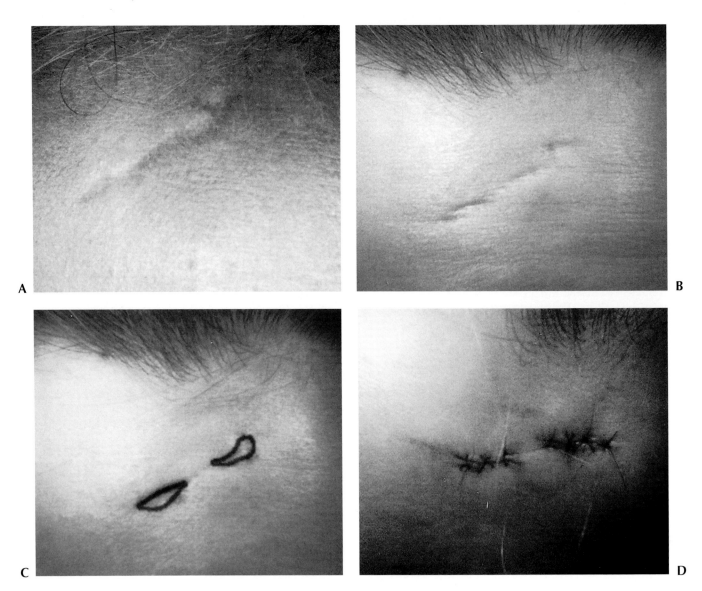

Figure 15-1 (*A*) Slantwise scar on the forehead of a young woman. (*B*) Patient raising her eyebrows and the direction of the scar changes. (*C*) Marking of the scar to change the direction of the scar. (*D*) Sutures in place creating a more linear and broken line scar, making it much less noticeable.

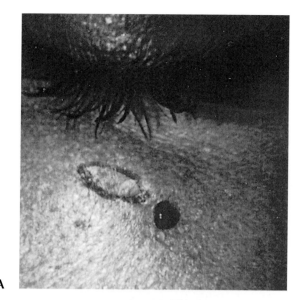

A

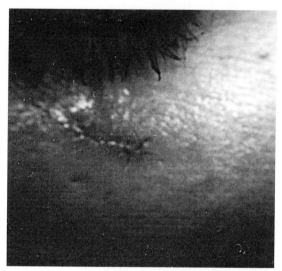

B

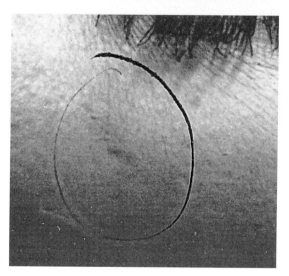

C

Figure 15-2 (**A**) Clustered acne ice-pick scars. (**B**) The excision of these scars and the creation of an S-plasty. (**C**) Postoperative result.

excess tension on the skin margin. Multiple simple interrupted or running interlocked removable sutures are used for final approximation of the epidermis. Hyperreversion of the wound edges has also been used to try to prevent widening after revision. This can only be achieved after well-placed deep sutures hold all the wound tension away from the skin surface.

Keloid treatment may start with injection of intralesional triamcinolone (IL-TAC) 1.5 to 25 mg/mL every month for 3 months. Surgical excision plus postoperative IL-TAC at 3 months followed by early suture removal at 5 to 7 days may further improve keloids (*Fig.* 15-3*A* and B). IL-TAC can be repeated every 4 to 6 weeks one or two times, then every 1 to 3 months for at least 2 years as needed to prevent recurrence of the keloid. Recurrences of aggressively treated keloids have been reported out to 2 years. Recurrence rate of keloids can approach 50 percent even after the aggressive combination regimen of IL-TAC plus surgical excision described above. The patient must undergo regular reevaluation and repeated IL-TAC or radiation therapy to optimize the outcome.[13] Reexcision should be considered only as a last resort, since the keloid can become unpredictably worse as a result of surgical reexcision. It is not uncommon for keloid-prone young adults to "grow out" of the tendency to form keloids in later life, so surgical intervention may be more successful later on.

DEPRESSED SCARS

Varicella zoster classically leaves depressed scars, as does cystic acne. The color match of the scar with the surrounding skin may help direct therapy. For depressed scars of similar color to the surrounding skin, filler substances can be used to raise the depressed area to the plane of the surrounding skin, thus improving cosmesis. Collagen, human cadaveric or recombinant collagen or fascia, or autologous fat transplantation may be moderately effective in bringing the base of the depressed scar closer to the plane of the surrounding skin. For mildly depressed scars, bovine collagen can be injected into the papillary dermis to improve the appearance of the scar. Human collagen or particulate fascia can be used similarly if the patient is at risk of allergic reaction to bovine collagen. For deeply depressed scars, autologous fat transplanted to the subcutaneous fat beneath the depression may be more useful in improving cosmesis.

If the base of the depressed scar is adherent to the structures beneath, subscision with a dissection instrument may be attempted to release the underlying adhesion and simultaneously create a plane into which the autologous fat may be injected to fill the depression.[14,15] A depressed scar may be revised by excising a small wedge of tissue at the lateral borders on either side of the depression and advancing the wound edges over the platform to raise the depression.[16]

For small depressed scars, punch excision with primary closure or with punch graft, with or without dermabrasion, can improve the overall texture of the face with pitted acne scarring (Fig. *15-4*A *through* C).[17] Although dermabrasion can be performed at any time, optimum scar improvement is generally achieved at 2 to 8 weeks after wound occurrence.

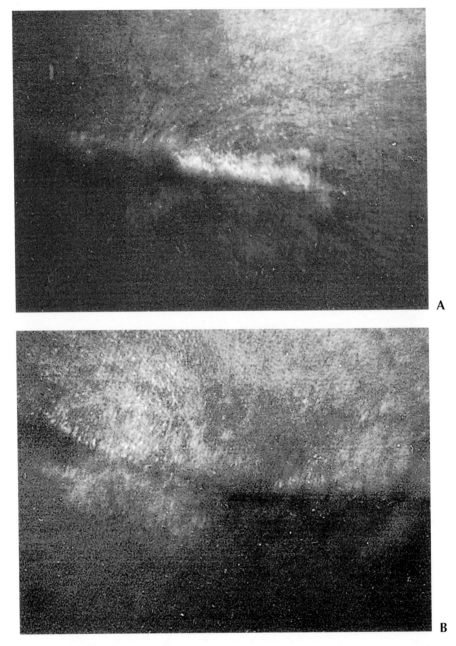

Figure 15-3 (**A**) Keloidal scar. Excision was recommended. (**B**) Six months later, a postoperative photo reveals a markedly diminished scar.

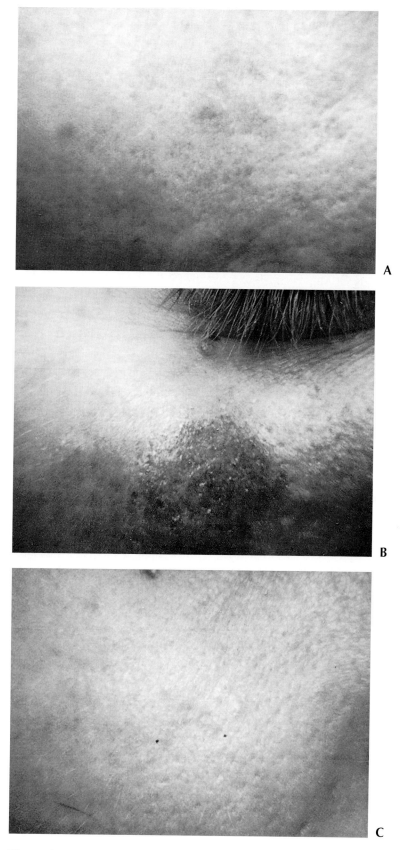

Figure 15-4 (*A*) Patient seen after an acne punch graft for an ice-pick scar. (*B*) Patient after dermabrasion. (*C*) Patient after the site has fully healed, 4 months postprocedure.

DISCOLORED ATROPHIC SCAR

Camouflage makeup is highly effective in covering flat scars, especially in those patients accustomed to applying makeup and who prefer not to undergo more aggressive therapy. Medical-grade tattooing can be used to camouflage hypopigmented scars. Accents or the Enhancer II micropigmentation systems can be used at 60-rps mode between settings 4 and 5. Mixing skin tones, white, black, and shades of brown to achieve a slightly darker tone than the patient's surrounding skin may give the best results.[18] However, differential pigment fading occurs over time and may leave the residual coloring significantly mismatched. Risks and alternatives of tattooing should be discussed with the patient prior to the procedure. Limitations include inexact color match, background skin color variation with seasonal sun exposure and tanning, as well as a predictable fading of the tattoo pigment over time.

HYPERPIGMENTED ATROPHIC SCAR

A combination of topical retinoids and topical hydroquinone bleaching cream with or without a topical glucocorticoid cream (modified Kligman formula) can be variably effective when applied twice a day to dark areas of a scar for 6 to 8 weeks. Also, a series of microdermabrasion treatments may be a helpful adjuvant for epidermal hyperpigmentation. A Wood's light can be used in scar evaluation to delineate epidermal hyperpigmentation prior to formulating the treatment plan.

Laser Treatment of Scars

In brief, lasers may be selected based on their emission wavelength to target epidermal or dermal pigment chromophores within scars. This makes them useful in treating hyperpigmented scars. Ablative, vaporizing, or resurfacing lasers may be selected to plane an elevated scar. However, elevated scars submitted to complete vaporizing, ablative resurfacing with the CO_2, argon, and Nd:YAG lasers tend to recur (see Chap. 14).

The 585-nm flashlamp-pumped pulsed-dye laser (PDL) may be effective alone or in combination with the high-energy pulsed CO_2 laser. The PDL with 7- to 10-mm spot size is used at 3 to 7 J/cm^2 for two to four treatments of hypertrophic scars or for two to six treatments for keloid scars and at 2.5 to 4.5 J/cm^2 for one or two treatments for striae. The high-energy pulsed CO_2 laser is used for one or two passes at 500 mJ and 5-W power, with a 3-mm collimated handpiece used not to completely ablate the hypertrophic scar but to deepithelialize and shrink the scar collagen either before or after use of the PDL (Fig. 15-5A through D).[19] The SPTL-1 candela flashlamp pumped-dye laser at 585 nm, 450-ms pulse duration, and energy fluence between 6.5 and 6.75 J/cm^2 without overlapping may be effective alone for improving red hypertrophic scars by 57 to 63 percent after one or two treatments.[20] The same laser type at similar settings except on a 5-mm spot size with 10 percent overlap and 6.0 to 7.5 J/cm^2 gave 77 percent improvement of erythematous hypertrophic scars after an average of 1.8 treatments, and improved postinflammatory hyperpigmentation at 510 nm and 2.0 to 2.5 J/cm^2 by 80 percent after an average of 1.45 treatments.[21]

Erythema, pliability, and texture of hypertrophic burn scars from chemical peels, CO_2 laser procedures, and accidental thermal injury were improved after an average of 2.5 treatments using the 585-nm PDL at a pulse duration of 450 to 1500 ms, 5.0 to 6.5 J/cm^2 fluence, and 7-mm spot size without overlap.[22] Early intervention to prevent unfavorable scars using the PDL has been advocated.[23] Depressed atrophic scars have been treated with a combination of high-energy pulsed CO_2 and erbium:YAG lasers with 80 to 88 percent improvement at 3 months.[24]

Summary

Multiple modalities exist for modifying and revising the appearance of scars. A combination of nonsurgical and surgical modalities can be custom-combined for each individual's unique scar. This chapter gives an overview of some of the more useful techniques available to the dermatologic surgeon for the correction of unacceptable scars.

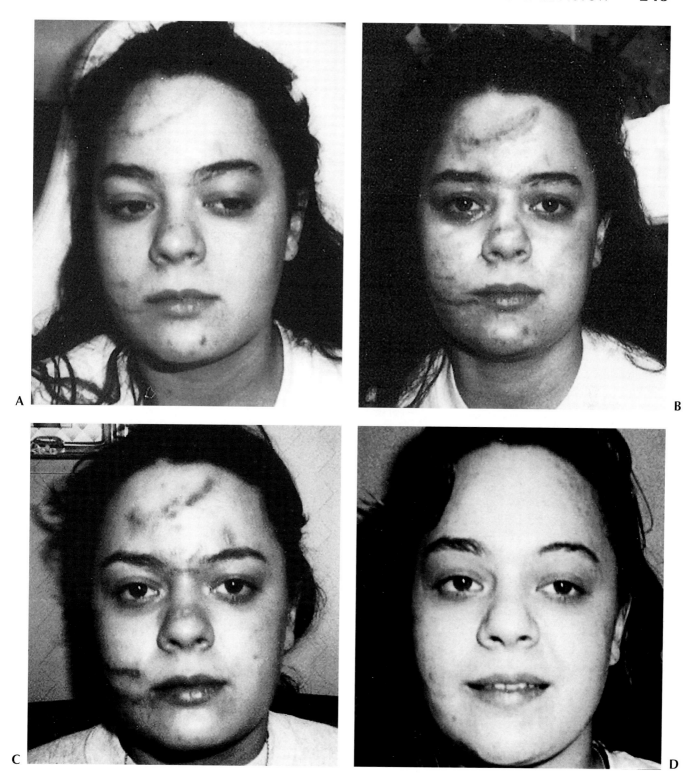

Figure 15-5 (**A**) Patient with scarring after a motor vehicle accident. (**B**) Patient having undergone CO_2 laser resurfacing. (**C**) Patient 4 weeks after CO_2 laser. The patient underwent flash pump/PDL laser therapy. (**D**) Patient 6 months after the completion of treatment.

References

1. Ferguson MJW. Scar formation: The spectral nature of fetal and adult wound repair. *Plast Reconst Surg* 1996; 97(4):854–859.

2. Fisher D. Scar evaluation. *Med Trial Tech Q* 1973; summer:41–47.

3. Goslin JB. Physiology of wound healing and scar formation. In: Thomas JR, Holt GR, eds. *Facial Scars: Incision, Recision and Camouflage*. St. Louis: Mosby; 1989:10–21.

4. Braumann LS, Spencer J. The effects of topical vitamin E on the cosmetic appearance of scars. *Dermatol Surg* 1999; 25(4):311–315.

5. Jackson BA, Shelton AJ. Pilot study evaluating topical onion extract as treatment for postsurgical scars. *Dermatol Surg*; 25(4):267–269.

6. Williams C. Cica-care: Adhesive gel sheet. *Br J Nurs* 1996; 5(14):875–876.

7. Yang JY. Intrascar excision for persistent perioral hypertrophic scar. *Plast Reconstr Surg* 1996; 98(7):1200–1205.

8. Engrav LH. A comparison of intramarginal and extramarginal excision of hypertrophic burn scars. *Plast Reconst Surg* 1988; 81(1):40–43.

9. Kaplan B, Potter T, Moy RL. Scar revision. *Dermatol Surg* 1997; 23:435–442.

10. Webster RC, Smith RC. Scar revision and camouflaging. Symposium on Plastic Surgery of the Face. *Otolaryngol Clin North Am* 1982; 15(1):55–75.

11. Izaguirre H, Navarro C, Rhomboid-to-"W" technique for excision and closure of facial skin lesions. *J Maxillofac Surg* 1983; 11:207–210.

12. Wolfe D, Davidson TM. Scar revision. *Arch Otolaryngol Head Neck Surg* 1991; 117:200–204.

13. Sherris DA, Larrabee WF, Murakami CS. Management of scar contractures, hypertrophic scars, and keloids. *Otolaryngol Clin North Am* 1995; 28(5):367–370.

14. de Benito J, Fernandez I, Nanda V. Treatment of depressed scars with a dissecting cannula and an autologous fat graft. *Aesthet Plast Surg* 1999; 23(5)367–370.

15. Schuller-Petrovic S. Improving the aesthetic aspect of soft tissue defects on the face using autologous fat transplantation. *Facial Plast Surg* 1997; 13(2):119–124.

16. Harahap M. Revision of a depressed scar. *J Dermatol Surg Oncol* 1984; 10(4):206–209.

17. Mancuso A, Farber GA. The abraded punch graft for pitted facial scars. *J Dermatol Surg Oncol* 1991; 17(1):32–34.

18. Guyuron B, Baughan C. Medical-grade tattooing to camouflage depigmented scars. *Plast Reconstr Surg* 1995; 95(3):575–579.

19. Alster TS. Laser treatment of hypertrophic scars, keloids, and striae. *Dermatol Clin* 1997; 15:419–428.

20. Alster TS. Improvement of erythematous and hypertrophic scars by the 585 nm flashlamp-pumped pulsed dye Laser. *Ann Plast Surg* 1994; 32:1890.

21. Dierckx C, Goldman MP, Fitzpatrick RE. Laser treatment of erythematous/hypertrophic and pigmented scars in 26 patients. *Plast Reconstr Surg* 1995; 95:84–90.

22. Alster TS, Nanni CA. Pulsed dye laser treatment of hypertrophic burn scars. *Plast Reconstr Surg* 1998; 102:2190–2194.

23. McCraw JB. Prevention of unfavorable scars using early pulsed dye laser treatments: A preliminary report. *Ann Plast Surg* 1999; 42:7–14.

24. Cho SI, Kim YC. Treatment of atrophic facial scars with combined use of high-energy pulsed CO_2 and Er:YAG laser: Practical guide of the laser techniques for the Er:YAG laser. *Dermatol Surg* 1999; 25:959–964.

Patient Information

Scar Revision

What Is in a Scar?

Scars are the result of the skin's repair of wounds caused by accident, disease, or surgery. This is a natural part of the healing process. The more the skin is damaged and the longer it takes to heal, the greater the chance of a noticeable scar.

Typically, a scar will appear more prominent at first, then gradually fade. Many actively healing scars that seem unsightly at 3 months may heal quite satisfactorily if given more time.

A scar's appearance will depend on its color, texture, depth, length, width, and location. How the scar forms will also be affected by an individual's age and the scar's location on the body or face. For example, skin over a jawbone is tighter than skin on the cheek and will make a scar easier to see. If a scar is depressed, it will make skin seem shaded, and if it is higher than surrounding skin, it will cast a shadow. A scar that crosses natural expression lines will be more apparent because it will not follow a natural pattern, and a scar that is wider than a wrinkle will stand out because it is not a naturally occurring line.

Any one or a combination of these factors may result in a scar that, although healthy, may be improved by treatment.

What Can and Cannot Be Done for Scars?

Several techniques can minimize a scar. Most of these are done routinely in the dermatologist's office with local anesthesia. Only severe scars, such as burns over a large part of the body, require general anesthesia and a hospital stay.

Surgical scar revision can change the length, width, or direction of a scar, raise depressed scars, or lower elevated scars. However, no scar can ever be completely erased, and no magic technique will return skin to its uninjured appearance. Surgical scar revision can provide improvement in the appearance of the skin while leaving another—though less obvious—mark. In addition, a scar's color cannot be altered; as it gets older, it usually fades and can often be hidden with makeup, but a certain difference in pigmentation will usually remain.

The most important step in the treatment of scars is careful consultation between patient and dermatologist—finding out what bothers a patient most about a scar and deciding the best treatment. Physicians stress that each scar is different and each requires a different approach.

Surgical Treatment with Scar Revision

The surgical removal of scars is best suited to wide or long scars, those in prominent places, or scars that have healed in a particular pattern or shape. Based on the ability of the skin to stretch with time, surgical scar revision is a method of removing a scar and rejoining the normal skin in a less conspicuous fashion. Wide scars can often be cut away and closed, resulting in a narrower, less obvious scar, and long scars can be shortened. Dermatologic surgeons may use a technique of irregular or staggered incisions to form a broken-line scar, which is much more difficult to recognize. Sometimes, a scar's direction can be changed, so that all or part of the scar crosses a natural wrinkle or line falls into the wrinkle, making it less noticeable. This method can also be used to move scars into more favorable locations, into a hairline or a natural junction (for instance, where the nose meets the cheek).

Best results are obtained when the scar is removed and wound edges are brought together without tension. Accordingly, scar removal is planned with great care, keeping in mind the structure of the muscle layers.

Scar Revision Preoperative Instructions

Please do not wear makeup to the office; if it is worn, please plan to remove it upon arrival.

To minimize the chance of bruising, please plan on doing the following:

Avoid aspirin or aspirin-containing products once you are scheduled for the procedure.

Preferably stay off aspirin or aspirin-containing products for 10 days prior to your treatment.

Avoid alcohol for 24 hours prior to the procedure.

Be sure to discuss with the doctor any bleeding tendencies and current medications being used.

Ice will be applied immediately following treatment. If you normally bruise easily, plan to go home and apply ice to the treated area(s) for an extra few hours.

Get a good night's sleep before the procedure.

Eat a light meal (breakfast or lunch) the day of treatment prior to the appointment.

Although the treatments are well tolerated by most patients, to minimize any discomfort you may apply a topical over-the-counter anesthetic agent (Ela-max 4%) to the area(s) to be treated for 1 hour prior to your visit. This product may be purchased at your local pharmacy; follow the application instructions packaged with it.

Scar Revision Setup Tray

Patient

1. Cape or drape (optional)
2. Clean hat

Doctor and Staff

1. Visor mask
2. Sterile gloves

Materials

1. Betadine solution
2. Sterile surgical ellipse tray
3. Clean gauze
4. Gentian marker
5. 1- and 3-mL syringes
6. One 30g metal hub needle
7. 1% Lidocaine with epinephrine, buffered
8. Alcohol wipe
9. Saline bottle
10. Thermometer and cover
11. Suture/skin closures, Glustitch as appropriate
12. Polysporin
13. Telfa, gauze, tape
14. Mastisol (optional)
15. Steri-Strips (optional)

Scar Revision Postoperative Instructions

You may use Tylenol or Extra-Strength Tylenol for any discomfort. It is best not to take aspirin or alcohol for 24 hours after the procedure.

Keep the Band-Aid or dressing dry for ____ hours and then remove.

Using a Q-tip, gently cleanse the wound with tap water or saline solution once a day. Do not use hydrogen peroxide, alcohol, or soap.

Pat the wound dry; liberally apply antibiotic ointment twice daily, in the morning and at bedtime.

Wear a Band-aid or nonstick dressing during the day. This will keep the area clean and covered.

At bedtime, apply a thin layer of ointment. You may leave it uncovered.

If you have had "stitches" placed, do wound care as above the entire time they are present. You will be given further direction when you return for stitch removal.

Should minor bleeding occur, apply firm, constant pressure for 15 to 20 minutes. It is not unusual for mild, red-tinged drainage to occur up to 48 hours after surgery.

Should you have any questions or problems with infection, pain or discharge, please call (___) _____.

Consent for Scar Revision*

Patient Name _____

Date_____

I hereby authorize _____ and/or the surgical team to perform the following operative procedure _____
_____.

I have been informed, to my satisfaction, of the above-mentioned procedure(s), why it is being done, and that the alternative of no treatment at all poses no risk to my health. I understand that, after scar revision, it may take many months to see the results, that additional revisions may be necessary, that little or no overall improvement may be gained, and that my condition may actually be worsened as a result of this surgery.

I understand that this will be a surgical procedure and that it will be performed under local anesthesia, possibly with adjunct IV sedation. I have previously had no allergy to these agents. I realize that this procedure will be an operation done with a scalpel, which is performed to cut out and remove irregular scar tissue. In doing so, some normal tissue may be removed and a new scar will be formed. I give permission to my doctor to do this procedure in the manner the doctor considers to be best for me. The doctor has my permission to make the best possible cosmetic closure; however, I understand that the final, resulting scar represents an attempt to improve my current condition, and I realize that no scar is completely invisible.

I have been made aware that there are certain risks inherent to the performance of any surgical procedure—such as loss of blood; infection; bruising; reactions to anesthesia; the formation of thick, painful, or otherwise objectionable scars; numbness; and/or loss of muscle function—and that these may be permanent. Additionally, I acknowledge that the doctor has made no promises to me, oral or written, in connection with the operation. I recognize that every surgical procedure involves uncertainty and that no result can ever be guaranteed. I understand and accept the possibility that the procedure may have to be repeated or revised multiple times to achieve optimal results.

I understand that no significant improvement may occur, or that the scar may actually be worsened.

I give permission to have any tissue removed during the procedure be sent for histologic examination by a pathologist.

*Information adapted from the "What Is in a Scar?" brochure produced by the American Academy of Dermatology.

I release the doctor from responsibility for any condition that arises as a natural complication of the procedure. I also realize that it is my responsibility to keep postoperative appointments and perform postoperative care as instructed. If I feel that any problems exist, such as bleeding or infection, or if I have any doubts, I am to contact the doctor as soon as possible.

Initial_____

ACKNOWLEDGMENT

- I understand that the two sides of the body are not the same and can never be made to look the same in all regards. I understand that bone and muscle structures help create overall shape and are never identical on both sides of the body, and that these will remain unchanged by the surgery.

Initial_____

- I have been satisfactorily informed of the possible experiences, benefits, and risks of the surgery and, if applicable, the administration of anesthesia, as well as the possibility of a lengthy recovery time (sometimes 18 months or longer) until improvement is noted.

Initial_____

- I have been given the opportunity to ask any and all my questions have been answered to my satisfaction.

Initial_____

- I give permission to _____ to take still or motion clinical photographs with the understanding such photographs remain the property of the center. If in the judgment of the center medical research, education, or science will be benefited by their use, such photographs and related information may be published and republished in professional journals or medical books or used for any other purpose which the center may deem proper. It is specifically understood that in any such publication or use, I shall not be identified by name.

Initial_____

- For the purpose of advancing medical education, I consent to the admittance of authorized observers to the operating room.

Initial_____

My signature indicates that I have read this "Consent for Scar Revision" and understand and accept the risks involved with this surgical procedure. I hereby authorize _____ _____ and/or the surgical team to perform this surgical procedure on me.

_____   _____
Signature (Patient/Responsible Party)   Date

_____   _____
Signature (Witness)   Date

_____   _____
Signature (Parent/Guardian)   Date

CHAPTER 16

Liposuction

History of Liposuction

Liposuction originated in the early 1970s in France and Italy and has since gone through many permutations. It has been transformed into what is now best referred to as "reduction liposculpture." Liposuction has become the most sought after cosmetic procedure, accounting for 16 percent of cosmetic procedures in women and 20 percent in men.[1] The technique of tumescent liposuction revolutionized the procedure by allowing significant volumes of fat to be safely removed without the need for blood transfusion. More than 250,000 liposuction procedures are currently performed every year.[2,3]

The instrumentation for liposuction has varied over the years among various surgeons. A more recent adaptation is the vacuum pump; however, many experts believe that it offers no advantage. The cannulae have varied in their port designs, gauges, and lengths. In addition, the cannulae can be augmented with the use of ultrasound, and a recent addition has been a reciprocating or vibrating power source. However, these are probably physician-oriented rather than patient-oriented devices. Others have attempted to improve results by using external ultrasound, but there has been no proven benefit. Our preferred method is syringe-assisted liposuction, which we have found to be versatile, precise, and extremely safe. It also has the added benefit of being quiet. Some surgeons, however, have found the need for syringe emptying to be cumbersome. Nevertheless, it has been our experience that the time from initiation of the syringe-assisted procedure to completion is, on average, the same as an equivalent procedure with the use of the vacuum pump.

This chapter reviews the step-by-step approach to setting the stage for safe and effective facial and body liposuction. Emphasis is placed on basic prerequisites, equipment, anesthesia, patient selection, and consultation. An understanding of the anatomy of fat in the key cosmetic units is essential to achieving a successful liposuction procedure (see Chap. 7). The intraoperative techniques, preoperative and postoperative care, and complications and their management and prevention are all outlined.

Liposuction has been performed by three different methods:

1. The *dry technique* involved liposuction without prior fluid infiltration. This was the original method of per-

forming liposuction under general anesthesia. However, significant morbidity and mortality relating to large volumes of blood loss made it fall out of favor.

2. The *wet technique* involved liposuction using a low volume of dilute lidocaine (0.2 to 0.5%) and epinephrine (1:100,000 to 1:400,000). Although this technique was better than the dry technique, it was limited to low volumes of aspirated fat and was associated with greater patient discomfort.

3. The *tumescent technique* involves a large volume of saline infiltrated into the liposuction area. Its mixture includes epinephrine (1:1,000,000) and lidocaine (0.05 to 0.1%) with 1 percent of the total volume consisting of bicarbonate (8.4%). Some solutions also include triamcinolone acetonide (10 mg/mL) at less than 0.1% of the final mixture.

Setting Up for Liposuction

CREDENTIALING

In an effort to standardize the many approaches, the American Academy of Dermatology—along with the American Society of Liposuction Surgery (ASLSS) and the American Academy of Cosmetic Surgery (AACS)—has recently offered guidelines for performing liposuction.[4,5]

Appropriately performed liposuction is safe and effective, and current fashion trends have led to its increased popularity. The increased demand for slender bodies has been met by an increased supply of physicians attempting to perform liposuction. Unrealistic patient expectations in a milieu lacking in proper regulation of the procedure has opened the door to many poorly trained physicians who perform liposuction with little knowledge of how to avoid complications and how to deal with them if they arise. In turn, this has led to increased patient dissatisfaction, morbidity, and even mortality in a field of elective surgery. An appropriate physician movement has come about to regulate the credentialing of liposuction in order to decrease its untoward effects. Various cosmetic groups have begun to formulate guidelines, and even some state medical boards, such as those in California and New Jersey, have started to set standards for credentialing surgical procedures including liposuction (see Chap. 3).

EQUIPMENT

The surgical suite should preferably be an ambulatory center approved by the state or credentialing organization (e.g., AAAHC) (see Chaps. 1 and 2) of ample size to allow the surgeon and two or more assistants to work comfortably. A power table (preferably leg-operated) is needed that allows positional changes during liposuction and the ability to produce a Trendelenburg position if needed. Patient monitoring equipment (Fig. 16-1)—including a pulse oximeter, electrocardiographic (ECG) equipment; continuous blood pressure and pulse recorder that may be set to give readings at least every 5 min, and a crash cart equipped to manage emergency situations (see Chap. 7)—should be part of every surgical suite. A "cuff infuser pump," a mechanical or a pressure infusion pump (Fig. 16-2), and tubing connecting the pressure infusion machine to the infiltrating cannulae are needed for the infusion of the tumescent anesthesia fluids (Figs. 16-3 and 16-4). A vacuuming device to aspirate and evacuate the fat is needed; it can be electrical or manual. We have found that the Fournier and Toledo[6] manual syringe assisted by the

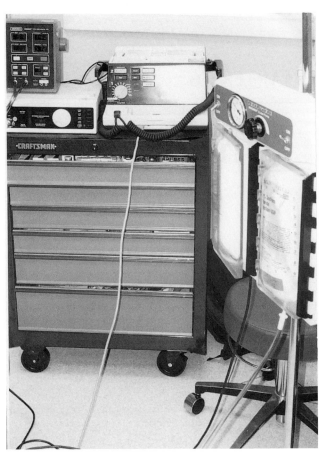

Figure 16-2 The double-chambered unit at the right of the photo is a pressure infusion pump allowing for the concurrent delivery of 2L of tumescent fluid for anesthesia.

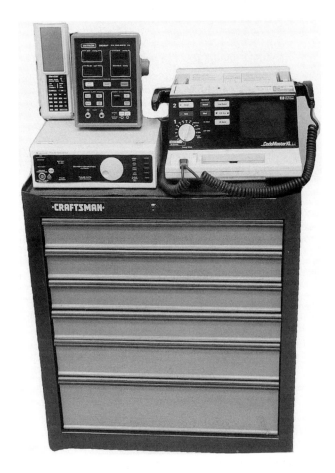

Figure 16-1 Patient monitoring equipment with continuous electrocardiographic equipment, blood pressure monitor, pulse oximeter, oxygen defibrillator along with automatic propofol delivery pump.

addition of a horseshoe lock to maintain the vacuum is a convenient, quiet, reliable, and safe device for aspirating fat. If a syringe breaks, it can be replaced by another without the need for a backup vacuum unit. Additionally, there is no possibility of aerosolization of aspirate.

The cannulae come in different sizes, diameters, lengths, and tip shapes, with differing numbers of openings, or ports, along their shafts. The tulip-shaped cannulae are available to fit the Toomey hub (Fig. 16-5). The type of cannula used is determined by the body location, the thickness and density of the fat, and the presence or absence of scarring and fibrosis. It is important for the surgeon to get a feel for the different type of cannulae and their implementations during surgery. This improves the surgeon's ability to choose the cannula that is most appropriate for each specific procedure in order to provide safe and efficient liposculpturing for the specific body area. There has been a recent trend in dermatology toward the use of increasingly smaller-sized cannulae, owing to claims that smaller cannulae allow for finer contouring. However, finer cannulae, even though blunt, can increase the risk of perforation and possible embolization.[7]

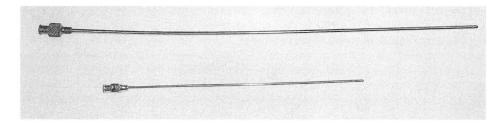

Figure 16-3   The Zaki (Byron, Phoenix, AZ) infusion cannula for pretunneling and delivery of tumescent fluid.

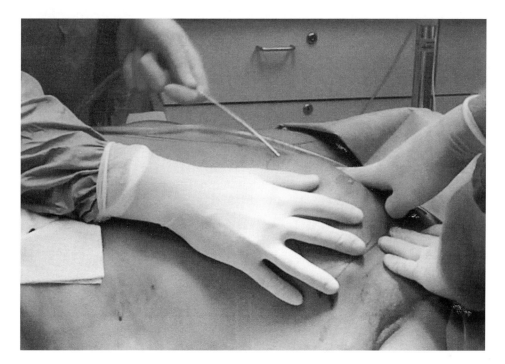

Figure 16-4   The Zaki cannula attached to tubing from pressure infusion pump infiltrating local anesthesia.

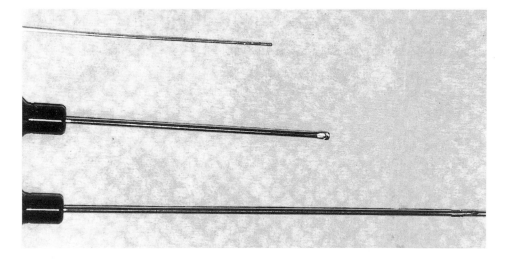

Figure 16-5   The tulip cannula for attachment to the Toomey hub.

In our practice, we have used 3- to 6-mm cannulae and occasionally 8-mm cannulae for large-bulk liposuctions without encountering any major complications and have achieved excellent result in more than 6000 procedures over the past 10 years.

Table 16-1 lists the equipment needed for liposuction procedures.

ANESTHESIA AND FLUID REPLACEMENT

Patient comfort and safety are pivotal to good anesthesia (see Chap. 8). Anesthesia influences the patient's overall sense of the procedure and of the surgeon. A decrease in pain and the time spent in surgery increases the comfort and thus acceptance of the procedure. Increased acceptance improves the likelihood of a patient's undergoing additional cosmetic procedures and his or her likelihood of recommending to others the procedure and the surgeon.

The type of anesthesia selected during liposuction depends on the patient, the doctor, the body area operated on, and the volume of liposuction (higher volumes mean longer procedure times, and greater patient awareness and may increase the likelihood of discomfort and infection). Recently, the type of anesthesia used has also come to depend on individual state regulations. Since the advent of tumescent infiltration, the choice of types of anesthesia available for liposuction

procedures has expanded. Available anesthesia can be divided into three groups, based on the Ramsey sedation scale.

In the first group, the patient senses no sharp pain but is completely aware of his or her surroundings (Ramsey level 1 or less). This level includes local anesthesia; local anesthesia with sedation, which may include oral or intramuscular (IM) routes of administration; and regional nerve blocks. Sedation using an IM route is difficult to reverse in case of an emergency; in our opinion, these patients should be appropriately monitored.

The second group involves conscious sedation, which is defined in Chap. 8. This group corresponds to Ramsey levels 2 to 3. This is a form of monitored anesthesia that allows the patient to undergo a painless procedure void of memories while also permitting him or her to respond to commands and maintain the airway. It allows for a rapid onset of safe sedation, which provides comfort for both patient and physician. It also makes for a rapid recovery to a clear-headed state. In our opinion, integral to its use is its administration in an ambulatory surgery setting with proper patient selection and an anesthesiologist or experienced certified registered nurse anesthetist (CRNA) performing the patient monitoring.[8]

The third group comprises general anesthesia, corresponding to Ramsey levels 5 to 6. It should be performed in a hospital or a properly equipped ambulatory surgery

Table 16-1
Equipment Needed for Liposuction Procedure

Patient
1. Cape
2. Photo pants

Doctor and Staff
1. Surgical hats
2. Mask
3. Sterile gloves
4. Sterile gowns

Materials
1. Three sterile medium drapes
2. One large sterile bath towel
3. Sterile Socks
4. Sterile huck towel
5. Handle cover for sterile light
6. Syringes
   A. 2, 60 cc Luer-Lok (if hand infusing) or 1 and 2 rapid infusion tubing (open only 1)
7. 2- and 60-mL Toomeys
8. 1- and 30-gauge 1-inch metal-hub needle
9. 1- and 21-gauge 1-in. needle

10. 1- and 3-mL syringes
11. Four fat boxes
12. Steri-Strips, ½ in.
13. Mastisol
14. Two 4-0 Vicryl P2 (open only 1)
15. Sterile liposuction tray
16. Cannulae
    A. 2 long infusion cannulae
    B. Two harvesters (usually 4 mm or 6 mm)
17. 3 mL lidocaine 1% with epinephrine, buffered
18. Local anesthesic mixture (Kline's solution)
    A. 1 L normal saline
    B. 50 mL lidocaine 2% plain
    C. 5 mL sodium bicarbonate
    D. 2 mL epinephrine
    E. 1 mL triamcinolone acetonide 10 mg
19. Compression garment
20. Black marker
21. Povidone-iodine solution
22. No. 15 blade

center. The risk of general anesthesia may not be warranted for an elective procedure.

It is our policy that irrespective of the anesthesia selected, fluid replacement should be carried out in every patient undergoing liposuction. Operative fluid loss occurs from three different sources: the volume of fat extracted, the percentage of blood in that volume, and the third-space loss postoperatively. Restricted fluid intake prior to sedation as well as normal metabolism also correlate with the fluid deficit. An average of 5 to 10 percent of blood has been found in the total volume of fat removed. It is possible for a healthy person to lose 10 percent of his or her blood volume safely as long as the fluid volume is replaced. For calculation purposes, it can be estimated that 75 mL/kg of body weight in a man and 65 mL/kg of body weight in a woman is blood.[9] For fluid replacement purposes, the estimated third-space loss is 50 percent of the volume extracted.

If the patient is given nothing by mouth for 8 h, an average man (weight, 65 kg) would initially require 1000 mL of replacement crystalloid fluids to begin with. This would be followed by continuous crystalloid infusion to match the volume of fat extracted plus an additional 10 percent of fluid to account for possible blood loss. After the patient is in the recovery room, he or she completes the fluid replacement, which amounts to 50 percent of the fat volume extracted (replacing the estimated third-space fluid loss). In addition, the intravenous (IV) access is important for any patient undergoing liposuction to allow a quick access for the introduction of medications in an emergency.

TUMESCENT TECHNIQUE

The tumescent technique involves infiltrating large volumes of dilute lidocaine and epinephrine into the targeted fat for a minimum of 10 to 15 min before liposuction on that area is begun. It enables one to perform many liposuction procedures while patients are under local anesthesia without any sedation. In addition, the tumescent technique allows for the expansion of the fatty compartment, thus providing an increased safety zone from superficially localized neurovascular and lymphatic bundles.

The amount of tumescent fluid infused is limited by the maximum dose of lidocaine that can be safely used. We use a conservative limit of 35 mg/kg; however, some have reported using higher levels, such as 50 to 60 mg/kg, safely.[10–13] The tumescent concentration is made of a 1-L bag of lactated Ringer's solution to which is added sodium bicarbonate ($NaHCO_3$)- 10 mL plus adrenaline chloride solution 1:1000 (1 mL) plus 2% lidocaine without epinephrine (50 mL). This is translated into a solution of 0.1% lidocaine with 1:1,000,000 epinephrine. A single milliliter of 0.1% lidocaine contains 1 mg of lidocaine. Therefore, in a healthy 70-kg person, one can infiltrate 2.5 L of 0.1% lidocaine using the limit of 35 mg/kg or 3.5 L for the 50-mg/kg lidocaine limit.

INDICATIONS

Liposuction is indicated for the treatment of patients with localized fat deposits. It cannot remove scars, stretching, dimpling, or cellulite. It is not a technique for weight loss; rather, it is a sculpturing procedure that helps to change the body's contour. Liposuction can be used for conditions other than cosmetic body contouring, including localized solitary or multiple lipomas or hematomas, lipodystrophy, gynecomastia or pseudogynecomastia, or axillary hyperhidrosis. It may also assist in flap elevation, debulking, or movement.[14] It has been used in many cosmetic procedures, in which it helps decrease the final scar length, such as breast reduction and abdominoplasty.[15]

The Consultation

UNDERSTANDING YOUR PATIENT

The success of the procedure relies on proper patient selection as much as on the proper execution of the operative procedure. During the first encounter with the patient, it is important for the physician to adjust the patient's expectations from the surgery to the realities of his or her body. An open-ended question such as: "What would you want to achieve from liposuction?" can help the physician focus on the areas the patient wants to address and may help weed out those individuals who expect the impossible (e.g., expecting to become a changed person based on the procedure; see Chap. 5).

PATIENT EVALUATION

After the physician and patient arrive at a realistic view of the probable results, the patient's eligibility for liposuction must be assessed. The patient's general health, age, weight, and skin tone must be evaluated, as well as the location of the dysmorphic fat. While the patient is in a standing position, his or her body contour is evaluated. The skin is examined for its elasticity, tone, and redundancy. Stretch marks, scars, cellulite, dimpling, sagging, and muscle tone are best assessed by making the patient contract the underlying muscle (e.g., to examine his or her abdomen, the patient should be asked to lean forward). All these observations should be well documented. Although preoperative clearance by the family doctor is one of the requirements, one should always examine the patient's abdomen for the presence of hernias or scars that may hide an incisional or umbilical hernia. If any doubts exist about hernias, a preoperative ultrasound or computed tomography (CT) examination should be scheduled. The patient must be made aware that the procedure will improve contours but not decrease weight. Inches will be lost, but liposuction will not remove cellulite, stretching, or dimpling.

Three different manipulations performed during the evaluation can help decide whether the patient can benefit from liposuction or may need a lifting procedure such as abdominoplasty. The "pinch test" is used to evaluate a bulging mass or any area to be improved upon by liposuction. If pinching the skin leads to a substantial amount of subcutaneous tissue being grasped between the fingers before liposuction, then liposuction may benefit the area (Fig. 16-6). If the fingers can almost touch each other before the procedure, then the visualized bulge may be caused by muscle flaccidity, bone protuberance, submuscular fat, or simply excess skin.

While the pinch test is being performed, the "muscle contraction test" can also be performed. This test pulls away

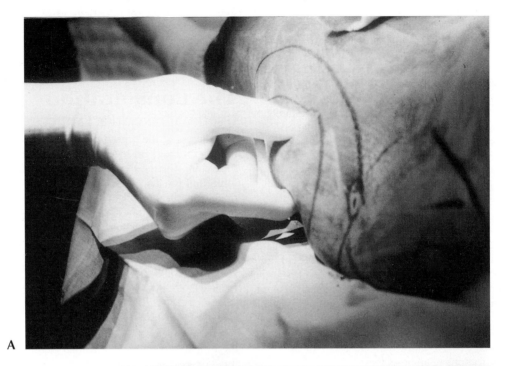

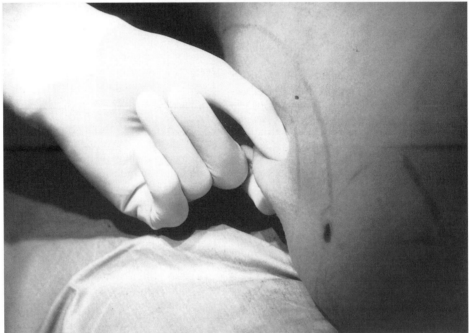

Figure 16-6 (*A*) The pinch test revealed a substantial fat pad present before liposuction. (*B*) The same patient's pinch test with the completion of liposuction. The digits nearly touch, revealing the complete removal of the fat pad.

any muscle grasped by the pinch, leaving only subcutaneous fat and skin in the grasp. In this way, one can differentiate between muscle laxity and subcutaneous fat. It can also help evaluate areas as the lateral thighs. By contracting the gluteal muscle, the buttock is elevated, relieving its pressure on the lateral thighs. If a considerable change in the shape of the thighs occurs, then both the lateral thigh and the buttock should be treated as a cosmetic unit. The "lifting test" helps evaluate the effect that simple skin excess has on the body's dysmorphism. Just as with face-lift or eyelid lift, the lifting test requires pulling up skin and its subcutaneous tissue in the opposite direction to gravity and examining the contour of the body part. If mere pinching is not enough to achieve the desired appearance and a lifting test shows the patient's desired improvement, then the excess skin needs to be addressed.

PRIMING YOUR PATIENT

A common method helpful to patients is the use of visual aids. Some surgeons like to use computer-modified images (see Chap. 4) to help patients visualize how they may look after completion of the procedure. Many facilities use digital imaging as well as "before" and "after" photographs of previously treated patients. The reaction of the patient to the photographs should be noted as an index of his or her expectations. If the patient appears to have a realistic perspective, an information packet that details the procedure and offers background on the surgeon is given to the patient, along with a medical clearance form. If the patient is ready to set a date for the procedure, available dates are discussed by an assistant, and both pre- and postoperative appointments are made.

The medical clearance includes a complete physical examination as well as superficial musculoaponeurotic system (SMAS), complete blood count (CBC), pregnancy test, urinalysis, prothrombin (PT) and partial thromboplastin times (PTT), bleeding time, fibrinogen, TSH, and T4 levels. An ECG and chest radiograph must also be obtained. Several days before the set date, the patient is seen again by the physician, at which time the blood tests, diagnostic studies, and medical clearance form are evaluated and the consent form is signed. In addition, the patient's weight and the dimensions of the areas to be treated are recorded. It is important to stress to the patient that he or she should not make any special preparations for the procedure other than engaging in mild exercise or walking. Exercise and diet can also aid the improvement after recovery is complete. Preoperative and postoperative information for coming several weeks is given to the patient, who also is told to avoid tobacco, alcohol, and aspirin-containing products for at least 2 weeks before the procedure.

THE COSMETIC BODY UNIT

A patient may often request that a specific body part be altered, such as "love handles" or a double chin, or may simply ask "to look younger again." It is the responsibility of the surgeon to translate the patient's desire into a realistic plan. When needed, the surgeon should tactfully point out other body areas involved in the same or adjacent cosmetic units that may be integral to achieving the desired cosmetic outcome. He or she should explain the effect an incompletely treated cosmetic unit will have on the body's contour (see Chap. 7).

Liposuction of the Face and Neck

Aging is generally defined as involving wrinkling and sagging of the skin (see Chap. 6). These signs are readily apparent on the face and neck. Liposuction has simplified the earlier, tedious open procedures and allowed for closed intervention with limited side effects, especially in the face and neck. We have found that facial and neck liposuction with the use of small instruments—cannulae of 2.1- to 4-mm gauge and a 10- or 60-mL syringe—further limits complications and achieves excellent results.

ANATOMY

Liposuction of the face and neck is limited to the superficial anatomic structures from the skin to the fascia—the reticulum cutis. The bony and surface landmarks are reviewed before the procedure is begun. The body is organized so that each of the cuticular and subcuticular skeletal structures is ensheathed by an investing or covering fascia. These linings have been divided into superficial and deep fascia. The superficial musculoaponeurotic system (SMAS) is a thick layer of fascia deep to the subcutaneous fat. There are numerous connections made up of fibrous septa between the SMAS and the overlying dermis. The SMAS is then a broad fibrous fascia enveloping and interlinking the muscles of facial expression into a functional unit. Liposuction of the face and neck is performed on fat superficial to the SMAS layer.

In liposuction of the face and neck, the major nerves and blood vessels should be consciously noted after a review of surface topographic landmarks. The specific depth and arrangement of important structures is predictable. For example, the branches of the seventh nerve are superficial beyond the border of the parotid and are lightly covered by the SMAS. The superficial temporal vessels and auriculotemporal nerve run approximately 2 cm above the zygomatic arch before becoming more superficial in the subcutaneous fat. The superficial cervical fascia invests the platysma and adheres to the deep fascia in the pretragal and mastoid prominence. This layer is continuous over the sternocleidomastoid muscle. The external jugular vein and greater auricular nerve are not covered by platysma in the superior lateral neck; therefore they are vulnerable. Injury to the motor nerves, greater auricular nerve, and external jugular vein can be avoided by remaining in the plane superficial to the SMAS.

INDICATIONS

The process of aging is a dynamic phenomenon that involves changes in the physiologic function and morphology of the skin—specifically the dermis and the supporting adipose, and SMAS tissue. In contrast to the youthful face, the aged face has little ability to resist gravity. The youthful face is "full of fat" (see Chap. 6). This fat drapes the pillars of the face (i.e., the bony skull, malar eminence, and chin). Combined, these provide the structural underpinnings of the face over which the skin is "draped." Aging is, in the esthetic sense, largely defined by changes in the reticulum cutis.

The surgeon, therefore, must evaluate the patient's skin tone, facial contour, and facial fat distribution before recommending facial or neck liposuction. The esthetic considerations of greatest importance include a distinct mandibular border, the neck-chin angle, cheek contour, nasolabial mounding, and malar fat pads. We believe that early intervention, when tone is good and the "aging" changes are just becoming apparent, yields the best results (see Chap. 6).

TECHNIQUE

Preoperative marking of the sites to be treated should be carried out with the patient in the sitting position so as to accentuate the sagging and redundancy (Fig. 16-7). These markings should take into account the surface anatomy, with particular attention to the branches of the facial nerve (see Fig. 16-7). The liposuction procedure can be done under local anesthesia or in combination with presedation, depending on its planned scope. The site to be treated is first incised in a beveled fashion with a no. 11 blade sufficiently to allow for the entrance of a blunt 2-mm infusion catheter attached to a 10-mL syringe. Next, diluted lidocaine plus epinephrine is systematically infiltrated into the subcutaneous layer and this action hydrodissects the tissue plane (Fig. 16-8).

The cannula is then introduced, with its opening pointed downward (Fig. 16-9). The syringe's plunger is withdrawn and stabilized with the two digits of the surgeon's "power" hand. To guide the extraction, the other hand pinches the tissue to be treated. The area near the beveled incision should be done initially because the syringe's vacuum is lost toward the end of the procedure. Fat is seen to flow through the syringe. While filling the syringe, one can readily cap it and maintain this adipose tissue poised for fat transfer. The varied sites of incision for different areas are noted in Fig. 16-10. Both the submental and jowl areas can be approached through the same incision. At the completion of the procedure, if it was performed under local anesthesia, the patient is returned to the sitting posture and the symmetry of the removal is assessed. The sites of the incision are covered with Steri-Strips; suturing is not required. A facial neck garment is applied and should be worn for a minimum of 1 week.[16] The patient is discharged to a responsible person to be accompanied for the first several hours and transported home.

The standard setup we use for face and neck liposuction is depicted in Fig. 16-11.

DANGER ZONES

In performing liposuction on the face and neck, one must stay above the SMAS layer and its neck extension (the platysma) to avoid damage to such important anatomic structures as facial nerves and blood vessels. The facial artery and vein and the branches of the facial nerve, specifically its marginal mandibular nerve branch, are at highest risk for injury. The facial artery and vein cross the mandible medially to the medial edge of the masseter muscle and are most vulnerable at this point. These structures can be felt

clinically if the patient bites tightly while the surgeon palpates along the mandible at the medial edge of the masseter muscle. The marginal mandibular nerve runs underneath the SMAS along the mandible and is most vulnerable over the jowl liposuction area, where the SMAS is thinnest, at a 2-cm radius drawn over the midmandible 2 cm posterior to the oral commissure.[17]

Malar Fat Pad

The malar fat pad is located over the maxillary prominence, below and lateral to the infraorbital rim. This fat is triangular in shape, with its base lying over the nasolabial fold. It lies immediately below the skin and over the orbicularis oculi muscle, which is the extension of the SMAS at this layer. Beneath the orbicularis oculi muscle at this level is the suborbicularis oculi fat pad (SOOF), which extends laterally over the zygoma. The infraorbital foramen, with its infraorbital nerve, and the zygomatic branch of the facial nerve course underneath the SMAS and orbicularis oculi muscle. The angular artery, which is the extension of the facial artery, courses medially to this fat pad.

Submental Fat Pad

The submental fat pad is located in the submental area in a triangular fashion extending from the midline of the mandible to the hyoid bone, superficial to the platysma. The position of the hyoid bone determines the point of slope where the neck meets the mandible and thus the naturally available horizontal distance of the mandible. This is an important fact to mention in the patient's consultation. On its lateral edge, the submental fat pad becomes confluent with the submandibular triangle. The important layers in this area include skin, superficial fat, platysma, subplatysmal fat pad, superficial layer of investing fascia, digastric muscles, and sternohyoid muscle. With aging, the platysma becomes more atrophied and care must be taken not to perforate it, especially between the medial platysmal bands, where the fascia is deficient and one may inadvertently penetrate into the fat between the digastric muscles.

DISCUSSION

The aging of tissue is related to tissue involution and migration. The loss or gravitational drag that causes the "sagging" of this tissue is responsible for many of the esthetic changes that occur over time on the face and neck. The morphology of aged skin shows an overall thinning of the epidermis; otherwise, the alterations in aged epidermis are slight. However, the dermal aging changes are marked and have greater physiologic consequences. There is a flattening of the dermal–epidermal junction because of retraction of epidermal papillae, as well as the microprojections of basal cells into the dermis. The major alteration is in the aged dermis and concerns the architecture of the collagen and elastin networks. Both fiber components appear more compact because of a decrease in spaces between these fibers resulting from a loss of ground substance. Collagen bundles appear to unravel, and elastosis of elastin fibers occurs. The net effect is a dermis that is more lax and prone to wrinkling.

(text continues on page 260)

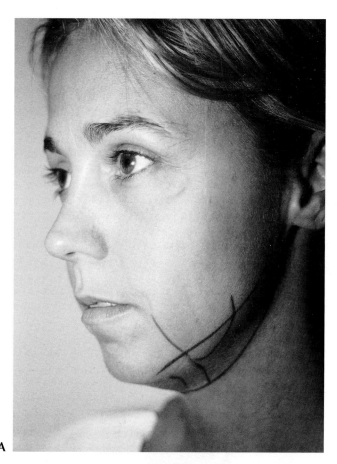

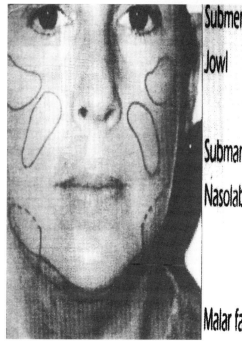

Figure 16-7 (*A*) The patient is marked in a seated position using a gentian violet pen, which accentuates the jowl and neck. (*B*) The entry points for facial liposuction and the direct fat pads.

Submental incision	Jowl, neck, chin
Jowl	In smile crease or inferior to earlobe
Submandibular	Submental, inferior to earlobe
Nasolabial mound	Smile crease or nasal vestibule, lateral nasal vestibule, lateral nasal ala
Malar fat pad	In "crow's feet"

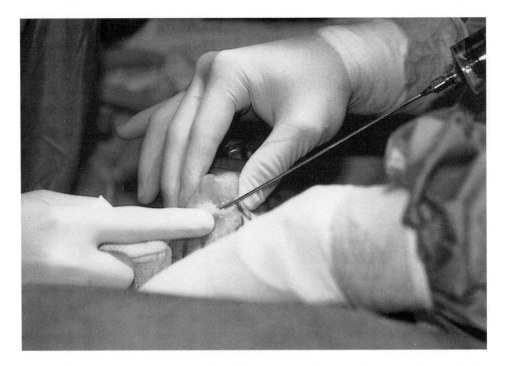

Figure 16-8 Cannula insertion for neck liposuction for infusion of tumescent fluid, which hydrodissects the tissue plane.

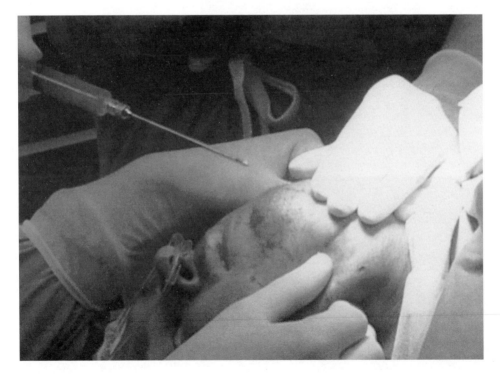

Figure 16-9 The cannula removed containing fat. This is a 3-mm neck harvester. It will be followed by a 4-mm spatula tip to further dissect the plane.

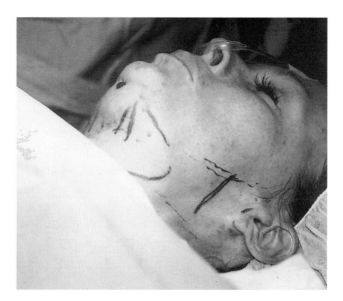

Figure 16-10   The marking on this patient in the pre-auricular area is the preferred area for the jowl. It can be approached for the submental area, but care must be taken not to injure the marginal mandibular branch of the facial nerve.

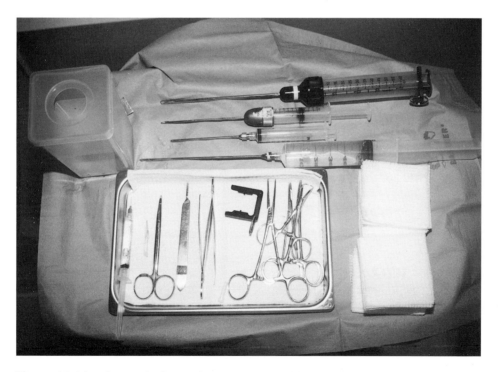

Figure 16-11   The standard setup for syringe-assisted liposuction of the face and neck. From top to bottom; the 4-mm spatula-tip syringe; the jowl harvester 3-mm syringe; the 3-mm neck harvester with three ports down to prevent subdermal fat injury; and the infusion cannula. The ring lock for the syringe appears with the surgical instruments on the tray.

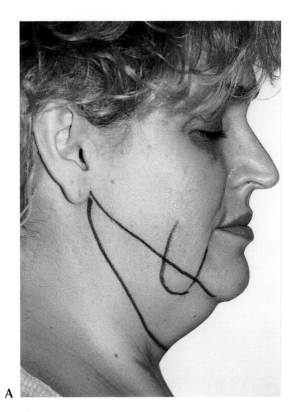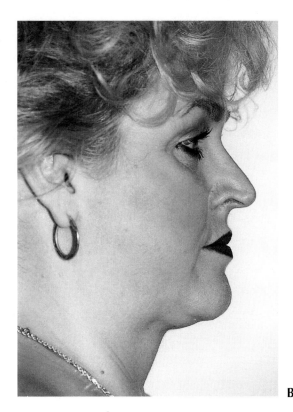

A   B

Figure 16-12 (*A*) A patient marked before liposuction of the jowl and neck. (*B*) The same patient 6 months after liposuction.

Not only does the skin become wrinkled and redundant, but the subcutaneous soft tissue also involutes. The underlying SMAS, which is uniquely related to the skin of the face and neck by its fibrous septal attachments (containing the adipose tissue), becomes stretched, losing its tone and elasticity. Therefore, advanced cosmetic surgical interventions not only mobilize and remove excess skin but also shorten and strengthen the underlying SMAS (see Chap. 17). It does appear, however, that early correction of sagging by the closed technique, using facial liposuction with a small cannula, yields exceptional results by causing wound contraction, producing a certain amount of skin tightening with healing (Figs.16-12 to 16-15).[16]

Body Liposuction

Before the procedure, the patient is marked in the standing position, with a surgical pen outlining the areas to be sculpted (Fig. 16-16). It is important to mark the patient while he or she is standing because positional changes can accentuate or minimize dimples or push fat and dimples in different directions, leading to incorrect intraoperative sculpting. Different marking methods are adopted by different physicians. Regardless of the method, the marking should be consistent and should outline the "hills" and "valleys," as well as danger zones and dimple areas of the cosmetic unit (see Chap. 7). Circles or ovals are drawn around the fat pads, with long, continuous lines to outline the areas to be feathered to avoid

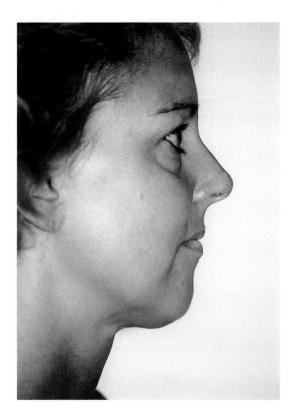

Figure 16-13 A patient marked in Fig. 16-7 seen 6 months after liposuction.

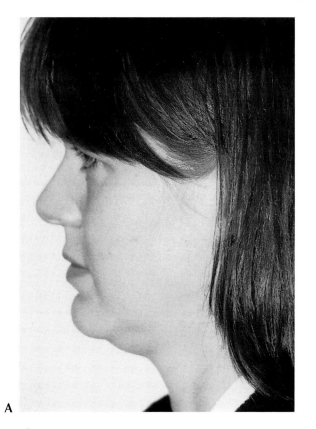
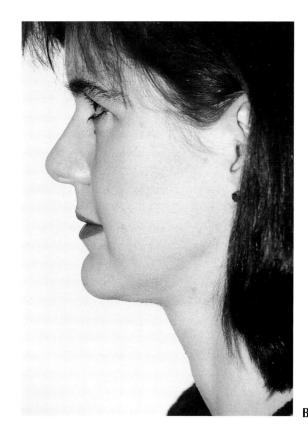

Figure 16-14 (*A*) Before neck and jowl liposuction. (*B*) After neck and jowl liposuction.

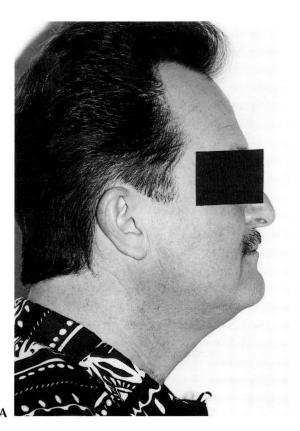
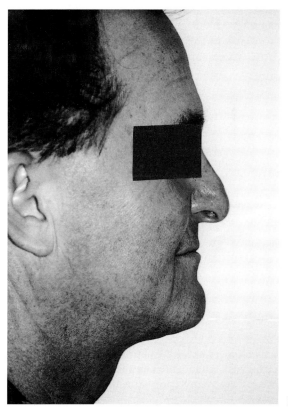

Figure 16-15 (*A*) Before neck liposuction. (*B*) After neck liposuction.

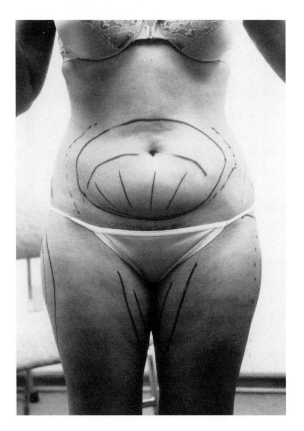

Figure 16-16   The patient is marked in the standing position for lower abdomen and outer and inner thighs. The dashed lines represent areas to undergo peripheral meshing. The solid lines indicate the discrete fat pads.

Local anesthesia consisting of 1% lidocaine with epinephrine is infiltrated into the epidermis over the incisions. A no.15 blade is then used to puncture, in a tangential direction, the skin adjacent to the body areas to be treated. With the "showerhead" infiltrating cannula, the tumescent fluid is infused into the areas to be treated at the same time, allowing pretunneling and hydrodissection and disrupting the fatty lobules (Fig. 16-21).

The sculpting is carried out with the cannula connected either to a syringe or to the tubing of a continuous suction machine. The cannula port is usually turned down toward the deep tissues except when liposuction is performed under the nipple or umbilicus. The surgeon's dominant or "power" hand drives the cannula in a radial criss-cross, "spoke-wheel" pattern with long in-and-out movements, first in the deep levels and then in the more superficial ones (Fig. 16-22). Some surgeons use smaller-diameter cannulae at the superficial levels. The nondominant hand is used as an ever-present guide to help stretch the skin evenly over the liposuction area. The nondominant or "smart" hand helps confirm the correct placement of the cannula tip as well as intermittently

a sharp drop-off between the treated and the surrounding untreated skin (Figs. 16-17 and 16-18). The highest points are outlined with an inner circle, and the incisions are marked by circles of about one-quarter inch. The valleys are outlined as dashes. This outlining is performed before the patient is brought to the surgical suite and allows for a last-minute review with the patient of the areas to be treated and the incision or entrance sites (Fig. 16-19).

The patient is brought into the operation room or other office-based surgical area and IV access is established. The patient is scrubbed with a povidone-iodine solution (Fig.16-20) and transferred onto a table draped in sterile fashion, generally in the supine position. With proper assistance, all areas of the body can be reached without moving the patient into a prone position.

The photographs of the patient's preliposuction contour are positioned and mounted for the surgeon's easy reference and the patient is connected to the monitoring equipment. If conscious sedation is used, it is administered via the IV line at this point.[8] The patient generally receives intraoperative IV antibiotics prophylactically.

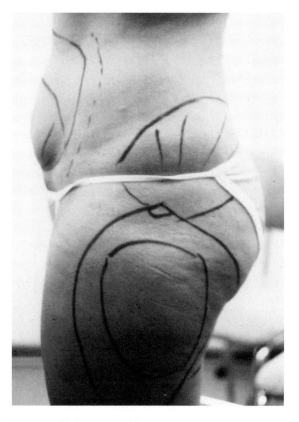

Figure 16-17   The patient in Fig. 16-16 in the lateral view. The solid circle within the greater circle or lateral thigh indicates the maximum amount of fat. The smaller circle between the thigh and high hips is the entry point for both sites for liposuction.

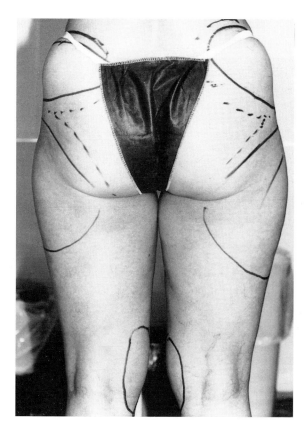

Figure 16-18 Marking representing the avoidance of the "Bermuda triangle" while still accomplishing some liposuction of the buttock, lateral thigh and knee.

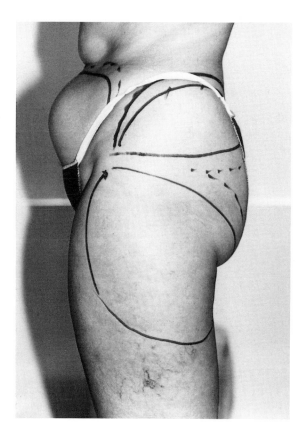

Figure 16-19 Marking representing the handling of this liposuction procedure as dictated by the cosmetic unit of the abdomen, high hips, buttock, upper and outer thigh.

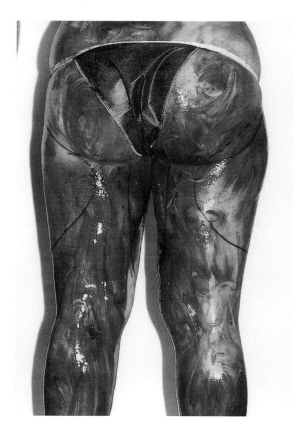

Figure 16-20 A patient fully scrubbed with povidone-iodine before a liposuction procedure.

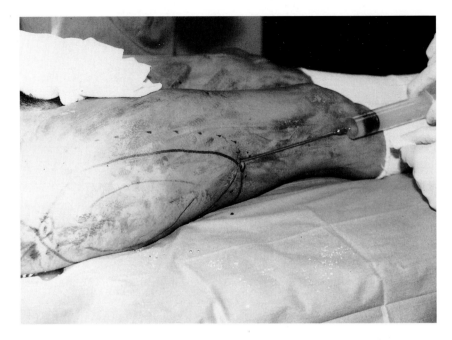

Figure 16-21 The manual infiltration of tumescent anesthesia as opposed to the use of expensive pressure or mechanical devices and tubing.

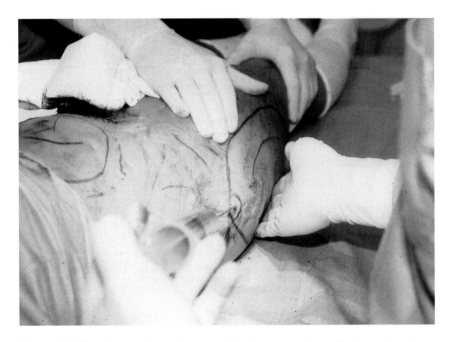

Figure 16-22 Liposuction under way, with the surgeon's nondominant hand as a guide placed on the skin, which helps confirm the correct placement of cannula. The trabeculation of the liposuction is powered by the surgeon's dominant hand.

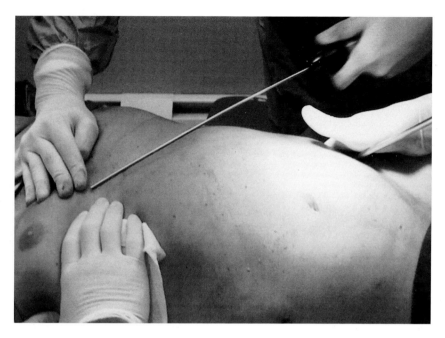

Figure 16-23 The surgeon's nonworking, nondominant hand validates proper placement and insertion of the cannula in the chest to avoid submuscular placement.

performing the pinch test, allowing the surgeon to verify the degree of subcutaneous fat remaining (Fig. 16-23).

To achieve uniform removal of adipose tissue, tunneling is generally created by treating the same area from two different ports, which allows a criss-cross overlap of the treated area. Tunneling straight in and withdrawing straight out is done in long strokes. Each stroke is redirected into a different track along the same plane within the layer of fat, almost as if elevating a flap yet leaving some fibrous septa intact. Wrist movements with short strokes can create the sense of movement of the cannula and, in fact, may result in the overtreatment of a singular site. Arching by lifting the cannula while pushing it further into the fat should also be avoided unless one is certain that the cannula is not traversing into other fat planes penetrating deeper structures.

Although some surgeons use cannulae that are no greater than 3-mm gauge, we find 4- or 6-mm gauge cannulae when performing liposuction on the body in the deep planes to be quite effective.

Feathering of the edges is performed by simply meshing the fat beyond the marked skin areas, without cannula suction or with the syringe's plunger only partially withdrawn for milder vacuum pressure. This breaks down the surrounding fat, allowing for a more uniform contour with the avoidance of a "cliff drop" deformity after liposuction. Suturing of the incision sites is accomplished with 4.0 absorbable suture with a reverse-cutting P2 needle, and the appropriate garment is applied. The technique as presented here is essen-

tially the same for each cosmetic unit treated. Our standard liposuction tray appears in Fig. 16-24.

THIGHS AND BUTTOCKS

The thighs and buttocks are examined in the standing position. Each area of the thighs and buttocks should be evaluated from the lateral, medial, anterior, and posterior directions, with the surgeon's eye at the same level as the area to be corrected. A common complaint in women is cellulite over the thighs and buttocks. It is important to stress to the patient that liposuction will not improve this condition.

The lateral outer thigh, the "saddlebag area," is of most common concern to women. Ideally, the female outer thigh should conform to a single smooth curve. This curve begins at the waist, curves over the iliac crest and greater trochanter, and terminates at the knee.[18]

The lateral thighs tend to become heavy some time after puberty, usually in the late teens to mid-thirties. This can result in significant topographic discrepancies between the upper and lower parts of the body—a condition that can significantly benefit from liposuction (Figs. 16-25 to 16-27). In other patients, the body habitus is relatively balanced; however, the upper posterior lateral thigh along with the inner thigh and outer buttocks seem to be unresponsive to diet and exercise (Fig. 16-28). These patients are greatly aided with liposuction of the outer and inner thigh (Figs. 16-28 and 16-29).

(text continues on page 269)

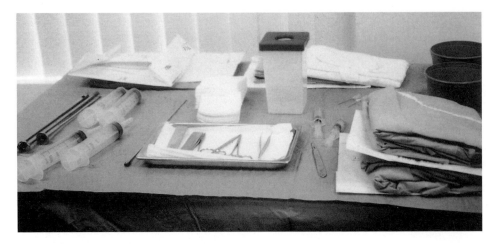

Figure 16-24   The standard setup for syringe assisted liposuction.

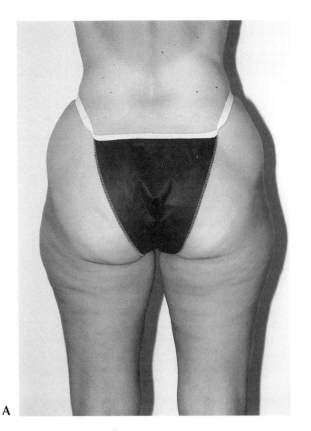

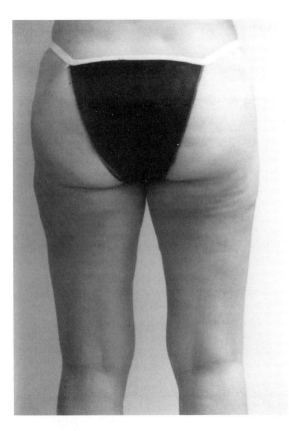

A

B

Figure 16-25   (**A**) Before liposuction. Note the discrepancy between girth of the waist and that of the buttock and thigh. This is sometimes termed the *violin deformity.* (**B**) The same patient after liposuction. Note the much more balanced upper trunk and lower body.

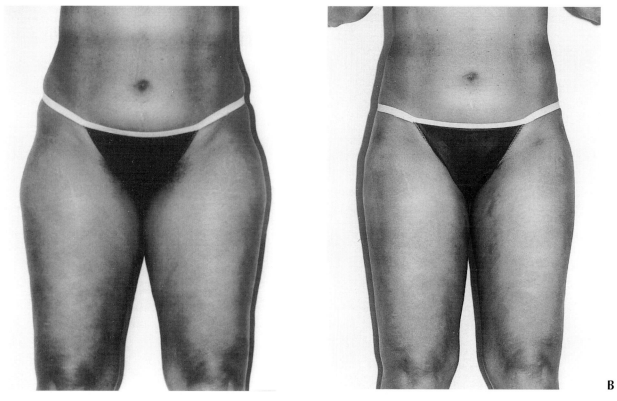

A   B

Figure 16-26   (*A*) Before liposuction. Note the discrepancy in balance between waist, high hips and lateral thighs. (*B*) After liposuction. Note the nice balance, establishing a harmonious silhouette.

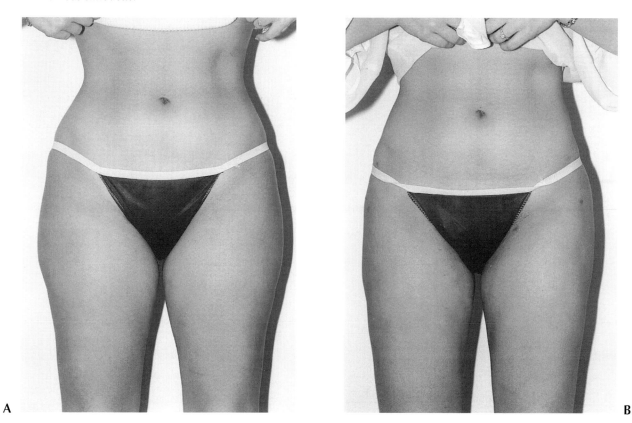

A   B

Figure 16-27   (*A*) Before liposuction. Note the narrow waist and the square lower cosmetic unit. (*B*) After liposuction, a more balanced contour is noticed.

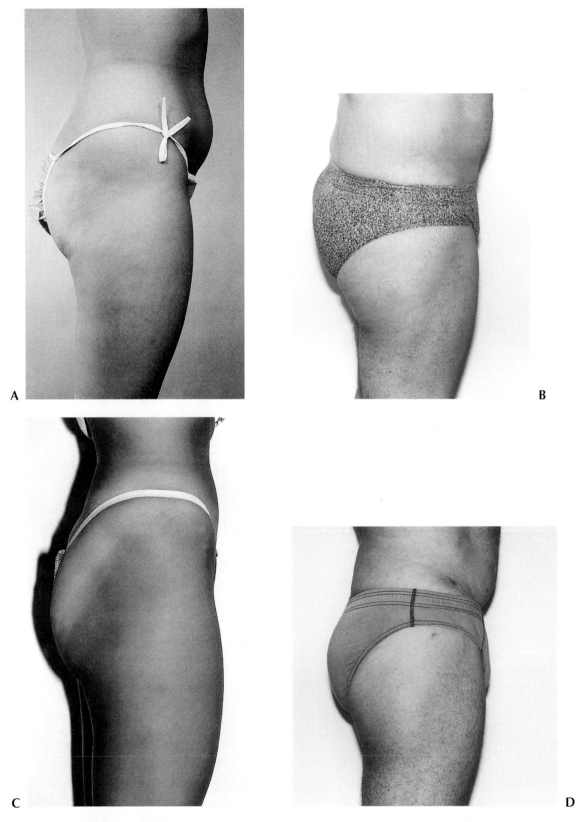

Figure 16-28   (*A* and *B*) Before liposuction. Note the relatively balanced habitus except for the fat pads prominent on the upper posterior thigh to the buttock "banana fold" region. (*C* and *D*) After liposuction. The simple elimination of the pads for the thigh and buttock fold produces a balanced silhouette.

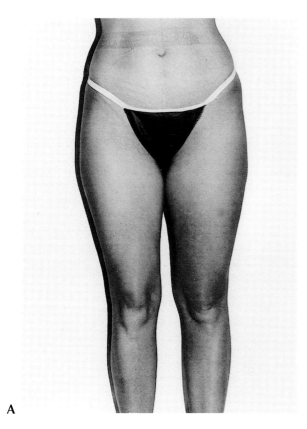 A

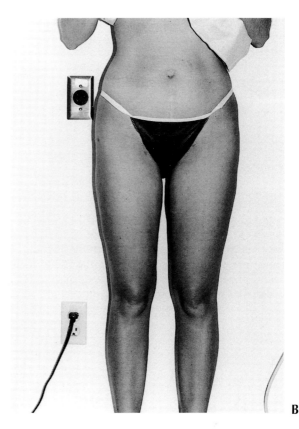 B

Figure 16-29 (**A**) Before liposuction. The cosmetic unit of the lower trunk to midthigh is not in proportion; therefore, the high hips, buttocks, and lateral and inner thighs require liposuction to come into balance. (**B**) After liposuction. The form is now well balanced.

In suctioning the buttock, it is important to avoid the area termed the "Bermuda triangle." This area comprises the medial gluteal triangle, an equilateral triangle, with its base inferiorly at the infragluteal fold, its lateral edge at the lower posterior trochanters bilaterally, and its tip at the coccyx superiorly. Suctioning of this area may result in serious complications that produce not only an unnaturally appearing buttock but also the possibility of neurologic injury.

An anterior projection of the medial thigh often represents muscle more than fat, and suction in this area can be very unforgiving. It should be approached only by those with extensive experience.

ABDOMEN AND FLANKS

The abdomen can be divided into upper and lower sections by an imaginary line passing between the iliac crests through or just above the umbilicus. It also can be divided by the linea alba into right and left mirror images. The outer limits of the abdomen are defined by the anatomic landmarks of the xiphoid and costal margins superiorly and pubis and

superior iliac spine connected through the inguinal ligament (Poupart's ligament) inferiorly. The fatty layer of the abdomen is bordered dorsally by the rectus abdominis fascia, external oblique and internal oblique aponeurosis, and rectus abdominis muscle dorsomedially. It originates from the fifth to eighth ribs and extends down to the pubis.

The upper half of the abdomen is composed of a superficial fatty layer, often somewhat fibrous in nature, and is usually less extensive in having a localized fat deposit. The lower half of the abdomen contains the bulk of localized fat, but the appearance of size may be skewed. Caution must be used in the lower abdomen because of the superficial epigastric artery, which originates from the femoral artery and courses bilaterally within the superficial fascia of the rectus abdominis muscle over the inferior anterolateral abdominal wall toward the umbilicus.

Generally, two incision sites (1 to 1.5 cm) are placed just superior to the mons pubis.[19] Some use four incision sites, two midline and superiorly to Poupart's ligament and the other two at about the level of the sixth rib over the border of the rectus muscle.[20]

The abdomen as a region can be resistant to diet and exercise, and the surgeon must determine the appropriate technique for dealing with it. Reduction by liposuction can vary from a finesse case to a staged bulk removal of tissue. Various pre- and postoperative photographs demonstrate the varied results that are attainable (Figs. 16-30 to 16-35).

It has been our experience that male fat is generally more fibrous, especially in the upper and lower abdomen, and liposuction therefore more difficult. However, a significant improvement can be attained in appropriately selected patients (Figs. 16-36 and 16-37).

The lateral flanks are extremely responsive to liposuction in both men and women. This area is referred to as "love handles" by men and "high hips" by women. Here the subcutaneous fat overlies the external oblique muscle and its fascia.

It is important to treat this area with the abdomen as a cosmetic unit. At the inferior border of the lateral flanks is the lateral gluteal depression. It may be seen in some patients as a deep concavity. It is formed by the connections between the superficial and deep muscular fascia systems. This area

may easily shift during liposuction and must be marked before the procedure with the patient in the standing position. To reach the dorsal extension of the waist, the patient should be turned to the lateral decubitus position and the liposuction extended to near the posterior midline (Figs. 16-38 and 16-39).

GYNECOMASTIA

Gynecomastia may represent a hypertrophy of the mammary glands (true gynecomastia) or localized fat deposits (pseudogynecomastia), but it usually represents a combination of hypertrophied fat and glandular tissue. It may be seen in up to 70 percent of pubescent boys, with peak incidence at age 14. In the majority of cases, it resolves in 1 to 2 years. Gynecomastia may be found in one-third of men, and most cases are idiopathic.[21–23] Still, it is important to have the patient examined by his or her family physician for the presence of endocrine diseases (e.g., thyroid, pituitary),

(text continues on page 275)

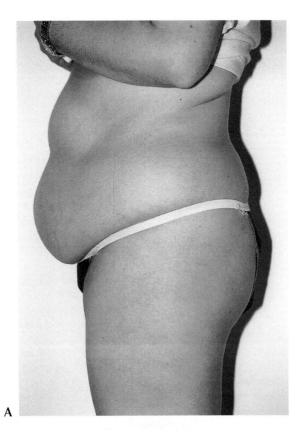
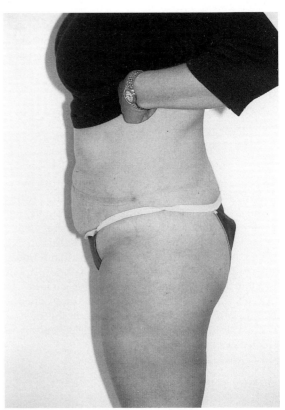

A   B

Figure 16-30   (*A*) The abdomen as a cosmetic unit, in this case, requires the fullness of the lower abdomen to be balanced with the upper abdomen as well as with the contiguous high hips. (*B*) After liposuction. The approach of dealing in cosmetic units (see Chap. 7) allows for quite a transformation in shape.

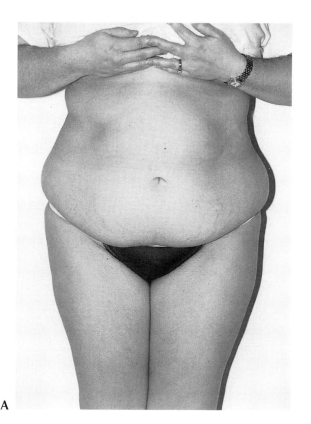
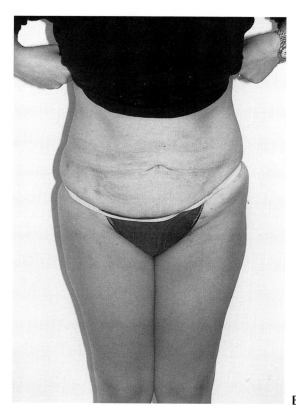

A

B

Figure 16-31 (*A*) In certain cases, it is apparent before liposuction that a procedure must be staged because we prefer to stay within the bounds of 5000 mL of total volume removed. Therefore, in this case, the cosmetic unit of the lower waist and high hips was treated as the first stage. (*B*) After liposuction. A dramatic reduction of the treated area is noted. The patient is scheduled next for liposuction of the upper buttock and inner and lateral thighs.

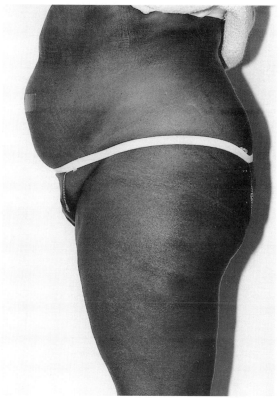
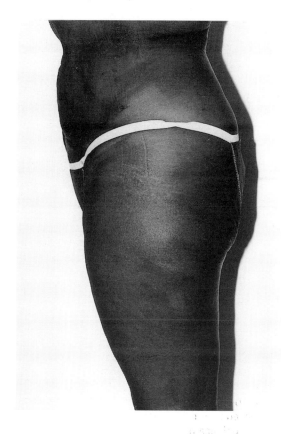

A

B

Figure 16-32 (*A*) Before liposuction. (*B*) After liposuction.

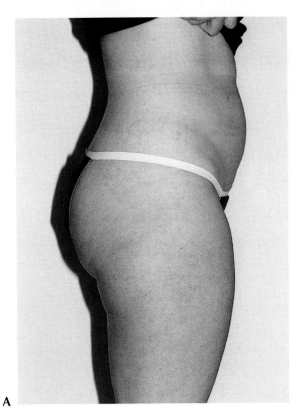
A

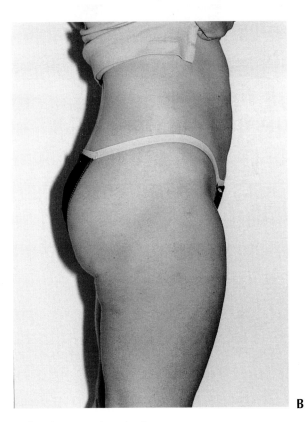
B

Figure 16-33 (*A*) Before liposuction. The lateral view demonstrates that the cosmetic unit of the thigh and buttock region (as well as the lower abdomen) is poorly balanced. (*B*) After liposuction. The area of the "banana fold" into the lateral thigh, as well as the lower abdomen into the high hips, was addressed, leading to a much more youthful-looking android habitus.

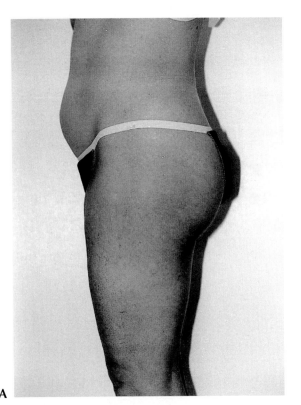
A

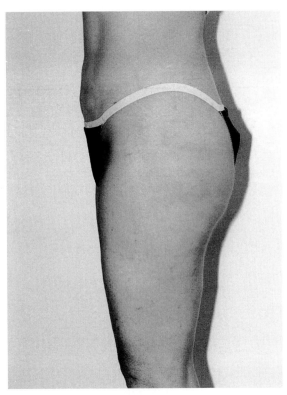
B

Figure 16-34 (*A*) Before liposuction. The cosmetic unit of abdomen to high hip was more pronounced than that in Fig. 16-33*A*. (*B*) After liposuction. The concentration on the upper cosmetic unit again creates the more favored android form (see Chap. 7).

272

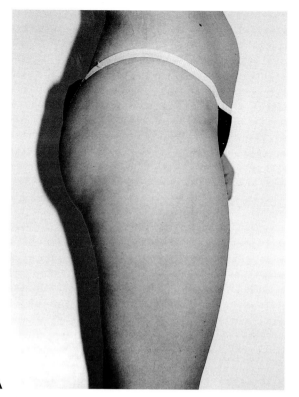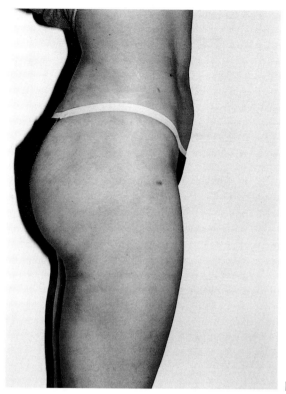

A
B

Figure 16-35 (*A*) Before liposuction. The buttock appears high and poorly rounded. The approach here requires a consideration of abdomen and high hip unit along with the thigh-buttock cosmetic unit. (*B*) After liposuction. The approach outlined creates a "lower" buttock that is sharply marginated and has a well-proportioned contour.

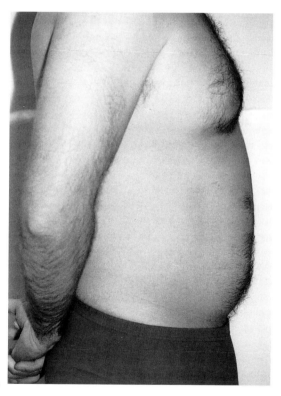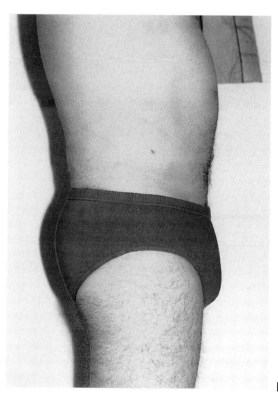

A
B

Figure 16-36 (*A*) Before liposuction in a man. Men usually have a more rounded abdomen with a less marked upper and lower division, as seen in many women. One must use the pinch test to be certain that the fat resides in the subcutaneous plane and not in the omental space (see Chap. 7). (*B*) After liposuction. An excellent result can be achieved if the fat lies in the appropriate plane. The pinch test before liposuction aids the surgeon in predicting and relating the probable results to the patient.

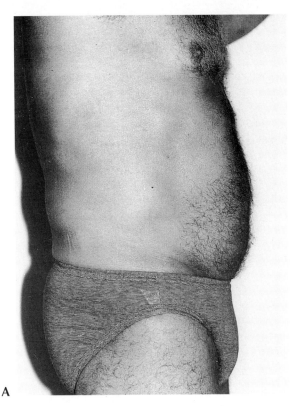
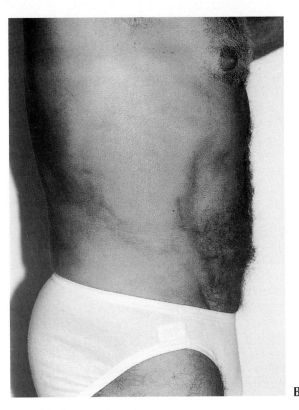

A

B

Figure 16-37 (*A*) Before liposuction. The cosmetic unit to be treated is the complex of the abdomen and high hips. (*B*) After liposuction. The improvement in shape and girth of the abdomen and waist is apparent.

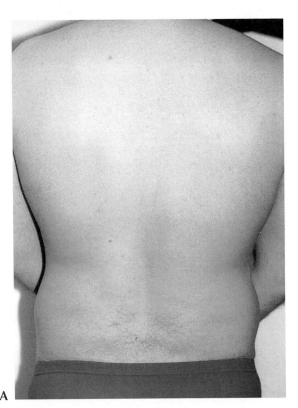
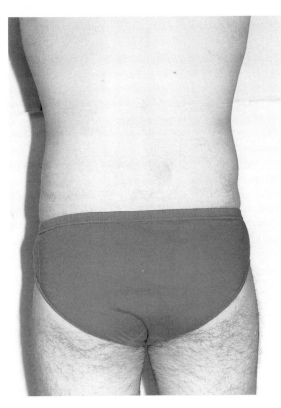

A

B

Figure 16-38 (*A*) Before liposuction. In this patient, the "love handles" have made the cosmetic unit of the waist to appear greater than the android trochanteric dimension, greatly reducing contour. (*B*) After liposuction. The contour is returned to balance as the waist cuts in and is smaller in diameter than the trochanteric and lateral thigh dimension.

274

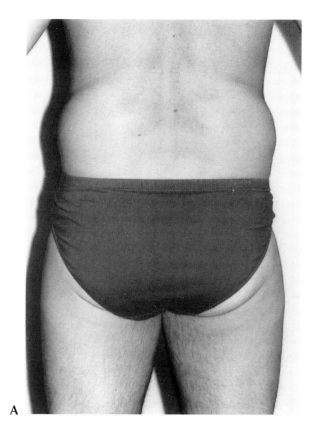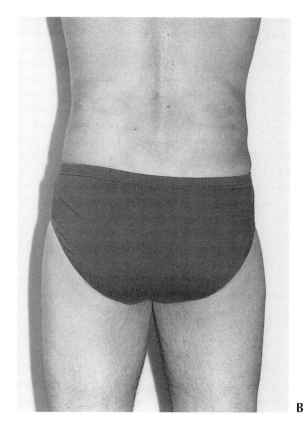

Figure 16-39 (*A*) Before liposuction. This patient is similar to the one shown in Fig. 16-38. (*B*) After liposuction. There is improved balance.

gonadal diseases (e.g., Klinefelter's syndrome), liver diseases (e.g., cirrhosis), malignant diseases (e.g., gonadal, adrenal, breast), or medication intake (e.g., hormones, antiepileptic agents). A thorough breast examination should also be performed by the surgeon with specific attention to the quality of the breast tissue, because diffuse softness corresponds to fat and can be approached with liposuction but localized, unilateral, fixed hard masses may need mammography or sonography for the presence of tumor along with possible biopsy.

Marking is done with the patient in the sitting or standing position. The extent of the gynecomastia is marked medially and laterally with the pectoralis muscle flexed and relaxed to help outline the liposuction boundaries. Access incisions can be made in the periareolar, inframammary, or axillary folds. We use a 4- to 6-mm cannula attached to a 60-mL syringe, which is introduced through the incision. The dissection is carried out in a spoke-wheel pattern. The cannula port is maintained in a downward direction except beneath the areola, where the port is turned upward to remove the subareolar tissue. A vest garment is worn by the patient

for approximately 4 weeks after the procedure.[23] Occasionally, the glandular component underneath the nipple is too fibrosed to be completely removed by liposuction alone. In such an event, the glandular component may be surgically excised after the liposuction procedure through a small periareolar incision.[24] When properly performed, liposuction of this area is quite gratifying to the patient (Fig.16-40).

ARMS

Anatomy and Danger Zones

The most often treated subunit is the posterior humeral area overlying the triceps. This area extends from the axilla to the olecranon. Tumescence creates a distance from most neurovascular bundles, but injury can still occur. Still, there are a few important structures that course outside of the muscular fascia in the deep fat layer which, and in muscular patients or with the use of a tourniquet, can be easily viewed through the skin. They include the basilic vein (a branch of the subclavian vein that exits the fascia three-quarters of the way distal on the biceps brachia) and the cephalic vein (which

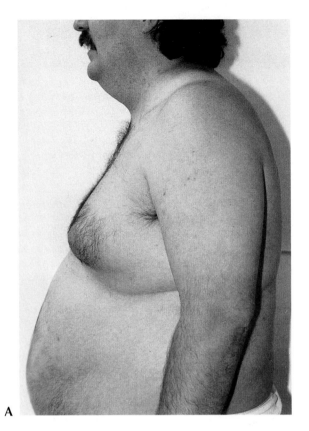

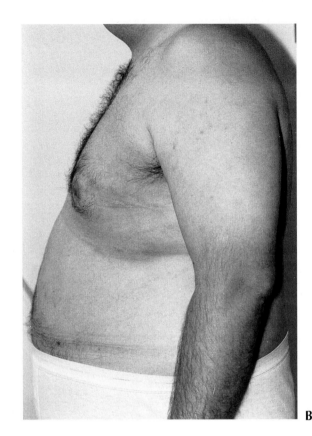

A B

Figure 16-40 (*A*) Before liposuction. This patient had bilateral breast enlargement, but his hormone evaluation was normal. However, because of a history of breast carcinoma in the family, a mammogram was performed, showing the specimen to be made up of normal adipose tissue. (*B*) After liposuction. A great reduction in mass is apparent. It is common to have a residual fibrosed breast bud; if this is problematic, a simple excision will remove this in a relatively bloodless field after healing from the liposuction procedure.

courses laterally and superiorly to the brachial fascia). Both can be tracked from the antecubital fossa medially when a tourniquet is applied. The brachial artery lies deeper to the basilic vein and is separated from the superficial fat by the muscular fascia in a sulcus between the biceps and triceps.

The medial antebrachial cutaneous nerve of the forearm originates in the medial cord of the brachial plexus and receives fibers from C8 and T1. It runs down the arm on the medial side of the brachial artery side by side with the basilic vein; it pierces the deep fascia in the cubital fosssa with the basilic vein and runs along the medial aspect of forearm, supplying the medial skin of the arm. The radial, ulnar, and median nerves all hug the humerus. The ulnar nerve becomes vulnerable only at the elbow (posterior to the medial epicondyle). The lymphatics course throughout the arm, with the superficial lymphatics concentrating around the basilic vein.[25]

The best way to evaluate the arms for fat and skin laxity is by having the patient raise his or her arms to 90 degrees with his or her body and bend the elbows upward. While in

this position, the "hanging portion" (lower third) of the arm is assessed for adiposity by the pinch test. In the youthful, well-proportioned arm, the ratio of the anterior to the posterior arm has been described as the coefficient of Hoyer.[26]

Some believe that the posterior arm skin can undergo significant retraction if vigorous liposuction of the posterior arm fat is achieved and that poor skin contour and contraction are caused by overly conservative fat removal.[27] However, caution is advised. The utilization of the pinch test in this setting is also helpful in determining skin flaccidity; if the skin does not retract at all, brachioplasty may be the only remedy.

Generally, the liposuction incision site is proximal to the elbow. Depending on the volume of fat, the cannulae may range from 3 to 6 mm. Some authors prefer specialized cannula with a bent swan-neck keel (3.7 mm, 30 cm long) and advocate multiple small incisions, as many as needed, to allow thorough, aggressive fat removal in all angles.[27] We have not found this to be an advantage.

The medial epicondylar fat pad may become more prominent after the surrounding fat is removed, and it is prudent to address it from the start. At this area, immediately proximal to the elbow, one often encounters fibrous fat; here, maneuvers using the "smart hand" to determine the extent of fat removal assist in achieving a more uniform liposuction.[27] The delicate zone of upper arm fat adjacent to the axillary fold must be cautiously yet adequately treated to ensure a good contour. The skin of the upper anterior arm is very thin and, as with the anterior upper thighs, should be approached only with extensive experience. In this region, treatment should be very conservative so as to avoid creating deformities (Fig. 16-41).

KNEES

Knee recontouring is ideally suited to an outpatient setting and can be done primarily under local anesthesia. Age is rarely a consideration in determining patient suitability, because the limited scope of knee recontouring produces little physiologic stress on the body, and excess skin over the inner and outer knee surfaces is virtually nonexistent. However, caution in this area is warranted. Despite good technique, the potential for excessive skin contraction overlying the genicular saphenous lymphatic drainage channel may rarely result in persistent low-grade edema of the foot. Even so, older patients who complain of their knees rubbing together when walking and younger individuals who complain of chubby knees can therefore be treated with equal success. Also, genu valgum, or "knock knee," can be esthetically improved with this relatively simple procedure.

The rate of healing after liposuction tends to be slower in the extremities than on the face, neck, and trunk. This differential must be taken into account in patient selection, instrumentation, wound care instruction, and limiting postoperative activities as well as estimating the time necessary to see results. Knee liposuction is aimed primarily at removing the bulge at the inner knee, which usually becomes unapparent in the seated position and may reduce to a mild concavity. Therefore it is important to examine the patient in both the standing and seated positions while applying the pinch test to the localized fat deposit of the medial knee. An over-aggressive approach here may create undesirable dimpling when the patient is seated. In addition, what may appear to be a baggy bulge above the knee in the standing position usually takes on a smooth and well-contoured form in the seated, flexed position. Therefore liposuction above the knee in the suprapatellar zone calls for extreme caution and is usually best avoided.

The major portion of the knee's localized fat deposits overlie the medial tibial plateau and may extend upward to the distal third of the inner thigh. In heavier patients, there is often extension downward to the anteromedian aspect of the leg, the medial-posterior popliteal zone, and a localized fat deposit can sometimes exist over the lateral knee. The patient must understand that the patella and the width of the tibial plateau contribute greatly to the contour of the knee and that the overlying fat is all that can be changed. Therefore the patient's expectations must be realistic, even though a substantial improvement can be achieved in most cases (Figs. 16-42 to 16-46).[28,29]

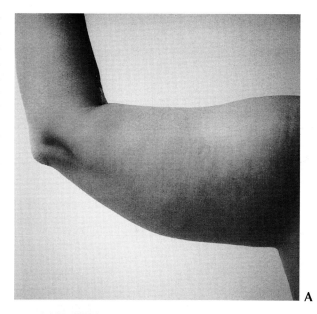

A

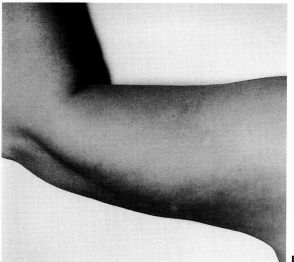

B

Figure 16-41 (*A*) Before liposuction. The medial epicondial fat pad was this patient's primary concern, but the patient's girth was an issue for the surgery team. (*B*) After liposuction. A definitive reduction in fat at the elbow was acomplished but the slope from elbow to axilla was made more linear.

CALVES AND ANKLES

The first recorded attempt to treat the legs was made by a French physician in the 1920s, who curetted the fat off the leg of a ballerina. It resulted in arterial damage that necessitated leg amputation. Today the area can be addressed with a good cosmetic outcome similar to that in the other areas mentioned.

In evaluating the calves and ankles, one must perform the pinch test to differentiate between musculoskeletal and

(text continues on page 281)

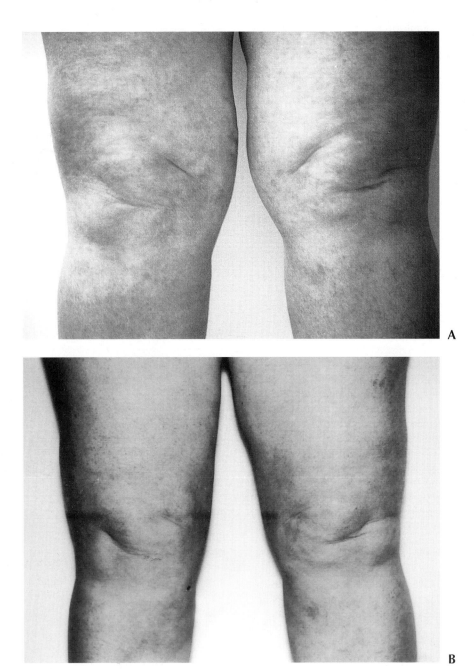

Figure 16-42   (*A*) Before liposuction. This patient complained that her knees rubbed together. A significant bulge was still present when the patient was seated. (*B*) After liposuction. There is now a nice contour in both the standing and seated positions.

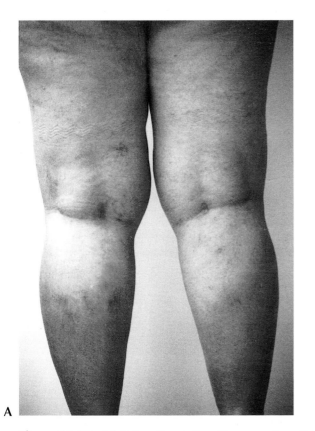
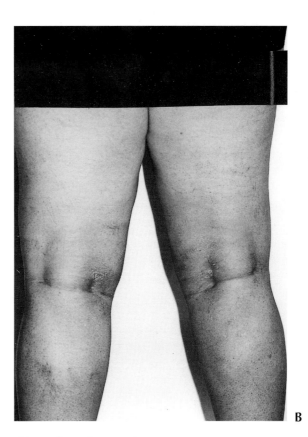

A   B

Figure 16-43   (**A**) Before liposuction. The cosmetic unit to be addressed was the complex
of the medial thigh and knee. (**B**) After liposuction. The cosmetic unit has a much more
linear, balanced appearance.

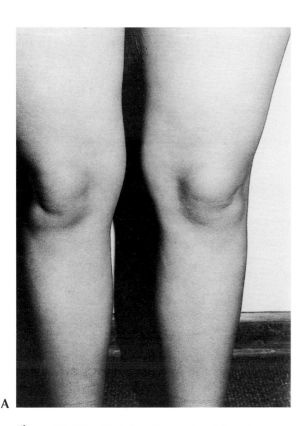
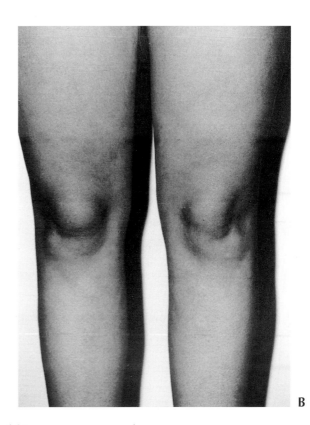

A   B

Figure 16-44   (**A**) Before liposuction. The primary concern of this young woman was her
"chubby knees." (**B**) After liposuction. A balanced cosmetic unit from the knee through inner
thighs has been achieved.

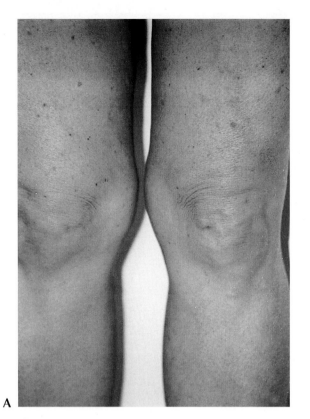
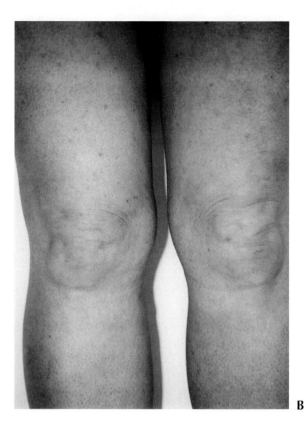

A   B

Figure 16-45 (*A*) Before liposuction. The knee has a prominent fat pad; however, the areas above and below the cosmetic units are quite linear. (*B*) After liposuction. The bulges have been reduced without producing a straight line from inner thigh to ankle.

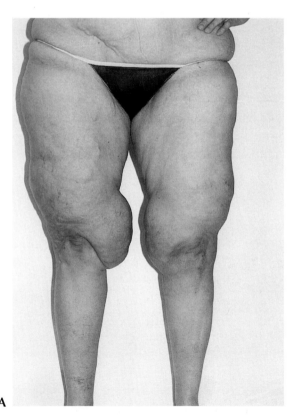
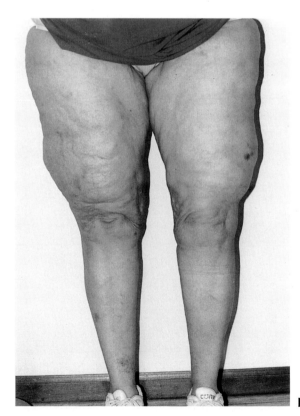

A   B

Figure 16-46 (*A*) Before liposuction. A pronounced lipodystrophy existed, and the patient's major concern was wearing a dress. (*B*) After liposuction. The inner thigh–knee complex is greatly improved.

turning posteromedially to the knee, running laterally to the outline of the gastrocnemius muscle, and winding anteriorly to the medial malleolus. The saphenous nerve joins the superficial course of the greater saphenous vein over the crural fascia in the superficial fat, below the medial knee area, and down to and including the ankle region. The superficial peroneal nerve exits the crural fascia and becomes vulnerable around the ankle area anterior to the lateral malleolus. Therefore, surgeons who perform liposuction must be experienced in approaching these areas. However, after these areas are properly treated, the results can be excellent (Figs. 16-47 and 16-48).

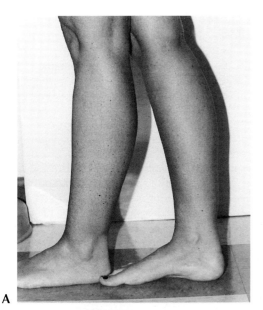

A

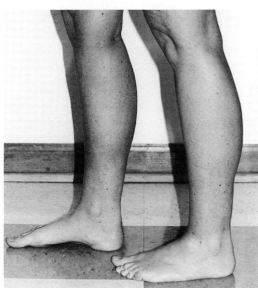

B

Figure 16-47 (**A**) Before liposuction. Note the "stovepipe" deformity at the lower calf and ankles. (**B**) After liposuction.

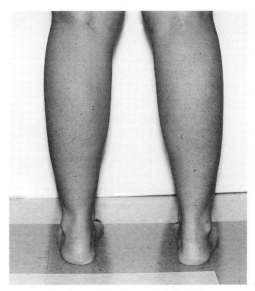

A

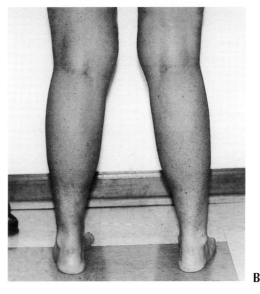

B

Figure 16-48 (**A**) Before liposuction. Posterior view of "stovepipe" preoperatively. (**B**) After liposuction. Posterior view of the area corrected by liposuction.

fat hypertrophy. The area is evaluated in the standing position, and the patient is asked to contract the calf muscles so the surgeon can better assess the contribution of muscle hypertrophy to the shape of the legs. Although most neurovascular bundles travel underneath the investing fascia of the calves and ankles, three danger areas should be avoided. The small saphenous vein exits the crural fascia at the distal end of the popliteal fossa; it runs in the midline of the posterior calf along with the sural nerve, over the crural fascia in the superficial fat, turning laterally to the Achilles' tendon, and winding behind the lateral malleolus. The greater saphenous vein runs along the medial thigh over the fascia lata,

At our facilities over the past 15 years, the syringe-assisted approach has been extremely effective. For physicians initiating a new practice, initial costs are greatly diminished, obviating the need for costly vacuum equipment and tubing. In our opinion, this overall simplification, along with greater control over the extraction process, favors the syringe-assisted liposuction technique.

Complications

SYSTEMIC COMPLICATIONS

Death

Although imperfect, surveys performed to assess the fatality rate from liposuction have revealed a higher number of deaths than those due to automobile accidents.[30] Fatality rates reported range from 0 percent,[31,32] 0.002 percent,[33] and 0.003 percent[34] to as high as 0.02 percent.[30,35] Some causes of death, such as anoxia secondary to inappropriate anesthesia, are indirectly related to liposuction.[31] Some deaths are related to severe pulmonary edema caused by fluid overload, incurred by patients receiving blood transfusions and fluid replacements in the hospital after a hemoglobin drop, from 12 to 6, following liposuction.[7]

The surgical dermatologic literature has not reported deaths from liposuction surgery; plastic surgeons, on the other hand, have a record of an extremely high death rate, as fatalities are reported to occur in 1 of 5000 patients undergoing liposuction in the hands of this group.[36]

The leading causes of death from liposuction include pulmonary emboli, perforated viscus, lidocaine toxicity, and hemorrhage (see below), accounting in a recent study[30] for 23 to 32 percent, 15 to 20 percent, 10 to 14 percent, and 5 to 7 percent, respectively. Others attribute these complications to the combination of multiple procedures in one session, thus prolonging operating time and increasing the likelihood of the mentioned side effects. Our experience, using conscious sedation along with tumescent anesthesia in 6000 patients, has been excellent, without a need for transfusion or hospitalization. The keys to safety lie in patient selection, conservative goals for total aspirate, short operative time, and proper technique.

Infection

Although some suggest that the tumescent anesthesia (specifically, lidocaine at 0.05% concentration) is bacteriostatic,[37] an effect augmented by bicarbonate, others fail to show such an effect.[38] It is likely related to the size of the bacterial inoculum and should not be relied on. A rate of 0.02 to 0.34 percent of postoperative infection was found in a retrospective questioner-based study (only 4 percent of polled doctors responded).[32] Another reported a 0.4 percent injection rate; this included cases in which an open procedure was combined with liposuction.[39]

Deaths and serious sequelae are possible from infection associated with liposuction. In a survey of the American Society of Aesthetic Plastic Surgery (ASAPS),[30] 7 of 93 (7.5 percent) deaths revealed in patients undergoing liposuction (some along with other procedures such as abdominoplasty) were due to massive infection, accounting for an overall rate of 0.001 percent. A review of the recent literature shows four cases of necrotizing fasciitis with disseminated intravascular coagulation (DIC) after liposuction,[40–42] one caused by intestinal perforation.[40] The other case resulted from contamination of the operative area, as is evident from the rapid postoperative symptom onset and culturing of *Staphylococcus aureus* from the wounds.[41] Toxic shock syndrome was clearly identified in two cases and associated with contamination of the surgical field[43] and, as suggested,[41] such contamination may well be involved in other reported infections. Although *S. aureus* is the most common organism, other organisms, such as *Mycobacterium fortuitum*,[44] should be suspected and proper coverage implemented after culturing is performed.

Meticulous attention to sterile perioperative technique as well as pre- and postoperative infection prophylaxis is of the utmost importance, but hospital-based liposuction is not the solution, because it, too, may be associated with serious infections.[42] In the event of an infection, early recognition is paramount. The early signs of a serious infection include severe pain out of proportion to the clinical finding as well as a foul-smelling or pus-containing discharge from the drainage sites, requiring an immediate response. The use of proper techniques, sterile fields, and prophylactic perioperative antibiotic agents is the best approach to avoiding infection.

Fat Emboli

The Task Force on Lipoplasty survey[35] revealed fat emboli to be responsible for 0.017 percent of deaths, almost matching thrombi as the cause of pulmonary embolus (six cases of thrombus and five cases of fat emboli).

Fat embolism syndrome (FES) causes acute respiratory distress syndrome (ARDS) and is different from pulmonary embolism. It was most commonly reported in cases where liposuction was combined with an open procedure such as abdominoplasty. In our review of the literature, it has been reported only in cases performed before 1990. FES may occur after a mechanical trauma to the bone marrow or could, as some believe, be caused by inflammatory mediators released in response to free fatty acids.

Pulmonary Emboli

The risk of pulmonary embolus (PE) in patients with deep venous thrombosis (DVT) is estimated to be between 0.07 and 8.0 percent. In patients at high risk (e.g., those with any of the following: age older than 40 years, male gender, obesity, history of malignancy, previous DVT, surgery >2 h, nephrotic syndrome, systemic lupus erythematosus, history of drug abuse, protein S/C deficiency), the incidence of DVT may be as high as 60 percent. In most cases, PE is asymptomatic and occurs in the perioperative period.[45] Teimourian has reported five cases.[15] All were performed before 1983 without tumescence; three were liposuction alone and two were liposuction combined with abdominoplasty. The diagnosis was made by a lung scan, and the patients survived after treatment with warfarin. No similar problems have been seen since in 10,000 patients. A 54-year-old, 225-lb woman was reported to have died 18 h after liposuction under general anesthesia; her autopsy revealed saddle and distal PE from a left calf DVT.[7]

Perforated Viscus

Although often blunt, the cannula may penetrate deep tissue, either if it is very small (which requires less force than with a larger cannula), because of poor technique (by not following the cannula tip with the nondominant hand), or by passing through adhesions from prior surgery or hernias. Reported perforations include multiple penetrations of the small intestine,[46] bilateral lacerations of the lumbar artery with secondary hemorrhage, and hemodynamic instability.[47]

Cardiovascular

Left bundle branch block (LBBB) discovered intraoperatively should lead to termination of the procedure. In the reported instance, the patient's recovery in the hospital was uneventful; the cardiologist believed that the LBBB was an idiosyncratic reaction.[31]

Blood Loss

Continuous bleeding at the incision site caused by an undisclosed known bleeding diathesis in a patient with normal preoperative bleeding studies has been reported.[31] It should be considered in the differential of a patient with hemodynamic instability; the source may be hidden.[47]

Before tumescent liposuction, blood loss accounted for about 45 percent of total aspirated fluid (includes estimated loss in tissue and in the aspirate, the latter ranging between 15 and 35 percent).[48] In our experience, the blood loss with the tumescent technique is minimal, usually ranging at 5 to 10 percent of the total aspirate (Fig. 16-49), with some report-

ing even lower rates of 1 to 2 percent.[49] With a more prolonged procedure, the likelihood of a greater blood aspirate increases as the effect of epinephrine in the tumescent fluid subsides. If the blood loss is expected or found to exceed 25 percent of the patient's estimated blood volume, transfusion should be considered.

Lidocaine Toxicity

Signs of toxic blood lidocaine levels begin as subjective changes (e.g., paresthesias, metallic taste in mouth, talkativeness). These signs progress to objective ones such as slurred speech, nausea and vomiting, and muscle twitching at 5 to 8 mg/dL. Then seizures and cardiomyopathy occur at 8 to 12 mg/dL, eventuating in coma and, finally, respiratory and cardiac arrest at levels above 12 mg/dL. Therefore it is very important to monitor the patient, maintain IV access, and follow up with the patient in the recovery period. In a recent survey,[7] two of four patients were presumed to die from elevated blood lidocaine levels. One had blood levels of 5.2 mg/L (but likely had a perforation, perhaps through an appendectomy scar, because the level of lidocaine in peritoneal fluid was 17 mg/L). The other had a lidocaine level of only 2 mg/L, with immediate desaturation upon being turned supine. Another patient, who died 13 h after liposuction, had a blood lidocaine level of 14 mg/L. The rate of infusion, as well as the vascularity of the infused area, is directly correlated with the rate of systemic absorption. Peak lidocaine levels range between 12 and 24 h for body and 4 and 5 h for face tumescent anesthesia infiltration.[50] It is also important to factor in other medications, such as midazolam, in patients undergoing this elective procedure, because such medications may decrease the metabolic rate of lidocaine by the cytochrome P3A4 system.

Although some believe that the previously mentioned deaths are secondary to conscious sedation or general anesthesia, the data on general anesthesia alone do not support this notion.[51] We believe that an important factor in our safety record has been the rapid infusion of tumescent fluid combined with efficient fat removal via 3- to 6-mm cannulae, which is allowed for by conscious sedation.

Other

One case of acute hearing loss after abdominal liposuction has been reported. It was presumed to be secondary to embolization or transient hypoperfusion associated with general anesthesia.[52]

LOCAL COMPLICATIONS
Contour Irregularities

Anywhere from 2[31] to 9.7 percent[53] of patients show persistent irregularities such as skin dimpling, depressions, divots or dents, waviness, asymmetry, or redundancy that require a second corrective procedure. Depressed grooves, if not present immediately after surgery, may represent inappropriate positioning of compression or girdle devices.[54] Poorly fitting or incorrectly worn girdles pulled too high over the thighs or riding down over the belly during postural changes may lead to depressions. These usually resolve spontaneously over time after the girdle or binder is removed. If the

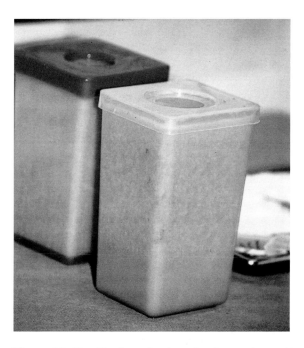

Figure 16-49   The fat collection after liposuction, with less than 5 percent of the total aspirate.

improvement is not to the patient's satisfaction, massage for 6 to 8 weeks may be beneficial. If no improvement is seen in 4 to 6 months, a touch-up procedure comprising of serial microlipoinjections to level off the depression can be performed (see Chap. 9). The best treatment is proper patient education to avoid this as well as early postoperative follow-up, at which time one specifically looks for such early skin irregularities.[54]

Effect of Weight Gain on Body Contour

In the breasts and buttocks, new weight gain may preferentially localize as other commonly involved fat storage areas are reduced or eliminated through liposuction. Because the number of lipocytes in adults is generally stable, weight gain results in the enlargement of the adipocytes' size rather than an increase in their number. There is no correlation between the areas treated or the amount of fat removed and the degree of breast enlargement.[55] It has been reported that 53 percent (16 patients) of a treated group experienced increases in breast fullness, with 11 (75 percent) noting an actual increase of one to two bra cup sizes.[55] A weight increase ranging from 2 to 5 kg was seen in about 50 percent of the patients with breast enlargement. Still, as others have noted,[15] the shape of the patient remains balanced unless a contour deformity due to constriction is present, which may lead to the accentuation of the contour deformity. Although liposuction does not appear to predispose a patient to weight gain, weight control is a factor that should be discussed with the patient and documented by preoperative measurements.

Hematoma or Seroma

Hematoma or seroma occurs in about 0.5 percent of cases.[31] Although bruising is seen in almost all cases, seroma is unusual. In the event of seroma formation, aspiration and evacuation with an 18-gauge needle is helpful to expedite healing and alleviate discomfort.

Paresthesia

Paresthesia is a common sequela of liposuction and occurs in about 0.2 percent of cases.[31] It is believed to be caused by the negative pressure of the vacuum pump and the blunt traumatization of cutaneous nerves. It usually resolves spontaneously but may persist for 6 months to a year.

Scarring

Scarring is most often a result of external forces.[56] Hypertrophic scarring or keloid formation can occur at the cannula incision site in scar-prone individuals. Friction bullae, from overlying trauma of the girdle, may lead to skin necrosis with subsequent hypertrophic scarring. The pain of the friction normally leads to cessation of the repetitive motion before severe damage occurs, but in patients who have undergone liposuction, the overlying skin is numb for a variety of reasons (e.g., from the tumescent anesthesia, which lasts for about 12 h after surgery, from analgesics taken after surgery, or from regional hypoesthesia directly from the liposuction). Therefore these patients may be susceptible to repeated motion injury. Scarring can also be seen in patients who are "pickers," who consciously or subconsciously pick at the stitched incision sites or other liposuction areas. Liposuction

that is too superficial, especially if the cannula port is turned toward the surface, may also lead to skin necrosis.

The early detection of skin sloughing is important because it may help prevent severe scarring and pigmentary irregularities. If sloughing occurs, the first step in care is to avoid friction, making sure that the area remains clean (free of bacterial or yeast infection; if there is doubt, skin cultures should be performed). Wound healing is accelerated by using topical antibiotic and Vaseline-impregnated gauze, changed daily. If a scar forms, it should be tackled aggressively with a combination of intraluminal (IL) triamcinolone injections, silicone sheathing, and pulsed-dye laser (see Chap. 15).

Hypopigmentation and Hyperpigmentation

The frequency of these sequelae is similar to that seen with other cutaneous surgeries, with a higher incidence noted in individuals with darker skin. To minimize this occurrence, many experts prefer the use of fewer incisions that are well hidden under clothing or between cosmetic borders.

Asymmetry

The patient's body is asymmetric to start with, however subtle the difference may be. It is important to discuss any pre-existing asymmetries with the patient and have preoperative photographs taken that can be used during surgery to determine where more fat needs to be removed to re-create symmetry. One aid to visual assessment is to compare the amount of fat removed from each area, which should be helpful when the same procedure is performed bilaterally. Proper marking is important, and it helps if the patient can be placed in a standing position during the marking procedure.

Superficial Skin Necrosis

Superficial skin necrosis usually occurs from the overlying tape and is seen in about 0.2 percent of cases.[31] Other causes include friction from poorly fitting compression garments; liposuction performed in the superficial plane in a large contiguous surface area; and, more recently, from the use of ultrasound-assisted liposuction, especially when it is implemented in the superficial plane.

Other

Talcum powder on the surgical gloves may cause a starch granuloma.[57] Although an uncommon occurrence, this can be easily avoided by using starch-free surgical gloves. Although liposuction removes fat, it may also introduce fat by traumatic implantation of fat cells into other areas, as seen in a recent case where a pseudolipoma was identified after abdominal liposuction. It was presumed to have occurred after traumatic opening of the external oblique aponeurosis by an overly aggressive liposuction technique.[58]

Ultrasound-Assisted Liposuction

Ultrasound-assisted liposuction (UAL) uses ultrasound energy in direct contact with the subcutaneous fat, leading to its emulsion and supposed "easier" aspiration. Debates exist concerning its benefits and whether these perceived or real benefits justify the equipment costs, the learning curve, and the associated increased complications.[59] Even those who specialize in UAL agree that it is not essential for producing better results.[15] UAL should be avoided in such areas as the face, neck, inner thighs, lower leg, and lower abdomen in combination with abdominoplasty.[15]

Power-Assisted Liposuction

A search to help treat fibrotic areas and ease operator fatigue has brought about the idea of power-assisted liposuction (PAL). The PAL device is offered by MicroAire Surgical Instruments. The cannula is powered by either medical-grade nitrogen (N_2) or by tanks of compressed air. The cannula has a 2-mm stroke and reciprocates at 2000 to 4000 cpm, a speed that can be adjusted by the surgeon.[60] A study by Fodor and Vogt[60] performed a patient- and evaluator-blinded comparison of PAL with traditional liposuction. In the study, one side of the body, randomly chosen, and its matching contralateral body area were suctioned on one side with traditional liposuction; the other side was suctioned with PAL. There was no difference in patient satisfaction, side effects, contraction of skin, postliposuction healing, or operator time. The only benefit of PAL over traditional liposuction was increased ease of suctioning fibrotic areas and thus less surgeon fatigue.[60] A microscopic examination of the harvested fat revealed that it was similar to that aspirated with traditional liposuction, making it useful for lipoinjection.[60] The additional cost and possibility of mechanical malfunction may negate the advantage of PAL for most surgeons.

It is important to give patients both pre- and postoperative instructions. A patient undergoing liposuction should be given an overview of the procedure and asked to sign a consent form. Pre- and postoperative instructions must also be given.

References

1. Klab C. Our quest to be perfect. *Newsweek* 1999; August 9:52–59.
2. Coleman WP, Hanke W, Lillis P, et al. Does the location of surgery or the specialty of the physician affect malpractice claims in liposuction. *Dermatol Surg* 1999; 25:343–347.
3. Lamberg L. Dermatologists debate sentinel node biopsy, safety of liposuction, and antibiotic prophylaxis [news]. *JAMA* 2000; 283:2223–2224.
4. Jackson RF, Carniol PJ, Crockett CH, et al. 2000 Guidelines for liposuction surgery. *Am J Cosmet Surg* 2000; 17:79–84.
5. Coleman WP III, Glogau RG, Klein JP, et al. American Academy of Dermatology Guidelines of Care for Liposuction. *J Am Acad Dermatol* 2001; 45:438–447.
6. Toledo LS. *Refinements in Facial and Body Contouring.* Philadelphia: Lippincott-Raven; 1999.
7. Rao RB, Ely SF, Hoffman RS. Death related to liposuction. *N Engl J Med* 1999; 340:1471–1475.
8. Abeles G, Warmuth IP, Sequaria M, et al. The use of conscious sedation for outpatient dermatologic procedures. *Dermatol Surg* 2000; 26:121–126.
9. Bisaccia E, Scarborough D. An overview of syringe assisted liposuction. *Cosmet Dermatol* 1991; 4:12–16.
10. Ostad A, Kageyama N, Moy RL. Tumescent anesthesia with a lidocaine dose of 55mg/kg is safe for liposuction. *Dermatol Surg* 1996; 22:921–927.
11. Hanke CW, Bernstein G, Bullock S. Safety of tumescent liposuction in 15,336 patients. *Dermatol Surg* 1995; 21:459–462.
12. Samdal F, Armand PF, Bugge JF. Plasma lidocaine levels during suction assisted lipectomy using large doses of dilute lidocaine with epinephrine. *Plast Reconstr Surg* 1994; 93:1217–1223.
13. Klein JA. Tumescent technique for local anesthesia improves safety in large volume liposuction. *Plast Reconstr Surg* 1993; 92:1085–1098.
14. Coleman WP III. Noncosmetic applications of liposuction. *J Dermatol Surg Oncol* 1988; 14:1085–1090.
15. Teimourian B, Adham MN: A national survey of complications associated with suction lipectomy: What we did then and what we do now. *Plast Reconstr Surg* 2000; 105:1881–1884.
16. Bisaccia E, Scarborough D. Facial liposuction—An office technique. In: Stucker F, ed. *Plastic and Reconstructive Surgery of the Head and Neck.* Philadelphia: Decker; 1991:181–187.
17. Seckel BR. *Facial Danger Zones: Avoiding Nerve Injury in Facial Plastic Surgery.* St. Louis: Quality Medical Publishing; 1994.
18. Pitman GH. Liposuction and Aesthetic Surgery. St. Louis: Quality Medical Publishing; 1993:337–411.
19. Sequeira M, Abels G, Scarborough DA, et al. Liposuction for the pendulous lower abdominal panniculus. *Cosmet Dermatol* 1997; 10:9–11.
20. Clark DP. Liposuction of the abdomen: An analysis of form. *Dermatol Clin* 1999; 17:835–848.
21. Matarasso SL. Liposuction of the chest and back. *Dermatol Clin* 1999; 17:799–804.
22. Bisaccia E, Scarborough DA. Liposuction for gynecomastia. *Cosmet Dermatol* 1991; 4:10–11.
23. Bisaccia E, Scarborough DA. Gynecomastia treatment via liposuction. Surgery: an alternative to traditional approaches. *Cosmet Dermatol* 1994; 7:10–11.
24. Gasperoni C, Salgarello M, Gasperoni P. Technical refinements in the surgical treatment of gynecomastia. *Ann Plast Surg* 2000; 44:455–458.
25. Moore KL, Dalley, AF. *Clinically Oriented Anatomy*, 4th ed. Philadelphia: Lippincott Williams & Wilkins; 1999.
26. Glanz S, Gonzalez-Ulloa M. Aesthetic surgery of the arm. *Aesthetic Plast Surg* 1981; 5:1–17.
27. Lillis PJ. Liposuction of the arms. *Dermatol Clin* 1999; 17:783–797.
28. Scarborough DA, Bisaccia E. Liposuction of the extremities: Part 1: Recontouring the knees. *Cosmet Dermatol* 1993; 16:11–13.
29. Lillis PJ. Liposuction of the knees, calves and ankles. *Dermatol Clin* 1999; 17:865–879.
30. Grazer F, Dejong RH. Fatal outcomes from liposuction: Census survey of cosmetic surgeons. *Plast Reconstr Surg* 2000; 105:436–446.
31. Bernstein G, Hanke CW. Safety of liposuction: a review of 9478 cases performed by dermatologists. *J Dermtol Surg Oncol* 1988; 14:1112–1114.
32. Hanke CW, Bernstein G, Bullock S. Safety of tumescent liposuction in 15,336 patients: National survey results. *Dermatol Surg* 1995; 21:459–462.
33. Jackson RF, Dolsy RL. Liposuction and patient safety. *Am J Cosmet Surg* 1999; 16:21–23.
34. Teimorian B, Rogers WB II. A national survey of complications associated with suction lipectomy: A comparative study. *Plast Reconstr Surg* 1989; 84:628–631.

35. ASPRS Task force on lipoplasty, J.G. Bruner (chair). *1997 Survey Summary Report*. Arlington Heights, IL: American Society of Plastic and Reconstructive Surgeons, 1998.

36. Hales D. You want a tuck or a lift . . . *Parade Magazine* June 20, 1999:10–11.

37. Klein JA. The antibacterial effect of tumescent liposuction fluid (letter; comment). *Plast Reconstr Surg* 1999; 104:1934–1935.

38. Craig SB, Concannon MJ, McDonald GA, et al. The antibacterial effects of tumesent liposuction fluid. *Plast Reconstr Surg* 1999; 103:666–670.

39. Gingrass MK. Lipoplasty complications and their prevention. *Clin Plast Surg* 1999; 26:341–354.

40. Gibbons, MD, Lim, RB, Carter PL. Necrotizing fasciitis after tumescent liposuction. *Am Surg* 1998; 64:458–460.

41. Umeda, T., Ohara, H., Hayashi O., et. al. Toxic shock syndrome after suction lipectomy. *Plast and Reconstr Surg* 2000; 106:204–207.

42. Brillo DJ, Cancio LC, Kim SH, et al. Fatal complications of liposuction *South Med J* 1998; 91:487–492.

43. Rhee CA, Smith, RJ, Jackson, IT. Toxic shock syndrome associated with suction-assisted lipectomy. *Aesthet Plast Surg* 1994; 18:161–163.

44. Behroozan DS, Christian MM, Moy RL. Mycobacterium fortuitum infection following neck liposuction: A case report. *Dermatol Surg* 2000; 26:588–590.

45. Few JW, Marcus JR, Placik OJ. Deep vein thrombosis prophylaxis in the moderate- to high-risk patient undergoing lower extremity liposuction. *Plast Reconstr Surg* 1999; 104:309–310.

46. Talmor M, Hoffman LA, Lieberman M. Intestinal perforation after suction lipoplasty: A case report and review of the literature. *Ann Plast Surg* 1997; 381:169–172.

47. Talmor M, Fahey TJ, Wise J, et al. Large-volume liposuction complicated by retroperitoneal hemorrhage: Management principles and implications for the quality improvement process. *Plast Reconstr Surg* 1999; 105:2244–2248.

48. Pitman GH, Holzer J. Safe suction: fluid replacement and blood loss parameters. *Perspect Plast Surg* 1991; 5:79–89.

49. Klein JA. Tumescent technique for local anesthesia improves safety in large-volume liposuction. *Plast Reconstr Surg* 1993; 92:1085–1098.

50. Clark DP. Anesthesia. In: Ratz JL, ed. *Textbook of Dermatologic Surgery*. Philadelphia: Lippincott-Raven; 1998:31–40.

51. Rao RB, Ely SF, Hoffman RS.: Death related to liposuction (letter; comment). *N Engl J Med* 1999; 341:1001–1002.

52. Hecksteden K, Bucheler M, Bootz F. Acute hearing loss after liposuction. *Plast Reconstr Surg* 1999; 104:1534–1536.

53. Chang KN. Surgical correction of postliposuction contour irregularities. *Plast Reconstr Surg* 1994; 94:126–136.

54. Warmuth I, Bader RS, Scarborough DA, et al. Post liposuction skin depression. *Cosmet Dermatol* 1999; 12:22.

55. Scarborough DA, Bisaccia E. The occurrence of breast enlargement in female following liposuction. *Am J Cosmet Surg* 1991; 8:97–102.

56. Warmuth I, Bader RS, Scarborough DA, et al. Liposuction. *Cosmet Dermatol* 1998; 11:18.

57. Baruchin AM, Ben-Dor D, Eventhal D. Starch granuloma following liposuction—The persisting hazards. *Am J Cosmet Surg* 11995; 2:1665–1667.

58. Sharma S, Perrotti JA, Longaker MT. Traumatic abdominal wall pseudolipoma following suction-assisted lipectomy. *Plast Reconstr Surg* 2000; 105:2589–2591.

59. Fodor PB, Watson J. Personal experience with ultrasound-assisted lipoplasty: A pilot study comparing ultrasound-assisted lipoplasty with traditional lipoplasty. *Plast Reconstr Surg* 1998; 101:1103–1116.

60. Fodor PB, Vogt PA. Power-assisted lipoplasty (PAL): A clinical pilot study comparing PAL to traditional lipoplasty (TL). *Aesthet Plast Surg* 1999; 23:379–385.

Patient Information

Liposuction Through Suction Fat Extraction for Men and Women: Overview

HISTORY

Many years ago, European physicians began to develop a technique for the removal of body fat. This technique differed from past operations for body contouring in that it could be done without leaving significant visible scars. Prior procedures for this problem involved extensive operations that resulted in large scars that could be concealed only by clothing. Through these early efforts of French and Italian surgeons, a new technique of suction fat removal was pioneered. It has been improved and perfected over the past 20 years and has remained the top cosmetic procedure performed in the United States since 1989.

Utilizing a "tumescent technique" void of high-pressure vacuum suction, dermatologic surgeons are able to extract fat cells through tiny incisions. Although it is not a treatment for generalized obesity, this surgical technique is ideally suited for the removal of localized fat deposits in the face, neck, hips, buttocks, abdomen, flanks, knees, calves, and male breasts.

FACIAL SCULPTING

With time and gravity, fat may accumulate in the neck and jowl. Suction removal of facial fat is a simple procedure done either separately or combined with other cosmetic procedures. Fat located in the jowl or cheek is usually removed through a very small incision just in front of the earlobe. A special fat extractor is placed beneath the skin in these areas and fat is removed with low-power suction. For fat accumulations in the neck and chin area, the minute incision is made just below the chin and the fat is then extracted from the entire neck area.

These procedures may be done under local anesthesia or combined with light sedation, depending on the extent of surgery. After the operative procedure, small special tapes are applied and a facial elastic garment is worn for about 1 week.

THE MINIMAL-INCISION FACE- OR NECK-LIFT

Patients with excessive wrinkled or loose, hanging skin must have a combined procedure of jowl and neck fat suction and skin and muscle tightening. Combining liposuction with a face-lift decreases the length of the incisions necessary for a face-lift alone. The removal of fat in these areas gives the patient a much finer and more youthful postoperative appearance. The use of fat suction greatly enhances the esthetic results while minimizing the need for invasive surgical lifting procedures.

Fat extraction in the face and neck can be done in both men and women with no age limit whatsoever. This procedure is also done in teenagers who inherit a double chin. It is an extremely safe procedure posing no serious problems.

THE TUMESCENT TECHNIQUE OF FAT REMOVAL BY BODY SUCTION

The tumescent technique is not new in body sculpting surgery. As leaders in liposuction surgery, Your doctors have been performing tumescent liposuction for more than a decade. Its recent popularity results from tumescent liposuction being recognized as an extremely safe procedure. A local anesthetic or saline solution is gently infused into the fatty layer of the skin, producing light pressure, or "tumescence." This results not only in excellent numbing of the tissues but also greatly diminishes potential blood loss from the tiny capillary vessels interwoven with the fat. Thus, the need for blood banking, transfusions, and a long recovery time is eliminated. A special small fat extractor is then introduced through a tiny skin opening that is usually less than a half inch in length. Within minutes, the fat cells are loosened and removed. In less than 1 hour, the procedure is complete and self-dissolving sutures are applied.

Patients are required to wear special surgical garments over the treated area. These garments can normally be worn under clothing. They are kept in place for several days and are important in supporting the skin. After the first 1 or 2 days of recovery, patients are encouraged to walk and resume normal activities to assist in the healing process. However, strenuous exercise should be avoided during the first few weeks.

ADVERSE EFFECTS

The recovery period for such surgery is remarkably rapid. Pain is minimal and is usually controlled by nonnarcotic analgesic agents. Although some pain and bruising are normal, they are usually minimal and well tolerated. On occasion, there is temporary fluid or blood accumulation underneath the skin. However, this is easily treated and resolves with no long-term adverse effects. Slight numbness in the overlying skin may occur during the healing phase; however, it gradually resolves over 3 to 6 months.

SUMMARY

Although this procedure is relatively new in the United States, it has been performed in France and Italy since the early 1970s. It has proven to be a very safe and effective way to loose inches. As with any surgical procedure, there is a degree of variability in patient healing. A small number of patients may need a touch-up procedure for best results. There is, of course, a limit to how much fat can be removed. The technique is not meant for generally obese patients and is not a substitute for weight loss. Age limits depend on the patient's general physical health. This procedure is ideally suited for a younger patient whose skin elasticity is at its maximum. However, several years and thousands of cases at our facility have shown that we can successfully extend the procedure to many older patients who have good skin tone. In our office, liposuction has benefited patients from 14 to 87 years. This technique is truly individual, and patients must be examined to know the possible benefits and expected results of their individual cases.

FREQUENTLY ASKED QUESTIONS ABOUT THE TUMESCENT TECHNIQUE

WHAT AREAS OF THE BODY ARE TREATED BY SUCTION FAT REMOVAL?

Body contouring through suction fat removal is ideally suited for removal of fat deposits in the face, neck, male breasts, hips, flanks, buttocks, abdomen, legs (both inner and outer thighs), knees, and calves. The treatment is not for individuals with generalized obesity. This treatment is highly effective for shaping one's contour and losing some inches. Fat suction removal has been used for the removal of large lipomas or fatty skin tumors. Previous techniques for removal of fatty skin tumors required large incisions. By applying the suction technique for fat removal, many large (baseball- or grapefruit-sized) lipomas can be removed through incisions less than 1 inch in length. Patients with male gynecomastia (male breast enlargement) can be treated with fat suction surgery. The scars are much smaller than those used in traditional subcutaneous mastectomy, and some of the complications and undesirable results of the previous techniques are eliminated by using the fat suction techniques for male gynecomastia or breast enlargement.

WHERE ARE THE INCISIONS PLACED IN BODY FAT EXTRACTION?

Incisions that are approximately a half inch or smaller are made to insert the blunt extractor. For removal of fat collections in the abdomen, the incision is made within the lower half of the belly button or in the pubic area (or both). This incision heals in a fashion that can barely be seen. For removal of fatty deposits from the thighs and buttocks, the incision is made in the crease just below the buttock or just above the hip when the lateral thigh is to be contoured. This very short incision is barely noticeable when healed.

CAN BOTH MEN AND WOMEN BE TREATED BY THIS TECHNIQUE?

Suction fat removal has successfully removed localized fatty accumulations in both men and women. In male patients, the most common areas of sculpturing are the abdomen, waist ("love handles"), and breasts.

WHERE IS THE SUCTION FAT REMOVAL PROCEDURE PERFORMED?

All suction fat removal treatments can be done as outpatient procedures. The fat removal is performed with the patient sedated but not asleep. Local anesthesia is then given, and the skin may be cooled with ice. If large or multiple areas of fat are to be removed, more than one session may be necessary.

IS THE PROCEDURE PAINFUL?

The pain is minimal in the postoperative period and can usually be controlled by a nonnarcotic analgesic agent. There is surprisingly little discomfort.

HOW LONG WILL I BE OFF FROM WORK?

Individuals vary, as do their work tasks. Anywhere from 2 days to 1 week after surgery can be expected, depending on the extent of the surgery. Usually 1 week is more than enough for patients undergoing most procedures.

WILL I BE BANDAGED?

Tight elastic surgical garments are necessary so that the skin can be lifted and supported to a new level. The garment is removed after 3 days for showering but should be worn under clothes for a few weeks. The function of the garments is to help prevent fluid accumulations under the skin and support the skin as it recontours.

WHAT WILL HAPPEN TO THE EXCESS SKIN?

Skin is a dynamic organ that has elasticity and, in most cases, is able to accommodate to the new body contour. Liposuction is not a treatment for cellulite. In some cases, cellulite is improved, but the goal of liposuction is to lose inches.

WILL THE FAT REGROW?

Fat cells are developed in childhood and puberty. Theories concerning fat metabolism and obesity are based on the concept that no new fat cells are produced after puberty. It is believed, according to this theory, that the fat cells existing at the time of puberty can either swell or shrink depending on weight gain or loss. When these fat cells are removed from the treated areas, it is believed that they are not re-formed or reproduced. On the other hand, individuals who abuse their diets may regain weight in the treated areas in the fatty cells that are left behind. This theory is not a proven; however, it is well supported by the observations after many cases of fat-suction body sculpting.

CAN THE PROCEDURE BE REPEATED?

In some instances, it is necessary to treat the same area more than once. In other instances, when more than one anatomic area is being treated, it may not be possible to treat them all in one session. Sometimes also, it is necessary to do a later "fine-tuning" secondary procedure to achieve maximum improvement in contour.

ARE THERE ANY ADVERSE EFFECTS?

Current world experience indicates that, when done properly and on good surgical candidates, there are no long-term effects from liposuction. There may be temporary fluid or blood accumulation under the skin; however, this resolves with no long-term adverse effects. Temporary numbness in the underlying skin may occur in some patients.

IS FLUID OR BLOOD REPLACEMENT NECESSARY?

On the day of surgery, body fluids are adequately replaced during the operative procedure. With the tumescent technique, we have never had occasion to hospitalize or transfuse anyone.

IS THERE AN AGE LIMIT?

Chronologic and physiologic age vary considerably between patients. On occasion, in older individuals, there may not be complete shrinking of the skin because of decreased elasticity. These people may require surgical recontouring and removal of excess skin.

IS THERE A WEIGHT LIMIT?

This technique is not meant to achieve weight reduction or to remove generalized obesity. It is merely a body sculpting procedure used to shape and mold offending bulges. During the past several years, research has begun on the role of liposuction in moderately obese patients. Our office, like several other large liposuction practices around the world, is investigating the use of liposuction surgery in patients who are 30 to 60 pounds overweight. These patients must be very carefully evaluated, selected, and observed.

HOW SMOOTH IS THE CONTOURED AREA?

With abdominal sculpturing, the contoured area is remarkably smooth. Only rarely are there any irregularities. With the thighs, abdomen, and hips, a condition known as "waddles" or "waves" can occur. These are slight "hills" and "valleys" that are caused by variations in the healing process. They may or may not be objectionable to the patient. Unclothed, the patient can feel or see them, and he or she must understand that this condition can occur. Even when waves are present, clothing obscures them. Liposuction surgery is not intended to improve "cellulite" skin dimpling; in fact, such dimpling may be worsened by this procedure. The goal is to improve the overall contour so that the patient will look better in clothing. Inches will be lost, not pounds.

Preoperative Instructions for Patients Undergoing Liposuction

Liposuction surgery or body contouring or sculpting is the most popular cosmetic surgical procedure in the United States. It is a procedure performed under local anesthesia and mild sedation. It consists of the removal of tunnels of fatty cell tissue that results in the recontouring of the body outlines of the patients so that their appearance in clothing is improved. It therefore allows the patient to have a more evenly proportioned silhouette. Goals for this cosmetic procedure must be realistic.

Beginning at least 2 weeks before surgery, if you are not already exercising regularly, it is essential that you walk at a brisk pace for at least 1 hour continuously 3 or 4 times a week. Walking daily at an easy pace should be continued for at least 3 to 6 weeks after surgery. After 6 weeks, full exercise or a brisk daily walk is recommended for a minimum of 6 months.

Do not take any aspirin or aspirin-containing products for 2 weeks before surgery and 2 weeks after surgery. If a product contains salicylic acid or salicylamide, you may not take it. If you are in doubt about any product, feel free to call our office at (___) _____ to inquire about this or any aspect of your upcoming surgery. Tylenol may be taken, but do not take any other anti-inflammatory medicine (e.g., Advil, Motrin, Clinoril, Naprosyn, Anaprox) during this interval without checking with the doctor. *This is very important!!*

One day before surgery, begin your antibiotic if prescribed.

You may want to shampoo your hair the morning of surgery. There will be a 72-hour post-operative interval in which we will ask you not to shower.

Please arrange for a ride to and from the surgery center and for someone to be with you for 24 hours after surgery. This is an absolute requirement for having outpatient surgery.

BRING your pain medication with you on surgery day. You may take it after surgery, before you leave the surgery center for home.

If, before surgery, you develop a cold, fever, flu, etc., please call the office for proper instructions at (___) _____.

Do not drink alcohol or smoke for 2 weeks before or 2 weeks after surgery.

Please note that during the surgical procedure you will *not* be under general anesthesia but will be lightly asleep and unaware of the operation.

Please wear a washable sweat suit or loose-fitting clothing with a zip-up top to the office on the day of surgery. *Avoid pullover shirts and blouses as well as pantyhose.* Do not wear jewelry.

GARMENT: A special girdle/binder and possibly knee- or thigh-high medical support stockings will be provided for you on the day of your surgery. Seventy-two hours after surgery, you may remove your support garment for laundering and air-drying. It may be necessary to purchase a smaller garment (available from Sears, J.C. Penney, or our office) several days or weeks after surgery as the shrinkage of tissue progresses. (Again, your initial girdle will be provided at the time of surgery.)

NOTE: Male patients having abdominal liposuction surgery should plan to wear an athletic supporter for 10 days after surgery.

Please remove contact lenses before surgery. If you wish to remove them in the office, please bring your lens case.

If face or neck liposuction is planned, do not wear any face or eye makeup to the office the day of surgery.

Postoperative Instructions for Patients Undergoing Neck and Facial Liposuction

Swelling and discoloration are normal after liposuction surgery. The amount varies from person to person. The following instructions are designed to minimize discomfort after surgery. *Please remember that it takes time to see the results of liposuction surgery.* You may not see results for 6 weeks to 6 months after surgery.

You can expect soreness after surgery, which can be relieved by pain medication. For the first 2 to 3 days after surgery, you may feel rather weak. You can expect some swelling after surgery, which lasts approximately 6 to 8 weeks. This will gradually decrease and is not a cause for alarm. Sleep with your head elevated at least a 45-degree angle for the first 5 to 7 days. Because of the infusion of the large volume of dilute anesthetic or saline used in this procedure, there may be some red-tinged fluid drainage from the wounds during the first 48 to 72 hours. This is normal.

Garment

Your special facial binder (supplied by our office) is to be worn for 3 weeks, 24 hours a day for 10 days and then 12 hours a day for 10 days. When necessary, you may take it off long enough to wash and air-dry it.

Activity

You should rest in bed for the remainder of the day of surgery. You should have assistance when using the bathroom because you may experience dizziness and fainting spells when standing. The chance of this greatly diminishes after 24 hours after surgery. You may resume your "normal" activities after 24 hours.

Physical Exercise

Beginning the second or third day after surgery, you need to begin mild exercising. Walking is recommended, beginning with 1 mile per day and increasing to 30 minutes or 3 miles per day. Exercise is important to promote faster healing and reduction of swelling. Move carefully and avoid bending, lifting anything heavy, and so on for the first 2 weeks. Strenuous exertional exercise can be resumed 4 weeks after surgery. Daily exercise is recommended for 6 months after surgery.

Returning to Work

This depends mainly on two factors, the extent of your liposuction surgery and your job. You may be off work from 1 to 10 days. Discuss this with the doctor before your surgery. Remember, bruising and swelling may occur and possibly last up to 2 weeks. The elastic support garment will cover much of this.

Diet

Meals are not restricted after surgery. You should drink clear liquids to prevent dehydration, even if you are not thirsty. You are encouraged to drink plenty of water (*not* tea, soda, or coffee) for 3 days after surgery. This will reduce the possibility of constipation. During these 10 days, also maintain a low-salt diet.

Swelling

Fluid retention may occur after this type of surgery. Swelling and discoloration of the surgical sites are common after liposuction surgery.

Bathing

Try to keep the tapes applied to your chin dry for 3 days. Showering from the neck down is possible 24 hours after surgery, but the facial garment must be kept dry. It may be removed for light cleansing of the face and neck after the third day. You may shampoo your hair on the third postoperative day. You may want to wash and air-dry the garment at this time.

Dressing Removal

Remove gauze bandages after 72 hours. If Steri-Strips have been applied, keep them dry for 3 days. You may remove the Steri-Strips 2 weeks after surgery.

Medication

Take medications as prescribed. Do not skip or double up on medications. *Do not take aspirin or aspirin-containing products for 2 weeks.* Tylenol may be taken. You will be given an antibiotic, either during surgery or as pills to be taken before and after surgery. This is done to reduce the chances of infection, which might retard healing.

Pain

Some pain is to be expected and is well controlled by medications prescribed prior to surgery.

Stitches

At times, absorbable stitches are used; their removal is not necessary. Other types of stitches are removed in 5 to 10 days after surgery, at your first postoperative visit. You may clean suture lines with saline solution or warm tap water twice a day and then apply Polysporin ointment.

Numbness

This sensation is frequent in the surgically treated areas for 6 to 12 weeks. Please do not be alarmed, since this is normal during the healing process. There may also be hardness and lumpiness during this time where the skin is tightening down. This will gradually subside.

Appointments

You will return to the office 4 to 7 days after surgery if no other procedure was done in conjunction with the neck liposuction, again in 6 weeks, and finally after 6 months. Your first postoperative appointment date and time will be given to you on the day of your surgery. An important part of our commitment to patients is their postoperative care. This is necessary to ensure your continued well-being throughout the healing process. We ask that you allow time in your busy schedule to keep these appointments.

Problems or Questions

Call the office at (___) _____ any time, even on weekends. Our phones are monitored every weekend for calls. For emergencies, the doctor's home number is given on the postoperative appointment card. There is no charge for postoperative appointments related to your surgery, but other topics you wish to address will necessitate an appropriate office-visit charge.

Other

No alcohol or smoking for 14 days after surgery.

No hot-tub bathing for 14 days after surgery. The elevated temperature in hot tubs causes increased circulatory flow that could increase swelling and bleeding tendencies.

POSTOPERATIVE INSTRUCTIONS FOR PATIENTS UNDERGOING LIPOSUCTION

Swelling and a large amount of discoloration are normal after liposuction surgery. The amount varies from person to person. The following instructions are designed to minimize discomfort after surgery. *Please remember that it takes time to see the results of liposuction surgery.* You may not see results for 6 weeks to 6 months.

You can expect soreness after surgery, which can be relieved by pain medication. For the first 2 to 3 days after surgery, you may feel rather weak. You can expect some swelling after surgery, which will last approximately 6 to 8 weeks. This will gradually decrease and is not a cause for alarm. Sleep in the position that is most comfortable for you. Because of the infusion of the large volume of dilute anesthetic or saline used in this procedure, there may be a considerable amount of red-tinged fluid drainage from the wounds during the first 48 to 72 hours after surgery. This is normal. If your dressings become saturated, place an old towel over your support garment to absorb additional drainage.

Garment

Your special girdle or binder (supplied by our office) is to be worn for 3 to 6 weeks, 24 hours a day for 21 days and then 12 hours a day for 21 days. After the first 3 days, you may take it off long enough to wash and line dry only. Patients who have liposuction surgery are to wear a special girdle and thigh- or knee-high medical support stockings. The support stockings will also be provided for you. Plan to wear these during the day for 7 to 10 days after surgery. Also, it may be necessary to purchase a second girdle (available at Sears, J.C. Penney, or our office) several days to a few weeks after surgery as the shrinkage of tissue progresses. Your initial girdle will be provided at the time of surgery. *Note:* Male patients should plan to wear an athletic supporter for 10 days after abdominal liposuction surgery (this is not provided).

Activity

Patients should spend the remainder of the day of surgery mostly resting in bed. You should have assistance when using the bathroom because you may experience dizziness and light-headed spells when standing. The chance of this greatly diminishes after 24 hours. We encourage you to resume your low-key, normal activities of daily living the next day, but do not overdo it.

Physical Exercise

Beginning the second or third day after surgery, you need to begin mild exercise. Walking is recommended, beginning with 1 mile per day and increasing to 30 minutes or 3 miles per day. This walking exercise is important to promote faster healing and reduce swelling. Do not overdo it; gradually increase it as tolerated without straining or to the point of perspiring. A list of additional exercises may include light stair-step exercises or light activity on an exercise bike. Strenuous exertional exercise may be resumed 6 weeks after surgery. Daily exercise is recommended for 6 months after surgery.

Returning to Work

This depends mainly on two factors: the extent of your liposuction surgery and your job. You may be off work from 1 to 6 days. Discuss this with the doctor before your surgery. For the first few days, you may have less energy because your body is focusing on healing. A nap or two during the day may be in order.

Diet

Meals are not restricted after surgery. You should drink clear liquids to prevent dehydration, even if you are not thirsty. You are encouraged to drink plenty of water (*not* tea, soda, or coffee) for 3 days after surgery. This will reduce the possibility of constipation. During these 3 days, also maintain a low-salt diet.

Swelling

Fluid retention may occur after this type of surgery. Swelling and discoloration of the surgical sites are common after body liposuction surgery. The genital areas may be swollen and discolored after abdominal liposuction because of gravity drainage.

Bathing

Leave the girdle or support garment on for 72 hours after surgery. Drainage often occurs around the incision sites during the first few days; a small towel may be placed over the girdle to help absorb the dampness. A brief shower can be taken 3 days after surgery and daily thereafter. Showers should last no longer than 2 minutes for the first 2 weeks to ensure that the small tape strips overlying the wounds stay in place. The gauze pads taped over the wound may be removed before the first shower. Replace the support garment immediately after showering and be sure to position the inner-thigh hem as close to the groin as possible. You may want to wash and line dry your support garment at this time.

Dressing Removal

Remove gauze bandages after 72 hours, at the time of your shower. Keep all Steri-Strips covering your incisions in place. They may be removed 2 weeks after surgery. *Patients undergoing mini tummy tucks are not to remove or disturb their abdominal dressing until their postoperative appointment, at which time it will be removed by the doctor or nurse.*

Medication

Take medications as prescribed. Do not skip or double up on medications. *Do not take aspirin or aspirin-containing products for 2 weeks.* Tylenol may be taken. During the surgery, you will be given an intravenous antibiotic, which is used to reduce the chances of infection that might retard healing.

Pain

Pain is usually minimal and well controlled by medications prescribed before surgery.

Stitches

Absorbable stitches are usually placed; their removal is not necessary. They dissolve on their own in a few weeks. Other types of stitches are sometimes used and must be removed by the doctor or nurse 5 to 10 days after surgery.

Numbness

This sensation is frequent in the surgically treated areas for 6 to 12 weeks after surgery. Please do not be alarmed, because it is normal. There also may be hardness and lumpiness during this time, where the skin is tightening down. These sensations will gradually subside.

Appointments

You will return to the office 4 to 7 days after surgery, again in 6 weeks, and, finally after 6 months. Your first postoperative appointment date and time will be given to you on the day of your surgery. An important part of our commitment to patients is their postoperative care. This is necessary to ensure your continued well-being throughout the healing process. We ask that you allow time in your busy schedule to make and keep these appointments. There is no charge for postoperative appointments related to your surgery, but other topics you wish to address will necessitate an appropriate office-visit charge.

Problems or Questions

Call the office at (___) _____ anytime. For emergencies, the doctor's home number is given on the postoperative appointment card.

Other

No alcohol or smoking for 14 days after surgery.

No hot-tub bathing for 3 weeks. The elevated temperature in hot tubs causes increased circulatory flow that could increase swelling and bleeding tendencies.

Sexual intercourse can usually be resumed in 5 to 10 days.

Consent for Liposuction Surgery

Patient's name_____

Date_____

I am aware that fat suction surgery is a relatively new procedure. Dr. _____ and/or the surgical team have explained to me that much that has been written about this method in newspapers, magazines, television, etc., has been exaggerated and sensationalized. The nature, goals, limitations, and possible complications of this procedure have been carefully explained to me and alternative forms of treatment have been discussed.

I have had the opportunity to ask questions about the procedure and its limitations and possible complications.

I clearly understand and accept the following:

1. The goal of liposuction surgery, as in any cosmetic procedure, is improvement, not perfection.

2. The final result may not be apparent for 3 to 6 months after surgery and sometimes up to 18 months or longer.

3. In order to achieve the best possible result, a "touch-up" procedure may be required. There will be a charge for any such operation performed.

4. Areas of "cottage cheese" texture (i.e., "cellulite") will be changed little by the liposuction procedure.

5. Liposuction surgery is a contouring procedure and is not performed for purposes of weight reduction.

6. Strict adherence to the post-operative regimen (i.e., wearing an elastic support for several weeks or months, exercise, and diet) discussed by the doctor and the surgical team and staff is necessary to achieve the best possible result.

7. Liposuction is meant to help me look better in clothes.

8. There is no guarantee that anticipated results will be achieved.

Initial_____

Although complications following liposuction are infrequent, I understand that the following may occur (among others):

A. Bleeding that, on rare instances, could require hospitalization and blood transfusion. It is possible that blood clots may form under the skin and require subsequent drainage.

Initial_____

B. Skin irregularities, lumpiness, hardness, and dimpling may appear after surgery. Most of these problems disappear with time, but localized skin firmness, lumpiness, or irregularities may persist permanently. If loose skin is present in the treated area, it may or may not shrink to conform to the new contour.

Initial_____

C. Infection is unlikely but if it occurs, treatment with antibiotics, surgical drainage, or both may be required.

Initial_____

D. Numbness or increased sensitivity of the skin over treated areas may persist for months. It is possible that localized areas of numbness or increased sensitivity could be permanent.

Initial_____

E. Objectionable scarring is uncommon because of the small size of the incisions used in liposuction surgery. However, rarely, severe bruising or skin ulceration may result in scarring in the treated area.

Initial_____

F. Dizziness may occur during the first week after liposuction, particularly upon rising from a lying or sitting position. If this occurs, extreme caution must be exercised while walking and, if dizziness is present, one must not attempt to drive a car.

Initial_____

G. Occasionally, fluid may collect under the skin (seroma formation) during the first several weeks after surgery. Although this is not a dangerous condition, it may require repeated drainage.

Initial_____

H. A certain amount of bruising and swelling is expected. This usually dissipates over the first few weeks after surgery. Occasionally, dark brown, mottled hyperpigmentation (brown staining) may persist for many months over the treated area; it usually fades over 12 to 18 months. Rarely, it may be permanent. In dark-skinned individuals, loss of pigment may occasionally occur, leaving lighter areas where treated; rarely, this is permanent. Although extremely rare, permanent swelling of an extremity may result.

Initial_____

I. In addition to these possible complications, I am aware of the general risks inherent in all surgical procedures and anesthetic

Initial_____

For the purpose of advancing medical education, I consent to the admittance of authorized observers to the operating room.

I give permission to _____ to take still or motion clinical photographs with the understanding such photographs remain the property of the center. If in the judgment of the center, medical research, education, or science will benefit by their use, such photographs and related information may be published and republished in professional journals or medical books or used for any other purpose that the center may deem proper. It is specifically understood that in any such publication or use, I shall not be identified by name.

I understand that it is mandatory for me to have made prior arrangements to be driven to and from the doctor's office by a responsible adult.

I know that the practice of medicine and surgery is not an exact science and the doctor cannot guarantee results. I acknowledge that no guarantee or assurance, expressed or implied, has been made by anyone regarding the operation that I have herein requested and authorized. I realize that the procedure may not be successful and that the result may not be fully as I desire.

The effect and nature of the operation and the risks involved have been fully explained to my complete satisfaction. I have had sufficient opportunity to discuss my condition with the doctor or associates and all of my questions have been answered to my satisfaction. I fully understand that the success or failure of the operation depends in part on my assuming responsibility for certain facets of my postoperative care. This includes but is not limited to wearing the garments provided by the doctor for 6 weeks after surgery as well as resuming my usual duties and the exercises the doctor or surgical team have prescribed for me.

I understand that certain complications can and do occur with any type of surgery and that they include, among others, unusual reactions to medications and drugs, bleeding, infection, poor wound healing, scar formation, rippling or waviness of small or large areas of the sites operated, and puckering or indentations of certain areas of the body. Furthermore, I acknowledge that there will be discolorations of the tissues involved that usually disappear within a few months. Nerve damage that causes numbness or burning is usually temporary but can be permanent in small areas. Furthermore, asymmetry of the operated areas can occur. Some people need further surgery or treatment to further improve appearance or function. These may involve additional expense.

I hereby release the doctor and surgical team from any consequences or any physical, emotional, personality, or mental changes that might result from this surgery.

Initial_____

I understand that the two sides of the body are not the same and can never be made to look the same in all regards. I understand that bone and muscle structures help create overall shape and are never identical on both sides of the body and that these will remain unchanged by the surgery.

I understand that elective surgical procedures are most often delayed until after the termination of a pregnancy. My signature attests that, to the best of my knowledge, I am not pregnant at this time.

I agree to discontinue smoking entirely for a period of 2 weeks before surgery and 2 weeks immediately after surgery.

I have discussed this liposuction consent with the doctor or the surgical team or staff and I understand the goals, limitations, and possible complications of liposuction surgery and the anesthetic associated with the procedure; I wish to proceed with the operation.

The following procedures are to be done: _____
_____
_____
_____
                                          Initial_____

My signature indicates that I have read this "Consent for Liposuction Surgery" and understand and accept the risks involved with this operation. I hereby authorize _____ _____ and/or the surgical team to perform this surgical procedure on me.

_____   _____
Signature (Patient/Responsible Party)   Date

_____   _____
Signature (Witness)   Date

If patient is a minor, complete the following:
Patient is a minor _____ years of age, and we, the undersigned, are the parents or guardian of the patient and do hereby consent for the patient.

_____   _____
Signature (Parent/Guardian)   Date

CHAPTER 17

Face-Lift

Surgical management of the aging face has incorporated a wide range of new techniques and developments over the past few decades. Many authors have employed their own terminology in advocating a particular approach to the face-lift procedure. Numerous methods are described, including the large-flap sculptured face-lift, the extended supraplatysmal plane lift, midplane, deep-plane, biplane, triplane, superiosteal, endoscopic, vertical, transblepharoplasty, extended supraplaysmal, composite, etc., to name a few.[1–7] There can be no universal consensus as to the "best" approach, since each patient presents a unique challenge for his or her particular rejuvenation needs. However, cosmetic surgery is purely elective surgery done on healthy individuals. Therefore it is prudent to minimize the risks of a more invasive surgery when equivalent or superior results can be obtained with a less aggressive face-lift procedure for most younger individuals. When the extent of the tissue redundancy requires the raising of larger flaps, there may be a need for the larger conventional procedure. Our approach utilizes variations of the Webster superficial musculoaponeurotic system (SMAS) plication technique to achieve a result customized to the individual patient.[8–12]

General Considerations

In all cases, face-lift surgery addresses changes in the skin, muscle, and superficial musculoaponeurotic system, a distinct fanlike structure covering the face,[13] along with fat and subcutaneous tissue. The appropriate facial procedure will consider the extent of change in these tissues and attempt the appropriate esthetic corrections. The overall approach must consider the patient's desired endpoint and can range from a subtle to a dramatically younger-looking result. In an effort to address the various types of facial aging, our approach ranges in the extent of the skin incision and the amount of redundant tissue to be addressed. In a careful analysis, the patient's age-derived texture and contour changes are highlighted, and realistic goals are frankly discussed. The patient must understand the principles underlying a face-lift operation and weigh the recuperative time and expense involved against any anticipated degree of improvement. The patient most suited for the "lunchtime" lift or sutureless face-lift tends to be the patient with early mandibular angle blurring and subtle neck drooping, with a minimum of fat accumulation. It is a matter of degree to move to the "minilift" procedure, and in this case the patient has a somewhat more pronounced drooping of the mandibular-cervical area, which is often due to excessive local fat accumulation. In addition, these patients present with mild to moderate laxity of the neck skin. Patients with extensive skin laxity are not candidates for the minimal-incision procedure and require a more conventional form of face-lift surgery. Also, extensive cords in the neck, which represent anterior platysmal banding, will require a more extensive procedure, while patients with little to mild skin laxity but dysmorphic fat in the jowls and/or neck can benefit from simple facial and/or neck liposuction (see Chap. 6).

During the preliminary consultation, the surgeon must clearly define the appropriate procedure, outlining the expected results and possible complications. Therefore, careful patient evaluation, thorough knowledge, and solid experience are required to select the appropriate procedure (see Chap. 6).

The procedure selected is based on several factors: general health, age, asymmetry, dysmorphic fat, weight gain or loss, muscle tone, bony structure, skin tone, skin thickness, and patient expectations. Those with a full, robust face or neck may require only facial and/or neck liposuction. Early tissue sagging and mild rhytids, depending on the skin's elasticity, can be substantially helped by limited skin procedures. Heavy sun damage, previous trauma, acne or other scarring, and radiation changes requires an individualized approach. If a large degree of tissue involution and sagging is present, a more standard rhytidectomy procedure should be chosen. In the choice of the appropriate procedure, the patient's chronological age is less important than the general quality of the skin and supporting structures. As a rule, however, the younger the patient, the better the results of the more limited procedure.

Preoperative Evaluation

In the preoperative evaluation for facial plastic procedures, we prefer clearance by a medical doctor and to make sure that an electrocardiogram, chest x-ray, SMAS, complete blood count (CBC), urinalysis, bleeding time, platelets, prothrombin time (PT), partial thromboplastin time (PTT), T4, and fibrinogen level are obtained. Photographs and consents are obtained preoperatively. In preparation for surgery, the patient is instructed that tobacco, alcohol, aspirin, nonsteroidal anti-inflammatory drugs, and anticoagulant medications are not to be used for 2 weeks prior to the procedure. A thorough history of all previous and current medications as well as any allergies, illnesses, or previous surgeries is obtained.

Anatomy of the Face and Neck

The entire operation encompassed in the minimal-incision rhytidectomy is carried out above the SMAS plane. The incisions and the dissection, therefore, do not invade deeper levels, where the major arteries and nerves of the face reside. Even so, a prerequisite to this procedure for the surgeon is a comprehensive knowledge of facial anatomy.

Anesthesia—Cutaneous

The minimal-incision rhytidectomy can be performed entirely under local anesthesia or with presedation. The tumescent technique for dilute local anesthesia permits regional local anesthesia of tissue using large volumes of 0.1% lidocaine and 1:1,000,000/epinephrine in physiologic saline. This infusion procedure not only enhances the turgor of the tissue, facilitating the removal of fat in liposuction, but also helps to establish the proper plane for surgical dissection superficial to the SMAS.[12]

Techniques

All of our patients undergo cervicofacial rhytidectomy in an outpatient ambulatory surgical setting. Intravenous conscious sedation is employed to ensure a comfortable patient experience.[14] Patients are marked while seated in an upright position (Fig. 17-1). The extent of the cutaneous incision is dictated by the amount of redundant tissue to be removed. The intervention of the "lunchtime" lift procedure is for maintenance, where tightening the SMAS and careful skin removal will result in restoration of an oval jawline and well-defined chin and neck angle (see Chap. 6). For the older individual with perhaps advanced drooping of the neck and jowls, a more striking restoration is performed, yet the conservative undermining and thorough SMAS resuspension allows for considerable excess skin removal and redraping, with minimal risk of blood supply compromise or nerve impairment. The various approaches are described, where the major variation depends on the degree of undermining and redundant skin removal; however, our standard face-lift surgical setup and tray remains the same (Figs. 17-2 and 17-3).

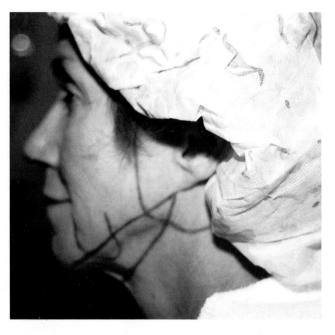

Figure 17-1 The patient is marked while seated upright—the preauricular marking projects the length of estimated undermining during the procedure. The jowl is outlined as in face-and-neck-liposuction. The platysmal band and neck are outlined to be swept during neck liposuction, to aid in creating the facial-neck flap as a cosmetic unit.

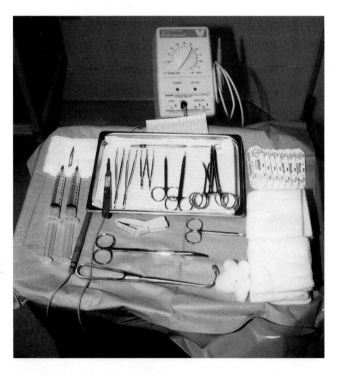

Figure 17-2 The face-lift tray (contents listed at the end of this chapter).

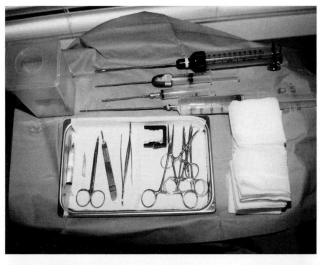

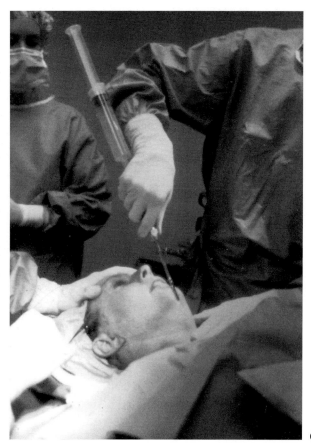

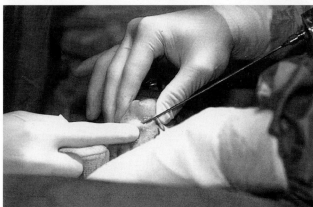

Figure 17-3   (*A*) Liposuction of the face and neck is part of the procedure to both remove fat and create the flaps (see Chap. 16). (*B*) Cannula hydrodissecting the plane of the neck. (*C*) Spatula cannula creating the flap while liposuction of the neck is under way.

After appropriate presedation, the patient is prepped and draped for sterility and a mixture of 3 to 5 mL of 1% lidocaine/ 1:100,000 epinephrine local anesthesia is infiltrated into the incision sites. The placement of the skin incisions can be undertaken for the particular rhytidectomy procedure. The incisions are initially a "nick" in the preauricular fold inferior to the tragus bilaterally; another "nick" with a no. 11 blade under the mentum in the midline; a 1-mm, "V"-shaped incision at the nadir point of attachment of the earlobe to help to appropriately realign and position the earlobe at the time of closure (Fig. 17-4); and a nick incision made on the posterior aspect of the auricle adjacent to the aricular sulcus the level of the tragus. Through these minute incisions, the hydrodissection is implemented via an infusion cannula (Fig. 17-5), entering the subcutaneous plane as in liposuction of the face and neck. The neck/jowls and periauricular zones

are then infused to produce a tumescent anesthesia, utilizing 150 to 1000 mL of 0.1% lidocaine/1:1,000,000 epinephrine in physiologic saline.

After this infusion through the submental incision , a 4-mm blunt spatula liposuction cannula is inserted. After expanding the appropriate plane by the use of hydrodissection, the cannula with syringe-assisted suction is moved radially, fully developing the cervical neck flap as in neck liposuction. After the neck flap has been developed in a blunt fashion, a facial liposuction of the jowls is accomplished using a 2-mm "tulip" liposuction cannula from the preauricular nick incisions. Caution is maintained during extraction of the jowl fat pads overlying the mandibular ramus to avoid possible nerve damage. The 4-mm cannula is then inserted into the preauricular incision and, in the minimal-incision rhytidectomy procedure, the undermining of tissue is extended along

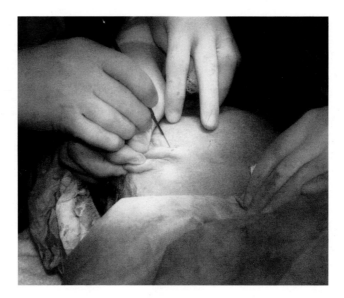

Figure 17-4   Marking of the incision at the nadir of the ear helps reposition the ear at closure. It essentially points to the position the ear should take to avoid "pixie ears" or a "Commander Spock" lower earlobe.

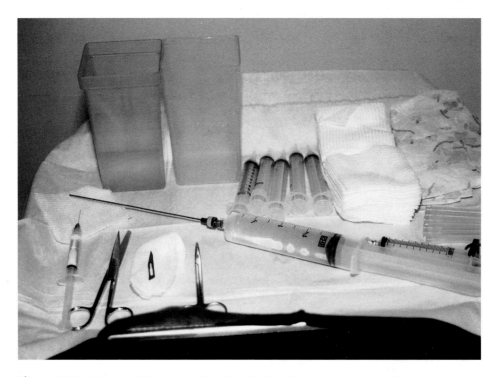

Figure 17-5   The "nick" incisions allow for this facial-neck infusion cannula to be passed to both anesthesized areas and begin to hydrodissect the tissue plane. The process in progress appears in Fig. 16-18.

the appropriate facial plane, staying superior to the SMAS. After that, via the posterior auricular incision, a nonsuction blunt radial dissection is carried out. The closed dissection is advanced with the use of the 4-mm spatula facial liposuction cannula, after which the incision defining the procedure is made. The multiple fibrous septa, separating the "tunnels" made by the passes of the cannula, are further dissected with the use of large Metzenbaum scissors (Fig. 17-6). In the lunchtime lift, the incision originates in the natural crease in the front of the earlobe just inferior to the tragus and extends downward through the original nick incision at the junction of the earlobe and cheek, after which it connects up with the minuscule V-shaped incision previously marking the nadir of the earlobe attachment. Then the incision rises, staying on the auricular side of the posterior sulcus, to end at the nick incision on the posterior auricle (Fig. 17-7). The length of the anterior incision length is approximately 1 cm and that of the posterior incision approximately 1.5 cm. In the minimal-incision rhytidectomy procedure, the extent of the incision is still conservatively small; therefore the area of dissection is accessed from limited surgical exposure (Fig. 17-8). A Foman retractor and small Allis forceps are helpful in carrying out the tissue dissection while opposing skin tension is maintained by an assistant. The underlying SMAS is then inspected and suctioned free of fat and debris.

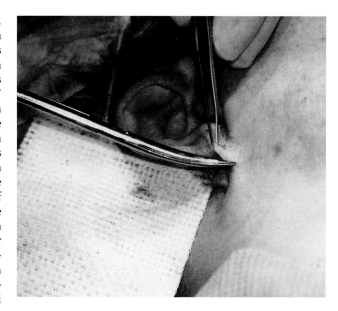

Figure 17-7 The "lunchtime" lift is an extremely small incision reaching only to under earlobe anteriorly and to the midpoint of the posterior sulcus of the ear.

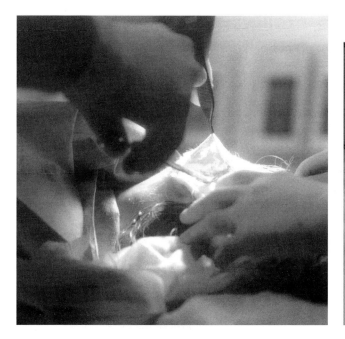

Figure 17-6 In the "minimal incision" face-lift, the undermining is not carried out nearly as far as for the full lift simply because the amount of tissue to be removed is less and therefore the new approximation of the remaining flap can be done over a shorter distance.

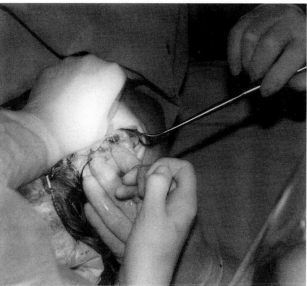

Figure 17-8 The limited access for plication is demonstrated. However, use of a Foman small retractor, along with opposing tension from the assistant, makes it possible to achieve an excellent result in the appropriately selected patient.

Plication

After the appropriate incision is made and bleeders are cauterized, the SMAS tissue is folded over itself and pulled up with the use of nonabsorbable suture. The number of plication sutures may vary depending on the degree of access and tension; however, we generally use four plication sutures. The first plication stitch runs from the angle of the mandible to the underlying point of the earlobe attachment, drawing together a span of approximately 2 to 6 cm, depending on the procedure being performed (Fig. 17-9A and B). This is a key positioning suture for posterosuperior lifting of the tissue. Additional sutures are placed along appropriate vectors in the posterior and preauricular area to achieve the desired upward force and esthetic results. The plication of the SMAS significantly reduces the overlying skin tension.

Correction of the facial skin redundancy is then accomplished. The trimming of the skin flap in this procedure can be especially difficult. The skin redundancy in the lunchtime procedure can only be redraped over a rather short distance. In this approach, the overlapping skin of the inferior lobe area is brought behind to the highest point of the posterior incision. The skin is relaxed and fanned out to approximate the closure and the earlobe delivered to its natural position through an anteroinferior bisection of the skin flap. The redundant tissue is then pulled posteriorly and superiorly and secured by the placement of one or two staples in the posterior sulcus. The earlobe is appropriately positioned with 4'0 absorbable buried sutures and the skin is approximated with Derma bond skin glue (Fig. 17-10). Light pressure is applied up to 2 h, after which, often, no dressing is required. In the minilift, because of the somewhat larger access, a greater tightening of the midface, jawline, and neck can be accomplished by the redraping of the SMAS layer in a posterosuperior direction. The skin flap is then drawn along the same posterosuperior vector under limited tension and fixed in place above and below the ear with two Ethicon skin staples (Fig. 17-11). The earlobe is delivered by bifurcating the skin flap with Metzenbaum scissors along the mandibular line marking, taking care to ensure that the previously made "V" of the delivered lobe rests just on the end of the bifurcation incision without excessive tension (Fig. 17-12). Excess skin is then trimmed to fit the anterior ear contour. The posterior redundant skin is dealt with by extending the incision posteriorly, horizontally into the hairline, with Metzenbaum scissors. Excess skin is trimmed to fit and affixed with Ethicon skin staples (Fig. 17-13). The preauricular incision is then closed with 5.0 Prolene suture, taking care to thin the tragal flap and preserve tragal contour. The difference in closure is related to the amount of redundant tissue removed and the distance over which this tissue must be lost, e.g., lunchtime mini or full lift (Fig. 17-14A and B). The same surgical sequence is then carried out on the opposite side.

The only variation for the full lift is that the superior extension of the incision rises above the ear and swings posteriorly 3 cm and then is carried in a linear direction temporally within the hair. After appropriate dissection, the elongated flaps and its redundant tissue is pulled superiorly, trimmed, and secured with staples (Fig. 17-15A and B).

The posterior incision is carried into the hairline to the extent necessary for smoothing after removing redundant neck skin.

Postoperative Care

Because of the utilization of Derma bond, the lunchtime lift requires no dressing. The other procedure's incisions are cleaned and dressed with antibiotic ointment and covered with nonstick gauze. A facial elastic garment is applied and the patient is kept in the recovery area until all discharge criteria are met. Initial postoperative instructions are reviewed with the patient's attendant, and the patient is discharged to a responsible adult. Upon return the next day, the head and neck areas are inspected and the dressings changed. Topical antibiotic ointment is applied twice daily, and the wounds are kept dry for 5 to 7 days. The patient is advised to avoid bending and lifting and instructed to sleep 30 to 45 degrees upright so as to minimize swelling. Sutures are removed in 7 to 10 days, at which time wearing of the facial elastic garment decreases from 24 to 12 h per day. Walking is encouraged for the first few weeks; aerobic activities may be resumed in 3 to 6 weeks.

Complications

A review of the complication rates in several large series demonstrates that hematoma is the most frequent complication of traditional cervicofacial rhytidectomy. The incidence ranges from 0.9 to 6.6 percent.[15] The hematomas tend to occur within the initial 12 h postoperatively. Pain is the most frequent complaint of patients with hematoma. This pain tends to be inordinately intense and constant. If the hematoma is expanding, it will require prompt drainage. To minimize compromising the skin flap in the standard technique, effective monitoring of pain postoperatively is essential, along with the prevention of nausea and hypertensive episodes. Hematoma could rarely occur with the minimal-incision technique and would require prompt drainage. However, aside from mild to moderate bruising, we have not had a problem with hematoma formation. Skin loss as a result of undue tension occurs in approximately 5 percent of cases in the more standard rhytidectomy procedure. In the minimal-incision lift, the skin flap is small and broad-based, which limits the possibility of sloughing. Facial nerve injury associated with traditional facioplasty occurs with an incidence from 0.4 to 2.5 percent. This can be limited by the use of blunt dissection, attention to the appropriate plane, and staying conservative in the extent of the dissection.

Sensory defects can occur, including injury to the greater auricular nerve, but more commonly transient sensory deficits occur around the ear. Bruising with or without pigmentary changes can occur. Temporary or, rarely, permanent alopecia can occur in standard rhytidectomy when incisions extend into the hairline. Infection and scarring are also risks. Skin or contour irregularities related to improper defatting, plication, or skin redraping may occur in all techniques.

(text continues on page 305)

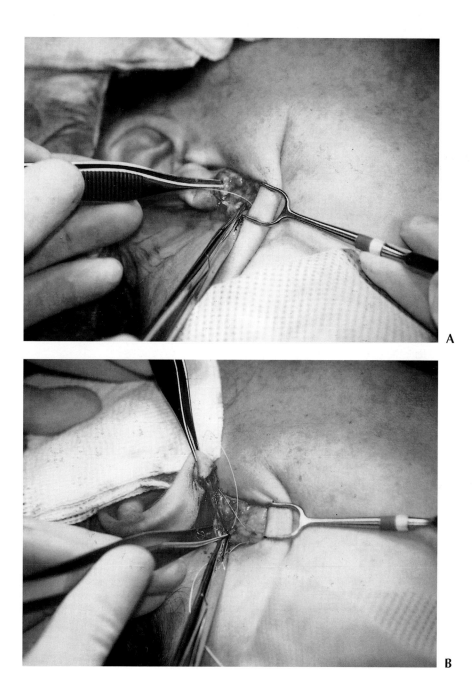

A

B

Figure 17-9   (*A*) The surgeon has reached into the dissected area with an Addison forcep, lifting the SMAS fascia and platysma first at the greatest distance available from access. It is then carried back to be secured in the posterior masseter fascia with 2/3′0 Mersilene. (*B*) The earlobe is lifted from the field while traction is moved posteriorly to facilitate the "lifting of the neck" by the placement of a suture.

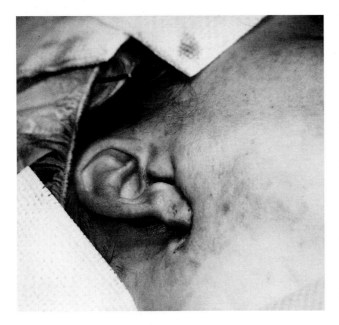

Figure 17-10 In the "lunchtime" version of this lift, the redundant skin is pulled and trimmed posteriorly and superiorly and secured with one or two staples adjacent to the posterior sulcus. Then the ear is repositioned utilizing the "V"-shaped incision tip of the ear and secured with a 4-0 Monocryl buried suture. Next, the reapproximated earlobe is closed with acrylic glue (Derma bond).

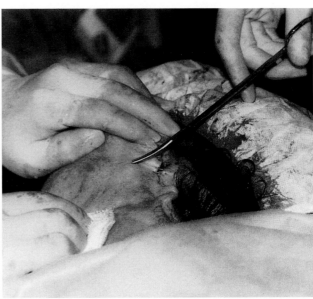

Figure 17-12 The earlobe is delivered by bifurcating the skin with a Metzenbaum scissors along the mandibular line that was marked initially, while the patient was seated. The bifurcation ends at the appropriate point, ensuring that the previously marked "V" rests just at the end of the bifurcating incision.

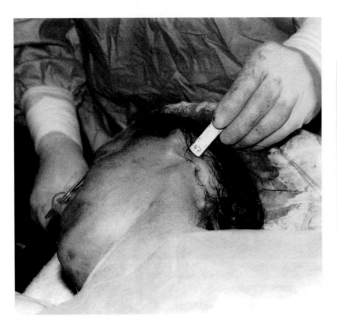

Figure 17-11 In the minilift, because of the larger incision and better access, a longer flap can be created. After neck plication, this is pulled over the ear and secured posteriorly by two skin staples.

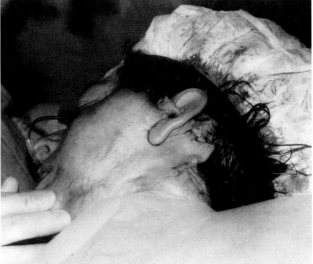

Figure 17-13 The redundant skin posteriorly is redraped by extending the incision horizontally and posteriorly into the hairline, where it is trimmed to fit.

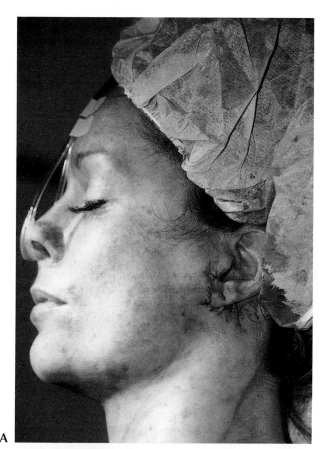

Figure 17-14 (**A**) The minilift with a much less aggressive incision, nicely approximated at the completion of the procedure. (**B**) In the full lift, the extent of the flap requires a posterior hairline closure along with an anterior closure. The anterior incision and hence closure is at the auricular canal interior portion of the tragus. The flap must be trimmed to maintain an esthetic tragal contour.

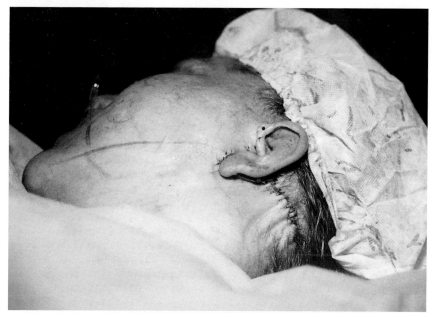

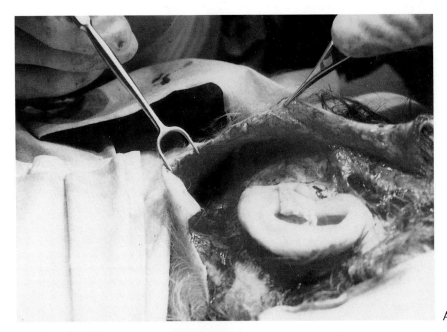

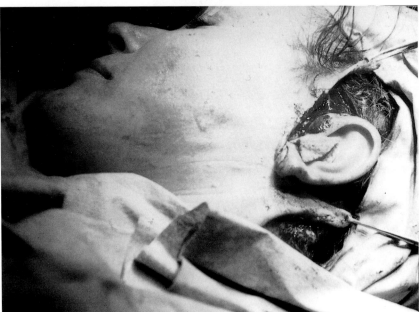

Figure 17-15   (**A**) The flap developed in the full lift can be extensive and requires precise approximation. (**B**) After lifting the skin, all is redraped by pulling the flap superiorly and posteriorly. It is secured with staples after redundant temporal tissue is trimmed to match the horizontally directed initial incision and posteriorly as in Fig. 17-13. The posterior redundant tissue is trimmed and secured by extending the incision and closure into the hairline.

Discussion

The dynamic process of facial aging results in a varied spectrum of tissue changes. Modern face-lift surgery addresses changes in the skin, fat, subcutaneous tissue, SMAS, muscle and bone, utilizing standard and innovative approaches. It is well understood that not all patients display the same degree of change in these tissues. Fat redistribution in the mandibular line as well as the submental and anterior cervical areas may contribute to a sagging appearance in the presence of minimally lax skin. In such cases, direct approaches or liposuction alone have been successfully employed to remove and recontour subcutaneous fat with excellent results.

The various approaches to rhytidectomy presented here are designed to correct the appearance of patients with excessive submandibular and submental fat, who, in our experience, will not completely respond to liposuction alone. These patients have mild to significantly redundant skin and some demonstrate a degree of anterior platysmal banding. One way to determine the extent of skin redundancy is to sweep the lower face and neck upward along the direction of the mandibular line. In general, if excessive skin is estimated to be present bilaterally with little or no fat compartment, the patient is probably a candidate for one of these approaches rather than simply for facial liposuction. In our experience, if the jowl and neck skin is pinched and the skin returns immediately upon release to the prepinched location, facial-neck liposuction will yield excellent results. However, if this does not occur, these patients benefit substantially from some type of face-lift procedure (Figs. 17-16A through D, 17-17A through D, 17-18A through D, 17-19A through D, and 17-20A through D).

Various depths and extents of tissue plane undermining employed in the approach to face-lift surgery have been promulgated through the years. Webster established, years ago, that it was not necessary to undermine skin flaps widely to achieve adequate short- and long-term results.[8–11,16–23] He showed—in many demonstrations during surgery and in procedures performed on fresh cadavers—that extensive undermining allows no more skin to be removed than is permitted by more conservative undermining.[9,10] Many years ago, he reported a series of patients in whom one side had essentially twice as much undermining as did the other.[11,12] The removable skin on each side was equal in amount, and long-term results were essentially the same on both sides. Burgess et al.[24] confirmed that skin closing tension was lower in SMAS suspension procedures than in non-SMAS plication procedures. He later conducted a cadaver study to determine the effects of skin-flap undermining and SMAS plication on wound-closing tension.[25] Results indicated that closing tension was significantly decreased with SMAS plication. The surprise was that the tension-reducing effect of SMAS plication was decreased with wider skin-flap undermining. It is logical that conservative undermining has certain advantages over radical undermining, since very wide undermining increases the danger of necrosing significant amounts of skin if the wound is closed under tension. Unless more radical undermining provides better results than does conservative undermining, it would seem unwise to continue use of the most dangerous approaches.

A renewed interest in the superficial plane face-lift approach has been called for by Duffy and Friedland.[26] On the basis of their experience in 750 patients, they reported long-lasting and predictable results with a minimum of complications when this approach was used. Beeson[27] delineates the advantages of effective management of the SMAS as an alternative to composite rhytidectomy for the majority of patients, and Lassus[28] implores surgeons to avoid the trend toward increasingly aggressive face-lift techniques, since—with the appropriate indications—the simpler superficial plane technique gives good and predictable results. However, amid the multitude of techniques currently used for performing face-lifts, there may never be a general agreement among surgeons as to which is the most effective. Kamer[29] undertook a retrospective chart review over a 6.5-year period of 634 patients who electively underwent either a SMAS or deep-plane rhytidectomy. He found that the deep-plane group underwent a "tuck" procedure 71 percent less frequently than the SMAS group (11.4 and 3.3 percent, respectively). If the assumption is made that the need for a tuck procedure implies a less than optimal face-lift, then the data of this study suggest that the deep-plane technique is more effective that the SMAS lift. However, too many variables entered into this retrospective study (such as initial patient selection criteria for each group, lack of a procedure protocol, which may have allowed for variations in skin removal and skin tension within each group, etc.) for any convincing conclusions to be reached.

For a time, it was hypothesized that radical undermining yielded a more significant "sheet of favorable fibrosis," which would help prolong the surgical result by providing long-lasting support. Webster's studies gave no substantiation for that theory, and he discredited it, since a more favorable long-term result could not be shown on one side over the other where both undermining techniques were used. To further cast doubt on that theory, Owsley[30] observed that, in performing a secondary lift, the scar density and adherence at the sub-SMAS—platysmal plane was significantly less fibrotic than that encountered at the subcutaneous plane—to his pleasant surprise.

A recent addition to the face-lift, which as a point of discussion has dramatically enhanced results, has been the addition of CO_2 laser resurfacing (see Chap. 14). This resurfacing combined with the short-flap lunchtime minilift has enhanced results quite dramatically.[12] The ability to combine multiple procedures in an attempt to achieve maximum cosmetic improvement is the ultimate goal of cosmetic surgeons and their patients. The key issue is to be conservative yet reach the appropriate result (Fig. 17-21A and B).

(text continues on page 311)

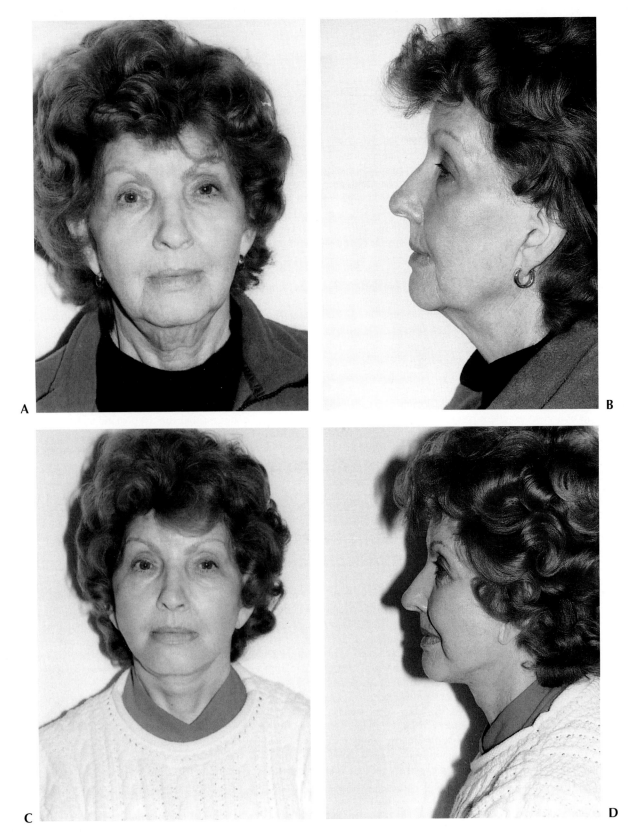

Figure 17-16   (*A*) The preoperative moderate extent of redundancy of skin documented by the pinch test (see Chaps. 16 and 17) required the minilift procedure. Note the "U"-shaped face. (*B*) Lateral preoperative shot documenting the lax skin. (*C*) The postoperative frontal view, revealing the return of the "V"-shape (see Chap. 6). (*D*) The lateral postoperative view, revealing a more youthful-looking neck and improved earlobe positioning.

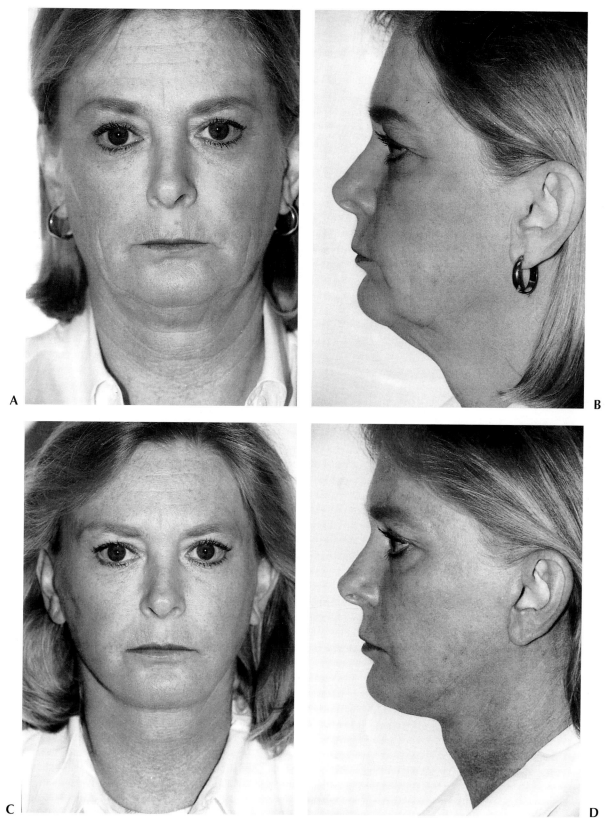

Figure 17-17   (*A*) Preoperative view of a patient to undergo minilift frontal view of "U"-shaped face. (*B*) Preoperative lateral view of same laxity in skin, along with a fat pad requiring some excision to achieve good results. (*C*) Postoperatively the "V" shape has returned to the face. (*D*) There is now a good profile and natural-appearing ear.

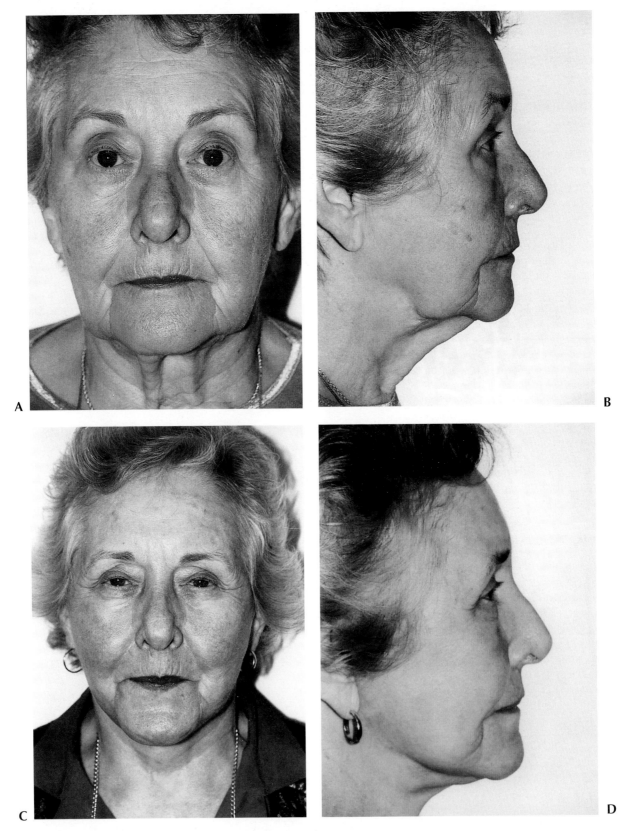

Figure 17-18 (**A**) Preoperatively, very lax skin that requires a full lift is seen; the "U" shape more obvious. (**B**) Preoperatively, there is a "turkey neck," which requires a full lift. (**C**) Post-operatively, the face's "V" shape has returned, with an excellent frontal mandibular definition. (**D**) A good mandibular angle is now seen, with an average improvement in "turkey neck."

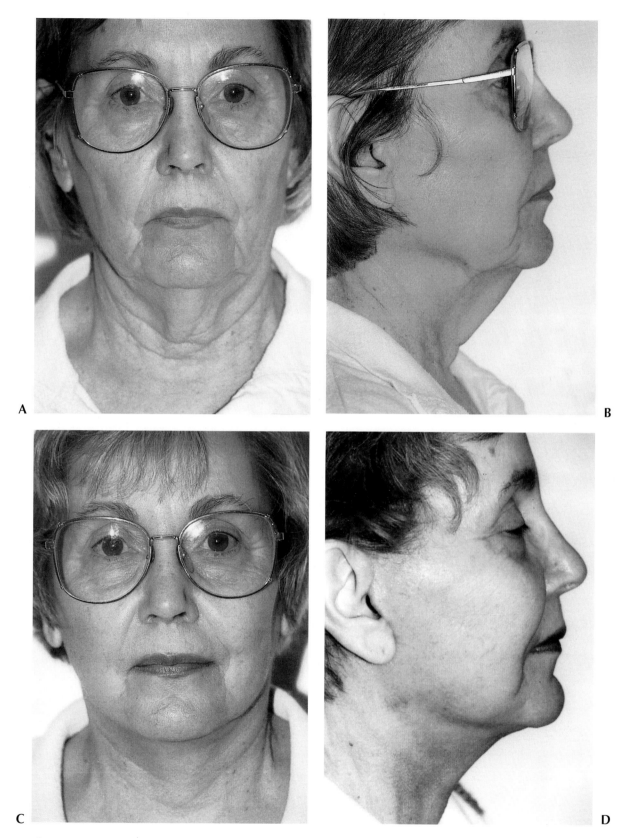

Figure 17-19 (*A*) Preoperative frontal view of full lift. (*B*) Preoperative frontal view of lateral lift. (*C*) Postoperative frontal view of frontal lift. (*D*) Postoperative frontal view of lateral lift.

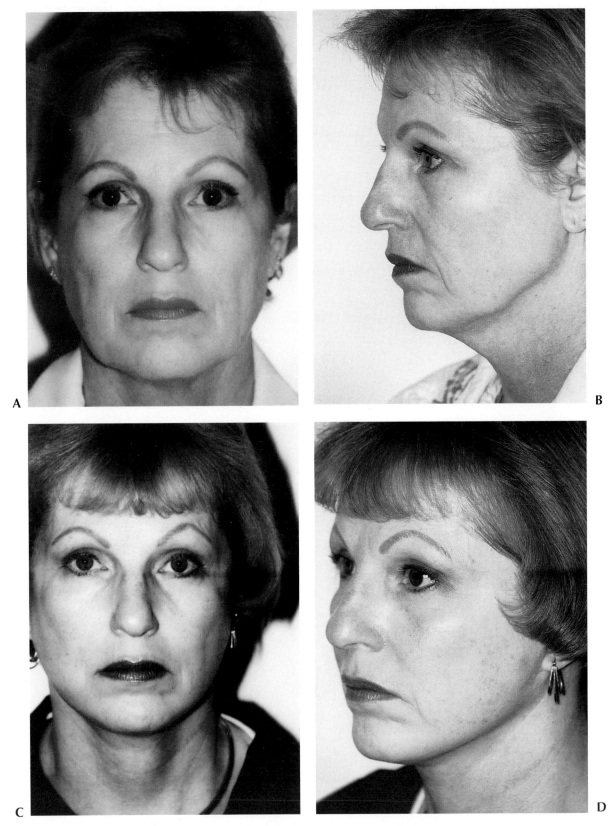

A

B

C

D

Figure 17-20 (*A*) Preoperative view of "lunchtime" lift. (*B*) Preoperative view of lunchtime lift. (*C*) Postoperative view of lunchtime lift. (*D*) Postoperative view of lunchtime lift. The natural earlobe position and tragus definition enhance the esthetic result of this procedure.

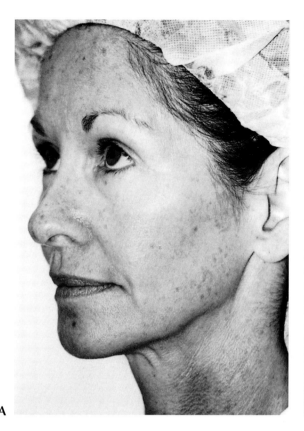

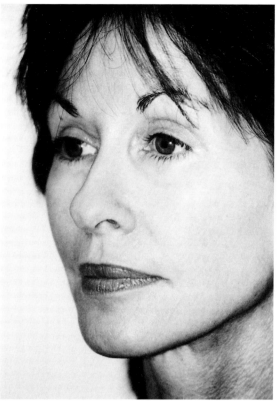

A

B

Figure 17-21 (*A*) Preoperative frontal view of patient prior to lunchtime lift and CO_2 laser resurfacing and blepharoplasty. (*B*) Postoperative view. Note the sharpened mandibular angle, skin finish, and upper lid definition.

References

1. Shire JR, Johnson CM Jr, Orr JB. The large flap sculptured facelift. *J Dermatol Surg Oncol* 1988; 14(12):1352–1356.

2. Hoefflin SM. The extended supraplatysmal plane (ESP) face lift. *Plast Reconstr Surg* 1998: 101(2):494–503.

3. Mitz V, Leblanc P, Maladry D, Aboudaram T. Results of biplane face lifts and maximal skin underlining and vertical SMAS flap. *Ann Chir Plast Esthet* 1996; 41(6):693–712.

4. Baker SR. Triplane rhytidectomy. Combining the best of all worlds. *Arch Otolaryngol Head Neck Surg* 1997; 123(11): 1167–1172.

5. Teimourian B, Delia S, Wahrman A. The multiplane face lift. *Plast Reconstr Surg* 1994; 93(1):78–85.

6. Aiache AE. Endoscopic facelift. *Aesthet Plast Surg* 1994; 18(3):275–278.

7. Hamra ST. *Composite Rhytidectomy.* St. Louis: Quality Medical Publishing; 1993.

8. Webster RC. Conservative facelift surgery. *Arch Laryngol* 1976; 102:657–682.

9. Webster RC, Davidson TM, Nahum AM. Facelift, part I. In: *San Diego Classics in Soft Tissue and Cosmetic Surgery.* San Diego CA: American Academy of Facial Plastic and Reconstructive Surgery; 1976.

10. Webster RC, Davidson TM, Nahum AM. Facelift, part II. In: *San Diego Classics in Soft Tissue and Cosmetic Surgery.* San Diego CA: American Academy of Facial Plastic and Reconstructive Surgery; 1976.

11. Webster RC, Brown CA, Hilger PA, Smith RC. Comparison between short and long term results in face lifts. *Aesthet Reconstr Facial Plast Surg* 1978; 5:1–98.

12. Bisaccia E, Sequeira M, Magidson J, Scarborough D. Surgical intervention for the aging face: Combination of mini-facelifting and superficial carbon dioxide laser resurfacing. *Dermatol Surg* 1998; 24:821–826.

13. Stuzin JM, Baker TJ, Gordon DA. The relationship of the superficial and deep facial fascias: Relevance to rhytidectomy and aging. *Plast Reconstr Surg* 1992; 89:441–449.

14. Abeles G, Sequeira M, Swensen RD, et al. The combined use of propofol and fentanyl for outpatient intravenous conscious sedation. *Dermatol Surg* 1999; 25(7):559–561.

15. Owsley JQ. The unfavorable result following face and neck lifting. In: Goldwyn RM, ed. *The Unfavorable Result in Plastic Surgery.* Boston: Little, Brown; 1984:597.

16. Cohen SR, Webster, RC. Primary rhytidectomy—Complications of the procedure and anesthetic. *Laryngoscope* 1983; 93(5):654–656.

17. Webster RC, Smith RC, Smith KF. Facelift, part I: Extent of undermining of skin flaps. *Head Neck Surg* 1983; 5(6):525–534.

18. Webster RC, Smith RC, Smith KF. Facelift, part II: Etiology of platysmal cords and its relationship to treatment. *Head Neck Surg* 1983; 6(1):590–595.

19. Webster RC, Smith RC, Smith KF. Facelift, part III: Plication of the superficial musculoaponeurotic system. *Head Neck Surg* 1983; 6(2):696–701.

20. Webster RC, Smith RC, Smith KF. Facelift, part IV: Use of superficial musculoaponeurotic system suspending sutures. *Head Neck Surg* 1984; 6(3):780–791.

21. Webster RC, Smith RC, Smith KF. Facelift, part V: Suspending sutures for platysmal cords. *Head Neck Surg* 1984; 6(4):870–879.

22. Webster RC, Hamden US, Smith RC. The considered and considerate facelift, part I: Conservative undermining, role of limited redraping, and choice of direction of pull. *Am J Cosmet Surg* 1985; 2(3):1.

23. Webster RC, Hamden US, Smith RC. The considered and considerate facelift, part II: SMAS plication vs. imbrication, theory of SMAS anatomy and dynamics, and conservation of the platysma. *Am J Cosmet Surg* 1985; 2(4):65.

24. Burgess LP, Lau P, Glenn M, Goode RL. Wound tension in rhytidectomy. A preliminary report. *Arch Otolaryngol Head Neck Surg* 1988; 114(11):1280–1287.

25. Burgess LP, Casler JD, Kryzer TC. Wound tension in Rhytidectomy. Effects of skin-flap undermining and superficial musculoaponeurotic system suspension. *Arch Otolaryngol Head Neck Surg* 1993; 119(2):173–177.

26. Duffy MJ, Friedland JA. The Superficial-plane rhytidectomy revisited. *Plast Reconstr Surg* 1994; 93(7):1392–1405.

27. Beeson WH. Effective management of the superficial musculoaponeurotic system as an alternative to composite rhytidectomy. *Facial Plast Surg* 1996; 12(3):223–230.

28. Lassus C. Cervicofacial rhytidectomy: The superficial plane. *Aesthet Plast Surg* 1997; 21(1):25–31.

29. Kamer FM, Frankel AS. SMAS rhytidectomy versus deep plane rhytidectomy: An objective comparison. *Plast Reconstr Surg* 1998; 102(3):878–881.

30. Owsley JQ. Aesthetic facial surgery. Philadelphia: Saunders; 1994.

31. Ivy EJ, Lorenc ZP, Aston SJ. Is there a difference? A prospective study comparing lateral and standard SMAS face lifts and extended SMAS and composite rhytidectomies. *Plast Reconstr Surg* 1996; 98(7):1135–1147.

Patient Information

The Face-Lift

Telltale signs of aging begin to appear on our face and neck as we reach our mid-thirties to early forties. Because our skin becomes less elastic as we age, we may develop loose and unsightly skin folds and wrinkles around the chin, jaw line, and neck. When this happens, we look older and much less attractive.

The face-lift, also known as a rhytidectomy, is a remarkable procedure that corrects the effects of aging and restores a youthful appearance. During this procedure, your facial skin and muscles are tightened, and your surgeon removes any loose, excess skin. The rhytidectomy is often combined with other cosmetic procedures, like liposuction and eyelid surgery, to help patients look years younger.

Patients who are just beginning to experience major signs of aging may wish to have a minilift. This procedure is similar to the full facelift, but not as extensive. It is helpful in improving the neck-chin angle and restoring the tight jaw-line definition usually found in the youthful face.

Cosmetic surgeons help people develop and maintain a healthy, more attractive, and younger appearance. Our skilled surgeons specialize in face-lifts and minilifts and have used their knowledge, skill, and experience for more than a decade to help numerous patients look younger and more attractive.

The Procedure

The cosmetic surgeons will perform this procedure in an outpatient setting. There, you will be given a light sedative and local anesthesia prior to the surgery.

During the procedure, your surgeon makes tiny incisions in front of your earlobes and near your temples. If you are having facial liposuction done at the same time, as many people do to remove fat deposits around the facial area, your surgeon will make a small incision beneath your chin. He then inserts a surgical instrument called a cannula into the fat layers below your skin and gently suctions the sagging, excess fat from your jowl and chin areas. After this fat is removed, your surgeon extends the incisions in front of your earlobes and slightly up, around, and behind your ears. Your loose skin is gently pulled up and back and the loose underlying tissues are tightened. Any excess skin is removed, and your incisions are closed with tiny sutures. Both the incisions and sutures leave relatively subtle lines that fall into the natural facial creases and hairline. The procedure generally takes from 2 to 3 hours, depending upon your skin condition.

Immediately after surgery, you will have to wear bandages and will need to apply cold compresses to your face and neck areas several times a day for the first 24 to 48 hours. Some swelling and discoloration may occur, which will often disappear within 10 days. Any discomfort you may experience can be minimized with cold compresses or medication.

The Results

Most patients who have had face-lifts are delighted with their more attractive and youthful appearance. Ask for a consultation to find out how the face-lift can help you look younger.

Five days following surgery, your doctor will remove your sutures. Any slight marks resulting from the incision are hidden in your natural skin creases and hairline and will fade significantly over time. Sometimes patients may experience a slight tightness or numbness around the treated areas; this, too, will diminish over time.

The final results of your face-lift will not be fully apparent for several weeks. During this time, you should avoid the sun and wear a sunscreen at all times when you are outdoors to protect the healing skin.

CONSENT FOR FACE AND NECK LIFT AND/OR FOREHEAD LIFT

Patient's name_____

Date_____

I hereby authorize _____ and/or his surgical team to perform a surgical operation for excision of the excess skin on my face and neck (except forehead lift wherein excess forehead and/or scalp skin will be removed), which also includes a change of appearance in my face. The doctor has explained the procedure to me and I completely understand its nature and consequences.

I understand that every surgical procedure involves certain risks and possibilities of complications, such as bleeding, infection, poor healing, scarring, nerve damage, muscle weakness, etc., and that these and other complications may follow even when the surgeon uses the utmost care, judgment, and skill. These risks have been explained to me and I accept them.

Initial_____

The following points have been explained in detail:

A. Bleeding will occur and in rare instances, may require hospitalization and blood transfusion. It is possible that blood clots may form under the skin and require subsequent drainage. Bleeding after surgery may

313

require reoperation. Smokers, drinkers, aspirin users, and male patients are at higher risk for postoperative bleeding. I understand all this and accept the risks.

Initial_____

B. Skin irregularities, lumpiness, hardness, and dimpling may appear postoperatively. Most of these problems disappear with time, but localized skin firmness, lumpiness, and/or irregularities may persist permanently. If loose skin is present in the treated area, it may or may not shrink to conform to the new contour.

Initial_____

C. Infection is unlikely but, should it occur, treatment with antibiotics and/or surgical drainage may be required.

Initial_____

D. Numbness or increased sensitivity of the skin over treated areas may persist for months. It is possible that localized areas of numbness or increased sensitivity could be permanent.

Initial_____

E. Objectionable scarring is uncommon but, rarely, severe bruising or skin ulceration may result in scarring in the treated area. This scarring may be painful.

Initial_____

F. Dizziness may occur during the first week following liposuction surgery, particularly upon rising from a lying or sitting position. If this occurs, extreme caution must be exercised while walking. Do not attempt to drive a car if dizziness is present.

Initial_____

G. The face will be swollen and bruised after surgery and may require several weeks to fully recover. It will be worst for a few days postoperatively and will usually improve greatly over 1 to 6 weeks. It may be 3 to 6 months before the final result is apparent.

Initial_____

H. All incisions and resultant scars have been fully outlined to me. I may require a later revision of such scars when my healing is complete.

Initial_____

I. The improvement from a face-lift varies greatly among patients. I understand it can never eliminate all wrinkles or signs of aging. I understand that the two sides of the face are not the same and can never be made to look the same in all regards. I understand that bone and muscle structures help to create the body's overall shape, that they are never identical on both sides of the body, and that they will remain unchanged by the surgery.

Initial_____

J. Numbness will occur after surgery and will improve gradually. Rarely, it can be permanent.

Initial_____

K. Facial nerve injury can occur in spite of good technical surgery.

Initial_____

L. Hair loss and/or scarring in the hairline, although unlikely, is possible.

Initial_____

I have an understanding of the operation, which includes but is not limited to the above items. I understand that secondary revisions may be required in some cases. I also understand that should revision be required, charges will be made for the use of the operating room, whether in the office or the hospital. I agree to be responsible for these charges.

I am aware the practice of medicine and surgery is not an exact science and I acknowledge that no guarantees have been given to me as to the results of the operation and procedures, nor are there any guarantees against unfavorable results.

I give permission to _____ to take still or motion clinical photographs with the understanding such photographs remain the property of the center. If in the judgment of the center, medical research, education, or science will be benefited by their use, such photographs and related information may be published and republished in professional journals or medical books or used for any other purpose which the center may deem proper. It is specifically understood that in any such publication or use, I shall not be identified by name.

I understand that the two sides of the face are not the same and can never be made to look the same in all regards. I understand that bone and muscle structures help create overall shape and are never identical on both sides of the body, and that these will remain unchanged by the surgery.

I understand it is mandatory for me to have made prior arrangements to be driven to and from the doctor's office by a responsible adult.

For the purpose of advancing medical education, I consent to the admittance of authorized observers to the operating room.

I understand that elective surgical procedures are most often delayed until after the termination of a pregnancy. My signature attests that to the best of my knowledge I am not pregnant at this time.

I agree to discontinue smoking entirely for a period of 2 weeks prior to surgery and 2 weeks immediately following surgery.

I have been given the opportunity to ask questions and all my questions have been answered to my satisfaction.

Initial_____

My signature indicates that I have read this "Consent for Face and Neck and/or Forehead Lift" and I understand and accept the risks involved with this operation. I hereby authorize _____ and/or the surgical team to perform this surgical procedure on me.

Mini Face-lift Preoperative Instructions

Use no aspirin, vitamin E, or drugs containing aspirin (Bufferin, Anacin, Empirin, Stanback, Excedrin, Fiorinal, Darvon compound, APC, and salicylates), or alcohol 2 weeks prior to surgery. Use only Tylenol instead. *Very Important!!*

No smoking 2 weeks prior to surgery and for 2 weeks postoperatively.

Get plenty of rest the previous night.

Wear clothes that either zip or button and do not have to be pulled over your head.

Arrange for a ride home.

Do not wear any eye makeup 48 hours prior to surgery. Wear no makeup to the office on the day of the surgery.

Do not wear any jewelry to the office on the day of surgery.

Be sure to scrub face thoroughly, and shampoo the hair prior to surgery.

Bring pain medication with you on surgery day.

Take all preoperative medications directed.

Please note that during the surgical procedure you will *not* be under general anesthesia but will be slightly asleep and unaware of the operation.

Day-of-surgery diet guidelines: No solid food or milk after midnight on the day of surgery.

Unlimited clear liquids from the list below may be taken up to 3 hours before the scheduled time of surgery. After that time, only oral medications may be taken. Oral medications should be taken with no more than 1 ounce of water up to 1 hour before surgery.

ONLY ACCEPTABLE CLEAR LIQUIDS

Water
Black coffee or tea
(no milk, cream, or nondairy creamer)
Apple juice (clear)
Club soda, ginger ale, Seven-Up, cola

Contact lenses must be removed before surgery. If you wish to remove them in the office, please bring your case.

Minilift Setup Tray

Patient

1. Sterile surgical hat
2. Cape

Doctor and Staff

1. Mask
2. Surgical hat
3. Shoe covers
4. Sterile gowns
5. Sterile gloves

Materials

1. Sterile minilift tray and large green retractor
2. One no. 11 blade, one no. 15 blade
3. Purple skin marker
4. Betadine solution

5. Bobby pins
6. Three sterile medium drapes
7. Two sterile fat boxes
8. Small sterile bath towel
9. Approximately 400 mL tumescent solution
10. Syringes
    A. Four to six 10-mL Luer-Lok (if fat transfer) or three
       10-mL Luer-Lok (if no fat transfer)
    B. Two 60-mL Luer-Lok
    C. One 60-mL Toomey
    D. One 12-mL Toomey
11. Two 30-gauge 1-in. metal-hub needles
12. One 21-gauge needle
13. Cannulas
    A. Small infusion
    B. Small accelator or neck harvester
    C. 4-mm tulip spatula
    D. Small gold tulip (open if needed)
14. Hyfrecator with foot pedal
15. Sterile light-handle cover
16. Kenalog 40 mg/mL 1 mL IM before procedure
17. Sutures
    A. Four packages of 2-0 Mersilene
    B. Three or four packages of 5-0 Prolene P3
       (open 2 to start)
18. Polysporin ointment
19. 2 medium Telfa pads
20. One 5 × 9 in. Surgipad
21. Facial support garment
22. ¼-in. Brown Steri-Strips
23. Sterile Mayo-stand cover
24. Mastisol
25. Tape
26. ½-in. Brown Steri-Strips
27. Four sterile cotton balls (if not on minilift tray)
28. Two 15-shot skin staplers

Mini Face-lift Postoperative Instructions

Swelling and discoloration may be present following facial surgery. The amount varies from person to person. The following may help minimize swelling and discoloration after surgery.

Activity

Do not drive until *after* your first postoperative appointment.

You should be resting in bed the remainder of the day of surgery. *Elevate* your head at all times for 2 weeks and either sleep on two pillows at a 45-degree angle or sleep in a recliner or lounge chair. Sleep with your head straight, and *do not* roll on your side.

Cold compresses in plastic bags should be applied to the face and neck at frequent intervals (especially for the first 4 hours). Remember to put the compresses into plastic wrappers to keep the bandages dry. Continued use of cold compresses for 30 minutes four to six times a day for the first few days will reduce swelling.

You may return to reasonable activity 24 hours after surgery. You may resume light exercise after 1 week. Avoid excessive bending or straining. After exercising, you may get some swelling; if so, resume the application of cold compresses.

Appointments

You will have to return for a dressing change 24 hours after surgery. Please arrange for a ride to and from the office for this appointment. In 5 to 7 days, you will have to return for suture removal. Please make sure that you arrange all of these appointments.

Diet

Let all liquids and foods cool to lukewarm. You should eat soft foods and do no hard chewing for 3 days. Drink clear liquids to prevent dehydration (four to six 8-ounce glasses of water a day).

Bathing

Try to keep the tapes applied to your chin dry for 3 days. Showering (lukewarm water) from the neck down is possible after 24 hours following surgery, keeping the facial garment dry. It may be removed for light cleansing of the face and neck after the third day. You may shampoo your hair on the third postoperative day. You may want to wash and dry the garment at this time.

Medications

Keep a record of the times medications are taken. Take medications as prescribed. *Do not* "hold back" or "double up" on medications without checking with the doctor. Do not overmedicate yourself. Instead, use elevation of your head and cold compresses for relief of mild discomfort. *No alcoholic beverages* or *smoking* is allowed for 2 weeks. This may be an ideal time to stop smoking for good, and we would be pleased to assist you with this.

Covering Discoloration

Cover creams may be used to camouflage discolorations. Do not put cover creams on sutures or incisions until they are healed (no crusting or moisture present). The nurse may instruct you on cover creams.

Avoid

Sunbathing or tanning booths for at least 6 weeks.

Care of Stitches and Skin Staples

Cleanse these areas twice a day using a Q-Tip and saline or warm tap water, followed by an application of Polysporin ointment. Do not clip or shorten any of the stitches.

You may *shampoo* your hair gently on the third day after surgery. Remember to keep facial/neck tapes *dry*. Shampoo in the sink if necessary.

Numbness

This sensation is frequent in the surgically treated areas for 6 to 12 weeks. Please do not be alarmed, since it is normal during the healing process. There also may be hardness and lumpiness during this time where the skin is tightening down. This will gradually resolve.

CHAPTER 18

Blepharoplasty

Blepharoplasty is a crucial procedure in the management of the aging upper third of the face. This oculoplastic procedure is indicated for the treatment of excess eyelid skin (dermatochalasis) and overrelaxation of eyelid skin (blepharochalasis). The indications may be strictly cosmetic, to restore a more youthful appearance to the eyelids, and also functional, in cases where excess upper eyelid skin results in hooding and decreased visual fields. Mastery of this technique requires a prior knowledge of eyelid anatomy, indications for the different surgical techniques, complications, and their management. This chapter reviews the surgical consultation, skin flap and skin-muscle flap techniques for correction of the upper and lower eyelids, as well as the transconjunctival approach. Finally, the postoperative course, complications, and their management are discussed.

The initial surgical consultation is the ideal setting to learn why the patient seeks surgery as well as to educate the patient on the procedure and its indications. The ultimate decision as to whether the patient indeed is a candidate for blepharoplasty will be made based on realistic expectations, motives, past medical history, and physical examination.

It is always wise to hand the patient a mirror and ask him or her to point to the areas that are bothersome as well as to state their reasons for seeking improvement. This maneuver will immediately reveal if the surgical goals are attainable and will allow the surgeon to address the patient's individual needs. During the initial encounter, a thorough past medical history should be obtained, with emphasis on possible contraindications to the procedure. The patient should be asked about his or her general physical health, allergies, medications, previous history of condition such as thyroid disease, chronic eyelid edema, history of bleeding disorders, psychiatric disorders, thyroid disease, diabetes, and previous procedures and complications.

The next step is a meticulous examination of the eyebrows and eyelids. The patient is assessed while sitting in a relaxed position, preferably with the surgeon sitting directly across at the same level. The patient is asked to raise the eyebrows to determine the integrity of the frontalis muscle and the temporal branch of the facial nerve. Any asymmetries are noted as well as the presence of eyebrow ptosis. Inferior displacement of the eyebrow or ptosis results from aging and can give the illusion of excess upper eyelid skin (pseudoblepharochalasis).[1] Identifying this condition is critical, as a blepharoplasty repair in the absence of eyebrow elevation may worsen the condition. The ideal eyebrow position in a male is horizontal at the level of the supraorbital rim. In females, the eyebrow arches above the supraorbital rim until it reaches a vertical line tangential to the lateral limbus or lateral canthus; then it tapers laterally.[2] The distance from the central upper eyelid to the inferior mid brow edge is about 10 mm. The amount of eyebrow ptosis can be quantified by aligning the zero mark of a ruler with the superior mid-eyebrow, then raising the eyebrow to the desired location and measuring the elevation on the ruler. The same measurement can then be obtained nasally and temporally.

The eyelids are evaluated next for excess skin texture, herniated fat, level of supratarsal crease, ptosis, lacrimal gland position, and lower eyelid laxity. Excess eyelid laxity can be very marked, manifest by redundant skin overhanging the eyelid, or subtle, with just a slight obstruction of the supratarsal fold. The distance from the upper eyelid to the eyelid crease or supratarsal fold averages between 9 and 11 mm.[2] This fold is an important landmark in establishing the inferior excisional margin when excess upper eyelid skin is being removed. In addition to its position, the visibility of the eyelid crease is very important cosmetically. A high crease typically is considered esthetically pleasing in women but can be feminizing in males. A very high crease may suggest disinsertion of the levator aponeurosis and should be referred to an ophthalmic plastic surgeon for repair. A very low crease may require excision of excess fat and deep fixation to the levator aponeurosis to recreate the fold. Certain ethnic groups, such as Asians, have epicanthal folds and may have an absent eyelid crease, the creation of which is more complex.[3,4] The crease should be placed lower than in Caucasians for its best esthetic effect; if the surgeon lacks expertise in the procedure, it is best to refer the patient to an ophthalmic plastic surgeon.

The presence of herniated fat is easily assessed by gently pushing on the globe through the lower eyelid to determine excess upper eyelid fat or through the upper eyelid to determine if there is an excess on the lower lid. Sometimes a hypertrophied orbicularis oculi muscle may give the impression of excess lower eyelid fat, and this can be better distinguished by the previous test as well as by evaluating the eye while the patient smiles. Fullness of the temporal eyelid may represent a prolapsed lacrimal gland, as there is no temporal fat compartment in the upper eyelid. Fat is present only medially and centrally. The surgeon must be very careful not to remove the lacrimal gland, as this would result in a chronically dry eye. Repositioning of the lacrimal gland is best left to the ophthalmic plastic surgeon.

Determination of lower eyelid laxity is the next step of the eye examination. It can be accomplished by pushing on the central aspect of the lower lid both medially and laterally and observing the extent of displacement of the medial and lateral canthi.[2] The lower eyelid can also be pinched away from the globe; if the apex can be retracted more than 6 mm, laxity exists. Laxity can also be tested by how quickly the eyelid retracts back to its natural position after it is pulled away and released. Last, the texture of the eyelid skin is evaluated for signs of excessive wrinkling or dyschromia. The patient may require carbon dioxide resurfacing or chemical peeling in addition to surgery to achieve the desired improvement.

If, after the initial evaluation, the surgeon feels that the patient is a candidate for the procedure, the preoperative and postoperative course can be discussed. This is the part of the consultation that can be greatly aided by "before" and "after" photographs of previously treated patients. The pictures can help to outline incision sites as well as the possible correction. The patient can be educated on details of the operation itself. Medicolegally, it is important not to guarantee results. The preoperative and postoperative instructions are then reviewed one by one and all questions are answered. The patient can take the instructions and consents home for further review prior to signing them. Fees can be discussed at this point. Ultimately, if the patient is sure that he or she wants to proceed with the operation, then he or she is referred to an ophthalmologist for baseline visual acuity tests, visual field maps, fundoscopic examination, and a Shirmer test to determine tear secretion.[2] It is critical to obtain these tests to ensure that any perceived visual change on the part of the patient is not blamed on the operation itself.

We like to schedule a second preoperative visit to evaluate the results of these tests as well as to answer any additional questions. The consent forms should be signed then, and preoperative photographs obtained. The photographs should be standardized to include shots of the patient looking straight ahead, with upward and downward gaze and with the eye closed. Oblique and lateral views of each eye should also be included. Once these photographs have been obtained, the patient is free to leave but will be quickly reevaluated just prior to the operation. Although the intent of this chapter is not to be a comprehensive review of orbital and facial anatomy, certain anatomic structures that may be compromised during blepharoplasty surgery are described. Many texts on this subject are available.[4–6]

The eyelids are divided into anterior lamellae consisting of skin and orbicularis muscle and posterior lamellae that include the tarsal plates and conjunctivae.[5] The eyelid skin is very thin and overlies the orbicularis muscle, which is concentrically divided into an orbital part (extending beyond the orbital rim), a preseptal part (overlying the orbital septum), and a pretarsal part (overlying the tarsal plates). The orbital septum is a fibrous layer that extends from the orbital rim and attaches to the levator aponeurosis several millimeters above the tarsal plate on the upper eyelid and to the inferior border of the tarsal plate on the lower lid after fusing with the lower eyelid retractors. The tarsal plates are made of fibrous and elastic tissue and give support to the eyelids. The conjunctiva is adjacent to the posterior border of the tarsal plate. The upper eyelid retractors consist of the levator muscle and Müller's muscle. The levator muscle originates from the orbital roof and extends inferiorly, eventually becoming a band (levator aponeurosis) that attaches to the anterior surface of the tarsal plate. Müller's smooth muscle arises from the inferior division of the levator muscle and attaches also to the superior border of the tarsal plate posterior to the levator aponeurosis.

The attachment of the levator aponeurosis to the orbicularis muscle and subdermal skin helps create the eyelid crease. An inferior attachment as well as presence of subcutaneous and lower preaponeurotic fat contribute to an absent crease in some Asians.[4] The lower eyelids retractors are formed from the inferior rectus muscle sheath and consist of the capsulopalpebral fascia and Müller's muscle. The two fuse about 5 mm before inserting into the inferior tarsal plate.[7]

Preaponeurotic fat pads separate the orbital septum from the levator aponeurosis. In the upper eyelids, there are two fat pads, a small medial one and a larger central one. There is no lateral fat pad. Typically, a prolapsed lacrimal gland may give the incorrect impression of herniated fat laterally. The novice surgeon must be very aware of this fact. The lower eyelid has three fat pads: medial, central, and lateral (temporal). The inferior oblique muscle separates the medial and central fat collections and must not be injured, especially during a transconjunctival blepharoplasty. The preaponeurotic fat pads are very vascular and great care must be taken when excising them so as to control bleeding and prevent serious complications such as retrobulbar bleeds.

Surgical Techniques

The surgical techniques can be individualized to each patient depending on the specific physical findings and the necessary correction. Patients may require excision of excess skin alone, skin and fat, or skin, fat, and muscle. The skin flap approach will address the first two cases, whereas a skin/muscle flap approach will be needed in the latter. In patients with just lower eyelid excess fat and good skin tone without excess skin, the transconjunctival approach would be most beneficial. In some cases, in the event of slight excess skin, this approach can be combined with superficial laser resurfacing.

rhytid, if present, just beyond the extent of lateral hooding. A toothed forceps is then used to pinch the excess skin between the supraorbital fold and the proposed upper surgical margin. The correct position is that which will remove the excess skin and still allow the lids to close. The correct position is determined medially and laterally, the points marked, and again connected with a line that extends downward medially and upward laterally to connect with the inferior surgical margins. It is important not to extend the incision markings not medial to the punctum, as skin webs may form over this concave area.[2] An approach we have found helpful is to pull the redundant lid skin in a downward direction and then bifurcate the tissue to help avoid overcorrection. Afterward, the bifurcations can be connected and excised (Figs. 18-2 and 18-3). Next, the muscle layer is resected, the redundant fat is either resected or desiccated. If too much skin is present medially, a small triangle can be removed from the upper margin lateral to the punctum. The process is repeated again on the opposite upper eyelid. It is important to obtain exact measurements of the ellipse of skin to be removed as well as the position of the surgical margins in relation to the eyelid margin. The final results should be symmetrical.

If a lower eyelid blepharoplasty is planned, the surgical margins of the lower lid are then drawn. The line extends 1.5 to 2 mm below the lashes from just lateral to the punctum to 2 mm lateral to the canthus and then slightly downward on a smile line until the orbital rim is reached. There should be

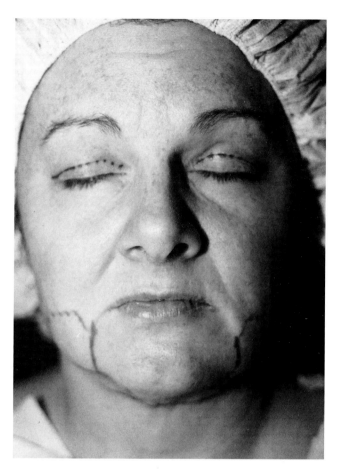

Figure 18-1   The planned surgical incisions are marked while the patient is seated. The upper lid marking is the existing crease; however, at the time of incision, the incision must be measured against opposite eyelid incision for symmetry. This patient is also marked for a face-lift.

UPPER EYELID SKIN FLAP TECHNIQUE

This technique is used to excise excess skin and fat; it is relatively simple and the risk of complications is low. The orbicularis muscle is not excised by this approach. Prior to initiating the procedure, the patient is told to wash her face with cetaphil cleanser if she has forgotten to remove any makeup. The hair is covered with a surgical cap and the face cleansed with an antiseptic surgical prep or providone-iodine. The planned surgical incisions are marked with a gentian violet pen while the patient is in a sitting position (Fig. 18-1). For the upper eyelids, a dot is placed on the supratarsal fold at a point along the midpapillary line, typically 8 to 10 mm above the eyelid margin. Second and third points are marked along the supratarsal fold medially above the upper eyelid punctum and lateral canthus. A line is then drawn that curves slightly along the supratarsal fold, connecting all the points. Laterally, the line is extended at 45 degrees upward along a

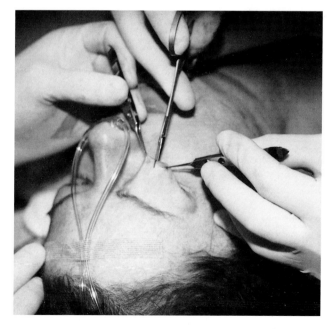

Figure 18-2   The incision has already been made and the upper lid is stretched over the lower lid to be bifurcated, to help ensure that the excision is not overly aggressive.

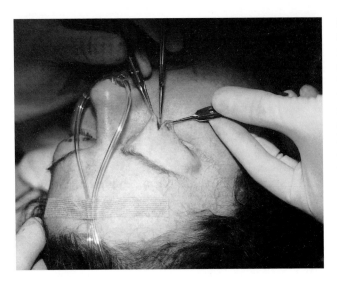

Figure 18-3 The bifurcation has been completed. Next, the lateral and medial bifurcations are made somewhat at the midline's length and the lid skin is simply excised, connecting the areas of bifurcation.

a distance of 5 mm between the lateral upper and lower eyelid incisions to avoid edema.[2] Once this step is completed, one or two drops of tetracaine 0.5% ophthalmic solution are applied to anesthetize the conjunctiva. A medium sized corneal shield is lubricated with bacitracin ophthalmic ointment and placed. Some surgeons avoid this step owing to fear of damaging the cornea; this can be prevented by proper lubrication and gentleness. The upper eyelid is anesthetized next with 2 to 3 mL of 1% lidocaine with 1:000,000 epinephrine, starting on the superior surgical margin, then the progressing to the inferior surgical margin. The opposite eyelid as well as the lower eyelids are then anesthetized. Any small hematomas at the injection sites can be controlled with gentle pressure. After waiting 10 min, the skin incisions are initiated. A no. 15 blade is used to incise the skin, first nasally to temporally along the supratarsal fold (lower surgical margin) and then along the superior margin. It is critical for an assistant to apply traction medially with a cotton tipped applicator to keep the skin taut while the incisions are made. Countertraction can be applied by the surgeon's finger laterally; otherwise the skin will tend to roll, resulting in a irregular surgical line. The lateral end of the ellipse of skin to be excised is then picked up with a Bishop-Harmon forceps and a small blunt-tipped scissors is used to undermine the skin superior to the orbicularis muscle. Once the skin has been removed, any bleeders are controlled with a bipolar cautery or battery-operated cautery device.

If any fat was identified during the preoperative evaluation, it should be removed next. Gentle pressure is applied on the closed eye or lower eyelid and the bulging areas of fat are identified. A small incision is made parallel to the fibers of the orbicularis muscle and orbital septum with a fine, sharp pointed scissors. The fat should herniate easily. A cotton-tipped applicator can be used to gently encourage the fat to prolapse. A few drops of anesthetic are injected at the base of the protruding fat to further anesthetize it. The fat is then clamped with a fine curved hemostat and any excess—with the exception of a small amount overlying the hemostat—is cut with a fine curved scissors. The remaining cut edges of fat are then cauterized with a bipolar current. Once hemostasis is achieved, the fat below the hemostat is grasped with a Bishop-Harmon fine forceps prior to releasing the hemostat. The cuff of fat at the base is inspected and, if necessary, further cauterized prior to allowing it to retract into the orbital septum. Gentle pressure can then again be applied to the closed eye to ascertain that no excess fat has been left behind. The same procedure is repeated over the central fat compartment if present. It is important to avoid placing too much traction on the herniated fat so as to prevent bleeding, and it is critical to inspect the herniated fat prior to cauterizing it to prevent damage to the levator aponeurosis, which can result in ptosis. It is also wise to place the excised skin as well as the fat from each compartment in a saline-soaked gauze, which can be used as a rough comparison to the amount of tissue to be excised from the opposite eyelid. Once the skin and fat is excised and the bleeding fully controlled, the wound is closed with running 6-0 or 7-0 nylon sutures, from medial to lateral. The running suture is easily removed 5 days postoperatively. Some surgeons prefer interrupted sutures as well as other suture types, such as 6-0 silk or 6-0 fast-absorbing plain gut. The last two, however, result in more postoperative cysts. The entire procedure as described is again repeated on the opposite eyelid. The postoperative care is as previously reported.

UPPER EYELID SKIN/MUSCLE FLAP TECHNIQUE

This technique is indicated in the setting of excess orbicularis muscle as well as in re-creation of the supratarsal crease. The procedure is similar until the point where the undermined skin is excised, exposing the orbicularis muscle. At that point, a 5- to 6-mm strip of orbicularis muscle is excised just above the interior wound margin, exposing the orbital septum and levator aponeurosis.[5] Some surgeons prefer to dissect the skin and orbicularis together.[6] Beyond that point, the fat is excised as previously described. The closure is completed as previously described if the supratarsal crease is at an acceptable level or with deep fixation if the supratarsal crease is being re-created. If such is the case, interrupted 6-0 nylon sutures are used to fix the skin to the underlying levator aponeurosis.

LOWER EYELID SKIN FLAP TECHNIQUE

This technique is used to excise excess skin or fat from the lower eyelid. The patient is prepped as previously described. The surgical margins are drawn using a gentian violet pen 1.5 to 2 mm below the lashes just lateral to the punctum to 2 mm beyond the lateral canthus, then slightly downward on a smile line until the orbital rim is reached. The corneal shields are applied, as previously described, and the skin is anesthetized with 1% lidocaine with 1:100,000 epinephrine. The injection should be in the plane between the skin and the orbicularis muscle. After waiting 10 min, the skin incisions are initiated from medially to temporally with traction placed on the medial skin by the surgical assistant and laterally by the surgeon's nondominant index finger. A small, blunt-tipped scissors is used to undermine the skin superior to the orbicularis muscle to the level at the orbital rim. Hemostasis is achieved with a bipolar or battery-operated cautery. If any fat was identified during the preoperative evaluation, it should be removed next. Gentle pressure is applied on the upper eyelid of the closed eye and the bulging areas of fat are identified. Using Bishop-Harmon forceps, the surgeon and surgical assistant can pick up the orbicularis occuli muscle and place slight traction superiorly and inferiorly while a small incision is made parallel to the fibers of the orbicularis muscle and orbital septum, just superior to the inferior orbital rim, in the sites overlying the central, medial, and temporal fat pads. The herniated fat is excised as previously described and hemostasis is again meticulously achieved. The skin is elevated and draped over the lid margin while the patient looks up and opens his or her mouth The excess skin overlying the lower eyelid incision is excised laterally to medially and, finally, the triangular piece of excess skin overlying the lateral incision is trimmed. The skin is then closed, initially with an interrupted key suture placed in a lateral and upward direction at the level of the temporal and horizontal incision, which places greater traction side to side as opposed to up and down. The horizontal margin is then closed with a running 6-0 nylon suture from the medial direction until the lateral canthus. The lateral component of the incision is closed with interrupted sutures.

LOWER EYELID SKIN MUSCLE FLAP TECHNIQUE

This technique is effective in the treatment of younger patients with excess fat and minimal excess skin. The skin is prepped, marked, and anesthetized as previously described. The skin incisions are initiated as in the skin flap approach (Fig. 18-4). Traction is placed superiorly and inferiorly along the incision margin on the central lower lid by the surgical assistant. A blunt-tipped scissors is used to penetrate the orbicularis muscle to the suborbicularis space. The incision is extended parallel and through the fibers of the orbicularis muscle medially and laterally until the plane just below the muscle. Bleeding is controlled with a bipolar cautery or battery operated cautery. The muscle is dissected bluntly from the orbital septum to the orbital rim. The fat is then excised as previously described and hemostasis is meticulously achieved. The skin is elevated and draped over the lid margin while the patient opens his or her mouth and gazes upward. The excess skin and muscle overlying the incision (vertically) is excised. Typically, only minimal skin should be removed by this technique. The lateral triangular excess is excised last. The skin is then closed, as previously described.

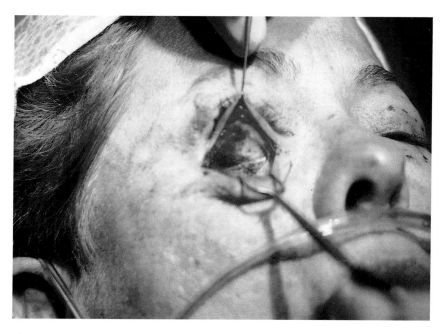

Figure 18-4 The skin muscle flap is incised. The assistant separates the superior and inferior aspects to expose the underlying orbital septum.

If there is any difference in the thickness of the superior and inferior incision margins, the excess muscle at the inferior or superior end is excised and the edge beveled until it apposes nicely prior to closure.[2] Care must be taken not to excise too much skin, as this will definitely result in an ectropion. When a lower eyelid blepharoplasty is being performed, irrespective of technique, too much laxity in the lower eyelid must be corrected by either a lid-shortening procedure, a medial canthal tendon plication, or lateral canthal sling to prevent an ectropion. The easiest correction is to take a full-thickness pentagonal wedge perpendicular to the lower lid edge corresponding to the excess skin. The bleeding is stopped with a battery operated cautery, then the defect closed. Vicryl sutures (6-0) are used to close the tarsal plate, the orbicularis, and subcutaneous tissue, and the skin is superficially closed with 6-0 silk. One suture should be placed at the lid margin at the level of the lash line and the ends tied inferiorly with another suture to prevent contact with the cornea or conjunctiva. The suture at the eyelid margin is removed 1 week later, whereas the rest can be removed at 5 days. It is suggested that the reader become acquainted with the other two surgical options, which are beyond the scope of this chapter.

TRANSCONJUNCTIVAL TECHNIQUE

This technique avoids a cutaneous incision and therefore is cosmetically ideal. It is indicated in patients with excess fat and minimal excess skin. Because there is no skin excision and downward traction from sutures, a resulting ectropion is rare. It is also an excellent procedure for patients who have undergone transcutaneous blepharoplasty in the past and seek a revision. The patient is prepped as previously described. Two drops of tetracaine 0.5% ophthalmic solution are applied to the conjunctiva. The inferior eyelid is injected below the plane of the orbicularis muscle with 1% lidocaine and 1:100,000 epinephrine (2 to 3 mL). A few drops of anesthetic are injected subcutaneously on the central inferior eyelid skin where a 4.0 Vicryl traction suture is placed through the skin, muscle, and tarsus. The lower eyelid is then retracted with a Foman retractor applied by manual pressure or a suture followed by gentle pressure applied on the closed eye to accentuate the fat pockets (Fig. 18-5). Additional anesthetic is injected subconjunctivally into each compartment and allowed to take effect for 10 to 15 min. The lower eyelid is again retracted and a superficial incision is made on the conjunctiva 3 or 5 mm below the tarsal edge from a line perpendicular to the cannaliculi to the lateral canthus with the assistant lifting the upper lid with a cotton-tipped swab or with a 5-0 silk suture applied to the inferior cut edge of the conjunctiva, which is retracted superiorly, covering the exposed cornea. This retraction suture may be held by the assistant or sutured to the superior eyelid margin and will serve to protect the eye if a scleral shield is not used. The level of the conjunctival incision is selected based on whether the preseptal or retroseptal transconjunctival blepharoplasty approach is preferred.[6] As pointed out in the discussion of the anatomy of the eyelid, the lower eyelid retractors (capsulopalpebral fascia and inferior tarsal muscle

or Müller's muscle) fuse with the orbital septum about 3 mm before inserting into the inferior tarsus. When the incision is made about 3 mm inferior to the tarsus, the preseptal space— a space between the orbicularis muscle and the orbital septum—is entered. This space must be dissected and the orbital septum penetrated, as previously described, by the transcutaneous approach to excise the fat. When the conjunctiva is incised about 5 mm from the inferior tarsus, the inferior tarsal muscle and the capsulopalpebral fascia are penetrated prior to fusing with the orbital septum; therefore the retroseptal fat is reached directly without cutting the septum. We find this approach to be easier. Care must be taken to incise the eyelid retractors very superficially, as the inferior oblique muscle separates the medial and central fat compartments, and it must be identified and avoided.

The conjunctival incision can be performed with a no. 15 blade, fine sharp scissors, battery-operated cautery, or Ellman radiosurgical needle.[7] The benefit of the last two is that bleeding is controlled while cutting. A central incision will expose all fat pads. Gentle pressure is applied to the globe on top of the upper eyelid, which exposes the fat. Several drops of anesthetic solution can be injected at the base of the fat pads. The three fat compartments are excised, as previously described. The medial and central fat compartments must be carefully examined prior to cutting and cauterizing to avoid damage to the the inferior oblique muscle. Hemostasis is critical to avoid retrobulbar bleeds, which can result in

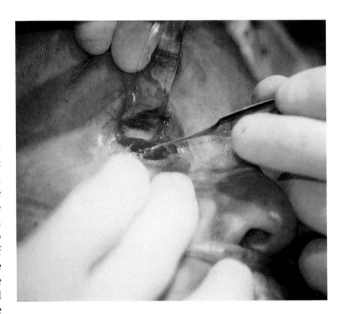

Figure 18-5   The transconjuctival approach. The incision has been made with light pressure on the globe with the assistant's digit on the skin above the globe (while holding the protective shield). This will reveal the fat through the incised septum.

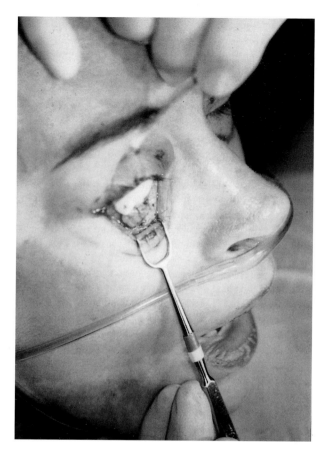

Figure 18-6 The shield is in place. The orbital fat is removed and the field is scanned to be certain that adequate hemostasis has been achieved.

blindness. The excised fat from each compartment should be placed in a saline-soaked gauze and saved for comparison with that excised from the opposite eyelid, in order to achieve symmetry. Only the fat that, with gentle pressure on the globe, protrudes over the orbital rim should be excised. When an adequate amount of fat has been excised and bleeding controlled, the traction suture placed on the inferior conjunctiva is released (Fig. 18-6). The apposition at the conjunctiva is checked and the lower eyelid returned to its natural position. No sutures are needed. A Steri-Strip can be applied to the infraocular cheek for some added pressure. Postoperative care instructions are the same.

COMPLICATIONS

In an effort to limit complications, the procedure is carried out in a certified ambulatory facility with appropriate monitoring of anesthesia; conscious sedation is employed (see Chap. 8) (Fig. 18-7). Postoperative complications can be minor or severe. The ability to identify and manage these adverse events is crucial. A collegial relationship with an ophthalmologist should be established for those situations

when such expertise is needed. Complications include corneal irritation, milia, cyst formation, allergic reactions, chemosis, dehiscence, loss of eyelashes, lagophthalmos, overresection of fat, ectropion, ptosis, lacrimal gland injuries, diplopia, hematoma, and, rarely, retrobulbar hemorrhage with associated loss of vision.[8–10]

Corneal irritation may result from inadequate lubrication and exposure or inadvertent abrasions by dressings, corneal shields, or sutures. The corneal epithelium can be examined with fluorescent dye and a slit-lamp microscope. Microabrasions can be treated with ophthalmic ointments. However, if there is failure to heal after 24 h, the patient should be referred to an ophthalmologist.

Milia and minor cysts may occur along the incision sites, particularly if nonmonofilament sutures are used. The lesions are easily evacuated with a no. 11 knife and gentle side-to-side pressure.

Allergic reactions occur most commonly to medications, particularly topical antibiotics. Such sequelae may appear in the form of periorbital erythema, scaliness, pruritus, conjunctival redness, or chemosis. Chemosis is conjunctival edema. which can result from allergic reactions, surgery, exposure, or abrasions. It is treated with topical lubrication and may take months to resolve. If topical steroids are used longer than a week, intraocular pressures should be checked by an ophthalmologist. The contact allergen should be discontinued.

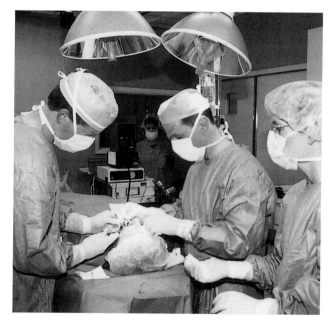

Figure 18-7 The procedure is performed in a certified operating suite with the attendant monitoring the patient, who is under conscious sedation.

Dehiscence of the wound may occur due to overexertion, delayed healing, or traction at the surgical site. If possible, the wound edges should be freshened and the site reapproximated. Although acceptable results may be achieved by secondary intention healing, scars will likely be more noticeable.

Loss of eyelashes may occur if the hair follicles are transected by an incision too close to the lid margin. The incision should be placed 1.5 to 2 mm below the cilia.

Lagophthalmos (inability to close the eyelids) may result from excessive upper eyelid excision. Minimal lagophthalmos improves as the postsurgical edema resolves.[2] Massaging the upper lid is also helpful. While the lagophthalmos persists, proper lubrication of the eye is absolutely necessary. If the condition is severe, a skin graft may be necessary to correct the defect. Overresection of fat in the upper eyelid may result in a deep superior sulcus; in the lower lid, it may lead to a tear trough deformity, which is an overaccentuation of the orbital rim.

Ectropion, or lower eyelid retraction, results in scleral show. It can result from overresection of eyelid skin or increased laxity of the lower lid. This problem can be corrected by lid shortening procedures, canthal plication or skin grafts. A discussion of these techniques is beyond the scope of this chapter. In many cases a simple wedge resection of the lower eyelid, as previously described, will correct the defect. Lateral bowing of the eyelid may occur when the fibers of the orbicularis muscle are transected laterally in the skin/muscle flap technique if too much skin and muscle are removed.[2] A suspension suture fixed to the periosteum may correct the problem.

Ptosis (droopy eyelid) can occur as a result of severing the levator aponeurosis during an upper eyelid blepharoplasty. It may also result from stretching of the upper eyelid retractors, as from a hematoma. Its correction entails reattaching the levator aponeurosis to the tarsal plate.

Injuries to the lacrimal gland may occur in the hands of the novice surgeon, who may mistake a lateral upper eyelid redundancy for excess fat. Damage to the lacrimal gland can result in a chronically dry eye.

Diplopia, or double vision, is a severe complication that may occur following an injury to the inferior oblique muscle. The advice of an ophthalmologist should be sought in these cases. The most common situation in which the inferior oblique muscle is damaged is during resection of the medial and central inferior fat pockets in the course of a transconjunctival blepharoplasty.

Anterior hematomas should be evacuated. When identified, the source of bleeding should be investigated and controlled. The best way to avoid this complication is to discontinue any drugs that may inhibit platelet aggregation at least 2 weeks prior to the procedure. Bruising is not considered a complication, as it is rather common. Severe ecchymosis, however, should be minimized by applying ice cold compresses, as described. The application of Steri-Strips in the area of the infraocular cheek also minimizes edema and bruising while also preventing any stretching of the skin that might otherwise result. Retrobulbar hemorrhage is the most feared complication of eyelid surgery as it can result in loss of vision. It results from bleeding into the orbital septum, with a resulting rise in intraocular pressure and possible central retinal artery occlusion and optic nerve ischemia. This complication occurs only when the orbital septum is penetrated to excise excess fat. That is why it is crucial to be meticulous in stopping any bleeding before allowing the cuff of the excised fat to retract back into the orbital septum. It is also important to be careful when cauterizing the fat, especially if a unipolar current is used, to avoid excessive tissue damage and possible ischemia. Signs of retrobulbar bleeds include pain, ecchymosis, and proptosis (bulging eye). The patient may already be experiencing some visual loss at the time of presentation, which may be reversible if immediate surgical and medical management is undertaken. A funduscopic examination should be performed to examine the optic nerve. Initially, the wound should be opened to help decompress the orbit and the bleeding source searched for and controlled. A lateral canthotomy and cantholysis will further relieve the intraocular pressure if necessary. The procedure entails making a horizontal cut from the lateral canthus to the orbital rim. The lid is then pulled medially to put the tendon on stretch. Once the tight band is identified, it is cut with sharp scissors. Medically, intravenous mannitol (1 to 2 g/kg over 30 min) and intramuscular acetazolamide (250 to 500 mg), followed orally by 250 mg every 6 h, may be instituted.[8,10] The patient should be referred immediately to an ophthalmologist who may further perform an anterior chamber paracentesis.

Last, if the globe is penetrated during infiltration of local anesthesia, the procedure should be stopped and the patient examined by an ophthalmologist. Scleral shields and injections at the proper plane should avoid this serious complication.

Conclusion

Periorbital surgery is of paramount importance in the rejuvenation of the aging face. The blepharoplasty technique is effective and can be mastered by the dermatologic surgeon who already is familiar with cutaneous surgical techniques. Knowledge of the anatomy of the eye and possible complications cannot be underestimated, and meticulous attention to detail will make the experience rewarding for both patient and physician (Figs. 18-8*A* and *B*, 18-9*A* and *B*, 18-10*A* and *B*, 18-11*A* and *B*, 18-12*A* and *B*, and 18-13*A* and *B*, 18-14*A* and *B*, 18-15*A* and *B*, 18-16*A* and *B*, 18-17*A* and *B*).

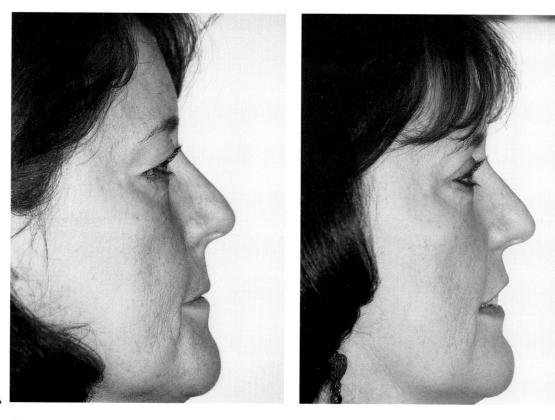

Figure 18-8 (*A*) Preoperative view of upper lids with the significant hooding. (*B*) Post-operative view, demonstrating well-defined upper lid skin.

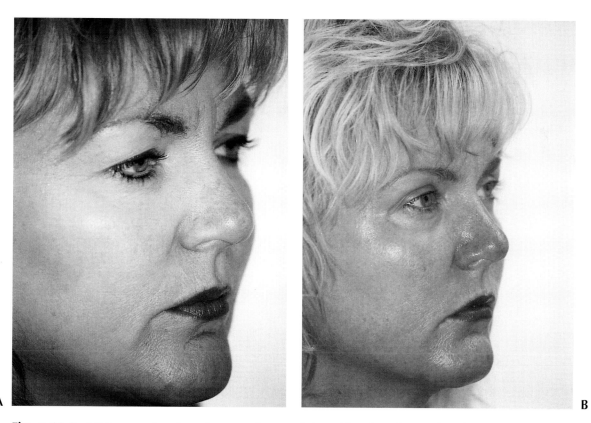

Figure 18-9 (*A*) Preoperative view, demonstrating mostly lateral hooding along with moderate rhytids on lower lids and skin. (*B*) Postoperative view of evenly exposed upper lid and decreased rhytids on skin. This patient also had a chemical peel.

325

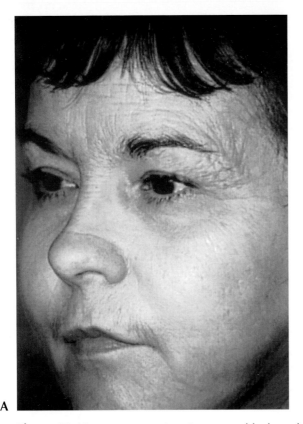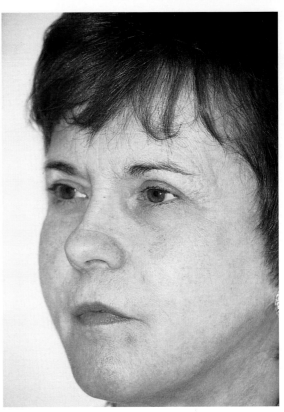

A   B

Figure 18-10   (*A*) Preoperative view: upper blepharoplasty. (*B*) Postoperative view of the same patient.

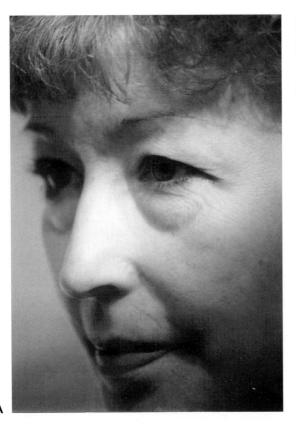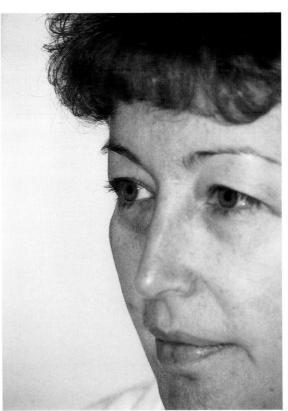

A   B

Figure 18-11   (*A*) Preoperative view; transconjunctival blepharoplasty. Notice bulging of fat, which is accentuated with pressure on the globe. (*B*) Postoperative view. The procedure does not leave any evidence of the cutaneous incision and the herniated fat pads have been removed.

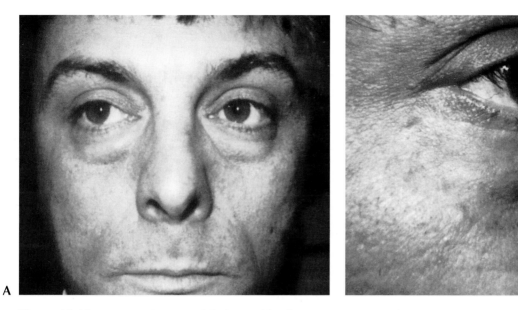

A   B

Figure 18-12   (*A*) Frontal view with bulging of fat (the incision was cutaneous). This is a skin muscle flap procedure. (*B*) Postoperative view. A fine incision line with excision below lower lid.

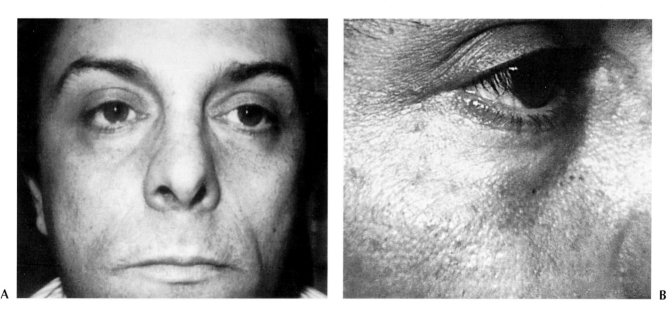

A   B

Figure 18-13   (*A*) Preoperative tangential view reveals a herniated pad. (*B*) Postoperative view. There is a marked reduction of herniated fat, with the lid incision from the cutaneous approach.

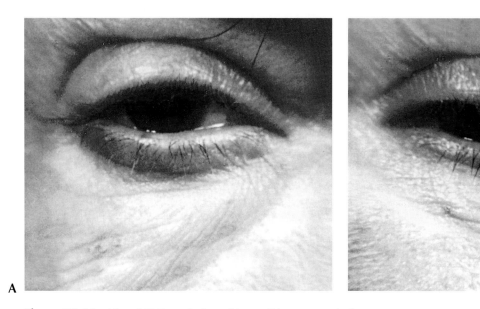

Figure 18-14 (*A* and *B*) Frontal view of lower lids preoperatively.

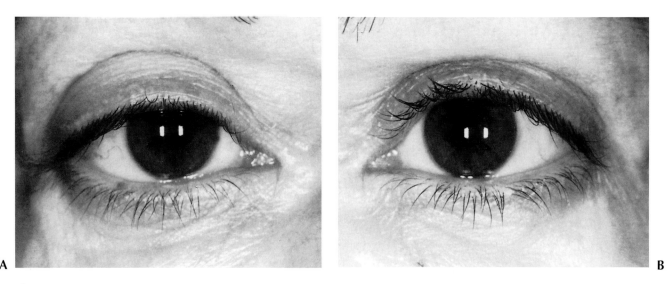

Figure 18-15 (*A* and *B*) Postoperative view of treated lower lids. This treatment was done by the transconjunctival approach, without cutaneous incisions.

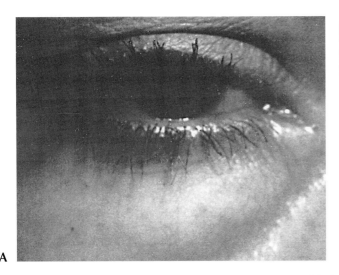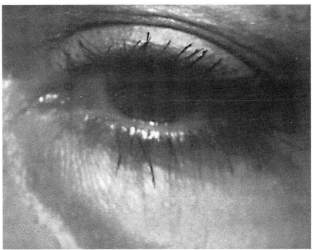

A   B

Figure 18-16   (*A* and *B*) Frontal view—more pronounced bulge.

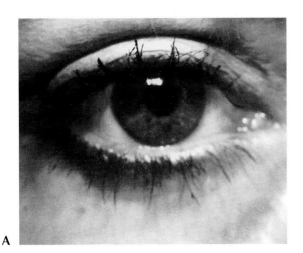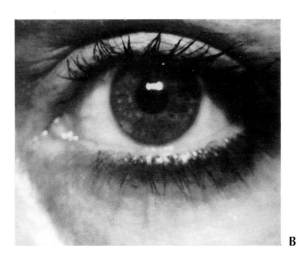

A   B

Figure 18-17   (*A* and *B*) After transconjunctival blepharoplasty. The fat has been removed.

References

1. Cohen SA, Baker SR. Management of the upper third of the aging face. In: *Advances in Otolaryngology—Head and Neck Surgery.* St. Louis: Mosby-Yearbook; 1994:69–90.

2. Alt TH. Blepharoplasty. In: Pinski JB, Pinski KS, eds. *Dermatologic Clinics.* Philadelphia: Saunders; 1995: 389–430.

3. Doxanas MT, Anderson RL. Oriental eyelids: An anatomic study. *Arch Ophthalmol* 1984; 102:1232–1235.

4. Chen WP. Upper blepharoplasty in the Asian patient. In: Putterman AM, ed. *Cosmetic Oculoplastic Surgery: Eyelid, Forehead and Facial Techniques.* Philadelphia: Saunders; 1999:101–111.

5. Tyers AG, Collins JRO. *Colour Atlas of Ophthalmic Plastic Surgery.* Oxford, UK: Reed Educational and Professional Publishing; 1995.

6. Asken S. Blepharoplasty. In: Coleman WP, Hanke CW, Alt TH, et al, eds. *Cosmetic Surgery of the Skin: Principles and Techniques.* St. Louis: Mosby-Yearbook; 1997:354–382.

7. Waldman SR. Transconjunctival blepharoplasty: Minimizing the risks of lower lid blepharoplasty. *Facial Plast Surg* 1994; 10(1):27–41.

8. Goldberg RA, Marmor MF, Shorr N. Blindness following blepharoplasty: Two case reports and a discussion of management. *Ophthalmic Surg* 1990; 21(2):85–89.

9. Baylis HI, Goldberg RA, Growth MJ. Complications of lower blepharoplasty. In: Putterman AM, ed. *Cosmetic Oculoplastic Surgery: Eyelid, Forehead, and Facial Techniques.* Philadelphia: Saunders; 1999:429–456.

10. Baylis HI, Goldberg RA, Growth MJ. Complications of lower blepharoplasty. In: Putterman AM, ed. *Cosmetic Oculoplastic Surgery: Eyelid, Forehead, and Facial Techniques.* Philadelphia: Saunders; 1999:411–428.

Patient Information

Eyelid Surgery

The eyes are among the first physical characteristics we notice about ourselves and others; they are also among the first areas in which we observe the inevitable aging process. As we grow older, wrinkles, deep lines, and "bags" begin to form around our eyes. Our upper eyelids may begin to sag as our skin loses its elasticity. In addition to being unsightly, this can impair our vision.

Bags or pouches under our eyes develop because the natural weakening of our skin and the supporting structures over time allows the fat that cushions and protects our eyes to protrude. These fat bags are the same in men and women and are often inherited. They are unrelated to weight and cannot be affected by dieting. These bags usually get larger as we age and cause us to look tired and older than we are.

Cosmetic eyelid surgery, also known as blepharoplasty, can correct sagging eyelids, bags beneath the eyes, and excess folds around the eyes. During this procedure, your doctor may remove the excess skin and fat from your upper and lower eyelids. The result is a more youthful and rested appearance. Blepharoplasty is often combined with other surgical procedures, such as the face-lift, to help erase years from your face.

Cosmetic surgeons help people develop and maintain a healthy and attractive appearance. Our skilled surgeons specialize in cosmetic eyelid surgery and have used their knowledge, skill, and experience for more than a decade to help numerous patients look years younger.

The Procedure

Blepharoplasty is usually performed in the surgeon's office. Patients are given a sedative to induce "twilight sleep" and a small amount of local anesthesia is administered around the eyes. There is usually only minimal pain or discomfort associated with the procedure.

During the surgery, your doctor follows the natural lines and creases around your eyes and makes tiny incisions in the upper and lower lids. He then removes excess fat and skin and closes the incisions with fine strips of tape and small stitches, which run along the incision line. These stitches dissolve on their own within 3 to 5 days. The entire surgical procedure usually takes 1 to 2 hours.

After surgery, ice compresses are applied to the eyelids. You will be sent home, where you will continue to apply these compresses to reduce swelling, which you can also alleviate by lightly elevating your head when you lie down. Any swelling or bruising that does occur will usually subside within 10 to 14 days. Sometimes you may experience some dryness of the eyes after surgery; this can be minimized with ointments your doctor will recommend. Your eyes may also be sensitive to light after surgery, and you should wear sunglasses whenever you are outside. Any discomfort you may experience can usually be controlled with a mild pain reliever.

Most patients resume normal activities within 2 to 3 days and return to work within a week. Contact lens wearers may wear their contacts 7 to 10 days after surgery. Women may use eye makeup 10 to 24 days after surgery.

The Results

Most patients are delighted with the results of eyelid surgery. Because bags, wrinkles, and deep lines are minimized, people who undergo blepharoplasty look rested and youthful. Most patients can reasonably expect the area around their eyes to look younger after surgery.

The results of blepharoplasty usually last from 5 to 15 years, depending upon your age and skin characteristics. Ask for a consultation to discuss how blepharoplasty can help you look years younger.

PREOPERATIVE INSTRUCTIONS

Take no aspirin, vitamin E, or drugs containing aspirin (Bufferin, Anacin, Empirin, Stanback, Excedrin, Fiorinal, Darvon compound, and salicylates) for 2 weeks before surgery. *Instead, use only Tylenol!!*

No alcohol for 3 days prior to surgery and avoid it while taking any post-operative medication.

Get plenty of rest the night before surgery.

Wear clothes that either zip or button and do not have to be pulled over your head.

Arrange for a ride to and from the office.

Do not wear any eye mascara or eye makeup for 48 hours prior to surgery. Wear no makeup to the office on the day of surgery. Makeup may be worn again 1 to 2 weeks following surgery.

Do not wear any jewelry to the office on the day of surgery.

Wash your face thoroughly and shampoo your hair on the morning of surgery.

Take all preoperative medications as directed.

Bring pain medication with you on surgery day.

Contact lenses must be removed before surgery. If you wish to remove them in the office, please bring your case.

A postoperative appointment card will be given to you as you check in on the day of surgery.

Blepharoplasty Setup Surgical Tray

Patient

1. Cape
2. Sterile surgical hat

Doctor and Staff

1. Sterile gloves
2. Sterile gown
3. Mask
4. Surgical hats

Materials

1. Sterile bleph tray
2. Ellman cart (for lower bleph only)
3. 5 mL Betadine solution
4. 5 cc Sterile water
5. Sterile medicine cup
6. Two sterile medium drapes
7. One sterile small bath towel
8. Two 6-0 gut sutures (upper bleph only)
9. ⅛-in. Sterile brown Steri-strips (1 pack, upper bleph only)
10. ¼-in. Sterile brown Steri-strips (1 pack, upper bleph only)
11. Syringes
    A. One 10-mL 0.9% sterile normal saline with 2-gauge needle (lower bleph only)
    B. Two 5 mL for lidocaine with epinephrine, buffered
12. Two 30-gauge 1-in. metal hub needles
13. One 21-gauge needle
14. Cold compress mask or pea packs
15. One 30-mL bottle saline (lower bleph only)
16. One 30-mL bottle lidocaine 1% with epinephrine, buffered
17. Mayo stand cover
18. Sterile light-handle cover
19. Tetracaine (keep refrigerated until needed)
20. Polysporin ophthalmic ointment
21. ½-in. brown Steri-strips (1 pack, lower bleph only)

Blepharoplasty

POSTOPERATIVE INSTRUCTIONS

After upper lid blepharoplasty, fine paper tapes are placed over the incisions. After the lower lid blepharoplasty, a wide paper tape may be placed under the lower eye area. *IT IS VERY IMPORTANT TO REFRAIN FROM PULLING AT ANY OF THESE TAPES!*

Immediately after surgery, dry gauze and a reusable ice pack will be placed over the sites in order to reduce swelling and minimize bruising. At home, this should be repeated for 30 minutes or more at least four times daily for the next 3 days.

You may return to most normal activities within 48 to 72 hours, engage in low-impact exercise after 2 weeks, and then return to full vigorous activity after 4 to 6 weeks.

Glasses may be worn. Do not wear contact lenses for 2 weeks following eyelid surgery. Do not wear swim goggles or a scuba dive mask for 6 weeks.

No lifting, bending, straining, sniffing, or nose blowing for 7 days postoperatively.

If you must sneeze, sneeze through your mouth.

Your head should be elevated at 30 to 45 degrees at all times for the first 2 weeks. For sleeping, consider using either a recliner or several pillows. Sleep with your head straight and *do not* roll on your side.

For lower lid blepharoplasty, prescription eyedrops may be prescribed by the doctor. Please use as directed.

Artificial tears (Refresh Saline Eye Drops) may be necessary for cleaning the eye of matter, blurred vision, or a "dry" scratchy feeling. This product is sold over the counter at your pharmacy.

Celluvisc may be used in the eyes at bedtime so that your eyes will not become dry while you are sleeping. This product is also sold over the counter.

You may shampoo your hair the third day following surgery. *Do not* bend over the sink. Please keep the eyelid tapes dry.

Take your postoperative medications as instructed, and please note that pain medications can produce nausea and vomiting, so take them only if you absolutely must. Occasionally blurred vision will be a problem with reading medicine labels. You may want to put a special mark on each bottle to help you identify your medications.

Stay out of the sun or hot places for at least 1 week.

Return for your postoperative check-up as instructed 4 to 7 days after surgery. You need to have a ride for your visit. Do not plan to drive until *after* your postoperative visit.

CONSENT FOR EYELID SURGERY

Patient's name_____

Date_____

I hereby authorize _____ and/or the surgical team to perform an operation upon me (or my _____ _____) to: (description of procedure)_____

_____

_____

1. The nature and effects of the operation, the risks and complications involved, as well as alternative methods of treatment, have been fully explained to me by the doctor and I understand them.

    Initial_____

2. I authorize the doctor to perform any other procedure that may be deemed desirable in attempting to improve the condition stated in paragraph 1 or any unhealthy or unforeseen condition that may be encountered during the operation.

    Initial_____

3. I consent to the administration of anesthetics by the doctor or under the direction of the anesthetist responsible for this service.

Initial_____

4. I understand that the practice of medicine and surgery is not an exact science and that reputable practitioners cannot guarantee results. No guarantee or assurance has been given by the doctor or anyone else as to the results that may be obtained.

Initial_____

5. I understand that the two sides of the human body are not the same and can never be made the same. I understand that bone, muscle, and support tissues are never identical on both side of the body, and that surgery cannot make my eyes identical.

Initial_____

6. For the purpose of advancing medical education, I consent to the admittance of authorized observers to the operating room.

Initial_____

7. I understand that as in any surgical procedure, despite the very best skill, technique, and judgment, there is a slight risk of possible complications associated with this surgery. These complications include but are not limited to:

a. Worsening or unsatisfactory appearance.

b. Blindness; this is extremely rare, but it has been reported in the medical literature.

c. Dry eyes; this normally may require the use of artificial lubricants (drops, ointment) for several weeks or months; rarely, it is permanent and may require discontinued use of contact lenses.

d. Drooping lids; this is rare but may result from damage to the eyelid muscle. Further surgery may be required. Very rarely, it may be permanent.

e. Ectropion (upper eyelids will not close, or lower lids assume an abnormally low position); this is rare but may require further surgery to correct. Very rarely, it may be permanent.

f. Unsightly scarring; often the scars are difficult to see; however, some people may develop whiteness, thickening, skin irregularity, or prominence along the incision lines.

g. Excessive tearing; this can occur for the first several weeks.

h. Blurred vision; this is common the first several days following surgery due to initial changes in tear flow. It generally resolves spontaneously, but may be permanent (extremely rare).

I have been made aware of these and other complications and accept this risk.

Initial_____

8. I give permission to _____ to take still or motion clinical photographs with the understanding that such photographs remain the property of the center. If in the judgment of the center medical research, education, or science will be benefited by their use, such photographs and related information may be published and republished in professional journals or medical books, or used for any other purpose which the center may deem proper. It is specifically understood that in any such publication or use, I shall not be identified by name.

Initial_____

9. I understand it is mandatory for me to have made prior arrangements to be driven to and from the doctor's office by a responsible adult.

Initial_____

10. The following characteristics were reviewed:

Initial

Brows	_____
Upper lid laxity	_____
Upper lid fat herniation	_____
Lower lid laxity	_____
Lower lid fat herniation	_____

I understand that eyelid surgery may not produce complete resolution of the above disorders, nor can it produce perfect symmetry.

Although uncommon, complications requiring further surgical corrections may occur with eyelid surgery.

I understand this, and that there may be an additional fee(s) for any subsequent corrective surgery.

Although uncommon, scarring of the incision lines may occur, resulting in white scar lines visible upon close inspection.

I understand that elective surgical procedures are most often delayed until after the termination of a pregnancy. My signature attests that to the best of my knowledge I am not pregnant at this time.

I agree to discontinue smoking entirely for a period of 2 weeks prior to surgery and 2 weeks immediately following surgery.

Initial_____

My signature indicates that I have read this "Consent for Eye Surgery" and I understand and accept the risks involved with this operation. I hereby authorize _____ and/or the surgical team to perform this surgical procedure on me.

_____ _____
Signature (Patient/Responsible Party)   Date

_____ _____
Signature (Witness)   Date

CHAPTER 19

Hair Restoration Surgery

History reveals that baldness has long been held undesirable. According to legend, Julius Caesar wore a laurel wreath at all times to cover up his hair loss because of the traditional belief equating hair or long hair with strength. To men in contemporary society, the loss of hair means not only the loss of youth but also often the loss of self-esteem. In more than 60 percent of men, physical maturity and aging are heralded by varying degrees of baldness. It is therefore no surprise that surgical intervention for male-pattern alopecia remains the number one cosmetic procedure in males. Also, about 10 percent of our hair transplant patients are women. For women, significant hair loss can be devastating. Next to wearing a hairpiece, the options in hair restoration include both hair transplantation and scalp reduction or lifting, pending the amount of donor tissue available.[1]

Hair Transplantation

HISTORY OF HAIR TRANSPLANTATION

The origin of hair transplantation lies in the 1939 report by the Japanese dermatologist Okuda[2,3] of using small hair-bearing skin grafts to remedy hair loss of the scalp, eyebrow, and upper lip areas, as outlined in his paper.[3] In 1953, Fujita[2,4] described eyebrow reconstruction in leprosy patients; his technique involved dissecting hair-bearing skin into small pieces for implantation. This is most akin to today's technique of strip harvesting to generate micrografts and minigrafts for insertion. Early experimentation with hair transplant surgery culminated in Orentreich's 1959 publication of his method,[2,5] in which he, much like Okuda, utilized small round punch grafts (4.0 mm) to obtain hair grafts and remove unwanted bald or scarring skin. The concept of using standard round punch grafting dominated for many years. Today's "gold standard" of combined micrografting with strip harvesting evolved owing to the contributions of several surgeons. The trend toward smaller grafts to establish a more natural look in hair restoration resulted in the use of small punches (1.5 to 2.5 mm); dividing the standard 4-mm plugs or grafts into quarters, halves, or single hairs; and utilizing islands left behind after total punch harvesting.[2] In 1968, Vallis[6,7] was the first to report strip harvesting of donor hair with the use of a double-bladed knife. This incisional strip of donor hair was placed into a thin slit along the frontal hairline. Then, in 1976, Coiffman[8,9] introduced a parallel scalpel to harvest tissue and a four-sided blade that he used to cut recipient sites to receive square grafts. Bisaccia and Scarborough further refined this technique and have been called the fathers of the multibladed knife.[10] Consequently, the concept of strip harvesting to create micrografts, minigrafts, and follicular-unit grafts with emphasis on a natural hairline developed throughout the 1990s to become the gold standard of hair transplantation.

CLASSIFICATION OF HAIR GRAFTS

Hair grafts are classified as standard and nonstandard. The standard round punch grafts (2 to 4 mm) introduced by Orentreich are now rarely used. Instead, nonstandard grafts have become the preferred type for hair transplantation. They consist of micrografts and minigrafts. Micrografts, or one- to two-haired grafts regardless of shape or method of insertion, are defined entirely by the number of hairs. Minigrafts, by definition, typically have a donor and recipient diameter of less than 2 mm; they can vary in shape (round, linear, or square) and number of hairs (generally two to four).[11] The term *follicular unit transplantation* comprises the use of hair grafts in which the follicular unit is left intact in the graft preparation (with the help of a microscope), whether it contains one or two hairs as in a micrograft or three or more hairs as in a minigraft.

INDICATIONS AND CONTRAINDICATIONS

Androgenetic alopecia remains the most common indication for hair transplantation. Less common indications include other forms of hereditary alopecia (high frontal hairline, high temples, alopecia triangularis) and cicatricial alopecia (due to face-lift, trauma, dermatosis, etc.).[12] Listed among the contraindications are bleeding diathesis and anticoagulant therapy (due to decreased visibility of the treatment site and expulsion of transplanted hair follicles), impaired wound healing, marked immunosuppression, and unrealistic expectations on the part of the patient.

PREOPERATIVE CONSIDERATIONS

As in any cosmetic procedure, proper patient selection remains paramount for successful results in hair transplantation. The consultation time provides the surgeon with an ideal opportunity to understand the patient's expectations and possible misconceptions. The goal of the consultation is an effective communication to allow the physician to navigate the patient's subjective expectations and hopes toward realistic expectations and facts. The patient has to realize that hair transplantation is aimed at providing a framework for the face that will soften the appearance of blatant baldness rather than restore a full head of hair. Numerous factors must be taken into account in screening candidates at the consultation visit. These include age, sex, family history, medical history, and psychological disposition as well as the amount, color, and quality of hair in the donor region. Also to be considered are the esthetic design of the anterior hairline and the extent of the patient's baldness as well as the possibility of beneficial adjunctive procedures such as scalp reduction.[13]

The patient's age and sex must be considered, as both have considerable influence on the outcome of this cosmetic procedure. Younger patients (age < 30 years) often have unrealistic expectations, and anything less than optimal results may be disappointing to them. Keeping the progression of alopecia in mind, the goal should be a mature adult hairline. This is particularly difficult for a young patient to deal with. If the patient's expectations do become more realistic in the course of the consultation, the outcome of hair transplantation would be unlikely to satisfy either the patient or the physician. Gender differences also play an important role. Women differ from men in their alopecia pattern and progression as well as their expectations and styling needs. In general, women are psychologically more severely affected by alopecia than men.[2] Yet in our experience, they are very grateful for any improvement.

In considering a patient for hair transplantation, it is important to review the family history, medical history, and psychological disposition. If there is a family history of balding, it may give the physician a clue as to the pattern of alopecia that might develop over time in a particular patient. This is helpful in evaluating how much a patient will benefit from a hair transplantation. Naturally, patients with a significant degree of balding are better suited than those in the early stages of genetic alopecia in terms of lasting satisfaction with the procedure, as rapid progression of alopecia will distort the results over time. The medical history should be focused on wound-healing ability (as affected by a history of diabetes, thyroid dysfunction, anemia, infectious diseases, and immunosuppression), bleeding tendency (bleeding diathesis and anticoagulant therapy), and scarring propensity so as to allow for optimal results. Finally, patients with uncontrolled depression and a hard-to-please attitude should be strictly avoided.

The amount and quality of donor hair plays a vital role in the success of hair transplantation. To begin with, an adequate density of donor hair is required in order to allow for a decent reconstitution of hair at the graft site. The quality of donor hair in terms of color and character determines the appearance of the newly created graft site. Donor hair that is light in color and fine in character simply makes less of a visual impression than hair that is darker in color and more coarse and curly in character, and it demands a higher hair density at the site of the grafting to obtain comparable results.[14] But this lighter, finer quality of hair lends itself better to creating a more natural-appearing hairline, since dark hair may contrast starkly with lighter skin shades, leading to a harsher hairline gradient (see Chap. 7).

Designing a framework for hair transplantation demands knowledge of the frontal forelock concept, the creation of a natural anterior hairline, and the potential usefulness of adjunctive surgical procedures. The idea of the frontal forelock is based on the ability to frame the face by placing even a limited amount of donor hair in the anterior-central region, thereby erasing the image of obvious baldness. To create a proper hairline, this hair should be placed at a mature height and should demonstrate an increasing gradient of hair density. The mature level of an anterior hairline is usually set 8 to 10 cm above the glabella or slightly higher, depending on the age of the patient and the extent of the alopecia. One to three lines of micrografts placed in front of several rows of minigrafts generate a natural-appearing transition zone. If the balding is quite extensive, hair transplantation by itself may not be sufficient to create the illusion of hair. Thus, adjunctive procedures such as scalp reduction or lifting may have to be considered as well.[15]

At the preoperative visit, the plan is again reviewed with the patient and any remaining questions are answered. Informed consent is obtained, baseline photographs are taken, preoperative medications are prescribed, and presurgical lab test samples are drawn.

HAIR TRANSPLANTATION TECHNIQUE

The patient is brought to the operative area and placed in the seated position. Preoperative vital signs are recorded and the appropriate marking of the donor and recipient zones is carried out. The donor site in the occipital scalp is selected and the hair is parted, wet down with providone-iodine, and stabilized with clips. The hair is then trimmed to accommodate the excision of a strip length predetermined as previously described on the basis of the necessary number of micro- and minigrafts. A 1% lidocaine solution with 1:100,000 epinephrine is diluted 1:1 with normal saline and is then infused into the posterior donor site until tumescence is achieved. This facilitates excision by enhancing skin turgor and separates the subcutaneous plane from the underlying occipital arteries, thus minimizing the possibility of their transection. The anterior recipient site is then anesthetized with a ring block utilizing a 1% bupivacaine solution with 1:100,000 epinephrine for prolonged anesthesia. The same solution is diluted with normal saline and is used to tumesce the site. Optional conscious sedation is available for the particularly anxious patient.[16] Once adequate anesthesia is achieved, the patient is ready to undergo the hair transplantation procedure.

It is convenient to employ two surgeons for this procedure. One "harvests" the donor tissue with a multibladed scalpel while the other creates the recipient sites (Fig. 19-1). Generally, the posterior scalp is incised with a four- or five-bladed scalpel with 1.5-mm spacers to a depth of 6 to 8 mm,

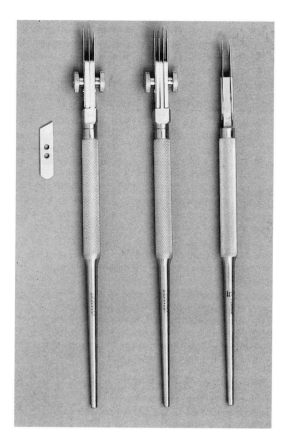

Figure 19-1 The multibladed knives with various-sized spacers.

just below the base of the hair follicle. The strip is cut in a smooth motion and the ends tapered with a no. 15 blade. An alternate approach is to harvest an ellipse of scalp with a no. 15 blade (Fig. 19-2). Next, a Metzenbaum scissors is employed to remove the donor tissue in an even fashion, typically taking about 1 mm of fat below the follicle while carefully visualizing the hair bulbs (Fig. 19-3). The donor strips are transferred in a two-handed approach to a petri dish moistened with saline. Depending on the scope of the procedure, the proper number of strips, each with a particular width, are taken and the donor site is closed with a 25-wide extension skin stapler (Fig. 19-4). Careful attention to the scalp anatomy can help to avoid transecting arteries. However, electrocautery or buried sutures may be required for hemostasis in the event that the occipital artery is transected. After closure of the donor site, one member of the two-surgeon team is delegated to the task of cutting the one or two hair micrografts and the three or four hair minigrafts from the harvested skin, utilizing a Personna surgical prep blade over an illuminated plastic surface or with a binocular scope (Fig. 19-5). To minimize trauma to the grafts, the blades are changed at the first sign of dullness and the grafts cut in a slicing motion rather than an up-and-down pressing motion. The prepared grafts are kept moist in a cold saline solution throughout the procedure to optimize their survival and thus the success of the transplantation procedure. At the same time, the second sur-

geon starts creating the recipient sites. While the recipient site can be prepared by a variety of instruments, we prefer the use of dilators over 16- or 18-gauge needles, Nokor needles, no. 11 and 15 blades, or punches. Dilators appear to minimize trauma to native hair follicles as holes are generated in a pushing fashion rather than by cutting or punching out skin, and they allow for superior hemostasis. The dilator helps in identifying the exact the sites that need grafting and in preventing "piggybacking" (the insertion of one graft on top of another). They also make it easier for members of our surgical team to insert the grafts (Fig. 19-6). Consequently, we utilize dilators to create the initial tract in one step from the medial-to-lateral direction, spacing the dilators 1 to 3 mm apart, depending on the density we are creating. To generate recipient sites for the minigrafts and micrografts, respectively, 20- and 25-gauge dilators are used. All the dilators are left in place until the process of graft insertion begins. This is easily accomplished by pulling the dilators, starting laterally with the nondominant hand and, with a curved jeweler's forceps, slipping the grafts into the recipient hole with the dominant hand (Fig. 19-7). The ideal placement proceeds by using the jeweler's forceps to grasp the fat at the bottom of the graft and insert it into the prepared slit, thereby causing the least possible degree of trauma to the follicles. Sometimes the end of a cotton-tipped applicator or the tip of the microdilator is used to help guide the the micro- and minigrafts into the recipient site. The process of graft insertion proceeds rapidly, as there is minimal bleeding, and the person inserting the grafts knows exactly which recipient sites are yet to be filled.[17]

The best results are achieved when the transplanted hair frames the face and gives a gradient of hair density true to a naturally occurring hairline. Thus a zone of micrografts is placed anteriorly to recreate a subtle hairline. The number of grafts and width of this zone will vary depending on the patient's pattern of thinning, his or her goals, and the characteristics of the donor hair (coarseness, curliness, and color).

POSTOPERATIVE CARE

Once the surgery is completed, several options exist; an acrylic glue (Derma bond) can be applied (Fig. 19-8) or a light compression garment—consisting of a topical antibiotic ointment, Telfa pads and an elastic wrap—can be placed over the transplanted area and changed the next day. This compression bandage helps to keep the grafts in place should any postoperative bleeding occur and prevents any mild, incidental trauma from dislodging the grafts. The patient is advised to make generous use of the antibiotic ointment and avoid picking at the crust. Ideally, the patient should not wash the scalp hair for one full week to allow the new grafts to settle. If necessary, the patient may use shampoo and a light stream of water to gently rinse the scalp hair surrounding the donor and recipient sites on day 3 after the transplantation. Vigorous activities are avoided for 2 weeks and donor-site staples are removed at 10 days. If the glue has been employed, the site requires little management and shampoo can be applied the next day. The glue seals the

(text continues on page 341)

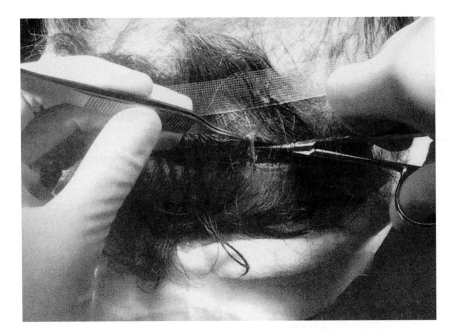

Figure 19-2 The alternate approach preferred by some surgeons is the ellipse excision, which is being harvested in this photo.

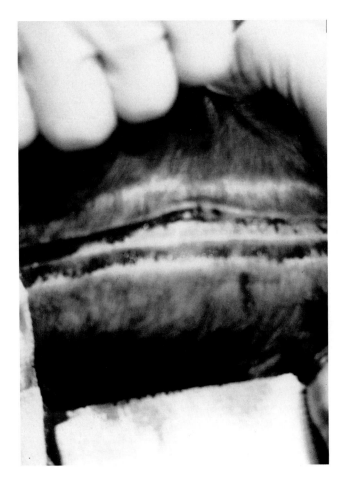

Figure 19-3 The hair bulbs are readily visible; care must be taken to avoid transecting the follicles.

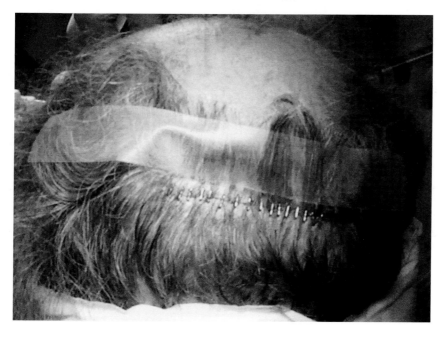

Figure 19-4   The donor area is closed with staples, which are removed between 7 and 10 days after the procedure.

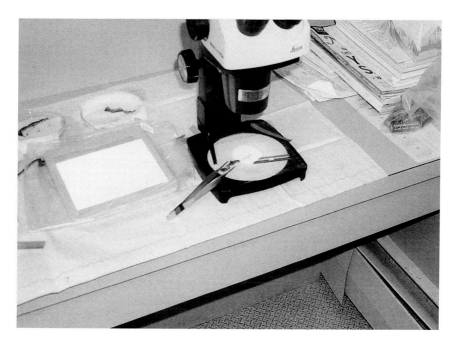

Figure 19-5   The donor strips/ellipse can be sectioned into grafts with the use of a lighted plate or the binocular scope.

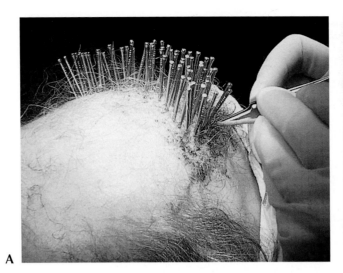
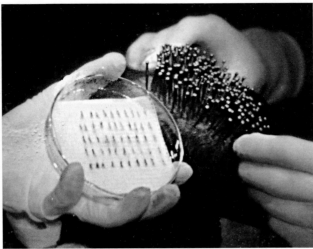

A

Figure 19-6 (**A**) The recipient-site incisions can be made in many different ways. This photo demonstrates the use of dilators, which are sharp at their tip and simply pushed in to create recipient sites. (**B**) The tray with harvested grafts is held by an assistant as the grafts are placed.

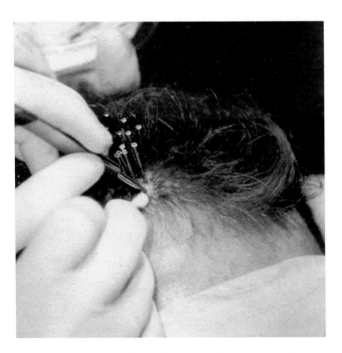

Figure 19-7 The grafts are being checked to assure for correct seating and orientation. Jeweler's forceps or the wooden tip of a swab is quite effective.

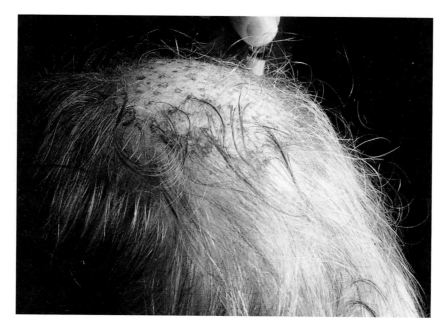

Figure 19-8   If the scalp is not very full of hair, acrylic glue (Derma bond) is a very patient-friendly means of securing grafts.

grafts and prevents epidermal water loss; and may also limit crusting (Fig. 19-9). The site of the transplant heals remarkably well with little evidence of the procedure (Fig. 19-10). The limitation is obviously that the area where the glue has been applied must be largely devoid of existing hair. With minimal care, the donor site heals well, and with repeated procedures the scar can be cut out and the patient left with an excellent cosmetic result at this site (Fig. 19-11).

COMPLICATIONS

While the list of potential complications is long, they are uncommon. Leading the list of complications in micro/minigrafting is cyst formation due to ingrown hairs (<10 percent), followed by bleeding at the donor site (<5 percent), infection (<1 percent), and reaction to medications (<1 percent).[18] Headaches as well as numbness and swelling of the scalp are routinely transient. Poor growth and take of grafts as well as scarring around grafts may rarely be seen. Telogen effluvium occurs on occasion; it necessitates reassurance of the patient. A complication unique to strip harvesting with micro/minigrafting is piggybacking or the insertion of one graft on top of another. This can be avoided with the use of dilators to control hemostasis and adequate lighting for good visualization during graft insertion. Other complications that are now rarely seen but were more commonly associated with the old method of punch grafting include arteriovenous fistula and aneurysm and hypertrophic scar formation. The former is treated with figure-eight suturing. The latter responds to intralesional triamcinolone acetonide (Kenalog).[19]

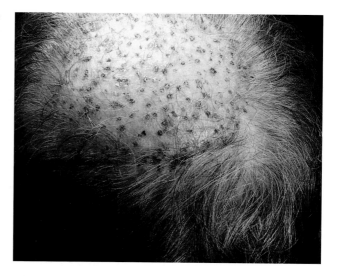

Figure 19-9   If acrylic glue is used, the patient requires no dressing and can shower the next day and comb his or her hair with no need for ointment, as the glue serves to prevent water loss transcutaneously. Hence the grafts do not crust significantly.

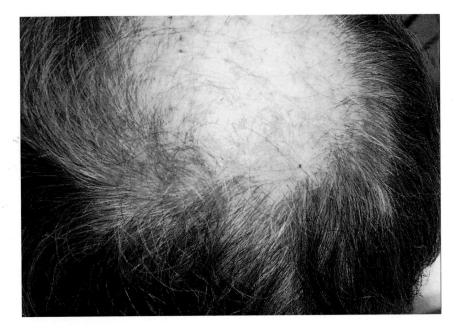

Figure 19-10 The patient in Fig. 19-9 is seen 2 weeks posttransplant, after the glue has fallen away.

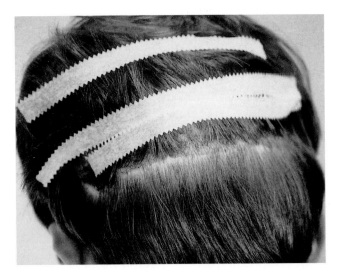

Figure 19-11 The donor-site hair is left with an excellent, cosmetically acceptable scar prior to growth of the transplanted hair.

CONCLUSION

Hair transplantation has changed significantly since its start in the 1960s. Standard punch grafting, which left the patient with telltale signs of transplantation, gave way to the current use of strip harvesting with micrografting, minigrafting, and follicular unit grafting. This allows for hair restoration in a nearly undetectable fashion, but the trade-off is that more sessions are required to produce a final density that approaches large graft coverage. In the hands of a physician dedicated to careful patient selection, good surgical technique, and vigilant postoperative care, hair transplantation is an effective tool (Figs. 19-12*A* through *D*, 19-13, 19-14, and 19-15).

Scalp Reduction and Lifting

HISTORY

Historically, the origin of scalp reduction may be attributed to the work of plastic surgeons in the 1930s who performed reconstructive scalp surgery for defects secondary to malignancies or cicatricial alopecia. The first report of scalp reduction is credited to Blanchard and Blanchard[20] in 1977, with their paper on "obliteration of alopecia by hair lifting." Shortly thereafter, in February 1978, Stough and Webster[21] and Sparkuhl[22] made their presentations on the topic at the International Hair Transplant Symposium at Lucerne,

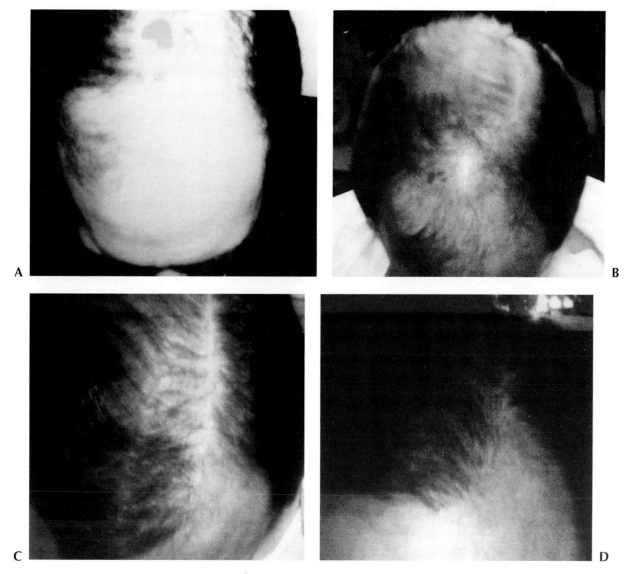

Figure 19-12   (*A*) Preoperative photo of patient prior to hair transplantation. (*B*) The same patient after the first session of 300 grafts. (*C*) The same patient after the second session of 400 grafts. (*D*) The same patient after the third session of 400 grafts.

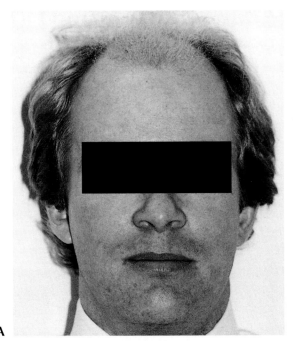

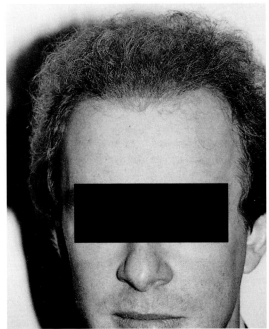

A

B

Figure 19-13   (**A**) Preoperative photo of patient prior to hair transplantation. (**B**) This same patient after 1500 grafts, with an excellent result.

Switzerland. It was not until the publication by Unger and Unger[23] in September 1978, in a widely read journal, that the subject of scalp reduction was exposed to a significant portion of the surgical community. Bosley et al.[24] wrote up a large series of scalp reduction cases in February 1979. Shortly after the initial use of the midline sagittal ellipse pattern, the para-median crescentic excision, as introduced by Alt,[25] and the Y pattern became popular. Brandy[26] contributed to these developments with his paper on circumferential scalp reduction in 1994.

Scalp lifting in its original form is credited to Marzola's lateral scalp lift,[27] a method he published in 1984. A few months later, Bradshaw[28] varied the Marzola incision by lengthening it from one sideburn, around the donor-dominant fringe, to the other sideburn while cutting both occipital arteries at the time of surgery. This method allowed for more extensive scalp lifting but had a 28.6 percent necrosis rate. After modifying several points in Bradshaw's method, including the need to ligate the occipital arteries several weeks prior to the actual scalp lifting to markedly decrease the necrosis rate, Brandy[29] reported the bilateral occipitoparietal flap in 1986. In short order, he introduced other variants of scalp lifting, namely the bitemporal flap, the modified bitemporal flap, and the frontoparietal advancement flap.[30–32]

CLASSIFICATION

Scalp reduction refers to the treatment of alopecia by surgical excision of redundant scalp tissue in areas of bald or balding skin. In essence, this procedure involves undermining the entire scalp above the nuchal ridge, followed by overlapping of the undermined scalp to determine a safe margin for surgical excision. Then, the excessive amount of bald skin is sur-

gically removed and the wound is sutured with a two-layered closure. While there have been many variants of scalp reduction, these can be classified into four basic types: (1) the midline sagittal ellipse or its variant, the lazy S; (2) the Y pattern, also known as the "Mercedes Benz" pattern or its variant, the double-Y pattern; (3) the paramedian pattern; and (4) the circumferential pattern, an adaptation of scalp lifting. Consequently, circumferential reduction is the only pattern of scalp reduction that does not require the undermining of bald skin.[2,19,33]

Scalp lifting differs from scalp reduction through its extensive undermining down to the hairline of the nape (beyond the nuchal ridge), which gives rise to 60 percent more stretch due to the lack of galeal restriction in this area. As this procedure does not involve the undermining of bald skin, it may pose less of a problem with stretch-back and slot formation. The five basic techniques of scalp lifting are classified as follows: (1) Marzola lateral scalp-lift; (2) bilateral occipitoparietal scalp-lift; (3) bitemporal scalp-lift; (4) modified bitemporal scalp-lift; and (5) frontoparietal scalp-lift.[19,28]

INDICATIONS AND CONTRAINDICATIONS

Androgenic and cicatricial alopecia are the common indications for scalp reduction and lifting, especially cases of more significant alopecia that might not have any notable benefit from hair grafting alone. The contraindications for both procedures consist of impaired wound healing, bleeding disorders, and anticoagulant therapy. Also, scalp reduction is of no help in marked posterior baldness, where scalp lifting does make a difference. And a high periauricular hairline speaks against scalp lifting, as this procedure does elevate that hairline.[19]

ADVANTAGES AND DISADVANTAGES

Scalp reduction and lifting may serve as adjunctive procedures to hair grafting in individuals with significant alopecia. However, both procedures are subject to certain limitations. Scalp reduction requires a certain amount of scalp laxity and is often associated with notable stretch-back and slot formation as well as some elevation of the periauricular hairline. While scalp lifting is not limited as much by lack of scalp laxity or by stretch-back and slot formation, it is associated with the following disadvantages: scar formation at the sideburns and vertex; permanent hypoesthesia at the vertex with a variable degree of resolution over time; periauricular hairline elevation; and the need for occipital artery ligations 2 to 6 weeks prior to lifting to minimize the risk of necrosis.[19,28]

CONTROVERSY

At first glance, scalp reduction and lifting seem almost miraculous in that they can help to provide coverage with good density in patients with advanced alopecia of the vertex and crown. However, both procedures involve significant stretching of the scalp skin, which results in several drawbacks. Of course, there is the stretch-back and slot formation associated with scalp reductions, as discussed above. Still, these limitations can be minimized by the use of tissue expanders and a posterior z-plasty, respectively. Less obvious drawbacks of both scalp reduction and lifting that are not correctable include the simultaneous decrease of donor density and scalp laxity. Consequently, less dense hair is obtainable for correction of frontal alopecia, the cosmetically most important area of the scalp, especially in view of the progressive nature of alopecia. Also, after repeated reduction in lifting procedures, the remaining scalp can be very thin due to stretching and may lack receptivity to grafting should fill-in be desired. Therefore, given the above considerations, scalp reduction and lifting are most compelling in the treatment of alopecia as an adjunctive procedure to allow a more efficient use of a limited amount of donor hair.[2]

PREOPERATIVE CONSIDERATIONS

The basis for any successful cosmetic procedure is proper patient selection. This process begins with a comprehensive evaluation, including a careful patient history and physical examination. In planning the patient's hair restoration, physicians must consider current needs as well as possible future needs, keeping in mind the progressive nature of alopecia. Numerous other factors must be taken into account, including the patient's psychological disposition, the extent of baldness, and the fine balance between improved coverage of crown and vertex versus decreased density of donor hair for transplantation to the cosmetically important frontal scalp.

The consultation time provides a chance for the surgeon and the patient to become familiar with each other. It is vital to talk about the patient's expectations of the proposed procedure as well as its limitations and possible complications. The nature of scalp reduction or lifting as an adjunct procedure to allow for more efficient use of a limited amount of donor hair grafts in patients with more extensive baldness of crown and vertex and the anticipated overall results should be reviewed. The patient needs to be enlightened on the possibility of unexpected events—such as scarring, infection, hematoma formation, and necrosis—which could affect the final results despite appropriate intervention. Finally, a schedule of the number of sessions of scalp reduction or lifting in association with transplantation procedures usually required to gain the expected results should also be outlined for each patient.

Finally, there is a preoperative visit during which any remaining questions are addressed and the expectations and limitations of the procedure are again reiterated. As unfulfilled expectations will invariably affect physician-patient relations in a negative manner and likely erode the patient's trust in the surgeon's ability, the time spent reviewing questions, answers, expectations, and limitations is well worthwhile. After this comes the time to obtain an informed consent, take preoperative baseline photographs, prescribe preoperative and postoperative medications (benzodiazepine for anxiety, antibiotics, antivirals, and hydrocodone bitartrate (Lortab) for postsurgical pain control), and order baseline presurgical tests (CBC with differential, hepatic panel, complete metabolic panel, thyroid function tests, PT, and PTT).

SURGICAL TECHNIQUE

On the day of the scheduled scalp reduction, the patient is prepped and draped appropriately. No shaving of the hair is performed. The surgical area is infiltrated with 1% lidocaine with 1:100,000 epinephrine at least 20 min prior to the surgical procedure. A ring block is employed. It is important to keep record of the amount of lidocaine injected and for it to be within physiologic limits, which for the average adult male would be less than 50 mL of this solution. Next, it is helpful to apply ice over the area for 10 to 15 min to enhance hemostasis. The incision for the scalp reduction may vary depending on the type of reduction that is planned. In alopecia reduction, the incision is generally placed in a line near the junction of the hair-bearing and non-hair-bearing scalp. In particular, this incision has to be placed so that the hair-bearing scalp margins of hair growth are not adversely affected, i.e., without transecting the hair bulbs. Once the incision is made, the scalp is undermined in the subgaleal plane using both blunt and sharp undermining techniques. This dissection can be aided by hydrodissection. The use of a 60-mL syringe attached to a small spatula liposuction cannula is helpful in carrying out the subgaleal saline hydrodissection. The undermining should be carried forward to allow for correction of possible "dog ears." Care must be taken to reflect on the anatomy and vascular supply of the scalp in performing procedures near the ear or nuchal line. After the dissection is complete, the redundant scalp is draped over the opposite wound margin with the help of towel clamps and is excised while under firm retraction. The area is irrigated with bacteriostatic saline and hemostasis is obtained with electrocautery. Then towel clamps are used to approximate the wound margins, holding off tension while the scalp is closed in two layers. Two-0 polydioxanone sutures (PDS) are used in the galea and staples are used in the skin, which are left in place for 12 to 14 days.[34] For scalps with limited mobility, tissue expanders may be used. Tissue expanders are employed several months prior to the actual scalp reduction by placement in from the incision, so that the scar and non-hair-bearing scalp are not expanded during the inflation process. Injection of the expander with bacteriostatic saline does not begin until 1 week after the staples are removed. Expansion with saline continues for a minimum of 6 to 8 weeks. Then, at the time of the expander's removal and reconstruction, the initial incisions are placed.[35]

Scalp lifting represents a more complex procedure than scalp reduction that allows for even more extensive removal of bald skin. The important first step prior to the actual scalp lifting procedure consists of bilateral occipital artery ligation 2 to 6 weeks ahead of time to promote development of collateral circulation, which is intended to keep necrosis of the scalp to a minimum. For this purpose a Doppler device is needed to identify and mark the location of each occipital artery. Following local anesthesia, vertical incisions down to the fascia at the identified sites will expose the occipital arteries and branches so that they may be ligated and transected. Then, the incision sites are closed with a 4/0 absorbable suture. In approaching the actual scalp lifting several weeks later, appropriate anesthesia is essential. Thus, intravenous sedation is ideal for this operation. After the patient has been sedated, local anesthesia with a proper mix of lidocaine and epinephrine is used to perform a "ring block" of the scalp and infiltration to below the nuchal ridge. Usually, the bilateral occipito-parietal (BOP) scalp lift is used as the initial procedure and may be followed some time later by a bitemporal scalp lift. Both temporal arteries must be identified with the Doppler device before proceeding with the actual incision of the BOP flap. This incision begins 1 cm behind the temporal hairline but clearly in front of the identified temporal artery; it then proceeds superiorly and posteriorly along the outline of the bald scalp in a bilateral symmetrical fashion, as previously illustrated.

The extensive undermining requires good visualization, which is obtained with the help of surgical assistants who perform the "lifting" maneuver. For the most part, this undermining follows the avascular subgaleal plane. However, the galea does not extend directly to the supraauricular, postauricular, and inferior occipital scalp. In these regions, the corresponding muscle must be split to reach the fairly avascular fascial plane and allow for optimal undermining. Next, a drain stab wound is made behind one or both ears to permit the placement of a drain. After meticulous hemostasis is obtained, the occipital scalp is advanced superiorly and the temporal scalp medially and anteriorly to determine the amount of excess bald skin. This is excised as a horseshoe-shaped crescent. Subcutaneous closure with deep galeal bites is achieved with multiple figure-eight PDS II sutures. The skin surface can be closed with staples or nonabsorbable synthetic sutures.[36]

POSTOPERATIVE CARE

Immediate postoperative care for both scalp reduction and lifting consists of a circumferential head dressing with Aquaphor, Telfa pads, and Curlex wrap. This dressing is removed the next day in the office, so that the physician may check the surgical site thoroughly for the development of complications. Also, the drains placed during the scalp-lifting procedure are removed. The patient is given another head dressing that he or she may remove at home the following day. Ideally, the patient should not wash the scalp until 3 to 5 days after the surgery. The second postsurgical follow-up occurs between days 10 and 14, at which point the skin-surface staples or sutures are taken out. Appropriate pain management is vital during this time. Initially, pain control is achieved with hydrocodone bitartrate and acetominophen 7.5/500 mg every 4 to 6 h. After the first several days, the patient is advised to use hydrocodone bitartrate and acetominophen only at night and to use extra-strength acetominophen during the day.

COMPLICATIONS

Potential complications of either scalp reduction or lifting are those that can be seen with any surgical procedure. These include infection, hematoma, hypoesthesia, scarring, and necrosis. Infections are exceedingly rare, which may be attributed to the excellent blood supply of the scalp; if an infection does occur; a culture must be taken before starting antibiotic therapy. The incidence of hematomas can be kept to a minimum by meticulous intraoperative hemostasis; when hematoma is detected, it should be treated by evacuation with a 16-gauge needle on a syringe and the application of pressure. Hypoesthesia of the crown, though it may improve over time, is an expected complication that the patient must be aware of prior to the surgery. While scar formation is implied with any surgical procedure, it is the development of hypertrophic scarring/keloids and excessive stretch-back that are considered actual complications; the former is treated with intralesional Kenalog injections; the latter is seen with scalp reduction and can be minimized with retention sutures and adequate closure of the subcutaneous tissue, including the galea. Finally, though necrosis as a complication is seen more commonly in scalp lifting, it does not occur often to a significant degree, especially due to the utilization of occipital artery ligation several weeks prior to scalp lifting to allow for the formation of a collateral circulation.[19,28]

Other complications related to the specific site of surgery, namely the scalp, are ingrown hairs, telogen effluvium, and slot formation. Ingrown hairs can be held to a minimum by carefully pulling out hairs caught in the skin closure site immediately after completion of the surgery. When ingrown hairs occur, they are treated with warm compresses. Telogen effluvium is discussed as a potential complication prior to surgery and, if it does happen, requires frequent reassurance of the patient. And slot formation seen with scalp reduction may be addressed with the posterior z-plasty (Frechet method).[37]

CONCLUSION

Despite some controversy surrounding scalp reduction and lifting, these represent important procedures that are useful in patients with balding so severe that it cannot be efficiently treated with hair transplantation alone. Hence, scalp reduction and lifting should be thought of adjunctive procedures that allow for more efficient use of a limited donor supply of hair grafts in this patient population (Fig. 19-16). These procedures may become obsolete in the future, when hair follicles can be cloned to provide an unlimited supply of grafts.

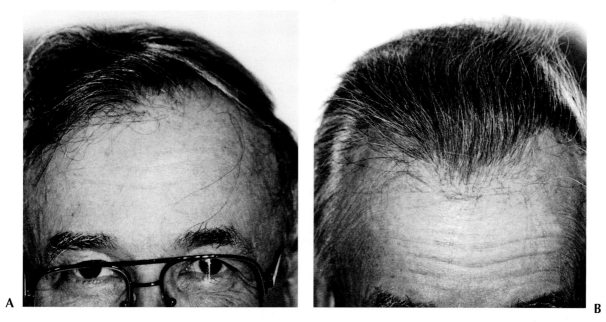

Figure 19-14   (*A*) Preoperative photo. (*B*) After hair transplantation.

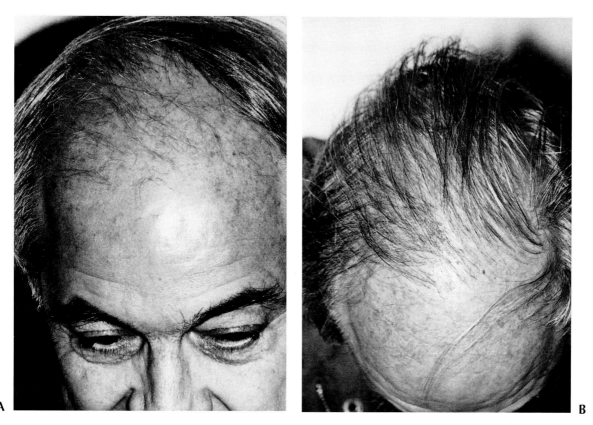

Figure 19-15   (*A*) Preoperative photo. (*B*) After hair transplantation.

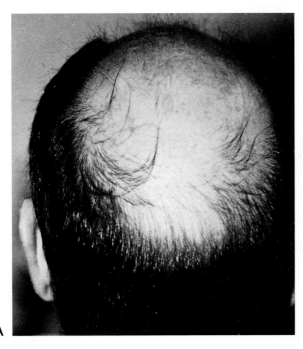 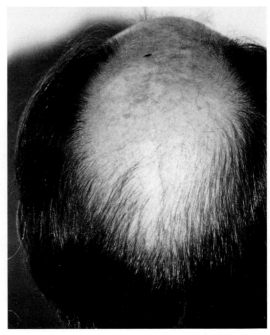

Figure 19-16 (**A**) Before scalp reduction procedure. (**B**) After scalp reduction procedure.

References

1. Scarborough DA, Bisaccia E. Geometric hair transplantation. *Cosmet Dermatol* 1995; 8:9–11.
2. Griffin EI. Hair Transplantation: The fourth decade. *Dermatol Clin* 1995; 13:363–387.
3. Okuda S. Clinical and experimental studies of transplantation of living hairs. *Jpn J Dermatol Urol* 1939, 46.135–138.
4. Fujita K. Reconstruction of eyebrow. *La Lepro* 1953; 22:364 (Japanese).
5. Orentreich N. Autografts in alopecias and other selected dermatologic conditions. *Ann NY Acad Sci* 1959; 83:463.
6. Vallis CP. Surgical treatment of the receding hairline. *Plast Reconstr Surg* 1968; 33:247.
7. Vallis CP. Surgical treatment of the receding hairline. *Plast Reconstr Surg* 1969; 44:271–278.
8. Coiffman F. Injertos cuadrados de cuero cabelludo. Presented at First Iberoamerican Congress of Plastic Surgery, Quito, Ecuador, 1976.
9. Coiffman F. Use of square scalp grafts for male pattern baldness. *Plast Reconstr Surg* 1977; 60:228–232.
10. Scarborough D, Bisaccia E. The multibladed knife for donor harvesting. In: Stough DB, Haber RS, eds. *Hair Replacement, Surgical and Medical.* St. Louis: Mosby–Year Book; 1996:117–122.
11. Stough DB, Bondar GL. The Knudsen nomenclature: Standardizing terminology of graft sizes. *Dermatol Surg* 1997; 23:763–765.
12. Halsner UEM, Lucas MWG. New aspects in hair transplantation for females. *Dermatol Surg* 1995; 21:605–610.
13. Bisaccia E, Scarborough D. Square grafting. In: Unger W, ed. *Hair Transplantation*, 3rd ed. New York: Marcel Dekker; 1995:485–497.
14. Pomerantz MA. Creating a hairline. *Dermatol Clin* 1999; 17:271–275.
15. Beehner ML. A frontal forelock/central density framework for hair transplantation. *Dermatol Surg* 1997; 23:807–815.
16. Scarborough D, Bisaccia E. Monitored anesthesia care as an adjunct to local anesthesia for scalp surgery In: Stough DB, Haber RS, eds. *Hair Replacement, Surgical and Medical.* St. Louis: Mosby–Year Book; 1996:97–103.
17. Sequeira M, Abeles GD, Scarborough DA, et al. The use of sharp microdilators in hair transplantation. *Cosmet Dermatol* 1998; 4:9–11.
18. Stough DB, Miner JE. Male pattern alopecia: Surgical options. *Dermatol Clin* 1997; 15:609–622.
19. Brandy DA, Brandy KL. Hair replacement surgery. In: Robinson JK, Arndt KA, LeBoit PE, Wintroub BU, eds. *Atlas of Cutaneous Surgery.* Philadelphia: Saunders; 1996:281–293.
20. Blanchard G, Blanchard B. Obliteration of alopecia by hair lifting: A new concept and technique. *J Natl Med Assoc* 1977; 69:639–641.
21. Stough DB, Webster RC. Esthetics and refinements in hair transplantation. The International Hair Transplant Symposium. Lucerne, Switzerland, Feb 4, 1978.
22. Sparkuhl K. Scalp reduction: Serial excision of the scalp with flap advancement. The International Hair Transplant Symposium. Lucerne, Switzerland, Feb 4, 1978.
23. Unger MG, Unger WP. Management of alopecia of the scalp by a combination of excisions and transplantations. *J Dermatol Surg Oncol* 1978; 4:670–672.
24. Bosley LL, Hope CR, Montroy RE. Male pattern reduction (MPR) for surgical reduction of male pattern baldness. *Curr Ther Res* 1979; 25:281–287.

25. Alt TH. Scalp reduction as an adjunct to hair transplantation, review of relevant literature, presentation of an improved technique. *J Dermatol Surg Oncol* 1980; 6:1011–1018.

26. Brandy DA. Circumferential scalp reduction. *J Dermatol Surg Oncol* 1994; 20:277–284.

27. Marzola M. An alternative hair replacement method. In: Norwood, OT, ed. *Hair Replacement Surgery*, 2d ed. Springfield, IL: Charles C Thomas, 1984:315–324.

28. Brandy DA. Scalp lifting: An 8-year experience with over 1,230 cases. *J Dermatol Surg Oncol* 1993; 19:1005–1014.

29. Brandy DA. The bilateral occipitoparietal flap. *J Dermatol Surg Oncol* 1986; 10:1062–1066.

30. Brandy DA. The Brandy bitemporal flap. *Am J Cosmet Surg* 1986; 3:11–15.

31. Brandy DA. The modified bitemporal flap for the treament of bitemporal recessions. *Aesthet Plast Surg* 1989; 13:203–207.

32. Brandy DA. A new surgical approach for the treatment of extensive baldness. *Am J Cosmet Surg* 1986; 3:19–25.

33. Pinski JB. Hair transplantation and bald-scalp reduction *Dermatol Clin* 1991; 9:151–168.

34. Bisaccia E, Scarborough D. Scalp reduction for the correction of vertex alopecia. *Cosmet Dermatol* 1992; 2:10–11.

35. Bisaccia E, Scarborough D. Tissue expansion for the treatment of alopecia. *Cosmet Dermatol* 1990; 3:15–17.

36. Swinehart JM, Brandy DA. Scalp lifting: Anatomic and technical considerations. *J Dermatol Surg Oncol* 1994; 20:600–612.

37. Frechet P. A new method for correction of the vertical scar observed following scalp reduction for extensive alopecia. *J Dermatol Surg Oncol* 1990; 16:640–644.

Patient Information

Hair Transplantation

The new millennium has ushered in a new age in hair transplantation. New techniques of mini- and micrografting allow for the restoration of a natural hairline.

The success of hair transplantation depends on the fact that hair follicle roots moved from their original location on the body to another area will behave as they did in their natural site. In common male baldness, for example, a horseshoe-shaped fringe of hair persists even in the most advanced cases. Hair follicles moved from this hair fringe to a bald area on the same patient's scalp will take root and grow. We routinely observe continuing hair growth in such transplants more than 10 years later, and studies document that these grafts will continue to grow for a lifetime. Many less common types of hair loss, in addition to ordinary male baldness, can be helped by this technique.

THE PROCEDURE

- The procedure takes place in the office and lasts about 1 hour. The donor area (the area from which the hair follicles will be taken) and the receptor area (the bald area into which hair will be grafted) are anesthetized by the injection of a local anesthetic. Anesthesia occurs very rapidly in almost all cases.

- A simple instrument called a dilator is used to bore tiny holes into the receptor area, into which the grafts will be placed.

- After clipping a small zone of hair close to the scalp surface in the donor area, it is removed from the scalp and grafts are created and trimmed to proper length. The clipped area can usually be covered over completely by surrounding hair, so that the donor site does not show, even immediately after the procedure.

- The prepared hair-bearing grafts are placed into the prepared sites on the bald scalp.

- The donor and receptor areas are dressed and often left unbandaged when micrografts are used, and the patient returns home.

Hair Growth in the Transplant

We transplant individual hairs or a rather small piece of scalp, each bearing a variable number of hair follicles. A crust (scab) forms over each graft shortly after the procedure and remains attached to the graft for 10 to 20 days, after which separates, leaving a clean pinkish mark to indicate the site of the transplant. Occasionally, some painless swelling on the forehead develops a few days after the procedure. This is harmless and disappears in a week. The hair stubs in the transplants do not grow but are shed between the second and eighth week after the procedure. Sometimes many of these hair stubs fall out attached to the separate crusts; sometimes they persist longer. Rarely, one or two of the transplanted follicles may not shed their hair stub at all, so that they continue growing immediately after the procedure. With these exceptions, the follicles rest for a period of 10 to 20 weeks after the operation, during which the stubs are shed and the grafts are bare. A new generation of hair is seen at the surface usually during the 12th week after transplantation, but this may occur slightly earlier or a few weeks later in the individual patients. These hairs grow at the same rate as they did in their original location.

Final Results

It is impossible to predict in advance precisely how many hairs will appear in any given transplant. The average number is between 1 and 4 hairs per micrograft, and 4 to 8 hairs per minigraft. It is extremely rare to encounter a patient who experiences only limited growth. The skin surface of the grafts usually blends in well with the surrounding scalp after a period of 3 to 4 months. In some patients, however, the grafts may be a shade lighter in color. The grafts are usually level with the surrounding scalp but occasionally are slightly elevated or depressed. Such grafts may be flattened down with an electric needle without interfering with hair growth. A second graft placed on the same site may replace individual grafts that prove to be unsatisfactory.

"Don'ts" of Transplantation

Don't disturb the grafts in any way during the first 10 days; don't comb or brush heavily over the graft sites. The scalp may be shampooed on the third day after transplanting, but without vigorous massage. Don't pick at the grafts—if they are itchy during the healing period, the doctor will recommend a soothing salve that may be applied gently. Don't attempt to pull off the crusts yourself, even if they have persisted longer than the 10 to 12 days. After this period, many of the crusts will be safely washed off in the shower.

Further Notes

Micrografts are often well hidden by the existing hair during the healing phase. Many patients return to work in 3 to 5 days. The number of transplant plugs that should be placed at one session and the frequency of transplant sessions depends on the characteristics of each case; these matters can be planned out in advance for each patient. Normal daily activities such as walking and driving are fine the day following surgery, but excessive sweating or vigorous exercise is not recommended for 2 to 3 weeks postoperatively.

DO NOT TAKE ASPIRIN-CONTAINING PRODUCTS FOR 14 DAYS BEFORE SURGERY AND AVOID ALCOHOLIC BEVERAGES FOR 72 HOURS BEFORE AND AFTER SURGERY.

Hair Transplantation Surgical Setup Tray

Patient
1. Cape

Doctor and Staff
1. Sterile gloves
2. Masks

Materials
1. Chair
2. Sterile light-handle cover
3. Two stools
4. One gooseneck lamp
5. Four white nonsterile drapes (two for chair, two for patient)
6. Comb
7. Bobby pins
8. Two Sani-pads, tied together on one side
9. Scissors
10. Syringes
    A. 2 to 10 mL LL
    B. 1 to 5 mL LL
11. Needles
    A. Three 27-gauge 1½-in.
    B. Two 30-gauge 1-in. metal hub
12. Marcaine 0.5% mixed in equal parts of lidocaine with epinephrine
13. Sterile bowl
14. One 30 mL bottle saline
15. One 30 mL bottle lidocaine 1% with epinephrine, nonbuffered
16. 1.5 mm HT scalpel handle
17. Four 1.5-mm spacers (occasionally 2.0 mm)
18. Five no. 15 blades
19. Three 3 × 4 in. Telfa pads
20. Two rolls Kling
21. One roll Coban
22. Polysporin ointment
23. Tape
24. Dilators
25. Skin staples no. 15
26. Alcohol
27. Betadine solution
28. Sterile medium drape
29. Kenalog, 40 mg
30. Hair transplant tray
31. Hair shaper blades
32. Bandage scissors
33. Clean gloves
34. Backlit screen

Hair Transplantation

PREOPERATIVE INSTRUCTIONS

Let your hair grow to a length of 2 to 3 inches on the back and sides.

Wash your hair the night before or the morning of the procedure.

Try to have 8 hours of sleep the night before the procedure.

Have something to eat, a *light* breakfast or lunch, before coming to the office.

Have someone accompany you to the office. You *will not* be allowed to drive yourself home.

Reserve a hotel room for the night of the procedure if you live out of the city. A list of hotels/motels close to our office is available upon request.

Bring your pain medication with you on surgery day.

Wear clothes that either zip or button and do not have to be pulled over your head.

Do not take any aspirin or vitamin E or drugs containing aspirin (Bufferin, Anacin, Empirin, Stanback, Excedrin, Fiorinal, Darvon Compound, and salicylate) for 14 days before the transplant procedure. Use only Tylenol instead. **THIS IS VERY IMPORTANT!!**

Do not drink any alcohol, take any drugs, or use marijuana for 72 hours before the transplant procedure.

If you are required to continue any medicines regularly, review these with the doctor at your preoperative appointment.

At your preoperative appointment:

You will have time to discuss any questions with the doctor.

You will be asked to sign surgical consent forms.

Preoperative photos will be taken.

A postoperative follow-up appointment will be arranged.

Hair Transplantation

POSTOPERATIVE INSTRUCTIONS

Immediately following your transplant and for the first day after, relax. Keep all activities to a minimum for 24 hours. Refrain from any vigorous activity. Do not jog, do not bend over, do not engage in sex, etc.

DO NOT, UNDER ANY CIRCUMSTANCES, REMOVE OR ALTER THE DRESSING DURING THE FIRST 24 HOURS.

When you get home prepare two ice packs; medium-size plastic bags with crushed ice will do quite well. (Be careful to seal the bags to avoid leakage.) Sit comfortably in a chair and cradle your head in a pillow. Carefully place one ice pack behind your head (donor site) and the other on top (transplant area). Keep these in place for at least 30 minutes, using extreme care not to move the pack, so that scraping across the graft sites is avoided.

Have something to eat after the ice pack routine. A light snack will help you relax. Avoid food that requires excessive or constant chewing. (For example: steak, gum, etc.) No alcohol is to be taken for 72 hours.

Take the medications prescribed by the doctor:

Antibiotics

Continue taking your antibiotics as directed to help prevent infection.

Sleeping Pills

You may be given sleeping pills to help you sleep comfortably for the first two nights following the procedure. If necessary, take one or two pills 30 minutes before retiring.

To avoid any movement of the dressing and avoid friction over the graft sites, sleep in a reclining chair, in about a 45-degree upright position, the first night. A reclining chair would be ideal, but not fully reclined. If there is no other recourse, settle in a comfortable living room chair or prop your head up on three or four pillows in bed. Do not roll to the side. In any event, keep your head elevated.

If you should notice any spotting of blood, do not be alarmed. Merely reapply an ice pack where spotting is observed. Ice applied for about 15 minutes with slight pressure should stop the bleeding. Please remain calm; anxiety is not needed and will only increase your blood pressure and the bleeding.

Your initial postoperative dressing will be changed in our office the next day. The donor site and recipient site will be cleaned. The doctor will check grafts and a lighter dressing will be applied to remain in place for another 24 hours. You may remove this dressing the following day.

Cleaning the Graft Sites

On the second postoperative day, remove the gauze dressing and clean the transplant and donor areas with warm tap water or saline solution. Moisten a thin, clean washcloth with the saline solution. Using a blotting motion, gently clean crusting or dried blood as well as the transplant and donor sites. Do this several times and then gently dry the transplant and donor sites with a clean soft dry towel using the blotting motion. Then liberally apply Polysporin ointment to transplant and donor sites. Continue both of these steps once daily (morning and evening) until all scabs fall off (normally 10 to 20 days).

Swelling

You were given an injection containing medication to combat the potential for swelling. Swelling and drainage are always a possibility, and with them there is some discomfort. Swelling may occur in a day or two around the forehead and eyes as a result of the local anesthetic. If it should occur, it usually resolves by the end of the first week. Cold compresses or ice packs, avoiding dietary salt, and keeping your head elevated will help.

Shampooing

Ideally shampooing of the hair is avoided until 10 days postoperatively. However, if you must, you may shampoo on the third day following surgery. Mix baby shampoo and water together. Pour the mixture over the scalp several times. Use a blotting motion over the transplanted area. Rinse the hair by pouring clean water over the scalp several times. With a clean soft towel, dry the scalp by blotting gently. Apply Polysporin ointment to both the donor and graft sites. Do not use a hair dryer. Do not shampoo more than once a day.

You will need to return to our office in 10 to 14 days so that we may remove the skin staples from the donor area.

The use of topical minoxidil (Rogaine) may be resumed once all crusts are gone.

The transplanted hair will start to grow in about 12 to 24 weeks and it will continue to grow at your individual growth rate. Haircuts do not require special instruments or attention. Your hair stylist or barber can tend to your needs. Occasionally, full growth takes 18 months.

We expect you to come back to our office in 6 months following your transplant to check your progress. Remember, this process takes time and not all grafts will begin hair growth at the same rate. If in the meantime you have any questions, do not hesitate to call.

Don't be alarmed if you think that a plug has fallen out. Occasionally you may find a scab with fine hairs attached, but this does not mean that the graft has fallen out. Remember to be gentle and do not traumatize the grafts when cleaning and shampooing, as outlined above.

ANY REDNESS, SWELLING, TENDERNESS, OR "PUS PIMPLES" SHOULD BE IMMEDIATELY REPORTED TO THE OFFICE AT (___) _____.

CONSENT FOR HAIR TRANSPLANTATION

Patient's name_____

Date_____

As a patient, you have the right to be informed about your condition and the recommended surgical, medical, or diagnostic procedures to be used, so that you may decide—after knowing the risks and hazards involved—whether or not to undergo the procedure.

I hereby authorize _____ and/or the surgical team to perform hair replacement surgery on me and any other medical procedures that, during transplantation, become medically reasonable and necessary.

1. I am aware that significant hair thickness and scalp coverage will depend in part upon my completing the necessary number of procedures, which usually take a minimum of one to six transplant sessions. Occasionally, many more sessions are necessary to achieve the desired result.

    However, because many variables exist, I have not been promised or guaranteed good results. I also understand that the quality and amount of my pre-existing hair is a major factor in the ultimate results. I understand that I will not have hair of the same thickness as I had prior to the onset of my hair loss.

    Initial_____

2. Prior to consenting to this cosmetic procedure, I state that I have read and discussed with my physician the informational literature supplied to me in the hair transplant folder, which includes the **pre- and post-operative instructions for hair transplantation and the patient self-check list.**

Initial_____

3. I fully understand the results that I may reasonably expect. A complete explanation of this procedure has been given to me. I do understand that I will not have a full head of hair after the procedure is complete.

Initial_____

4. **A transplant may look less natural on those with dark hair and light skin.**

Initial_____

5. I understand there will be slight scarring associated with this procedure. I understand that hair transplants are not perfect. Unsightly or objectional scarring, although rare, may occur.

Initial_____

6. I am aware that complications may occur. The more common complications and a partial list of rare complications of this surgery have been explained to me and I have reviewed a list of them, which I have initialed and dated. A copy of that list is attached to this request. Unforeseen rare complications, such as unanticipated reactions to medicine and anesthetics, uncommon infections, and unusual healing responses are a possibility. Every unforeseen complication may not have been discussed with me in detail, but I understand that such risks do exist.

Initial_____

7. I consent to and authorize the administration of such anesthetics as may be considered necessary by those performing the surgery on me.

Initial_____

8. For the purpose of advancing medical education, I consent to the admittance of authorized observers to the operating room.

Initial_____

9. I understand that I will be financially liable for the cosmetic surgery performed, regardless of the ultimate outcome.

Initial_____

10. I am entering this agreement of my own will. I believe I have been well informed. I understand that although good results are hoped for and expected, cosmetic surgery results cannot be guaranteed because of the nature of the human body, the healing process, and the risk of reasonable error in judgment and implementation, which is possible in any surgical procedure.

Initial_____

11. I give permission to _____ to take still or motion clinical photographs with the understanding that such photographs remain the property of the center. If in the judgment of the center medical research, education, or science will be benefited by their use, such photographs and related information may be published and republished in professional journals or medical books or used for any other purpose which the center may deem proper. It is specifically understood that in any such publication or use, I shall not be identified by name.

Initial_____

12. The pro/cons and alternatives to hair transplants have been explained.

Initial_____

13. **It has been explained to me that the amount and location of future hair loss on the scalp, including the sides or back area, cannot at this point in time be predicted. I do understand that it is possible to lose my existing hair at any point in time in the future. I do understand that this may affect the appearance of the grafted area. In the majority of men, some thinning of all areas occurs. Most men do not lose all of their donor (back of head) hair with age.**

A very thorough understanding of the above paragraph is required before a patient consents to hair restoration surgery. I have been given the opportunity to ask questions and all my questions have been answered to my satisfaction.

Initial_____

My signature indicates that I have read this "Consent for Hair Transplantation" and I understand and accept the risks involved in this operation. I hereby authorize _____ and/or the surgical team to perform this procedure on me.

_____ _____
Signature (Patient/Responsible Party)   Date

_____ _____
Signature (Witness)   Date

More Common Complications:

1. Nausea and vomiting from pain medication

Initial_____

2. Bleeding (Less than 5%)

Initial_____

3. Infection (Less than 1%)

Initial_____

4. Excessive swelling

Initial_____

5. Temporary headache

Initial_____

6. Temporary numbness of the scalp

Initial_____

7. Scarring around the grafts

Initial_____

8. Poor growth of grafts

Initial_____

9. Reactions to medications (Less than 1%)

Initial_____

10. Fainting (Less than 1%)

Initial_____

11. Occasional small ingrown hair causing a cyst (Less than 10%)

Initial_____

Rare Complications (*partial list only*)

1. Keloid formation

Initial_____

2. Complete failure of growth of transplanted hair

Initial_____

3. Persistent scalp pain

Initial_____

4. Total loss of donor hair

Initial_____

5. Permanent numbness of scalp

Initial_____

6. Noticeable scarring of donor area

Initial_____

7. Unnatural growth of transplanted hair

Initial_____

8. Loss of transplanted hair

Initial_____

9. Thinning of surrounding hair

Initial_____

I have read and understand the possible complications listed above, and understand there may be others.

_____   _____

Signature (Patient/Responsible Party)   Date

_____   _____

Signature (Witness)   Date

CHAPTER 20

Otoplasty: Treatment for Protuberant Ears

Otoplasty is a common cosmetic procedure for the treatment of protuberant ears. Like other forms of cosmetic surgery its goal is to enhance the patient's appearance. Specifically, it is aimed at making the protuberant ears less apparent by restoring them to a normal form and position in a symmetrical fashion. Several surgical specialties are performing otoplasty, including dermatologic surgeons. The skin rearrangement and cartilage excision techniques often employed are similar to those used in skin and cartilage removal surgeries secondary to skin cancer—procedures commonly performed by dermatologic surgeons.

Historical Background

In 1845, Diffenbach[1] reported the first surgical approach to the correction of prominent ears: He combined simple excision from the posterior sulcus with sutures subsequently fixing the ear cartilage to the periosteum of the mastoid. Variations of this surgical technique are still used and are called the *posterior approach*. The first description of surgical alteration of auricular cartilage to treat prominent ears is credited to Ely[2] in 1881. Subsequently, a multitude of surgical techniques for the treatment of excessively prominent ears and modifications thereof have been described; the literature reveals more than 170 techniques. They can be basically categorized into three groups: (1) leaving the cartilage intact and using only sutures to restructure the ear, as used in the permanent suture insertion of the Mustarde technique[3] and the incisionless otoplasty of Fritsch;[4] (2) incising the cartilage in order to make it more pliable but without resecting it (e.g., the Converse cartilage incision technique[5] and the anterior scoring described by Chongchet[6] and Stenstrom[7]); and (3) a technique that includes excision of cartilage. We favor this technique as it is simple and provides good results, with the deformity less apt to recur.[8]

There is also a relatively new nonsurgical approach that is perhaps better than surgical correction, with its associated risks. When the prominent ears are noted in infancy, the use of external temporary appliances to tape the ears in a corrected position for several months results in a successful permanent correction.[9–11] The only drawback with this method is that it takes highly motivated parents to follow the protocol.

Development of the Ear

At birth, the ear of a newborn shows a length of 66 percent and a width of 76 percent that of the adult ear. By the age of 3 years, the ear has attained 85 percent of its final size, and seven-eighths of the final growth occurs prior to age 7. Subsequent growth of the ear is not interrupted by otoplasty. Interestingly, between 30 and 80 years of age, the length of the auricle may increase up to 1 cm due to lengthening of the auricular cartilage. As a result, the auricular cartilage flattens, owing to reduced skin elasticity, and the lobule is elongated.[12,13]

Anatomy of the Ear

A thorough knowledge of the anatomy of the ear is essential for performing a safe and successful otoplasty. Below is a basic description of the intricate anatomy of the auricle.[14]

The external ear consists of the auricle and the external auditory canal. The helix arises anteriorly and inferiorly from a crus extending horizontally above the external auditory meatus, thus creating the outer frame of the auricle. The helix merges inferiorly into the cauda helicis and connects to the lobule. The anthelical fold lies between the anthelical crus and is also called the scapha. The anthelix extends upward from the cauda helicis medially to the helix until it bifurcates into the anterior superior and anterior inferior crura. The anthelix borders medially to the rim of the concha and the concha proper. The concha is composed of the conchal cymba superiorly and the conchal cavum inferiorly. These are separated by the helical crus and meet the anthelix at the anthelical rim. The conchal cavum anteriorly extends to the tragus and the external auditory meatus; inferiorly and posteriorly, it borders to the antitragus, which connects laterally with the anthelix. The tragus and antitragus are separated by the intertragal notch. The lobule does not contain cartilage and displays a variety of shapes and attachments to the adjacent cheek and scalp.

The arterial supply to the auricle and external auditory meatus is derived by the external carotid artery through the superficial temporal artery, which supplies most of the external ear canal and parts of the anterior auricle; the posterior auricular arteries provide blood flow to the posterior parts of the ear.

The sensory innervation involves several different nerves. They include the greater auricular nerve and the lesser occipital nerve, which are branches of the cervical plexus and the auricular temporal nerve, a branch of the mandibular division of the trigeminal nerve. A portion of the posterior wall of the external meatus is innervated by the auricular branch of the vagus nerve.

Indications

While prominent ears are considered a sign of good fortune in the Far East, western society looks upon prominent ears in a far less positive manner. In fact, a significant degree of morbidity is associated with this condition. Children with protuberant ears are often the subject of verbal and at times physical abuse by their peers, resulting in adverse psychological effects. In particular, Bradbury et al.[15] state that 10 percent of children on the National Health Service (NHS) waiting list for surgical correction of prominent ears had seen a child psychiatrist. Social distress entirely related to this condition was reported in 67 percent, starting as early as age 4. Thus, psychological concerns are the major indication for otoplasty. These psychological concerns often cause parents to be the first to initiate the step toward surgical correction, and the consulted surgeon will frequently concur with this request if it is based on an actual anatomic disproportion of the ear. However, it is very important to have the child voice its desire for this surgery, as the child is the best able to judge the degree of distress this condition imposes. Without the child's distinct wish for this cosmetic procedure, he or she is not a good candidate.

Once the patient and parents agree upon wanting to have the surgical correction done, the surgeon needs to evaluate the degree of deformity against potential surgical risks based upon the patient's medical history. If the patient has any pre-existent medical conditions that increase the risk of surgery an undue amount, it needs to be reassessed.

Finally, the patient's age plays an important role in the decision for or against surgery. As previously stated, 85 percent of the final size of the ear is achieved by age 3. Consequently, many surgeons prefer to correct ear malformations before 4 to 5 years of age or prior to school age.[7,16] Surgery before this age could result in marked inhibition of auricular growth. We restrict otoplasty in our office to patients who have achieved adolescence or adulthood without completely adjusting to their appearance, as they are more capable than

young children to describe the auricular features of concern to them and their desire for correction.[14]

Preoperative Considerations

A careful physical exam of the ears to determine the type of auricular anomalies present, as discussed below, is the first step in correcting these anomalies. This exam should also note the degree of symmetry between ears. These findings must be clearly documented in written form and with photographs. Standard photographs should show the right and left laterals, close-up views, as well as two frontal views with appropriate lighting. Second, it is important to discuss with the patient which auricular features are of most concern, as they may not be the same as the auricular anomalies noted by the surgeon. Patient satisfaction with the procedure is dependent on addressing these features. Next, it is vital to set realistic expectations for otoplasty. The surgeon must discuss with the patient what can and cannot be achieved with this surgery. The patient must understand that there is a range of improvement, not a guarantee for 100 percent satisfaction. Of course, potential complications, as with any surgery, need to be outlined verbally and in a written consent signed by the patient. Once the patient understands the surgery and its potential complications, has realistic expectations for improvement, and consents to surgical correction, preoperative clearance can be obtained. This should include a good physical and history by the internist or family physician as well as a normal electrocardiogram (ECG), chest x-ray, and standard laboratory tests. Finally, the patient is given the following advice: to avoid the use of aspirin and nonsteroidal anti-inflammatory agents for two weeks prior to surgery to minimize bleeding; to wash the hair the day before surgery, as this cannot be done for several days after the procedure; not to use cosmetics the day of surgery to simplify sterilization of the surgical field; and to take an oral benzodiazepine 1 h prior to surgery to decrease anxiety.

Surgical Technique

ANESTHESIA
Many of the surgical subspecialties prefer general anesthesia in performing cosmetic procedures, and others opt for conscious sedation. However, if the patient proves to be highly motivated, otoplasty can easily be performed with local anesthesia alone. In fact, it is the anesthesia of choice, whenever the patient has any medical contraindications to sedation or feels uncomfortable with the concept of sedation. Independent of the type of anesthesia chosen, light local infiltration with a mixture of 1% lidocaine and 1:100,000 epinephrine aids in hemostasis and outlining of the tissue planes.

EVALUATION OF THE DEFORMITY
Ear prominence is generally the result of one or more of the following anatomic malformations: (1) failure of anthelical folding, which commonly affects the upper and/or middle

thirds of the ear and presents as a wing-like defect; (2) concha enlargement and/or anterolateral rotation, such that the auriculomastoid angle exceeds 30 degrees or the distance between helix and mastoid at midauricle is more than 2.0 cm; (3) protrusion of the upper third of the ear as defined by an angle of over 40 degrees between the scalp and the root of the helix; (4) protrusion of the earlobe.[17–20] If the surgeon neglects to recognize and/or address all of the anatomic malformations contributing to the prominent ear, adequate correction may not be attained.

Surgical Correction of the Deformity

When a patient presents with all four deformities, they should be addressed in the following manner. First, the anthelical fold is created. Then, the concha is reduced and/or repositioned. The protrusion of the upper third of the ear and of the earlobe are often sufficiently corrected as part of the two procedures described above. If this is not the case, both can be individually corrected at the conclusion of the otoplasty.

The anthelical fold is created by lightly pressing the scapha onto the concha. The position of the fold is then marked on the anterior ear skin with a row of ink spots running just lateral to the anthelix from the superior pole of the superior crus down to merging point between anthelix and helix. Two ink spots are placed within the triangular fossa to mark the site of suture placement for reshaping the superior crus. The last set of ink marks run in the lateral concha just lateral to the newly created anthelical fold, noting the location of horizontal matress sutures to keep the reshaped anthelixes in place. Now, these ink marks are transferred from the anterior to the posterior skin of the ear and its underlying cartilage with the help of an abraded 25-gauge needle. This is done by passing the needle through the ink marks in order, and each time applying methylene blue at its distal end before withdrawing it. Next, a dumbell-shaped piece of skin is removed from the posterior surface of the concha. The larger the protrusion of the upper third of the ear and/or the earlobe, the wider the excision must be at the corresponding end and the further up and/or down along the concha should it be placed. Next, the posterior skin of the ear is dissected laterally close to the helical rim and medially to the postauricular sulcus and then the mastoid periosteum. Finally, we use 4-0 Mersilene on a noncutting needle to initially place and, thereafter, tie a number of horizontal mattress sutures: one from the triangular fossa to the upper scapha and at least four between the scapha and the lateral portion of the conchal cartilage.[12,21,22]

The conchal enlargement and/or anterolateral rotation is addressed by excising an adequate piece of cartilage from the midportion of the concha. The removed conchal strip is usually about 3-6 mm wide and 2.0 to 3.0 cm long, extending from the midconcha cymba down to the incisura terminalis auris. Conchal set back is then completed by placing multiple horizontal mattress sutures of 4.0 Vicryl between the conchal perichondrium and the mastoid periosteum. Finally, the skin is closed with several 4.0 Mersilene subcutaneous sutures and a running 5.0 Prolene suture on top, all of which is done in a tensionless fashion.[17,23]

Postoperative Care

After the surgical site has been cleansed, the reshaped auricle needs to be properly packed. For this purpose the dressing should be a molded bolster to effectively stabilize the positioning of the surgically corrected ears and avert hematoma formation. There are several different ways to achieve such a molded bolster; for example, use cotton-balls soaked in providone-iodine and shaped to fit the conchal bowl, scapha, and postauricular space. This mold is held in place with a light compression bandage. The patient returns the day after surgery to have the dressing removed and the ear examined closely for the formation of a hematoma. If the examination is normal, the dressing is reapplied and fixed with a standard head wrap for another week. Following dressing removal, the patient must wear an elastic headband nightly for at least 1 month. Postsurgically, typical follow up is scheduled at 1 day, 1 week, 6 weeks, 3 months, and 6 months to allow for the early recognition of complications and appropriate counteractive measures.

Despite lack of evidence for the use of prophylactic antibiotics in otoplasty, patients may be treated with cephalexin, a first-generation cephalosporin. Usually, the antibiotic is given as a one-time dose intravenously at the time of surgery as part of the conscious sedation protocol. If the procedure is done with local sedation only, a 1 week course of cephalexin postoperatively is recommended. Alternatively, ciprofloxacin may be used in the patient allergic to penicillin and/or cephalosporins.

Complications

Overall, the most common untoward outcomes of otoplasty include inadequate correction, contour distortion or an asymmetric correction.[22] These can result from an incomplete estimation of the type and number of malformations contributing to the individual patient's protuberant ears or a lapse of proper post-operative care. Even though some degree of retroprotrusion can be expected with most otoplasty techniques, it appears to be particularly common and significant with Mustarde's technique where permanent sutures alone are used to restructure the ear. In fact, Messner's and Crysdale's follow up on patients at least 1 year removed from Mustarde otoplasty revealed a return of the ear's final position to within 3 mm of the pre-operative state in up to 40 percent of patients, while only 14 percent remained with 3 mm of the immediate postoperative state.[24] These findings support the use of a cartilage removal or incising techniques aimed at a slight over correction to achieve a more permanent and pleasing results. Other causes of recurrence of the original ear deformity include insufficient removal or incising of cartilage to break the cartilage spring, failure to choose a non-cutting needle to avoid small cuts in the cartilage that make it more likely for sutures to tear through, and patient non-compliance with postoperative care.[21]

The "telephone ear" represents a specific surgical deformity following an otoplasty. It is due to an uneven set back of the ear and characterized by protuberance of the inferior and superior poles of the ear relative to its middle portion.

The use of a doughnut or dumbbell shaped excision on the posterior aspect of the ear will prevent this complication from developing.[23]

In the immediate post-operative period, hemorrhage or hematoma formation is the most common complication, occurring at about 2 percent in one extensive review of the morbidity of otoplasty.[25] It commonly affects the retroauricular space and requires immediate, meticulous treatment. Generally, if a patient complains of increasing, persistent pain under the dressing, a hematoma must be suspected. Subsequently, the dressing must be removed immediately, followed by careful inspection of the ear. If a tense, violet-bluish swelling is visualized in the retroauricular space with possible echymosis of surrounding tissue, a hematoma is present. Evacuation of the hematoma should be performed swiftly, and the patient should be started on antibiotics in order to avoid perichondritis. This last is an often encountered sequela of untreated hematomas, and leads to the destruction of cartilage, followed by severe deformities postsurgically. Resultant microtic ear deformities have been reported. Should significant hematoma formation occur past 72 h, prior to institution of antibiotics, a bacterial culture should be taken to confirm the choice of antibiotic.[14]

Severe, unrelenting unilateral pain as a sign of hemorrhage and its often encountered sequela of perichondritis are addressed in the above paragraph. The list of other causes of pain includes those easily prevented, such as excessive pressure on the ear or folding of the ear due to an improperly employed dressing. In addition, a contact dermatitis may manifest as pain, erythema, and pruritus due to sensitivity to the dressing material or applied topical materials.[21] Pain and tenderness of the ears following the surgery but unrelated to a specific treatable cause may occur up to 1 year postsurgery.

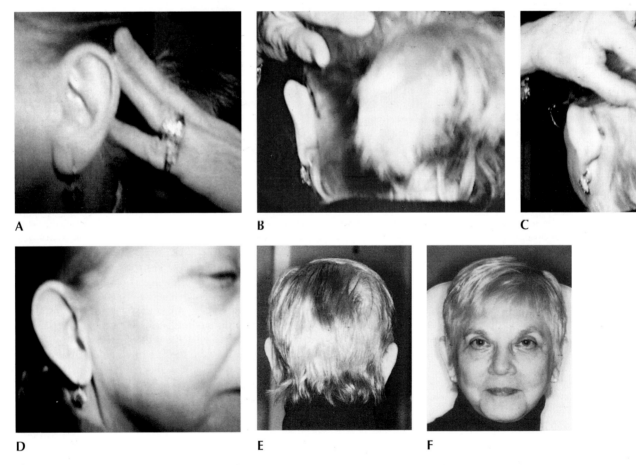

Figure 20-1 (*A*) Preoperative photo. Notice the posterior aspect of the upper helix folding outward, left more pronounced than right. (*B*) Postoperative photo. Notice the subtle tucking of the upper helix back toward the hairline. (*C*) Preoperative photo, left ear. These patients often do not want to wear short hair because of this cosmetic concern. The left ear in this patient bulges away from the scalp more conspicuously. (*D*) Lateral view of the right ear preoperatively. (*E*) Postoperative posterior view. The patient has an excellent result and is now comfortable with short hair. (*F*) Postoperative frontal view.

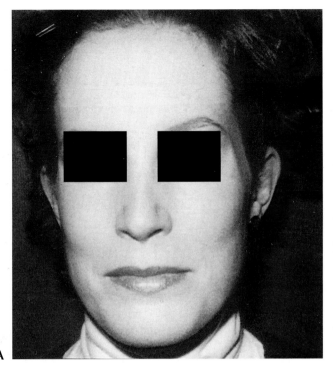 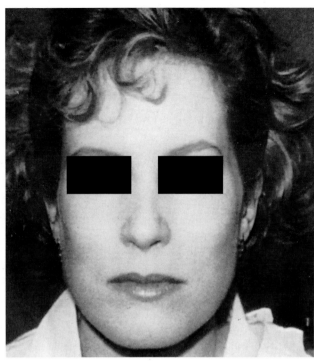

A B

Figure 20-2 Anterior view pre- and postotoplasty.

Apparently, the incidence for this postsurgical pain is significantly higher with the suture-only technique.[23,26]

Keloids and hypertrophic scarring are rarely encountered except in the Afro-Caribbean population. Lavy and Stearns suggest the use of a test incision in this population to assess scarring prior to surgery.[23] Of course, a prior history of keloids and hypertrophic scars raises the likelihood that this problem will recur with otoplasty and the patient should be made aware this possibility. Generally, this problem can be minimized by avoiding excessive tension during skin closure with proper technique. Faced with such scarring, the use of scar excision and intralesional steroid injections can usually restore a satisfactory result.

Skin necrosis is a relatively uncommon complication, probably due to the ear's excellent blood supply. The avoidance of an excessively tight dressing can avoid this problem and early post-surgical evaluation allows the surgeon to address its occurrence.

Conclusion

Young children with this common malformation often experience rejection and ridicule from other children, which can result in psychological trauma. Thus, successful otoplasty can be of significant help to a patient's self-esteem (Figs. 20-1*A–F* and 20-2*A–B*). Many surgical specialties perform this surgical correction, and dermatologic surgeons stand among them. In our opinion, dermatologic surgeons are innately qualified to perform otoplasty as they frequently deal with malignancies of the ear that require the excision of cartilage. The technique we use to correct conchal hypertrophy and anterolateral rotation is based on cartilage removal and easily done. And while many surgeons correct ear malformations before school age, we tend to limit otoplasty to adolescents and young adults, as they are more competent to state their wishes regarding the prominent ear and the degree to which it affects them.

References

1. Dieffenbach JF. *Die Operative Chirurgie.* Leipzig: FA Brockhaus; 1845. Cited by Tanzer RC. Deformities of the auricle. In: Converse JM, ed. *Plastic Reconstructive Surgery* 2d. Philadelphia: Saunders; 1977:1710.

2. Ely ET. An operation for prominence of auricles. *Arch Otolaryngol* 1881; 10:97–99.

3. Mustarde JC. The correction of prominent ears using simple mattress sutures: A ten-year survey. *Plast Reconstr Surg* 1967; 39:382–386.

4. Fritsch MH. Incisionless otoplasty. *Laryngoscope* 1995; 105:1–11.

5. Converse JM, Nigro A, Wilson FA, et al. A technique for surgical correction of the lop ear deformity. *Plast Reconstr Surg* 1955; 15:411–418.

6. Chongchet V. A method of antihelix reconstruction. *Br J Plast Surg* 1963; 16:268–272.

7. Stenstrom SJ. A natural technique for correction of congenitally prominent ears. *Plast Reconstr Surg* 1963; 32:283–293.

8. Bisaccia E, Scarborough DA. The surgical correction of the protuberant ear. *Cosmet Dermatol* 1990; 8:10–12.

9. Kurozumi N, Ono S, Ishida H. Non-surgical correction of a congenital lop ear deformity by splinting with Reston foam. *Br J Plast Surg* 1982; 35:181–182.

10. Matsuo K, Hayashi R, Kiyono M, et al. Nonsurgical correction of congenital auricular deformities. *Clin Plast Surg* 1990; 17:383–395.

11. Muraoka M, Nakai Y, Ohashi Y, et al. Tape attachment therapy for correction of congenital malformations of the auricle: Clinical and experimental studies. *Laryngoscope* 1985; 95:167–176.

12. Hell B, Garbea D, Heissler E, et al. Otoplasty: A combined approach to different structures of the auricle. *Int J Oral Maxillofac Surg* 1997; 26:408–413.

13. Balogh B, Millesi H. Are growth alterations a consequence of surgery for prominent ears? *Plast Reconstr Surg* 1992; 90:192–199.

14. Warmuth IP, Bader R, Scarborough D, et al. Otoplasty. In: Treatment of protuberant ears. *Cosmet Dermatol* 1999; 4:7–8.

15. Bradbury ET, Hewison J, Timmons MJ. Psychological and social outcome of prominent ear correction in children. *Br J Plast Surg* 1992; 45:97–100.

16. Elliott RA. Otoplasty. In: Regnault P, Daniel RK, eds. *Esthetic Plastic Surgery.* Boston: Little, Brown; 1984:245–274.

17. Burres S. The anterior-posterior otoplasty. *Arch Otolaryngol Head Neck Surg* 1998; 124:181–185.

18. Becker OJ. Surgical correction of the abnormally protruding ear. *Arch Otalaryngol* 1949; 50:541–560.

19. Elliot RA. Otoplasty: A combined approach. *Clin Plast Surg* 1990; 17:373.

20. Davis J. *Aesthetic and Reconstructive Otoplasty.* New York: Springer-Verlag; 1987:37.

21. Spira M. Otoplasty: What I do now—A 30-year perspective. *Plast Reconstr Surg* 1999; 104:834–840.

22. Ducic Y, Hilger PA. Effective step-by-step technique for the surgical treatment of protruding ears. *J Otolaryngol* 1999; 28:59–64.

23. Lavy J, Stearns M. Otoplasty: Techniques, results and complications—A review. *Clin Otolaryngol* 1997; 22:390–393.

24. Messner AH, Williams SC. Otoplasty: Clinical protocol and long-term results. *Arch Otolaryngol Head Neck Surg* 1996; 122:773–777.

25. Calder JC, Naasan A. Morbidity of otoplasty: A review of 562 consecutive cases. *Br J Plast Surg* 1994; 47:170–174.

26. Tan KH. Long-term study of prominent ear surgery: A comparison of two methods. *Br J Plast Surg* 1986; 39:270–273.

Patient Information

Otoplasty

Children with protruding ears have long been the victims of cruel nicknames, like "Dumbo" or "Mickey Mouse," which makes them likely candidates for otoplasty. Realistically, this surgery can be performed at any age after the ears have reached full size, usually around 5 or 6 years of age. Even if the ears are only mildly distorted, the condition can lead to self-consciousness and poor adaptation to school. When it comes to otoplasty, early intervention will have emotionally more positive results.

Adults may also benefit from this procedure, which improves self-esteem with relative ease. This surgery may also be done in conjunction with other cosmetic surgical procedures. Not only is it possible to "pin back" ears, but they can be reshaped, reduced in size, or made more symmetrical.

Successful facial cosmetic surgery is best achieved when there is good rapport between patient and surgeon. Trust, based on realistic expectations and exacting medical expertise, develops during the consultation before surgery, when you and your surgeon review specific questions about your special needs.

To help you decide if otoplasty is right for you, it is important to understand the surgery. Otoplasty does not alter hearing ability. Bringing the ears into proportion with the size and shape of the face and head is the main goal of your surgery.

In considering otoplasty, parents must be confident that they have their child's best interests at heart. Realistic expectations and a positive attitude toward the surgery are important factors in all facial surgeries, but they are especially critical when the patient is a child or adolescent.

Adult candidates for otoplasty should understand that the firmer cartilage of fully developed ears does not have the same molding capacity as this cartilage in children. Through a consultation with a cosmetic surgeon, parents can decide what is best for their child, not only esthetically but also psychologically and physically.

Selecting a qualified cosmetic surgeon is of paramount importance. During the consultation, the surgeon will examine the structure of the ears and discuss options for correcting the problem. Even if only one ear needs "pinning back," surgery on both ears may be recommended to achieve the most natural, symmetrical appearance.

Once, with the agreement of your surgeon, you decide that otoplasty is indicated, your surgeon will discuss the procedure and recovery time. After a thorough medical history, the surgeon will explain the type of anesthesia required, surgical facility, and costs. Typically, a local anesthetic combined with a mild sedative will be suggested for older children and adults. Under normal conditions, otoplasty requires approximately 2 hours.

Surgery begins with an incision just behind the ear, in the natural fold where the ear joins the head. The surgeon then removes the amounts of cartilage and skin required to achieve the most natural appearance. In some cases, the surgeon will trim the cartilage, shaping it into a more desirable form, and then pin the cartilage back, using permanent stitches to secure it. In other instances, the surgeon will not remove any cartilage at all, merely using stitches to hold the cartilage permanently in place. After sculpting the cartilage to the desired shape, the surgeon places stitches to anchor the ear until healing occurs, thereby holding the ear in the desired position.

Soft dressings are applied to the ears for a few days. Most patients experience only mild discomfort. If you are accustomed to sleeping on your side, your sleep patterns may be disrupted for a week or so because you cannot put any pressure on the ear areas. Headbands are sometimes recommended to hold the ears in the desired position for 2 weeks after surgery.

The risks are minimal. A thin white scar remains behind the ear after healing. Since the scar is in the natural crease behind the ear, it is barely visible. Anything unusual should be reported to the surgeon immediately.

Facial cosmetic surgery makes it possible to correct many facial flaws that can undermine one's self-confidence. By changing how you look, cosmetic surgery can help change how you feel about yourself.

Insurance does not cover surgery that is done purely for cosmetic reasons. Surgery to correct or improve birth defects or traumatic injuries may be reimbursable in whole or in part. It is the patient's responsibility to check with his or her insurance carrier for information on the degree of coverage.

Otoplasty

PREOPERATIVE INSTRUCTIONS

No aspirin, vitamin E, or drugs containing aspirin (Bufferin, Anacin, Empirin, Stanback, Excedrin, Fiorinal, Darvon compound, and salicylate) for 2 weeks before surgery. **INSTEAD USE ONLY TYLENOL!!**

No alcohol 3 days prior to surgery, and avoid it while taking any postoperative medication.

Get plenty of rest the night before surgery.

Wear clothes that either zip or button and do not have to be pulled over your head.

Arrange for a ride to and from the office.

Do not wear any jewelry to the office on the day of surgery.

Wash your face thoroughly and shampoo your hair on the morning of surgery.

Take all preoperative medications as directed.

Bring pain medication with you on surgery day.

A postoperative appointment card will be given to you as you check in on the day of surgery.

Otoplasty Surgical Setup Tray

Patient

1. Cape or drape (optional)
2. Clean hat

Doctor and Staff

1. Visor mask
2. Sterile gloves

Materials

1. Betadine solution
2. Sterile surgical ellipse tray
3. Clean gauze
4. Gentian marker
5. One 3-mL syringe
6. One 30-gauge metal-hub needle
7. 1% Lidocaine with epinephrine, buffered
8. Alcohol wipe
9. Saline bottle
10. Thermometer and cover
11. Suture/skin closures, Glustitch as appropriate
12. Polysporin
13. Telfa, gauze, tape
14. Mastisol (optional)
15. Steri-strips (optional)

Otoplasty

POSTOPERATIVE INSTRUCTIONS

Immediately following your surgery and for the first day after, *relax*. Keep all activities to a minimum for 24 hours. Refrain from any vigorous activity. Do not jog, do not bend over, do not engage in sex, etc.

When you get home, prepare an ice pack. A medium-sized plastic bag with ice cubes will do fine. (Be careful to seal the bag to avoid leakage.) Sit comfortably in a chair and cradle your head in a pillow. Place the ice packs over your ears. Keep it in place for at least 1 hour.

DO NOT, UNDER ANY CIRCUMSTANCES, REMOVE OR ALTER THE DRESSING DURING THE FIRST 24 HOURS.

Have something to eat after you arrive home. A light snack will help you relax. Avoid foods that require excessive and constant chewing. (For example: steak, gum, etc.) No alcohol is to be taken for 72 hours.

Take your medications as prescribed by the doctor.

Antibiotics

Continue taking your antibiotics as directed to help prevent infection.

Sleeping Pills

You may be given sleeping pills to help you sleep comfortably for the first two nights following the procedure. If necessary, take one or two pills 30 minutes before retiring.

Pain Medication

Take as directed every 4 to 6 hours, as needed, at the first sign of discomfort. The feeling of tightness will generally fade in 1 to 3 days.

To avoid any movement of the dressing, you must sleep in a sitting position the first night. A reclining chair would be ideal, but not fully reclined. If there is no other recourse, settle in a comfortable living room chair or prop your head up on several pillows in bed. Do not roll to the side. In any event, keep your head elevated.

If you should notice any spotting of blood on your dressing, do not be alarmed. Merely reapply an ice pack where spotting is observed. Ice applied for about 15 minutes with slight pressure should stop the bleeding. Please remain calm; anxiety is not needed and will only increase your blood pressure and the bleeding.

Remove the wrap on the day following your procedure. Please do this while seated, since on rare occasions momentary light-headedness may occur.

Cleaning the Surgical Site

Starting the first morning after surgery, you will clean the surgical site with saline solution or warm tap water. Take a thin, clean washcloth and dampen it with the cleaning solution. Using a blotting motion, gently clean the surgical site, then carefully dry with a clean soft towel, again using a blotting motion. After cleaning and drying, liberally apply Polysporin ointment to the surgical site. Do this morning and evening until all scabs fall off (normally 10 to 20 days).

Swelling

You were given an injection containing medication to combat the potential for swelling. Swelling and drainage are always a possibility, and also some discomfort. This may occur in a day or two around the ears as a result of the local anesthetic. If it should occur, it usually resolves by the end of the first week. Cold compresses or ice packs, avoiding dietary salt, and keeping your head elevated will help.

Shampooing

After 48 hours following surgery, you may shampoo your hair. Use baby shampoo and use a cup to pour water gently over the surgical sites. Pat dry with a soft towel. Do not use a hair dryer. Do not shampoo more than once a day. Continue cleaning the suture line with saline or warm tap water at least twice daily until the crusts have fallen off naturally.

Your first checkup will be in 10 to 14 days, when most of the crusts have fallen off. Sutures will be removed at this time.

Do not massage the scalp for 6 weeks following surgery.

We expect you to come back to our office 3 to 6 months after your surgery for an interim checkup. If in the meantime you have any questions, do not hesitate to call.

Problems or Questions

Call the office at (___) _____ anytime. For emergencies, the doctor's home number is given on the postoperative appointment card.

ANY REDNESS, SWELLING, TENDERNESS, OR "PUS PIMPLES" SHOULD BE IMMEDIATELY REPORTED TO US.

CONSENT FOR OTOPLASTY

Patient's name_____

Date_____

I hereby authorize _____ and/or the surgical team to perform an otoplasty operation upon me (or my _____) to: (description of procedure)_____

_____

_____

1. The nature and effects of this operation, the risks and complications involved, as well as alternative methods of treatment have been fully explained to me by the doctor and I understand them.

    Initial_____

2. I authorize the doctor to perform any other procedure that may be deemed desirable in attempting to improve the condition stated in Paragraph 1 or any unhealthy or unforeseen condition that may be encountered during the operation.

    Initial_____

3. I consent to the administration of anesthetics by the doctor or under the direction of the anesthetist responsible for this service.

    Initial_____

4. I understand that the practice of medicine and surgery is not an exact science and that reputable practitioners cannot guarantee results. No guarantee or assurance has been given me by the doctor or anyone else as to the results that may be obtained. I understand that complications may include the following:

    a. Bleeding, possibly requiring reoperation or prolonged compression dressing.

    b. Infection, possibly requiring prolonged use of antibiotics and resulting in scarring or disfigurement (rare).

    c. Unsightly scarring or disfigurement, reoperation may be necessary, and scarring may be uncorrectable or painful.

    d. No improvement or worsening of appearance.

    e. Need for touch-up procedure at some future point (additional costs of surgery will be the patient's responsibility).

    f. Numbness may occur, or the area may be overly sensitive; rarely, this can be permanent.

    Initial_____

5. For the purpose of advancing education, I consent to the admittance of authorized observers to the operating room.

    Initial_____

6. I give permission to _____ to take still or motion clinical photographs with the understanding such photographs remain the property of the center. If in the judgment of the center medical research, education, or science will be benefited by their use, such photographs and related information may be published and republished in professional journals or medical books or used for any other purpose which the center may deem proper. It is specifically understood that in any such publication or use, I shall not be identified by name.

    Initial_____

7. I understand that the two sides of the human body are not the same and can never be made the same. I understand that bone, muscle, and support tissues are never identical on both sides of the body, and that surgery cannot make my ears identical.

    Initial_____

8. I understand it is mandatory for me to have made prior arrangements to be driven to and from the doctor's office by a responsible adult.

    Initial_____

9. I understand that elective surgical procedures are most often delayed until after the termination of a pregnancy. My signature attests that to the best of my knowledge I am not pregnant at this time.

    Initial_____

10. I agree to discontinue smoking entirely for a period of 2 weeks prior to surgery and 2 weeks immediately following surgery.

    Initial_____

11. I have been given the opportunity to ask questions and all my questions have been answered to my satisfaction.

    Initial_____

My signature indicates that I have read this "Consent for Otoplasty" and I understand and accept the risks involved in this operation. I hereby authorize _____ and/or the surgical team to perform this surgical procedure on me.

_____   _____
Signature (Patient/Responsible Party)   Date

_____   _____
Signature (Witness)   Date

If patient is a minor, complete the following:

Patient is a minor _____ years of age, and we, the undersigned, are the parents or guardian of the patient and do hereby consent for the patient.

_____   _____
Signature (Parent/Guardian)   Date

Index

Note: Page numbers followed by *f* indicate figures; those followed by *t* indicate tables.